ALIVE AND WELL

ALIVE AND WELL

DECISIONS IN HEALTH

Arlene Eisenberg
Consultant in Health Education
Rockland Community College

Howard Eisenberg
Senior Editor
Medical Economics

McGraw-Hill Book Company

New York St. Louis San Francisco Auckland Bogotá
Düsseldorf Johannesburg London Madrid Mexico
Montreal New Delhi Panama Paris São Paulo
Singapore Sydney Tokyo Toronto

This book was set in Helvetica by Black Dot, Inc.
The editor was Alison Meersschaert;
the designer was Joan E. O'Connor;
the production supervisor was Dennis J. Conroy.
The drawings were done by J & R Services, Inc.
The cover photograph was taken by Janeart Ltd.
Von Hoffmann Press, Inc., was printer and binder.

See Acknowledgments on pages 623–626.

ALIVE AND WELL DECISIONS IN HEALTH

1 2 3 4 5 6 7 8 9 0 V H V H 7 8 3 2 1 0 9

Library of Congress Cataloging in Publication Data

Eisenberg, Arlene.
Alive and well.

Bibliography: p.
Includes index.
1. Health. I. Eisenberg, Howard, joint author.
II. Title.
RA776.E375 613 78-10910
ISBN 0-07-019113-1

To our parents
who taught us the importance of good health,
and our children
who taught us so much about today's
college student.

CONTENTS

PART V LOVE AND THE HUMAN LIFE CYCLE

IN APPRECIATION

It may well be true that a person can learn more from writing one book than from reading a thousand books. In writing *Alive and Well*, we learned from many sources:

- *Educational institutions* Georgetown University, the University of California, Pennsylvania State University, and Harvard Medical Area newsletters have been particularly informative.
- *United States government publications and releases* They have kept us up to date, and perhaps a bit ahead, medically.
- *Voluntary agencies* Organizations such as the American Cancer Society and the American Heart Association have been of considerable help.
- *Medical and social science journals and respected periodicals such as* The New York Times.
- *Medical schools and medical societies and specialty organizations* Special thanks to the American Academy of Family Physicians and its continuing education program.
- *Books that are currently popular and books that are classics in their fields* We are in debt to the National Library of Medicine, to Finkelstein Memorial Library, and to the Medical Economics and Medical World News Libraries for opening doors and drawers for us.

We learned a great deal, too, from those who graciously shared their knowledge and experience with us in personal and telephone interviews. In mentioning a few names, we risk omitting many others who helped, too, and to whom we are grateful. We especially wish to thank: obstetrician-gynecologist Henry Eisenberg; cardiologist Irving Levitas; internist Samuel Alhadeff; Drs. Irving Karel and Stephen Wotman of the School of Dental and Oral Surgery of Columbia University; Phyllis Karel, dental hygienist; Gilbert Goetz, pharmacist; William Gautiere, physiologist; Sonya Shapiro, educator; Claude E. Forkner, Sr., M.D., for his assistance and permission to use his Medical Passport; Harold Osborne and Irving Goldberg of the National Institutes of Health, as well as the various institute information people; the many at NIH who patiently sat still for interviews and for reviewing sections later (especially Drs. Basil M. Rifkind, Gio B. Gori, Heinz W. Berendes, and Benjamin T. Burton); people at the National Institute of Mental Health, the National Institute on Drug Abuse, and the National Clearing House on Smoking and Health who gave us assistance; Dr. Esther Krueger of Keane Community College, whose encouragement at a key stage was so valuable; and especially Irwin Polk, M.D., author and health columnist and good friend, who was always ready with answers to tough questions at a moment's notice.

We wish, too, to express our appreciation to the many students, present and past, who shared their thoughts about what a college health text should be.

There would probably be no book in hand at all if it were not for those who helped in its physical preparation from research through typing and fact checking: Esther Makower, Harry Scharaga, Barbara Wahl, Sandee Eisenberg, Evan Eisenberg, and especially Heidi Eisenberg who contributed in a hundred different ways. We thank Sandee, Evan, and Heidi, as well as our extended family, for their patience at times when *Alive and Well* usurped their places.

A very special thank you to our medical board: Keith Sehnert, M.D., Visiting Professor at Georgetown University and Case Western University and vice-president of Interstudy; and Harris Faigel, M.D., director of Student Health Services at Brandeis University. And to our reviewers, Beverly Barck, Golden West College; Andrew J. J. Brennan, Hunter College; Kenneth S. Clarke, Pennsylvania State University; Barbara Combs, City College of San Francisco; Janet Faurot, Long Beach City College; Roger Hough, Long Beach City College; Esther S. Krueger, Kean College; Gerald W. Matheson, University of Nevada, Reno; Helen Mountain, Lakewood Community College; Gene Norris, Trinity University; Terry W. Parsons, Bowling Green State University; Julius Shevlin, City College of New York; and Harold Slobof, Mankato State College, who patiently waded through manuscript drafts and offered guidance and suggestions.

Finally, thank you to someone who has been with us from the beginning, guiding us through the unfamiliar labyrinth of textbook writing, our editor Alison Meerschaert. You cannot tell a book by its cover, but if you can tell it by its editor, *Alive and Well* will be first rate.

In the pages that follow, we share with you what we have learned. We hope it will keep you *Alive and Well*.

Arlene Eisenberg
Howard Eisenberg

INTRODUCTION

> Every man [or woman] is a fluid that becomes a solid . . . a history in the making, a personality that is being created. And our progress, or our disintegration, depends on physical, chemical, and psychological factors, on viruses and bacteria, on physiological influences and, finally, on *our own will.*

The last three words of these lines penned in 1935 by Alexis Carrel, Nobel Prize winner in medicine and physics, point clearly to the rationale behind this health text. We are buffeted and shaped by an infinite variety of factors, many uncontrollable, that surround us. But in the end, the most influential factor is the human mind and how effectively we use it.

Many health authorities today agree that the individual can play a significant role in improving health care, reducing unnecessary and premature deaths, and controlling upward-spiraling health costs. Professor Eli Ginzberg of Columbia University has suggested that patients are an immense, untapped health resource, and that educating the American people to do more about their own health would be a lot more economical and effective than producing more doctors.

When it comes to health, then, we are to a great extent masters of our own destiny. It is to this concept that *Alive and Well: Decisions in Health* is dedicated.

This book does not stand alone. It is part of a virtual revolution in health care in the United States that is taking place in doctors' offices, hospitals, schools, clinics, and community centers throughout the country, and that is being spread by books, newspapers, TV, radio, programmed learning tapes, and records. The basic concepts of this revolution in health education are the major themes of *Alive and Well:*

- **Individual decision making** The decisions *you* make every day—about eating, drinking, loving, working, playing, exercising, as well as about specific medical questions such as when to take an aspirin or when to see a doctor—will have more impact on your health than anything the medical community does. *Alive and Well* not only gives you the information you need to make sound decisions, but examines the decision-making process as well.
- **Preventive medicine** An early "ounce of prevention" added to your daily life will do a great deal more to protect you from heart disease, many cancers, and a wide variety of other health problems than belated pounds of cure from a physician. Throughout *Alive and Well,* the emphasis is on prevention.
- **Health consumerism** As an alert consumer, you try to be as informed as possible before deciding to purchase an automobile, a house, or an appliance. As a health consumer, you should be similarly well informed. *Alive and Well* provides a wealth of health consumer information on everything from contact lenses to sex clinics, from food labels to nursing homes, to assist you in making educated health decisions. A variety of Health Consumer Tips appear throughout the text to guide you in becoming an aware health consumer. Who's Who in Health Care sections will acquaint you with the professionals best able to help you with various health problems.
- **The patient-physician partnership** With the revolution has come a decline in the medical mystique that put the physician on a pedestal and ignored the responsibility of the patient in making health care decisions. Today many patients recognize that they need to take a more active role in their own health care, in partnership with physicians, dentists, and other health care workers. When to Seek Help sections (covering everything from depression to respiratory ills) and Communicating with the Physician sections will help you develop a sound working patient-physician partnership.
- **Self-care** Many authorities believe that the patient-partner can take on many simple medical tasks: taking blood pressure, pulse, and respiration readings; doing simple examinations of skin, mouth, breasts, prostate, ears, and throat; handling common emergencies resulting from accidents, heart attacks, choking, and adverse drug reactions; and treating the up to 70 percent of illnesses that do not demand a physician's care (e.g., colds, upset stomachs, minor wounds). The numerous Self-Care sections in *Alive and Well* will help you to master many of these procedures. The Treatment sections of disease listings include simple remedies for illnesses responsive to self-care.
- **Open discussion** Health is an area of dynamic growth and, thus, constant ferment in which differing, sometimes conflicting opinions coexist. It is our belief that the informed health consumer—you—should be exposed to varying opinions. Thus we have attempted, where appropriate, to present balanced views of controversial issues. Absolute balance is, of course, impossible. At times it may seem that one or another view predominates. However, we hope that you will not automatically make it yours. Your views should be based on *your* values as well as on the facts, and should be reached through enlightened decision making (a process described in Chapter 1). For topics which are the focus of sharp controversy—such as abortion

and homosexuality—we have added Opinion sections that present major points of view.

Each chapter begins with a list of key questions entitled "What's Ahead. . . ." Look for the answers as you read, and you will more easily grasp the major objectives and concepts of *Alive and Well*.

Few courses you take in college have the potential to make as great a difference in your life as does a health course. As Dr. William Hettler, Director of the Wellness Center at the University of Wisconsin has suggested, what you learn in a health course can give you more vitality and more years for the things you enjoy most—friends, books, skiing, sex. We kept this suggestion in mind as we wrote *Alive and Well*. We hope you will keep it in mind as you read.

ALIVE AND WELL

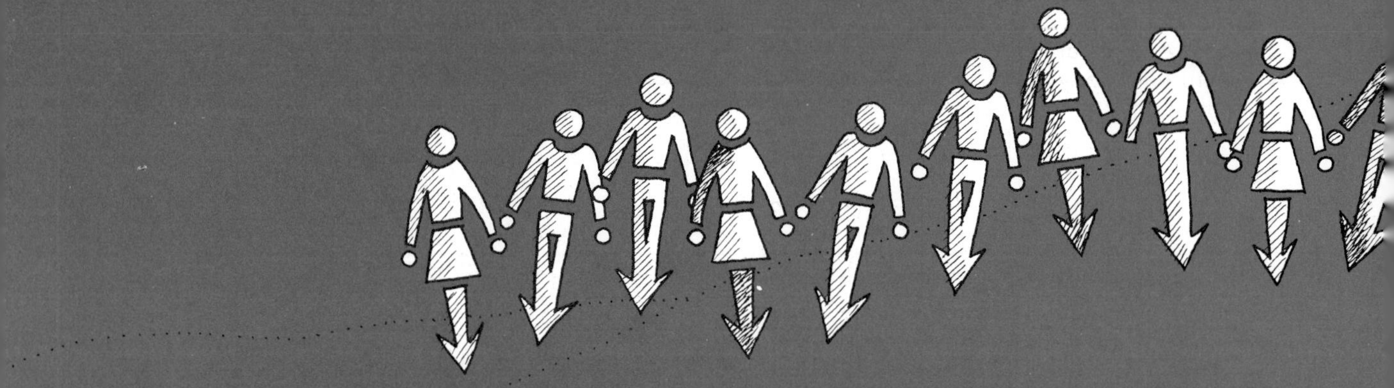

1 LEARNING ABOUT HEALTH

WHAT'S AHEAD IN CHAPTER 1 What is health? What does it mean to you? How can you achieve the kind of health you want? How do the themes of *Alive and Well*—preventive health care, personal and community decision making, and informed consumerism—affect your health and the quality and length of your life? How do they affect community health? Which segments of the community most influence the kind of health care Americans receive? Who has the *most* influence over your health?

Scene: A medical laboratory many years in the future. Woody Allen, quick-frozen and foil-wrapped in the 1970s, is thawed out.

DR. MELIK Well, he's fully recovered except for a few minor kinks.

DOCTOR Has he asked for anything special?

DR. MELIK Yes, this morning for breakfast. Er, he requested something called wheat germ, organic honey, and tiger's milk.

DOCTOR Oh, yes, those were the charmed substances that some years ago were felt to contain life-preserving properties.

DR. MELIK You mean there was no deep fat, no steak or cream pie or hot fudge?

DOCTOR Those were thought to be unhealthy. Precisely the opposite of what we now know to be true.

DR. MELIK Incredible.[1]

Humorist Woody Allen was being funny, of course, but he was also making a social comment. It is unlikely that cream pies, marbled steaks, and hot fudge sundaes will ever be considered health foods. Still, radical shifts in the acceptance of scientific data are not unusual. Note, for example, the implied

[1]Reproduced with permission of Jack Rollins and Charles H. Joffee Productions from United Artists' *Sleeper*.

medical endorsement in a cigarette advertisement, published in 1952, picturing a white-coated man and the headline: "More physicians smoke Camels than any other cigarette." Or the fact that in the 1950s obstetricians recommended that pregnant women gain no more than 12 or 13 pounds, while today so low a weight gain is considered "unsafe." Or that the preferred treatment for an enlarged thyroid 25 years ago was x-ray, though today this treatment is known to cause cancer.

But though new medical discoveries may modify or change accepted "truths," a personal philosophy of health can last a lifetime. As you will see in reading this book, you are to a great extent master of your own health. More than any new scientific breakthrough, the health decisions *you* make will be chiefly responsible for keeping you alive and well.

WHAT IS HEALTH?

"He's as healthy as a horse!" "Health is better than gold!" "I don't care if it's a boy or a girl, just so long as it's healthy!"

What do people mean when they use the word "healthy"? Does health mean the same thing to a 20-year-old as it does to someone at 85? Can a person have arthritis or diabetes, or be confined to a wheelchair, and still be healthy? What criteria does the physician use in judging health? What criteria do you use?

Is health, as eighteenth-century British philosopher-economist Jeremy Bentham described it, merely "the absence of disease"? Or is it more than that? Karl Menninger, the eminent psychiatrist, has described it as "the body in harmony with its environment." And Thoreau wrote, more lyrically, "Measure your health by your sympathy with the morning and Spring. . . . Thus you may feel your pulse."

How important is health to you? Michel de Montagne said, some 400 years ago: "Health is a precious thing and . . . without it life comes to be painful and oppressive to us. . . . As far as I am concerned, no road that would lead us to health is either arduous or expensive." Do you agree?

Or do you stand with Robert Alberra, who said early in this century: "If the road to 70 is too hard, I don't want to take it. I prefer to enjoy my pleasures—good food, good whiskey, and a good smoke."

What kind of health do you want for yourself and those you care about? How much effort are you willing to put forth to attain the benefits of good health? These are key questions to ponder as you read on and work at developing a philosophy of health. Also keep in mind three basic points: (1) the most important aspect of health care is prevention; (2) *you* make the most important decisions about your own health—on a personal level and as part of the community; (3) only an informed and active health consumer can

Some Other Definitions of Health

A state of complete physical, mental, and social well-being and not merely the absence of disease or infirmity.

World Health Organization

A relative state of ability to mobilize one's resources to respond effectively within one's environment to the stresses that come one's way. It facilitates the attainment of personal goals by enabling utilization of personal, physical, emotional, and intellectual attributes in a social setting.

Kenneth S. Clarke

Henri Dauman

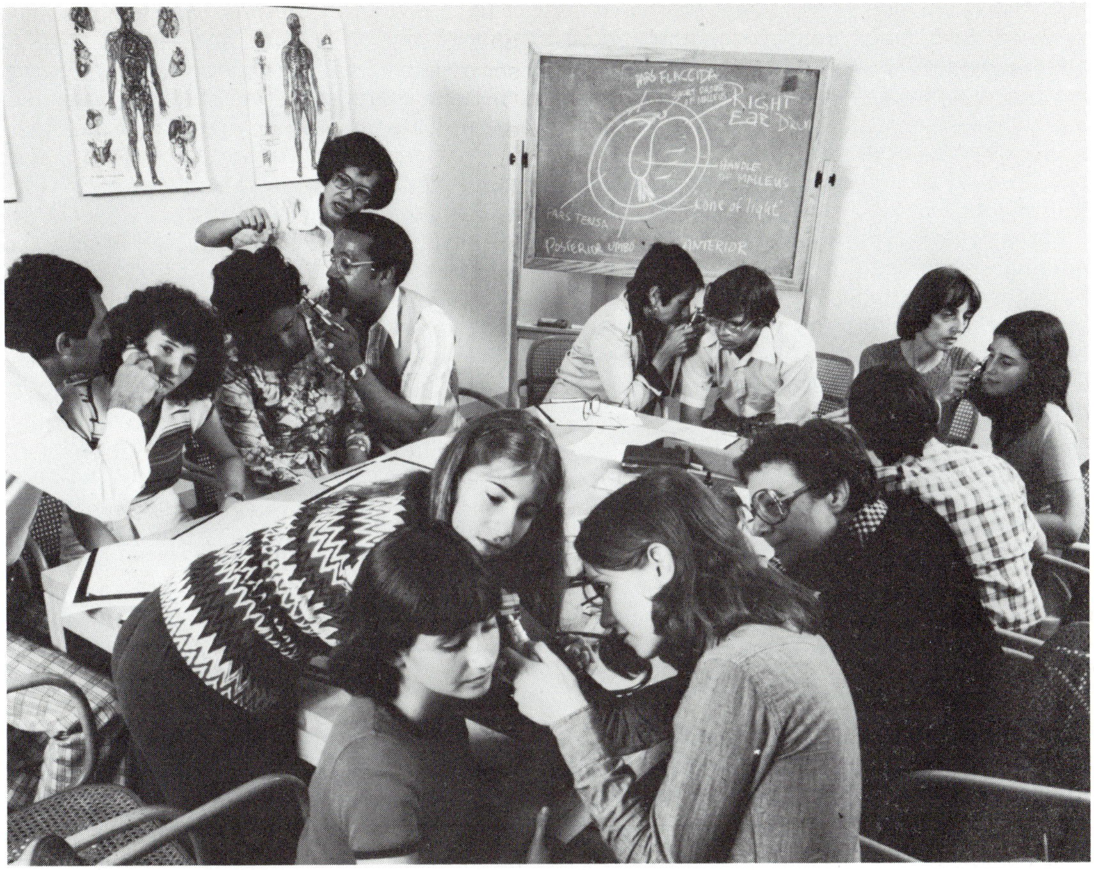

Programs such as this one at the Center for Medical Consumers and Health Care Information in New York City are in the forefront of the movement to improve consumer health education and increase self-care.

obtain full benefit from the health care system. Because of their importance, these three areas—preventive health care, decision making, and the active consumer—are the major themes of *Alive and Well.*

PREVENTIVE HEALTH CARE

Every year, thousands are disabled by diseases that are preventable or curable, or die prematurely from conditions that could have been controlled. Many factors have been suggested to explain our failure to utilize what we know to make life healthier and longer. Among them are: poverty; poor health education; inadequate dissemination of information on the latest advances in treatment and diagnosis to local practitioners and hospitals; economic interests that sometimes clash with health interests; personal lifestyles and philosophies that often put comfort and pleasure ahead of health and safety; a feeling of invincibility ("Bad things happen to other people"); a medical community oriented toward making sick people well rather than preventing sickness; and attitudes favoring instant solutions over day-in-day-out effort (taking pills instead of cutting calories in order to lose weight).

These factors, you will note, have little or nothing to do with major medical breakthroughs or shortages of medical facilities. Most of them fall into the area of *preventive health care*—health care that involves both the individual and the resources of the community in preventing illness before it begins and in keeping minor illnesses from becoming major ones.

How can preventive health care become a reality? Many authorities believe that three changes must occur:

1 *The medical community must become more prevention-oriented.* On your last visit to your doctor, did he or she take time to explain how you could avoid further visits, how your health habits might affect your future health, or how you could do self-examinations at home? Were you given a chance to discuss family problems that might eventually lead to mental or physical illness? If your physician is typical, the answer is probably no. Some private physicians, however, do preach and practice prevention and some hospitals and clinics sponsor patient education programs. School and college health education classes are becoming more prevention-oriented. Wellness centers, geared to prevention, are opening in some communities. But the number of persons being reached by programs such as these is still small.

2 *Major movers and shapers of society—government, business, the educational establishment, and the media—must cooperate in altering the physical and social environment.* Everything in our environment—the air we breathe, the water we drink, the food we eat, the noise that bombards our ears, the vehicles we drive, our jobs, our families, our friends, and so on—has some effect, positive or negative, on our health and well-being. Societal attitudes, parental and peer values, advertising and other merchandising techniques, films and TV, and books and magazines also have an effect by molding individual attitudes toward health.

Can these elements be altered in order to improve the health of Americans? There are indications they can be. For example: automobile and industrial emissions standards have reduced air pollution in some cities; nutrients have been added to some foods, hazardous additives removed from others, improving the quality of the foods we eat; media blitz education campaigns have been undertaken in a few communities with the result that individual health habits have been improved and risk of disease reduced.

Still, it is clear that our society is a long way from total commitment to the concept of improving health through prevention. Partly this is because of a split personality where health is concerned. Dentists warn that sugary snacks contribute to tooth decay, while children's TV shows push candy bars; we complain about air pollution, but drive when we could walk or bicycle; labels warn that cigarettes can be hazardous to health, but the government subsidizes tobacco growers. Partly this is because there is a limit to what we are willing to spend on health—compared with other necessities and luxuries—as you will see in Chapter 25.

3 *Individuals must become more involved in and responsible for their own health.* "The daily habits of people," says Dr. Lester Breslow, dean of the School of Public Health at U.C.L.A., "have a great deal more to do with what makes them sick and when they die than all the influences of medicine."

Observing a scientifically selected cross section of 7000 adults over an 11-year period, Dr. Breslow and colleagues found that risk of premature death was greatly reduced for persons who practiced seven fairly common health habits: (1) eating three meals a day at

TABLE 1.1 Expected lifespan according to number of good health practices

PRESENT AGE	NUMBER OF GOOD HEALTH PRACTICES		
	0–3	4–5	6–7
LIFESPAN OF MEN			
45	66.6	73.2	78.1
55	68.8	75.2	80.0
65	75.6	78.7	82.4
75	82.4	85.2	86.2
LIFESPAN OF WOMEN			
45	73.6	79.1	80.8
55	75.0	80.1	82.8
65	77.4	82.3	84.9
75	83.6	86.7	87.5

Source: Belloc, pp. 67–81.

regular times instead of snacking; (2) eating breakfast every day; (3) getting moderate exercise (long walks, biking, swimming) two or three times a week; (4) sleeping 7 to 8 hours a night; (5) not smoking; (6) maintaining moderate weight (less than 20 percent overweight; (7) consuming only moderate amounts of alcohol (no more than four drinks daily). (See Table 1.1.)

A Health Hazard Appraisal (see pages 8 and 9) developed by Dr. Lewis C. Robbins, based on the most common causes of death, suggests additional practices that adversely affect health: failure to use seat belts, use of nonprescribed dangerous drugs, uncontrolled high blood pressure or high cholesterol levels, failure to have regular rectal examinations after age 40, and women's failure to have regular Pap smears and breast examinations.

Further support for the importance of individual health habits comes from the fact that groups such as the Mormons that regulate many of these habits—diet, smoking, drinking, and exercise, for example—have fewer diseases and longer lifespans than the rest of the population. Scientific evidence that good diet, exercise, and other good health habits are the way to a longer, healthier life may disappoint those of us who have harbored the hope that the secret of long life would be found in the 95-year-old man who smokes, drinks, eats high-cholesterol steaks, and never does a lick of exercise. Or who have been waiting for an obscure college professor to come up with an elixir which, when sprinkled in our morning juice, would add years to our lives. Indeed, many scientists are hard at work searching for that elusive test-tube fountain of youth, and some of their work shows promise. But success—if it ever comes—is still a long way off. Meanwhile, the only available fountain gushes forth from our own intelligent lifestyles and from the informed, prudent decisions we make each day.

DECISION MAKING

Day in and day out we make decisions that affect our health: Should I get up early and jog, or sleep late and skip breakfast? Should I light another cigarette, or quit smoking altogether? Should I have fish for lunch and risk PCB poisoning, or a hamburger and overdose on cholesterol? Should I hitch a ride or walk the 2 miles to town? Should I buckle my seat belt and wrinkle my jacket, or leave it on the seat and risk wrinkling my skull? Should I stay up late studying and guzzling coffee, or get to bed early and hope I'll pass?

Very often we make major medical decisions that outweigh those of our health professionals: One family's physician is forever prescribing antibiotics for colds; the family believes such drugs should be reserved for serious illness and switches doctors. A middle-aged woman wants to take female hormones to ease the symptoms of menopause, in spite of her physician's warnings about the risks; she shops around until she finds a doctor willing to prescribe the hormone. A dentist urges periodontal treatment for a patient with gum problems; the patient decides not to seek this help.

In addition, we make a large number of vital

Health Hazard Appraisal: Are You Older Than Your Birth Certificate?

Directions: If uncertain, leave blank. Place scores on lines provided in the plus and minus columns. Add plus and minus columns to find the subtotals for each section. Follow the instructions for calculating your medical age at the end of test.

Part 1 Personal history	PLUS	MINUS
a Weight: "Ideal" weight at age 20 (was, is) ______. If current weight is more than 20 pounds over that, score +6 for each extra 20 pounds. If weight after age 20 is the same as at age 20 or less than 10 pounds more, score −3.	______	______
b Blood pressure: Under age 40, if blood pressure is above 130/80, score +12; over 40, if pressure is above 140/90, score +12.	______	______
c Heart murmur, but not an innocent type, score +24.	______	______
d Heart murmur with history of rheumatic fever, score +48.	______	______
e Cholesterol: Under age 40, if above 220, score +6; over 40, if above 250, score +6.	______	______
f If bacterial pneumonia more than three times in life, score +6.	______	______
g Asthma, score +6.	______	______
h Rectal polyps, score +6.	______	______
i Diabetes, adult onset type, score +18.	______	______
j Depressions that are severe, frequent, score +12.	______	______
k Regular medical checkup: complete, score −12; partial, score −6.	______	______
Subtotals	______	______

Part 2 Lifestyle and family or social history	PLUS	MINUS
a Disposition: exceptionally good-natured, easygoing, score −3; average, score 0; extremely tense and nervous most of time, score +6.	______	______
b Exercise: physically active, score −12; moderately active, score 0; sedentary, score +12.	______	______
c Home environment: unusually pleasant, better than average, score −6; average, score 0; unusual tension, strife, score +9.	______	______
d Job satisfaction: above average, score −3; average, score 0; discontented, score +6.	______	______
e Exposure to air pollution: substantial, score +9.	______	______
f Smoking habits: nonsmoker, score −6; occasional, score 0; moderate, regular smoking, 20 cigarettes, 5 cigars or pipefuls, score +12; heavy smoking, 40 cigarettes a day, score +24; marijuana, frequent, score +24.	______	______
g Alcohol habits: none or seldom, score −6; moderate, less than 2 beers, 8 ounces wine, or 2 ounces hard liquor daily, score +6; heavy, more than above, score +24.	______	______
h Eating habits: drink skim or low-fat milk only, score −3; eat much bulky food, score −3; heavy (three times a day) meat eater, score +6; over 2 pats butter daily, score +6; over 4 cups coffee/tea/cola daily, score +6; add salt at table, score +6.	______	______

i Auto driving: regularly less than 20,000 miles annually wearing seat belt, score −3; less than 20,000 per year, belt not always worn, score 0; more than 20,000, belt not always worn, score +12. ______ ______
j Drug habits: use of street drugs, score +36. ______ ______
k If father alive and over age 68, for each 5 years above 68, score −3; if alive and under 68 or dead after 68, score 0; if dead of medical cause (not accident) before 68, score +3. ______ ______
l If mother alive and over age 73, for each 5 years above 73, score −3; if alive and under 68 or dead after 68, score 0; if dead of medical causes (not accident) before 73, score +3. ______ ______
m Marital status: married, score 0; unmarried and over 40, score +6. ______ ______
n Home location: large city, score +6; suburb, score 0; farm or small town, score −3. ______ ______
Subtotals ______ ______

Part 3 For women only

a Family history of breast cancer in mother or sister, score +6. ______ ______
b Examine breasts monthly, score −6. ______ ______
c Yearly breast exam by physician, score −6. ______ ______
d Yearly pap smear, score −6. ______ ______
Subtotals ______ ______

Calculations

a Enter subtotals from part 1. ______ ______
b Enter subtotals from part 2. ______ ______
c Enter subtotals from part 3. ______ ______
d Add the three subtotals in each column. ______ ______
e Subtract minus column from plus column. ______ ______
f Enter current age. ______ ______
g Divide test total by 12, enter. ______ ______
h Add or subtract this figure from current age to find your medical age. ______ ______

Source: Sehnert and Eisenberg, pp. 131–135.

decisions as health consumers who spend billions each year on health care—for physicians' services, medications, surgery, hospitalization, and so on. But how well do we make these decisions?

Developing Decision-making Skills

Though humans have been making decisions since the first men and women walked the earth, decision making as a distinct organized process that can be learned is relatively new. Today the subject is being taught in many schools and colleges throughout the United States—though only a minority of students have as yet been exposed to it. These are the steps in the process of organized decision making:[2]

1 *Recognize and define the decision to be made.* Some people never get this far—they let things "just happen."
2 *Collect information about the subject on which the decision is to be made.* Some information—from past experience and

[2]Developed from Gelatt et al.

Rhoda Galyn/Photo Researchers

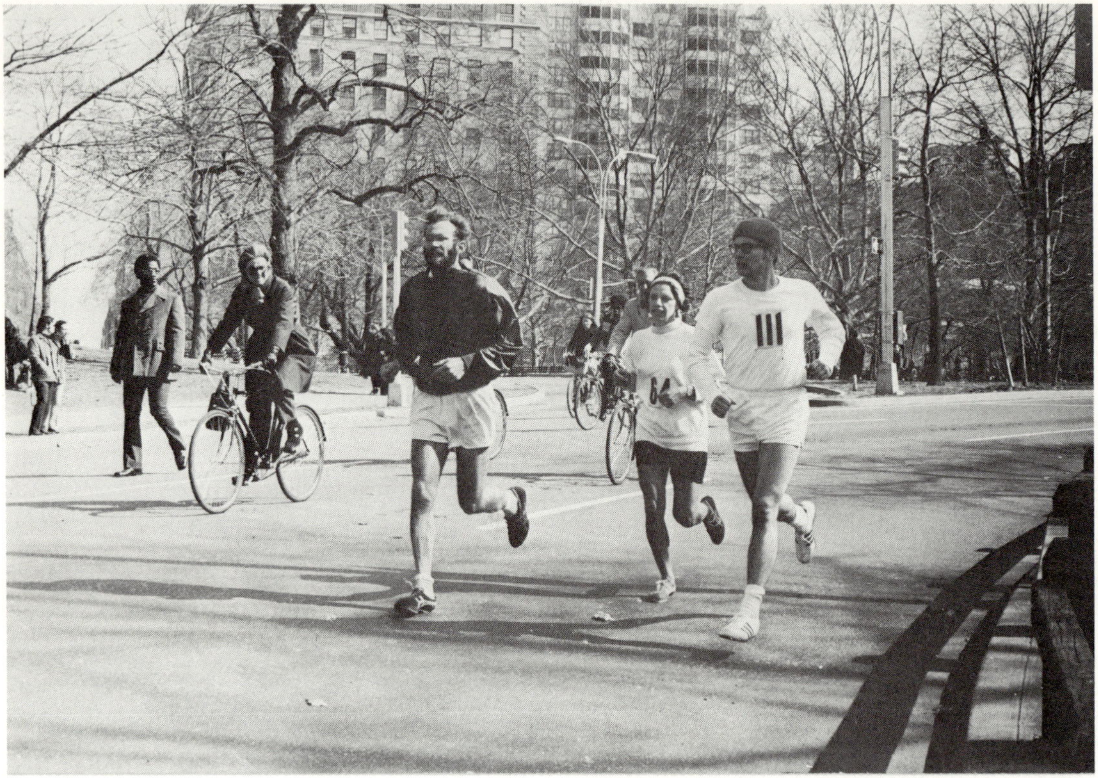

Barbara Pfeffer/Peter Arnold

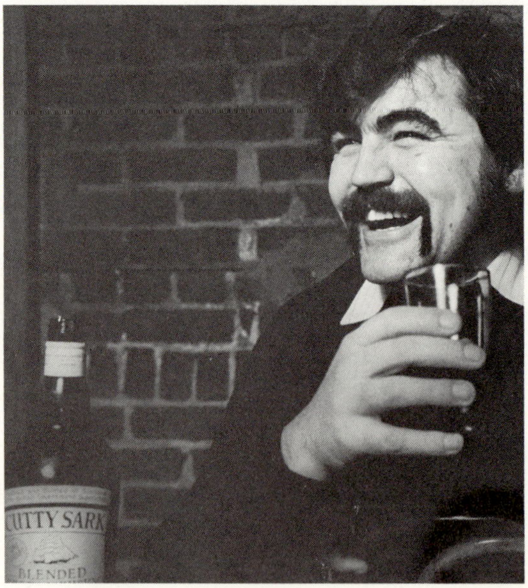

Day in and day out we make decisions affecting our health, many of them more important than any a doctor may make.

learning—you already have. Other material will have to be sought.

3 *Evaluate the information.* Sort out and eliminate information that is irrelevant or unreliable (see page 12).

4 *Outline the possible alternative solutions.*

5 *Define and weigh the risks, benefits, and possible outcomes of each alternative.* How will they affect you—and others?

6 *Know your values and goals.* What do you really want; what do you really think is good? Is health a number one priority? Or success? Or love? Or money? Or what others think? How do you choose between important but conflicting values? Such questions are basic to decision making; goals, after all, are what decisions are supposed to help us achieve.

7 *Develop a plan or strategy for decision making.* Although we all sometimes make decisions without conscious attention to strategies, every decision made uses a strategy. Sometimes the strategy is to postpone the decision pending more information; sometimes it is to avoid a decision entirely. Some other popular strategies include: the *wish strategy*, choosing what one desires most no matter what the risks—taking the long shot; the *safe strategy*, selecting the plan most likely to succeed even if the outcome will not be as rewarding—betting on the favorite; the *escape strategy*, selecting the plan that will avoid the worst outcome even if it will not bring the best—staying away from the races; the *combination strategy*, balancing desirability with safety—getting a chance at the big money without great risk of loss, hedging one's bets. This last strategy seems to offer the most, but it is also the most difficult to apply because it demands careful use of decision-making skills.

8 *Carry out the strategy.* No decision is complete until it is carried out.

9 *Accept responsibility for the decision.*

Weighing Risk against Benefit

Because no situation is without risk—not even crossing the street or staying in bed—using these decision-making techniques will not guarantee a good outcome; it will only improve the odds. The odds improve, too, when benefits we can expect from a particular decision outweigh the risks. When they do not, we can take steps to either reduce risk or increase benefits—or both. That's what daredevil Evel Knievel did several years ago in his attempted motorcycle leap across the Snake River Canyon. He increased his benefits by guaranteeing himself several million dollars, and decreased risk by using parachutes and other safety gear.

Anyone who consistently goes in for high-risk situations is playing Russian roulette. But no one is likely to be happy in a life without risk. The goal, after all, is not mere survival, but living, and living entails risks.

Most of us can be healthier than we are, but we are often unwilling to pay the costs—to give up the benefits we enjoy from cigarettes, or alcohol, or rich foods, or sexual adventurism.

THE ACTIVE, INFORMED HEALTH CONSUMER

Presently nearly $10 out of every $100 in the United States is spent on health care. Having sound information about health and knowing how to apply it—both in one's personal life and in community decision making—is crucial for those who want to be certain that the money is well spent.

Yet, when it comes to making decisions about health, many people feel ill-equipped. A course such as this gives an individual the tools for being an informed health consumer: basic information about health, basic concepts of how the body functions and interacts with its environment, how to find the health care that is needed, how to deal with health care professionals, how to handle simple medical problems, and how to understand and evaluate health care information, whether it comes from a physician, a TV anchorman, a magazine ad, or a well-meaning friend or relative.

HEALTH CONSUMER TIP

Questions to Ask in Evaluating Health Information

1 Who did the study? Did the researcher have scientifically respectable credentials and/or a proven track record? Has he or she been involved in any award-winning, pioneering, or otherwise significant work?

2 Where was the study done? Was it at a reputable institution—university, hospital, research center?

3 Who funded it? Was it the National Institutes of Health (NIH) or a major foundation? Or was it a commercial enterprise interested in marketing a product?

4 How many subjects were involved in the study? Studies based on small numbers cannot be considered conclusive.

5 Was the study merely anecdotal—a report of the experiences of one or several doctors and their patients, for example—or was it scientifically sound? Was there a *control group* getting a traditional treatment or none at all, as a comparison with the test group? Did physicians and subjects know who was getting which treatment (a condition that might bias the results)? Were the patients specifically selected for the test (which might also bias results), or were they selected at random?

6 How long did the study run? The effectiveness of a new antibiotic against strep throat could be demonstrated in a relatively short time; but effectiveness of an anticancer drug would not be confirmed until those who had been treated with it were cancer-free for a number of years.

7 If the study was epidemiological (an investigation of subjects in their natural state, their lifestyles unaltered), was follow-up carried out to be sure that a cause-and-effect relationship was really established? Just because all the people of Smalltown eat large quantities of strawberries and the population has a high rate of birth defects, we cannot conclude that strawberries cause birth defects. Such reports are merely suggestive and must be followed up by laboratory work and clinical trials.

8 Has the study been repeated successfully by another investigator? An accident, a mistake, poor design, or—very rarely—dishonesty in the original study could have caused inaccurate results.

9 Were the conclusions of the study appropriate to the sample? Sometimes the results of a small study are carelessly projected nationally. Surveys tell us something about the population being studied, but extrapolations—1 out of 10 freshmen at a small college take drugs; therefore 1 out of 10 freshmen college students in the United States take drugs—can be misleading.

10 Finally, what was the source of the information? A friend? A physician? A medical journal? A respected newspaper? A sensationalizing weekly? An ad promoting the product studied? A salesperson?

Statistics can be misleading:

The most dangerous thing a man can do is to go to bed, for more people die in bed than anywhere else.
Jacob Bigelow (1860)

Evaluating Health Information

In evaluating health information, it is necessary first to determine whether the information is *anecdotal*—somebody's personal experience—or whether it is based on sound scientific inquiry. Such inquiry is akin to Hercule Poirot methodically solving an Agatha Christie mystery—examining available evidence, advancing a theory, and then testing it out. The murder suspect has an alibi? The detective proposes another solution. False leads disturb him not at all. Testing them often adds to what is known, and is no waste of time. Finally, the mystery is solved—but a jury of peers must reexamine the facts and reach the same conclusion.

In health research that means other researchers must repeat the inquiry in the same way and achieve the same results before the theory can win acceptance in the scientific community. Even then it is not considered absolute truth, just the best information we have at the moment. Later information may alter what is accepted.

Often a theory is leaked to the public before it has undergone rigorous study. How can a health consumer decide whether a particular report heralds a great new medical advance, is a premature rumor of vague possibilities, or is outright quackery? One way is to ask your personal physician or other health professional. Another is to ask yourself some probing questions about the report—the kind suggested on page 12, in the first Health Consumer Tip.

Understanding Medical Language

One can hardly be an effective health consumer without understanding the language of the health field. Many of the purely medical terms may seem like Greek to you at first glance. That is not surprising since most are of Greek or Latin origin. But they are easy to decipher once you recognize they are constructed with building blocks of roots (often representing a part of the body), prefixes (word beginnings that further explain the word), and suffixes (endings that make an additional contribution to meaning). "Electroencephalogram," for example, is merely *electro* = electric + *en* = inside + *cephalo* = head + *gram* = record or writing, or an electrically made record of the inside of the head. Table 1.2 introduces some of the most common medical building blocks, many of which you will find frequently throughout the book.

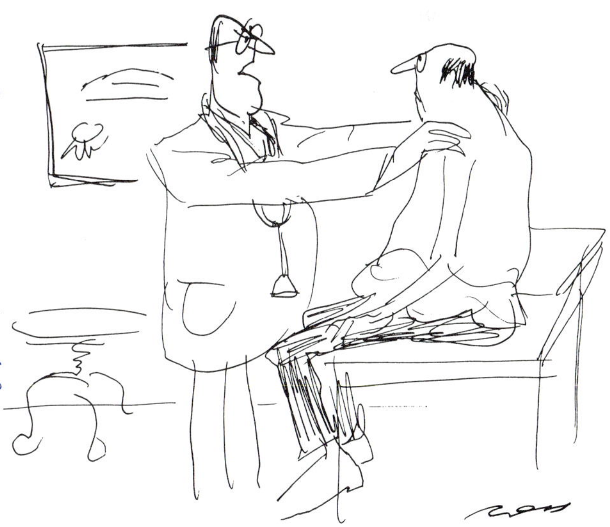

"Well, as near as I can tell, you have either logus of the bogos, the heebie-jeebies, or the jim-jam jeeters."

TABLE 1.2 Some common medical terms and how they are constructed

PREFIXES +	ROOTS +	SUFFIXES =	EXAMPLES
a = without	*meno* = month	*rrhea* = flow	amenorrhea
	pnea = air		apnea
ab = away from	*norm* = conforming to some standard	*al* = pertaining to	abnormal
an = without	*esthesia* = feeling		anesthesia
ante = before	*mortem* = death		antemortem
anti = against	*toxin* = poison		antitoxin
auto = self	*erotic* = sexually stimulating		autoerotic
bi = two		*ped* = footed	biped
di = two	*chroma* = color	*ic* = of, or pertaining to	dichromatic
dys = pain, difficult, abnormal	*phagia* = eating		dysphagia
en = in, inside, into	*cephalo* = head	*gram* = record	encephalogram
end(o) = within	*genous* = producing, caused by		endogenous
ex(o) = without, outside			exogenous
hyper = over, above	*glyc* = sweet	*emia* = condition of the blood	hyperglycemia
hypo = below, deficient			hypoglycemia
intra = within	*venous* = pertaining to vein		intravenous
inter = between	*dent* = teeth	*al* = pertaining to	interdental
macro = large	*cephalo* = head	*ic* = of, or pertaining to	macrocephalic
mal = abnormal, bad	*adapt* = adjust		maladaptive
mega = huge	*vita* = life	*amines* = group of chemical compounds	megavitamins
micro = small	*soma* = body	*ic* = of, or pertaining to	microsomatic
neo = new	*plasia* = growth		neoplasia
peri = around	*natal* = birth		perinatal
post = after			postnatal
pre = before			prenatal
tri = three	*dactyl* = digit, toe, finger		tridactyl
	carcino = cancer	*genic* = causing	carcinogenic
	gastr = stomach	*ostomy* = artificial opening	gastrostomy
	hepat = liver	*itis* = inflamation	hepatitis
	lapar = abdomen	*otomy* = cut into	laparotomy
	mast = breast	*ectomy* = cut out, remove	mastectomy
	myo = muscle *cardia(ium)* = heart		myocardium
	nephro = kidney	*sis (isis)* = condition	nephrosis
	neuro = nerve	*algia* = pain	neuralgia
	oto = ear	*scope* = instrument for viewing	otoscope
	phob = fear	*ic* = of, or pertaining to	phobic
	pneumo = lung, air, gas, breath	*pathy* = disease	pneumopathy
	psycho = mind *soma* = body		psychosomatic
	rhino = nose	*plasty* = shape, mold	rhinoplasty
	therm(o) = heat	*meter* = measure	thermometer

LOOKING BACK

REVIEWING CONCEPTS IN CHAPTER 1

- What scientists believe to be true may change as new information is discovered, but a philosophy of health developed by an individual can last a lifetime.
- Basic to such a philosophy is the understanding of three points: (1) Prevention is the most important aspect of health care. (2) *You* will make the most important decisions about your own health. (3) Only an informed and active health consumer can obtain full benefit from the health care system.
- A variety of public health measures have contributed to prevention of disease, but a great deal more needs to be done by the medical community, by the society at large, and most important, by the individual.
- Using appropriate decision-making skills improves the chances for "good" outcomes when we make health decisions. But no decision is risk-free, and we must weigh risks against benefits in each situation.
- The active, informed health consumer knows how to evaluate health information, and can differentiate between anecdotal reports and sound scientific studies that have been repeated by several investigators.
- Most common medical language is easy to decipher when you recognize the major building blocks—prefixes, roots, and suffixes.

I

HOW WE COPE--OR FAIL TO COPE--WITH LIVING

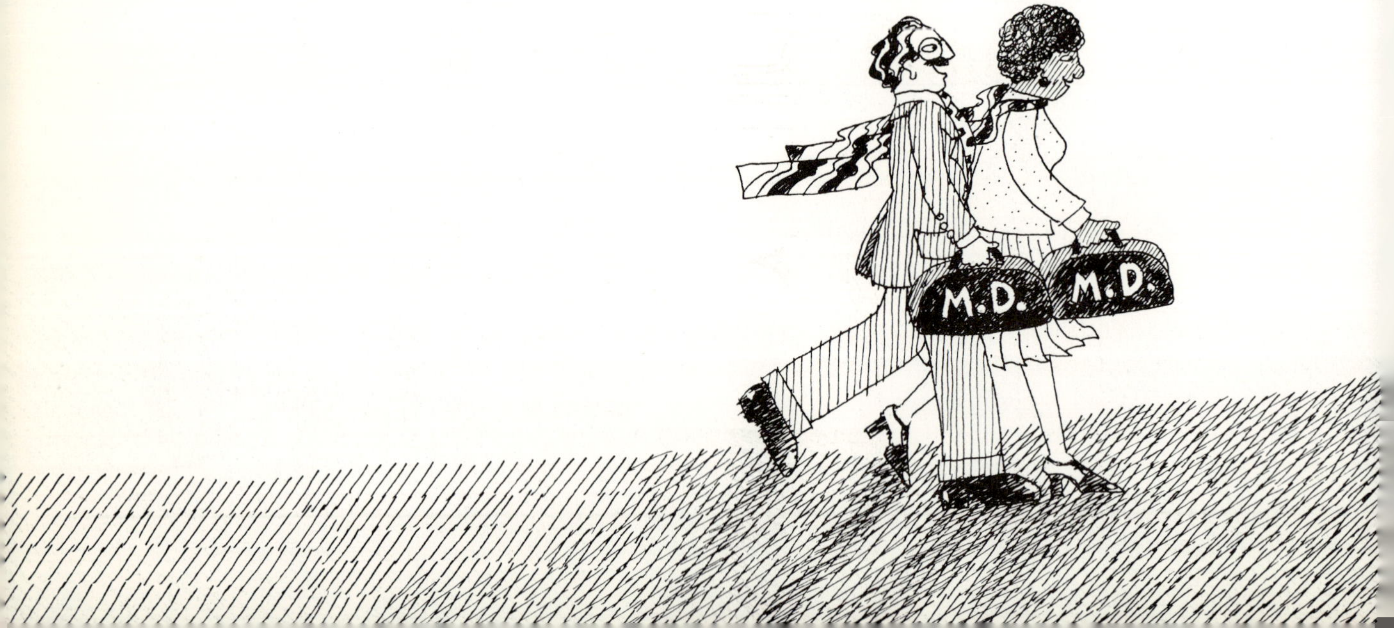

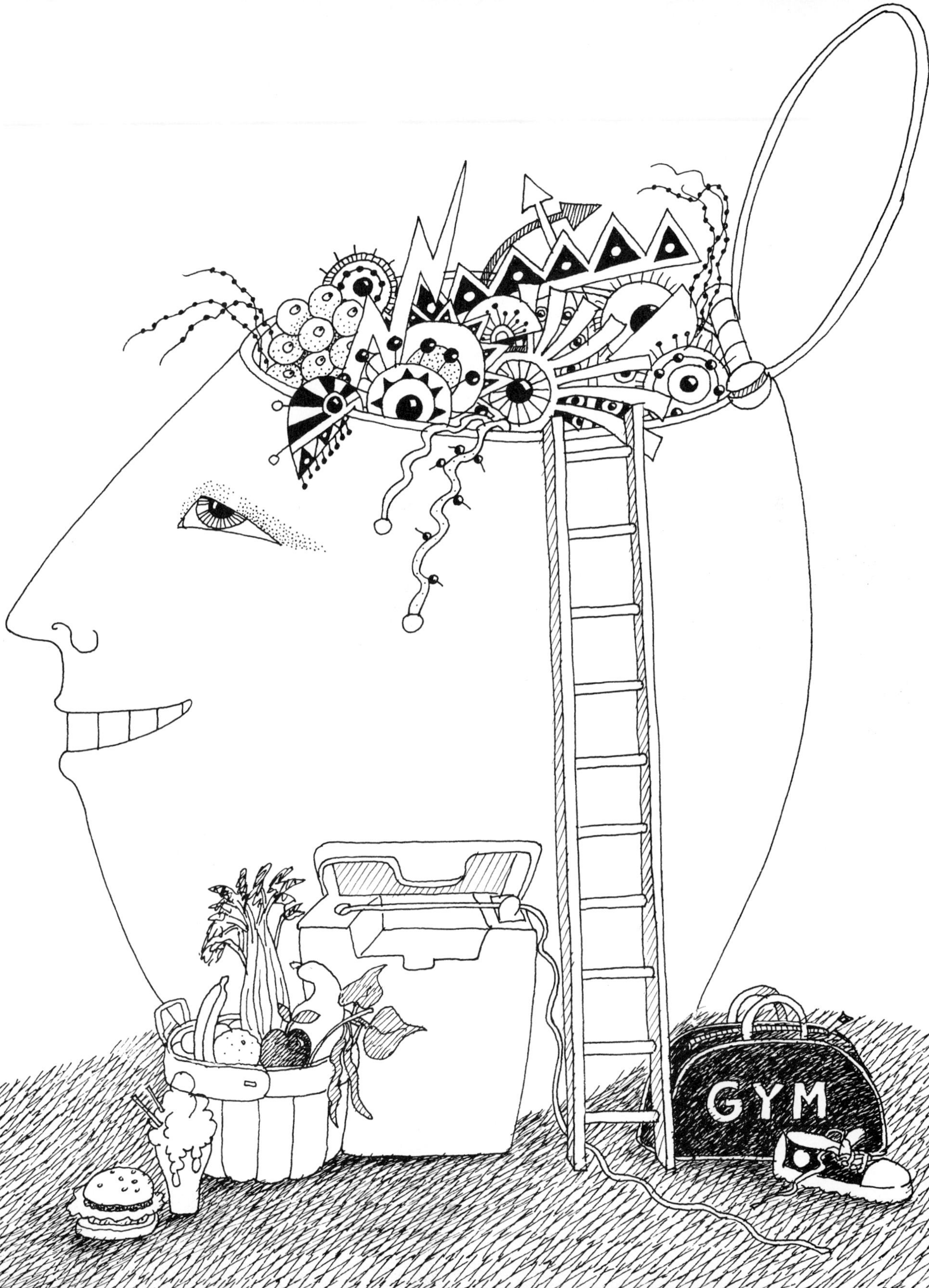
GYM

M.D.
M.D.

2
TOWARD GOOD MENTAL HEALTH

WHAT'S AHEAD IN CHAPTER 2 What is the search for identity? How does it affect your life and the lives of others? What is maturity? Can it be easily achieved? How do the striving for maturity, relationships with others, and a system of values and belief affect the development of good mental health? What is stress and how do humans respond to and deal with it? Are there more effective and less effective ways of handling stress? Can one learn to cope more effectively? What role does the balancing of work and play have in coping with college stress? How do relationships with parents change for the young student entering college? Can the student make these changes more positive? How can the special problems of students living with roommates for the first time, of those who commute to school, and of those returning to education after a break of many years best be resolved? How can students prevent fatigue? And how can they cope with it, once they are its victims?

Sept. 11. *My past seems to have died. I stand alone before my life-to-come, full of doubts and fears of inadequacy.*
Sept. 13. *College is vast and overwhelming. . . . I am somewhat awed at the brilliance around me.*
Sept. 14. *Last night at a college mixer I found myself lost and inadequate, terribly insecure. My status as a man was deeply shaken.*
Oct. 11. *I am obsessed and burdened with fantasies, thoughts, dreads. I feel a longing to return home and recapture a dead childhood. Help me!*
Nov. 10. *I have been quite depressed.*
Dec. 16. *I am going home for Christmas with horror at the social rejection and loneliness which is certain to engulf me at home. I am leaving college in fear. My past is suffocating me. Have I committed some crime which demands that I get air, air, air?*

Madison, p. 64

THE SEARCH FOR IDENTITY

This is not the diary of someone about to crack up from the stress of college life. Rather, it is the diary of a student in the throes of an identity crisis. This young man did find himself. In fact, he went on to be extremely successful not only in college and the professional career that followed, but in a happy marriage as well. The anxiety he exhibited was not an indication of mental illness, but a common sign of growth described as "acute postadolescent identity crisis." The more rapid the growth, the more intense the anxiety.

Of course, many young people find their identity on less troubled roads. A study of Vassar students found that although some sort of crisis may be necessary for dynamic growth, it is probably not necessary for achieving a stable and integrated life (Freedman). Erik Erikson (*b*, p. 14) has also suggested that "in some people . . . this crisis will be minimal."

Today it is recognized that such identity crises occur not just in young adulthood, but at many other periods of life as well. A housewife in her middle years going back to school and starting a new career probably experiences it; so does a man or woman going through a divorce, a middle-aged person trying to evaluate the past and the future, and an older person contemplating retirement.

Who Are You?

You are a million years of human development. You are countless genes inherited from your mother and your father, genes stretching back to the beginning of human history. You are the fetal environment of your mother's womb, the childhood environment in which you grew up, the adult environment in

Russian poet Yevtushenko described his steps toward adulthood:

I scarcely had one single care in the world,
my life, presenting no big obstacles,
seemed to have few or simple complications—
life solved itself without my contributions. . . .
I had no doubts about harmonious answers
which could and would be given to every question.
But suddenly this felt necessity
of answering these questions for myself. . . .
So there stood youth and there stood childhood together,
Trying to look into each other's eyes
and each offending, but not equally.
Childhood spoke first, "Hullo then.
It's your fault if I hardly recognize you.
I thought you'd be quite different from this.
I'll tell you honestly, you worry me.
You're still in very heavy debt to me."
So youth asked if childhood would help,
and childhood smiled and promised it would help. . . .

Yevgeny Yevtushenko, "Zima Junction,"
in *Selected Poems*, pp. 24–25.

Charles Gatewood

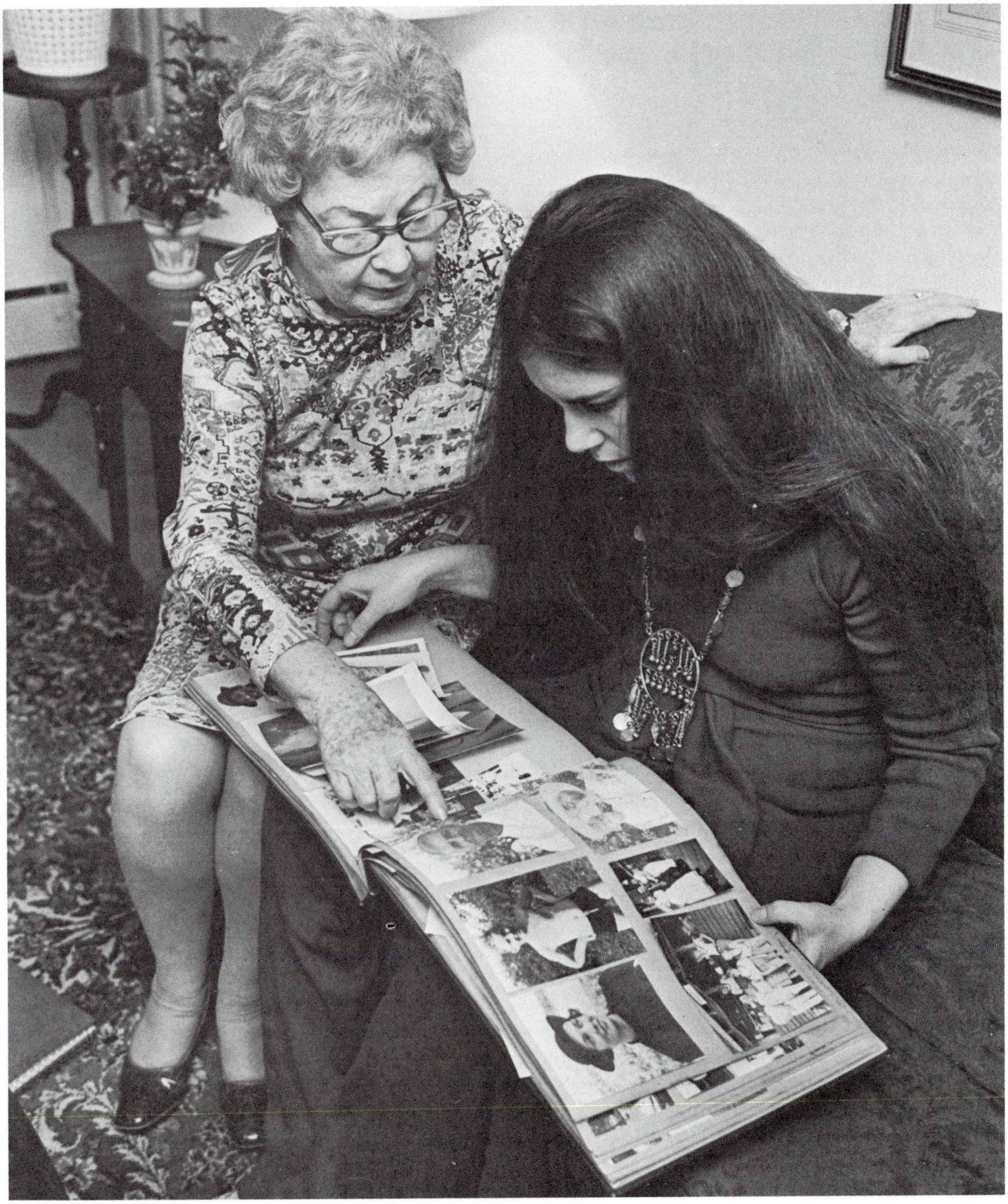

Who you are has been influenced by generations of genes, your childhood environment, parents, teachers, peers, your ethnic heritage, and the social, economic, and educational levels of your family.

Anatomy, History, and Personality are our combined destiny.

Erik H. Erikson (b, p. 285)

which you live, work, study. Your attitudes, feelings, concepts of the world, were influenced by your parents, your teachers, your relatives, friends, employers, and people you have never met but have seen on TV and in movies. You were shaped by major events in your life—births, deaths, marriages, divorces, illnesses, relocations, love relationships—and by minor ones—disappointments, slight injuries, praise, and criticism.

Who you are has also been shaped, from preschool through college and beyond, by your ethnic heritage; by the social, economic, and educational levels of your parents; by whether you are male or female; by the culture of your peers.

Your past will always be a part of you. But that is not all you are, and who you are does not remain static. You are always changing and developing. In his analysis of Martin Luther, Erikson describes the process as it occurs in the young adult:

> Each youth must forge for himself some central perspective and direction, some working unity, out of the effective remains of his childhood and the hopes of his anticipated adulthood; he must detect some meaningful resemblance between what he has come to see in himself and what his sharpened awareness tells him others judge and expect him to be. (*a*, p. 14)

College students, whether they are young adults or well into middle or even old age, face this challenge: to combine the past person and the present person to project a future person—a person unique in this world. This may mean breaking away from childhood and parents or from a previous adult lifestyle or previously held values. Or it may mean adopting a life much like that of one's parents, or keeping a familiar lifestyle that still feels comfortable, or recommitting oneself to earlier values. Successful resolution of the challenge does not always require change; but it does require independent choice.

Negative Identity

Sometimes the answer to the question "Who am I?" is "Nobody." When a child, an adolescent, or even an adult continually meets with belittling, hostility, lack of respect and praise, with low expectations and little opportunity for growth, independence, and freedom of choice from parents, teachers, employers, co-workers, peers, and others, then such a negative identity can develop.

A society that keeps the young in long-term dependence, deprives them of the chance to feel useful, responsible, or influential, and seems uncertain about when coming-of-age is actually reached (Is it when you can get a driver's license or a marriage license? Or when you can vote or legally drink beer?) can also contribute to a negative self-image. So can the apparent discrepancy between what young people have been told (ideals such as equality and plenty) and what they see (realities such as injustice, hunger, and disease) which leads to the question: "Am I—whom no one chooses to listen to, to respect, to give responsible work, to tell the truth about our society—a worthwhile person?"

Selecting a negative identity:

I was so unhappy with me, so dissatisfied with my image that any other one would do. I wanted to be anyone but me. So I started on drugs, then prostitution. I sank lower and lower.

A former prostitute-addict

Man . . . I'm tired of being a half-past-nothing. I've come into this stone world of street, with all its living, laughing, crying, and dying. A world full of backyards, rooftops, and street sets, all kinds of races of people and acts, of hustles and rackets, drugs and eyedroppers. A world of those who is and those who ain't.

I'm looking at me and no matter how I set my face, hard rock or soft sullen, I still feel the me inside rumbling low and crazy like, like I'm mad at something and don't know what it is. . . . What's the good of living in a present that's got no future, no nothing, unless I make something? I fell into this life without no say and I'll be a mother-jumper if I live it without having nothing to say. I'm tired of feeling like the invisible cat in the flick, walking all over the place, and the only time anybody looks at me is to say, "Get out of the way, kid." (Piri Thomas, pp. 46–48)

Minority Youth and Special Identity Problems

Minority college students—members of black, Spanish-American, Mexican-American, Indian, and other ethnic groups—have all the identity problems of other students plus the problem of living in a society that asks them to deny their ethnic identity: "Be like us, give up your ghetto or barrio or reservation ways, and you'll be accepted." Such attitudes are not likely to build self-esteem.

A student at a New York community college responded this way: "Identity is to me my race, my culture—me. Only in a raceless, classless, free society can one be judged by the content of his character, instead of by the color of his skin. And that we don't have"(Elisa, p. 53). Yet.

Piri Thomas, author and graduate of the ghetto who matriculated at Sing Sing Prison, urges that minority youth be provided with opportunities beyond learning about their heritages. These young people should have the chance to gain self-confidence and esteem through success—in school, in creative areas, in sports, in jobs: "Society must show them they can hope."

Appearance and Identity

An acceptable appearance generally leads to good feelings about oneself. Poor appearance can, on the other hand, become a vicious cycle: from depression about appearance to sloppiness in dress and grooming and inattention to interpersonal relations to less attractiveness and back to more depression.

Being born good-looking, however, does not automatically guarantee self-esteem. The attractive individual who gets through school and into a job with little effort may begin to wonder "Could I have made it without my looks? Do I have any other virtues?" He or she may fail to develop coping skills as well as ways of nurturing relationships with others.

Nor does an unattractive appearance always lead to lack of self-esteem. We all know people who lack perfect features, but are personable, interesting, and fun to be with. They have developed their assets rather than worrying about their shortcomings. Sometimes, however, a large nose, an almost absent chin, too much or too little breast development does damage self-esteem. In some instances new hairstyles, cosmetics, ways of dressing can camouflage the problem. Sometimes psychotherapy can help. In severe cases, the best solution may be cosmetic surgery, which, though it cannot solve deep emotional problems, can often have a dramatic effect on one's life. As Jean Cocteau once said: "A defect of soul cannot be corrected on the face, but a defect of the face, if you correct it, can correct a soul."

BECOMING MATURE

While seeking identity, the individual asks, "What kind of person should I be?" The Bible, the later Jewish, Christian, and humanist thinkers, and Greek and Eastern philosophers all defined ideals of what a human being ought and ought not to be. Today's psychologists and philosophers have continued trying to describe the perfect person and the ways in which individuals can reach a state of perfection. So far, no description has been acceptable to all. Ultimately, the question is one for philosophy. But science can help by studying those people generally considered to be successful at the art of living, and describing as scientifically as possible how they do it.

Researchers have come up with a variety of terms to describe the ideal state—"well-adjusted," "mature," "maturing," "mentally healthy," "self-actualized." We will use the word "mature," not because it is a better word than the others, but because it is most commonly used. The elements that researchers have suggested as components of maturity are even more diverse than the terminology. It is important to remember that these components are *goals* toward which we are always striving, rather than a state of being we can expect to reach at a certain point in life. Mature individuals do not expect to be perfect—but they keep trying. They continue to try to grow and mature, even into middle and old age.

Components of Maturity

We have already discussed such important components of maturity as knowing oneself and making choices. The following list[1] is not complete but is suggestive. Some of the areas overlap.

Sense of self The basis of a mature personality, of good mental health, is a strong sense of self-worth. When Jennie, who is always picking on herself for her shortcomings (overweight, difficulties with math), comes to realize that these are accompanied by positive qualities (an ability to develop close friendships, a flair for language), she is developing a sense of self-esteem. The person who has self-esteem, self-confidence, a sense of security, and a satisfaction with a personal value system is not threatened by the environment or by others—yet is not arrogant or unbending.

Independence or autonomy Independent persons make their own decisions and, more importantly, take responsibility for them. When Bob at 22 decides to become a mechanic—though his parents frown on the idea and society may not accord him high status—he has almost completed the gradual transition from the total dependence of infancy to the emotional independence of adulthood.

Interdependence Independence not tempered by the recognition that human beings are also *inter*dependent is *not* mature. When Randi is having marital problems, she shows maturity in being able to turn to others for help. She also shows maturity when she offers help to others having difficulties.

Adaptability or flexibility The mature person takes positions, but is ready to change them when new information is put forth or situations alter. Angie had always held a very strong position on one side of the abortion issue, but the experience of a close friend caused her to rethink her stand. She did so with an open mind.

Ability to accept and deal with reality Being mature means being able to admit that good and bad exist, and being at ease with imperfections. Steve is 5 feet, 5 inches tall. During his teens, he yearned for the height of his peers, and became obnoxious and belligerent to cover up his perceived inadequacy. But by the time he reached col-

[1]Adapted, in part, from Smitson, pp. 9–11.

lege, he could accept the reality of his short stature and found constructive ways to compensate for it.

Reality testing The mature person's reality is not that of the "authorities" or of "everybody else." When Lynn arrived on campus, she was advised to stay away from a group with a reputation for being "strange." But before she accepted this information, she did some evaluation and found that the group consisted of ordinary students, who had discovered that yoga helped them to relax.

Accepting others' perceptions of reality Mature thinking requires that we recognize that others may have different evaluations and perceptions. Though Brad really does not think he has been neglecting his family, he recognizes that his wife believes he has, and that her perceptions are as real for her as his are for him. So he acts to ease her concern and to build trust.

Having goals The life of the mature person has a sense of purpose. It is directed toward ends—education, marriage and family, career, and the attainment of human dignity. Contemporary philosopher John Rawls thinks of a person's goals as a "life-plan," which is: constantly revised and articulated; realistic; incorporating as many of one's goals as possible in a harmonious way; flexible enough to allow for changes in oneself and one's environment; and giving due weight to all parts of one's life, not imprudently choosing a smaller immediate gratification over a larger future one.

When plans are frustrated, the mature response is not to give up, but to retrench for further effort. When goals are clearly unreachable, the mature person will evaluate and reorder them—as Lea and Michael did when plans to defer having children until both finished law school were upset by an unplanned pregnancy. Neither wanted to abort, so they redesigned their life plan and timetables.

Delayed gratification Psychiatrist Dana L. Farnsworth (*b*) believes modern instant communications have contributed to the desire for instant gratification and the increase of impulsive behavior that have been observed in many young patients. Ralph is behaving maturely when he abandons the "I want what I want when I want it" attitude of childhood and is ready to put off immediate pleasure in order to reach future goals—skimping on movies, beer, and ski trips to save for a trip to Europe. He knows today's actions affect tomorrow.

Assertiveness Mature persons not only set goals, but are assertive in carrying them out. They neither behave like sheep, fearing to rock the boat, nor speak out so aggressively that they offend others and thus fail to reach their goals. They take positive, self-assured steps to get what they want—but without ignoring the feelings, needs, rights of others.

Responsiveness to others The development of "allocentrism" (an awareness of others and their needs), and a move away from "egocentrism" (interest in one's own needs exclusively) is an important sign of maturity (Heath). Smitson describes three types of people characterized by their responses to others: (1) those who are highly insensitive and show little or no response to the expressed or unexpressed needs of others; (2) those—the majority—who respond sensitively to the expressed needs of others, but do not pick up clues to unspoken needs; and (3) those who are highly sensitive, responding readily to both the expressed and the unexpressed emotional needs of those around them. This last group is attuned to catching little clues in language and body talk.

Empathy toward others Most societies have recognized the need to "put oneself in the other person's place." Sociologist Gisela Konopka quotes an old Chippewa proverb that says, "Never judge a man until you have walked a moon in his moccasins." Maslow speaks of an "identity, sympathy and affection for mankind." Mature persons feel themselves to be a part of humankind—part of family, community, country. They show both empathy (getting into another's shoes and then back into their own before acting) and sympathy (getting into another's shoes and staying there) (Clarke).

Ability to communicate The mature person is aware that we are always communicating—with words, with tone of voice, with silence, with eyes and facial expressions, with hand and body movements, by touching, even by the way we dress. A mature individual has a genuine desire to reach and be reached by others, and is both a good listener and a real communicator. The successful communicator generally is clear and specific, tries to be sure that minds have met, expects and accepts differences of opinion, accepts the feelings of another as real, gives the other a chance to save face, avoids sweeping problems under the rug, and avoids jumping to conclusions and destructive arguing (yelling, name-calling, exaggerating, etc.).

Giving to others Giving freely is often difficult. Gail shies away from it because she does not want to risk being hurt, rejected, or exploited. Andrew, on the other hand, is more mature. He readily tolerates the risks involved in a close, giving relationship. Dr. Hans Selye (*b*), authority on stress, points out that doing for others builds mental health because it gains us the love and esteem of others that is necessary to self-esteem.

Loving and being loved Without love—given and received—good mental health is not possible (Roberts). In psychiatrist William Glasser's view, inability to give and receive love is responsible for neurotic behavior. Psychiatrist Smiley Blanton suggests that love provides the strength, protection, and encouragement without which full human growth is impossible. We speak of all kinds of love—love of country, community, fellow human beings; love of parents, children, family; love of man for woman, woman for man; love of ideals; and not least, love of self, without which the other kinds of love are not possible. Eric Fromm said there are "certain basic elements common to all forms of love . . . *care, responsibility, respect and knowledge. . . . Love is the active concern for the life and growth of that which we love*" (p. 26).

Controlling emotions Mature persons are able both to express emotions and feelings—joy, love, excitement, anger, indignation—when appropriate, and to withhold them when they might hurt, embarrass, or offend. Their reactions are appropriate to a situation. A mature parent does not always blow up over a spilled glass of milk, but does express strong emotion when a toddler wanders onto a busy street. A teenager who feels like throwing things when not allowed to use the car may instead go out to play tennis, safely diverting negative energies into an overhead smash. Maturity means finding a balance between emotionality and rationality, neither permitting emotion to dominate behavior not omitting it from decision making entirely.

Systems of Belief, Moral Values, and Mental Health

Where do a system of belief and a set of moral values—be they based on religious faith or humanism—fit into the picture of the mentally healthy mature person? According to Abraham Maslow, they may be a major part of the picture "because ultimately the search for identity is, in essence, the search for one's own intrinsic, authentic values . . ." (p. 166). Psychiatrist Karl Menninger has expressed the belief that mental and moral health are identical, while William Glasser, developer of reality therapy, declares: "Morals, standards, values, or right and wrong behavior are all intimately related to the fulfillment of our needs for self-worth" (*b*, p. 11).

At three I had a feeling of
Ambivalence toward my brothers,
And so it follows naturally
I poisoned all my lovers.
But now I'm happy; I have learned
The lesson this has taught;
That everything I do that's wrong
Is someone else's fault.

Anna Russell, "Psychiatric Folksong,"
in Mowrer, p. 49.

Apparently, animals are incapable of even the most basic ethical choices. Comments psychologist Guy L. Roberts:

> Man alone adjudges the quality of his behavior, establishes value-goals, and transcends the immediate present and biological compulsion. . . . Man not only *can* make value choices, he *must* do so. . . . Lacking absolute knowledge, he sometimes makes wrong choices and suffers guilt pangs. . . . This negative voice of conscience, guilt, is man's guide to responsible living, to overcoming his anxiety. . . . The positive voice of conscience is joy and peace—a "well done, good and faithful servant!"—that wells up from within when man rises to the challenge and achieves in high proportion to his potential. . . . And the ratio of guilt to joy bears heavily on his state of mental health. (p. 177)

Where do we find a set of moral values? James Coleman, psychologist, suggests we can turn to four chief sources of understanding: (1) our culture and surrounding cultures, which tell us what others value; (2) science, which can help us better understand ourselves and the universe in which we live; (3) experience, which tells us, as individuals and as part of the group, what the consequences of various forms of behavior may be; and (4) religion, which helps us deal with the difficult-to-understand and gives us the opportunity to rise above the everyday, the mundane. No one of these sources seems sufficient in itself, nor—from the mental health standpoint—is any of them infallible.

Though belief in organized religion has ebbed and flowed during the past several decades, the interest in searching for meaning in life has remained constant. The route for some has been drugs; for others it has been through exotic religions of the East, groups on the fringes of Judaism and Christianity, pop-psychology cults such as est, Esalen, and Scientology. Some of these groups may offer a grain of guidance for the confused, but a number are responsible, according to Dr. Eli Shapiro, for a "sociopathic illness" spreading throughout the world. The symptoms include marked personality changes; a "million mile stare"; loss of personal identity; dropping out of school; adoption of unusual eating habits, clothes, names, and hairstyles; preoccupation with rituals and beliefs; estrangement from family, and complete dependence upon a charismatic leader who usually claims to be God or a divine messenger. Many cult members become incapable of making their own decisions and must be retrained to "grow up" again when they leave the group.

Of course, many people still find meaning in traditional biblical faiths. Armand M. Nicoli, in studying the phenomenon of religious conversion among collegians, found that turning to traditional religion leads to a strengthened sense of self; increased maturity levels; elimination of drug dependency; and improved impulse control, academic performance, interpersonal relationships, and communication with parents.

Students experiencing religious rebirth in college are a small minority. For many younger students, college is a time to question faith, to move away from dogmatic concepts and formalized religion (Chickering). A broad study found such students seeking a new religious view that accepts science and technology as legitimate ways of knowing and as contributors to social good, but which also recognizes that there is something more, that there are other ways of knowing—through God, revelation, intuition, and self-awareness. They believe in some sort of God, yet ad-

Yan Lukas/Photo Researchers

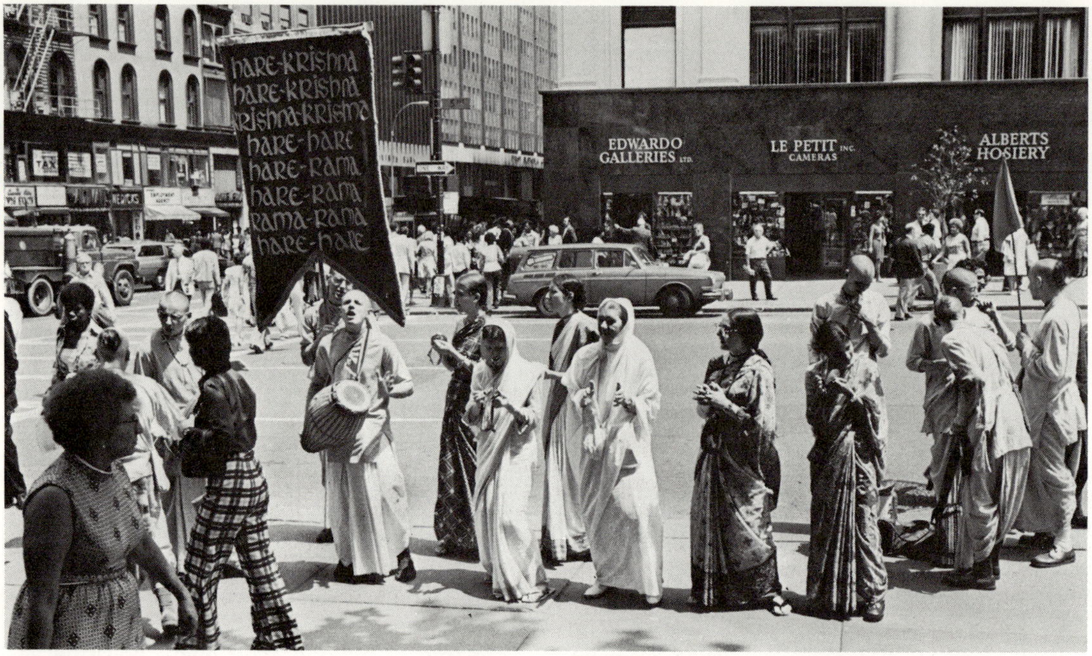

In a search for meaning, some young people have turned to religious cults.

mit doubt. And they see ethical action and concern for others as a crucial test of serious faith (Underwood). When organized religion appears to fail this test, many young people become cynical.

In addition to developing a set of values and exhibiting the other elements of maturity already discussed, the mature person has the ability to cope with problems.

RESPONSES TO STRESS AND ANXIETY

Michael, busy with baseball practice and fund raising for the team's trip to Florida, falls behind in his calculus class. As midterm exams approach, he begins to get the same queasy feeling in his stomach he used to get every morning when he was in first grade. The night before the calculus exam, he starts throwing up and is admitted to the infirmary. A sympathetic teacher exempts him from the exam, allowing him to stay on the team and make the trip. In June, he fails calculus.

Janet fails her English midterm. She blames the failure on the test, her teacher, the family responsibilities she must juggle with her studies. She makes no effort to do better. Blaming and excuses are her style. Comes the end of the semester, she fails the course and is put on warning.

Gwenn is afraid she won't pass psychology, and won't reach her goal of becoming a child psychologist. After a sleepless night, she gets up with new determination. She makes an appointment with the professor to try to figure out what her problem is. She revises her schedule, allotting more time to study and less to social activities. She and her roommate agree to limit company, so both can get some work done. Gwenn ends the semester with a B in the course, and a lot more confidence in herself.

We all cope with stressful situations according to our own life experiences and associations. Some ways of coping are successful, others are not. Competent coping is an important element in the mature personality. In order to understand coping, one must first understand the stresses that require coping response.

Stress

Stress is a condition or situation that demands that a person adjust. It can be physiological (a headache, a sprained ankle), psychological (an inner fear of not living up to childhood standards, a conflict between wanting to please parents and peer group), or a combination of both. Stress can also be caused by external events—exams, waiting for school acceptances, dental visits, a wedding or divorce, a new job, fear of war or of being mugged.

We cannot avoid stress in our lives. If we could, we would also avoid growth, because stress, called "the spice of life" by Hans Selye, is a necessary ingredient in learning and growing. Mild stress, properly handled, prepares us for more extreme kinds of stress later in life. As with medication, stress is needed in proper dosages. Inadequate amounts are not motivating enough; too much may be debilitating—especially over a long period of time. The proper dosage varies from person to person.

Timing is important, too. Studies have shown that those who handle stress best are those who met frustration and learned skills of mastery (driving a car, dating, etc.) at about the average age. Those who tried to learn mastery skills too early and met with too much frustration, as well as those who learned them too late and never encountered much frustration, are much less successful at coping with stress (Torrance).

Stress can be categorized by degree—from mild to severe. The duration of the stress is also an important factor. Mild stress that is prolonged—a job that is unpleasant, playing on a team under a coach who always seems to be needling, living with a nagging mate—may be harder to recover from than brief but intense stress. The relationship of stress to disease is discussed in Chapter 7.

> And no grand inquisitor has in readiness such terrible tortures as has anxiety. . . .
>
> Søren Kierkegaard

Anxiety

Anxiety is a key ingredient in the coping process. It is the alarm signal that sounds when we are faced with a difficult situation. If we ignore the signals, we may get into a lot of trouble. If we overreact to them and panic, we may not be able to respond at all. Take a situation as simple as crossing a busy street. If we did not feel a temporary sense of anxiety, we might just stroll right into an oncoming automobile. If, however, we felt too much anxiety, we might never be able to summon the courage to cross the street at all. Thus, anxiety, like stress, is not only essential, but essential in the right amounts.

For some, anxiety is felt as a nameless dread, a feeling of panic they cannot quite describe. For others, there is a "sense of uncertainty about the future," lack of appetite, tension across the back, gnawing in the pit of the stomach. A lump in the throat, butterflies in the stomach, headache, shortness of breath, rapid heartbeat, dry mouth, insomnia, and diarrhea are all physiological responses to stress. The effects of the emotions on the body are not imaginary; they are very real. They can lead to such psychosomatic (*psyche* = mind + *soma* = body) illnesses as ulcers, and can bring on asthma attacks.

Dealing with Stress: Copping Out

It is not the quality or quantity of stress we face in life that is important, but how we handle it. One approach is to use defense mechanisms—often a way of copping out. Sigmund Freud was the first to point out that we use defenses not just against physical attack but against attacks on our self-esteem as well. Common defense mechanisms include:

- *Denial* Protecting the ego from stressful situations by unconsciously refusing to recognize that they exist. (Riding in a car driven by a friend who is high on alcohol or drugs, one denies the possibility of an accident.)
- *Avoidance* Protecting oneself from a feared situation by avoiding it. (A person who is afraid of flying takes trains.)
- *Repression* Another form of denial, in which painful events are unconsciously blocked from the mind. (A young man may block the memory of early scoldings about masturbation, yet feel strangely uneasy about the subject as an adult.)
- *Rationalization* Denying reality by blaming others, environment, health—anything but oneself. ("The test was unfair." "The room was too hot." "We never studied that.") We are rationalizing, too, when we belittle what we can't have. ("I never really wanted to go to medical school.")
- *Regression* Resorting to the tactics of childhood when things go wrong. In the face of frustration, a person may throw a tantrum, pout, hurl objects, or run home to parents.
- *Fantasy* Escape from reality through TV, a movie, a book, or just daydreaming. When daydreaming substitutes for real-life achievement, it may interfere with functioning. (This is the Walter Mitty syndrome, in which one wins the hand of the beauteous superstar, shoots down more enemy planes than the Red Baron, etc.—but all in the mind.)
- *Other defense mechanisms* Humor, criticism, projection, attention seeking, substitution or sublimation, displaced aggression, and emotional insulation.

Defenses can be useful at times. Putting out of mind the thought that the world could be destroyed in 30 minutes by atomic warfare keeps the average person sane. Should world leaders put this out of their minds, however, it could lead to disaster. Rationalizing a failure now and then may help us to pick up the pieces and move on. If we do it all the time, failing to recognize and correct shortcomings, we may not rise above failure. A brief escape through denial, avoidance, or fantasy can be helpful when we lose a job, fail a course, or break an engagement, and need time before deciding what to do next.

Results of a long-term study of "normal" Harvard students indicate that some types of defenses (altruism, humor, suppression, anticipation, sublimation) are more mature than others (projection, schizoid fantasy, hypochondriasis, passive-aggressive behavior, acting out). Men who used mature defenses were, in the study, most likely to be happy and successful, both in careers and in personal lives (Vaillant).

Dealing with Stress: Coping

Though defense mechanisms can help a person adjust to a situation temporarily, they cannot solve problems. There is a more competent and positive approach to dealing with stress: problem solving, or coping. Coping is the skill and ability to *act* rather than *react*. Coping (from the French *couper*, to strike) has been described as:

> . . . adaptation to a stressful situation—to what is, and a working out of what should be. It does not mean total triumph over the environment, nor total surrender to it. Rather . . . a striving towards an acceptable compromise. . . . [The] goal of competent coping is to contain stress and maintain self-esteem, while realistically solving a problem. (Hoffman-La Roche, *b*, p. 14)

Development of coping behavior An infant who pushes back the blanket or shifts to a more comfortable position is coping with the environment. Another baby who cries because of hunger, a wet diaper, or loneliness, and gets a response from an adult, begins to have the satisfying feeling of competence, of control over the environment. This is the beginning, too, of a feeling of self-esteem: "I am somebody other people care about." However, the infant who cries and gets no response may not be able to establish self-esteem, may withdraw, become apathetic, develop a tendency to give up (Hoffman-La Roche, *c*). Sleep becomes an escape from problems.

As children grow, having opportunities to solve problems, make decisions, and "do for themselves" increases coping ability. They also learn how to cope—or not to cope—from parental example. The father who comes home from work and has a couple of drinks "to help me unwind" is teaching his children how to avoid coping by the use of alcohol or other drugs. Parents who face financial crisis by escaping to a winter vacation they cannot afford are also teaching a mode of reacting to problems.

Other factors influence coping behavior: genetic endowment, physical ability or disability, the coping styles of the culture in which one lives. Children in the lowest economic strata, for example, may see violence used frequently and adopt it as a coping style of their own. Self-esteem also influences the ability to cope. Children who find success in coping develop self-esteem which, in turn, makes future coping easier, and improves performance under stress. Conversely, children who lack early success have low self-esteem, feel incompetent, and show little ability to cope with stress (White).

Coping techniques For each individual and each situation, the exact approach to coping will be different. New situations require adapting and developing new techniques,

SELF-CARE

Basic Steps to More Effective Coping

1 Recognize your feelings: fears, hostilities, anxieties. Talk about them with someone you trust who is not emotionally involved. This can reduce stress.

2 Examine the problem causing the feelings. The Buddhist monk, learning to concentrate while sitting in an uncomfortable position, is told to think of his pain, not ignore it. In some way, when he concentrates on the pain, it becomes quite bearable. Look at—not away from—your problems. Making a written list of your problems may help.

3 Decide how to deal with the problem. The decision-making process discussed in Chapter 1 is a good way to proceed. But don't make a decision while feelings are disorganized by grief, confusion, anxiety. Take time to let your mind clear.

4 Keep your options open; don't become boxed in. There is a way out of every maze, but it may not be the one you originally hoped for.

5 Decide whether the stress—the job, the class, the marriage—is worth it. If it is, then ways of coping and improving the situation need to be found. If it is not, then don't be afraid to break away. But do it consciously. Don't let it "just happen."

6 Prepare for stress in advance when possible. Good planning—for example, collecting advance information on a new home, new school, or new job—lessens stress and anxiety.

7 Use some defense mechanisms when necessary as indirect and temporary aids in dealing with stress: rest and relaxation, hard work and hard play, time with friends, service to others.

broadening our problem-solving abilities. Creativity and inventiveness make for better coping. Torrance describes creative individuals who have coped under extreme conditions: Willard Millar, for example, who, in his escape from Korea, treated infections by crushing water purification tablets and applying them to his wounds, and created a natural alarm clock to keep himself from oversleeping by drinking a large quantity of water just before going to sleep.

When one feels overwhelmed by anxiety and unable to cope, then counseling or therapy may be needed to help restore old coping ways or devise new ones. How to obtain such counseling is discussed in Chapter 3.

COPING WITH COLLEGE AND THE CHANGES IT BRINGS

Whether students enter college straight out of high school or after a 10-year break, go away to college or stay in their own community, live with one or more roommates, with family, or alone, college presents a series of challenges to their arsenal of coping techniques. Some of the problems a student may face are described below.

The Pressures of College Work

Many college students would agree heartily with Dr. Ivan Koral and a report released by UNESCO suggesting that modern technological society requires us to store and deal with such great quantities of information that many of us suffer from "brain strain." Students who breezed through high school or have not been in a classroom in years often find the difficulty and volume of college work as well as the need for self-discipline and individual responsibility greater than expected. For students juggling jobs and/or family care, the pressures can be formidable.

Students react in several ways to the increased pressures: (1) They may push too hard, working all the time, never taking time out to relax. (2) They may panic and give up before they really start. (3) They may work out a balance in their lives between work and relaxation. Students choosing the last approach will usually be the most successful.

> Work is the grand cure of all the maladies and miseries of mankind.
>
> Thomas Carlyle (1795–1881)

> He that can take rest is greater than he that can take cities.
>
> Ben Franklin (1706–1790)

Balancing Work and Play

Both work and recreation are important elements in coping with life—not as solutions, but as temporary releases. They play other important roles in the development and maintenance of good mental health as well.

Play for the young child is "work." For an adult, play should be a break from work. The fisherman gardens on his day off, while the gardener goes fishing. Some people work so hard at play that they lose the pleasure of relaxation. The competitive business person who plays tennis to win and must be the best dancer on the floor "plays" too hard to get the needed change of pace and relaxation.

According to sociologist John L. Thomas (*b*), we need more time "to do nothing." In the United States the Puritan work ethic is so deeply engrained that we feel we should always be "doing something," and must justify such leisure activities as watching the sun rise or the waves roll in. The concept of the sabbath as a day of rest on which no labor is to be done has been lost. We have become a seven-hyperactive-days-a-week society.

The kind of balance to strike between work and relaxation is one of the major decisions we face today, whether we are college students, professors, presidents, construction workers, or textbook writers. The executive who is a parent, for example, must decide

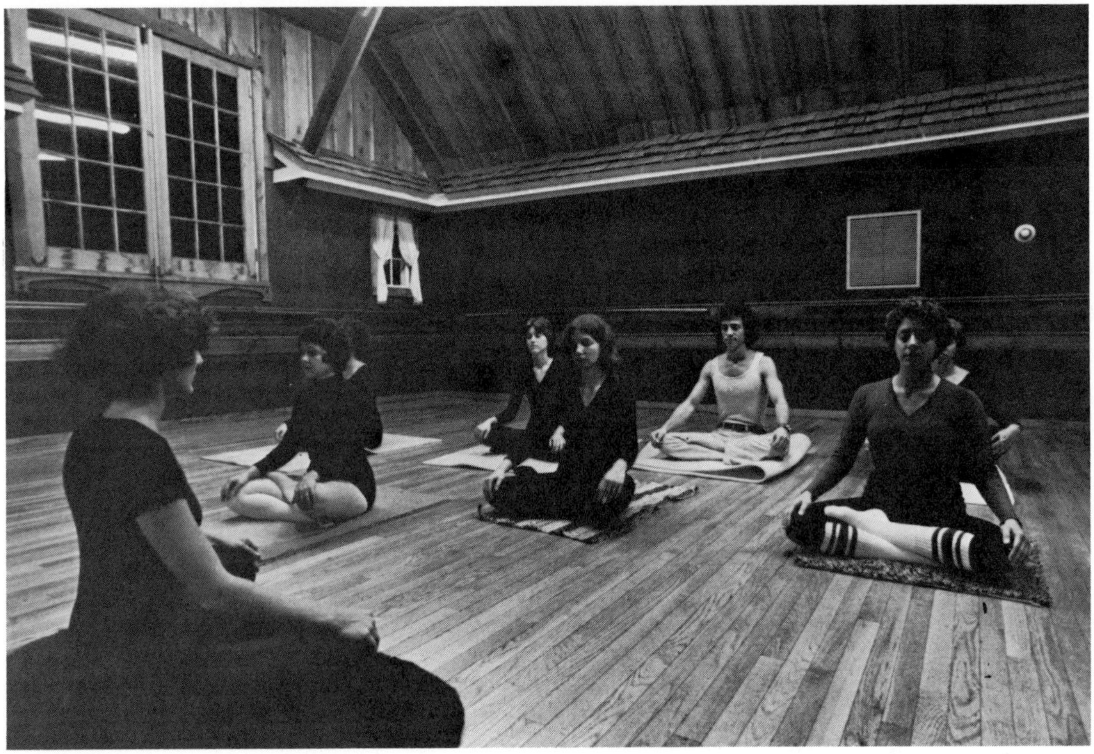
Mimi Forsyth/Monkmeyer

There are many routes to relaxation. Yoga is one. The Relaxation Response is another: Sit with eyes closed. Relax muscles starting with feet and working up to face. Breathe only through the nose. As you breathe out, repeat the word "one" silently to yourself. Continue for 10 to 20 minutes. (Benson)

whether he or she is willing to devote the time and single-minded energy demanded by the tough climb up the corporate mountain at the expense of family time. The college student must on occasion decide whether baseball practice or theater club is more important than a paper that is due and how much time to allot to each activity. We must all set our own priorities.

Fatigue

The premed student juggling studies and a lead in a school play who begins to lose weight, snap at her friends, and turn to cigarettes and alcohol for support; the veteran working at a monotonous assembly-line job by day and going to classes at night who finds himself exhausted, restless, even careless by day's end; the sophomore with a cough that has lingered all winter who finds her enthusiasm for life dulled, her energy dissipated; and the freshman loading furniture on weekends who returns home too tired to eat dinner, with aching muscles and throbbing head. All are suffering the symptoms of fatigue—mental, physical, or both.

Often fatigue results from a failure to

Children begin by loving their parents; as they grow older they judge them; sometimes they forgive them.
Oscar Wilde (1854–1900)

achieve a balance between work and relaxation. It is a warning that says slow down, change pace, relax, sleep. Symptoms vary widely, ranging from mild loss in timing (we burn the broccoli, strike the wrong typewriter keys) to physical aches and pains and psychological disorientation ("I'm so tired I don't know what I'm doing!").

Excitement, interest, and motivation may keep an individual going long after the point of fatigue, but the quality of performance continues to deteriorate. A break in a hectic schedule not only gives the body and mind respite; it may also lead to renewed vigor and accomplishment. It has been reported that many scientists find their creative ideas occur during breaks that follow periods of vigorous thought and activity. How fatigue can best be overcome—or prevented—varies according to the cause, as can be seen in Table 2.1.

Changing Relationships with Parents

For the student just out of high school, going to college represents a new stage in relationships with parents. The student's feelings are often ambivalent: "Parents try to do too much for us, to make decisions for us. Sometimes it's so stifling, you feel you've got to get away. But you don't want them not to care at all."

Parents feel equally ambivalent. They are proud to see their offspring going to college, exhilarated to know that it will not be long before they are entirely on their own. But whether the student rooms at home or goes away to college, parents have an uneasy feeling of loss, a sudden sense of emptiness and irrevelance. This reaction is particularly strong in mothers who have wrapped their lives in family and suddenly find the protective wrapper peeled away. Parents are also disturbed by the loss of control over their college-age children. Though they were the chief influence on the growing child, their direct influence is only a minor part of the life of the maturing collegian.

Young people often fail to recognize parental fears and loneliness, sometimes in part because they are trying to block out a separation anxiety of their own—an anxiety that is

Student on Parents

I've been away from my parents before college, but now, you know, you're away for a year and only go back on vacations. I think I appreciate my folks more. And I think of myself as more than just a son, sort of the difference between [me and] my folks in age and maturity is getting less and less.

College freshman (in Heath, p. 98)

Parent on Children

I feel my job with them is done. I don't have to discipline them any more, it's their problem. . . . I hope I can always be a mother, but we'll treat each other as adults. I have a much more relaxed feeling now.

Mother (in Lowenthal and Chiraboga, pp. 8–14)

SELF-CARE

TABLE 2.1 Overcoming fatigue

SOURCE OF STRESS CAUSING FATIGUE	POSSIBLE REMEDIES	PREVENTION
Heavy physical activity	Water or other fluids Rest Relaxation	Proper conditioning
Heavy mental activity (e.g., studying)	Physical activity (jogging, sports, etc.) Relaxation* Sleep if needed Food, coffee, cola	Pacing study or other mental activity with breaks Not letting work pile up
Monotonous activity or boredom (including long stretches of driving)	Physical exercise Mental stimulation (discussions, word games, etc.) Food, coffee, cola	Plan regular breaks (about every 2 hours) in activity
Lack of sleep	Various stimulants—food, drink, drugs, activity—are all temporary aids *Only* rest or sleep will relieve this fatigue	None but adequate sleep
Tension	Physical activity, sports Relaxation* Yoga, meditation Calming activities (knitting, solitaire, etc.) Warm bath	Improve coping techniques
General overwork	Rest, sleep Relaxation* Change of pace, getting away	Achieving balance between work and relaxation Pacing oneself
Poor working conditions (lighting, temperature, etc.)	Correcting conditions Taking frequent breaks	Correcting conditions
Illness	Rest, sleep Treatment of underlying disorder	Good preventive health care

*Relaxation includes doing nothing, listening to music, viewing entertainment, sports and so on, enjoying friends, as well as practicing specific relaxation techniques. (See photograph.)

perfectly legitimate and normal. If they do recognize the parental plight, they can help parents through this painful "weaning," and improve relations between the generations at the same time.

The fact that parents and college students share kindred feelings of loss and loneliness does not erase the differences between their generations. Individuals are very much the products of the world into which they were

Well . . . having your own personal convictions challenged every day by someone who is your best friend, and for whom you have a lot of respect, ah, can make you stop thinking that he's completely crazy and start checking your own values.

College freshman (in Heath, p. 191)

born. Worlds change. Parents forget this when they sermonize, "When I was your age. . . ." They think youth should always be the way they lived it. The conflicts and tensions that arise because of these differing world views are the fault of neither parents nor young people. Recognition of this by both generations can help narrow the gap.

Relationships with Peers

Friends are the greatest single influence on the development of a young student's personality and life direction during the college years. As Arthur W. Chickering, who directed a long-term study of personality development in college, put it: "A student's most important teacher is another student" (p. 253). Friends affect a student's values and sense of self, as well as the ability to express himself or herself. Friends help each other to become more independent and at the same time more "other-centered," more tolerant and accepting. Students are influenced not only by close friends, but by those with whom they share living quarters and by the overall school community.

Relationships with friends—as with family, mates, acquaintances—are more successful when one is assertive, and speaks up rather than suffering in silence. Hostility and smoldering resentment can arise from the failure to make clear from the beginning what you hold important. The foundation of a good relationship is clear communication and negotiations.

For the younger student, the first months of college, with their exposure to many new people from different backgrounds, are often a period of testing. A student should not feel limited to friends made then. Instead, he or she may move through several circles of acquaintances until a comfortable group is found. Rushing into deep relationships with members of either the same or the opposite sex can often be a mistake. The students who weather the difficulties of college change most easily will be those who are open to and willing to explore new values and lifestyles, but are at the same time wary of giving up their own without thoughtful decision making: examining risks, benefits, alternatives, outcomes.

Sharing Living Quarters

Each year hundreds of thousands of young Americans move out of home for the first time and into rooms or apartments shared with strangers or relative strangers. Sometimes the choice of living companions is their own, sometimes roommates are assigned by the college, and sometimes living arrangements are the result of a quirk of fate. Roommates from similar backgrounds often get along better than those from differing geographical or socioeconomic groupings. But they have less to offer one another in the way of opening up new ideas and horizons. The most exasperating roommate may be one who views college as an opportunity to suspend all rules and to peel off all the "restrictive" mores of family and community. Almost as taxing is the student who has not made a break with the past at all and still needs a nursemaid. The roommate is usually elected.

Some students find that rooming with a "best friend" is more wearing than rooming with an acquaintance. Others specifically advise against rooming with a good friend from high school. Explains one graduate student: "You're both going through so many changes

Kenneth Karp

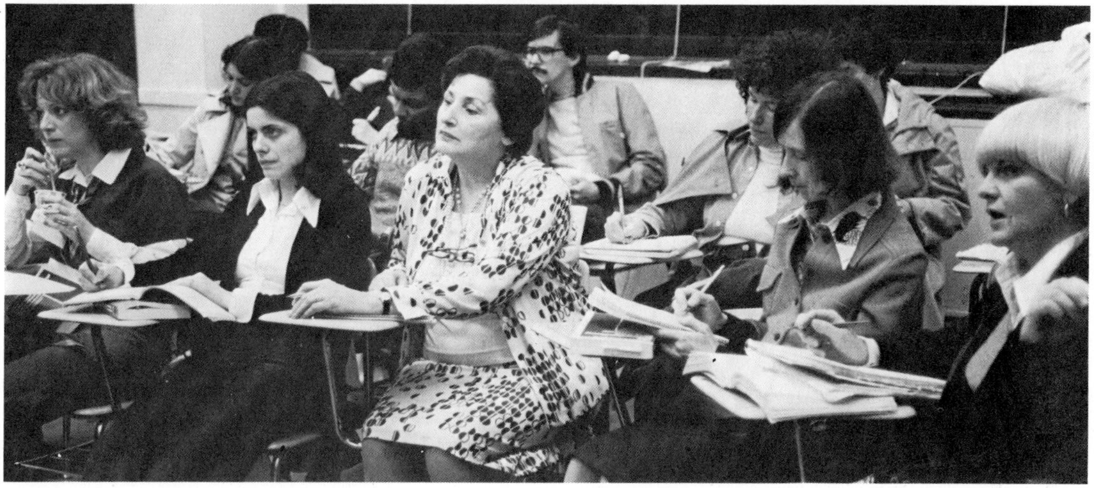

Though they face a variety of special adjustments to college life, older students do well. They make tangible contributions, often raising the academic effort of all.

that being together can stifle growth and cause friction. It's better to start fresh with someone new if you want to start building that new adult you." Roommate relationships can be kept more congenial if potential problems—cleaning, studying, borrowing, overnight guests, smoking—are negotiated in advance and new ones are discussed as soon as they come up.

Living Off Campus

Three out of four United States college students live at home or in apartments or rooms off campus. In the hassle of getting to and from school, making it home for dinner, and living two lives, commuting scholars frequently fail to take advantage of the variety of activities offered on campus. It is possible, however, for commuters to plan schedules so that they can use the library and other school resources: participate in clubs, teams, newspaper work, or student organizations; and attend seminars, lectures, dances, and sports events.

The student who lives at home must try more consciously than others to make new friends, to take advantage of career counseling, to be serious about study, and to move into a new stage of life. When the student leaves home to attend college, parents have no choice but to "let go." It is harder to make the break while living at home. A parent-student agreement on guidelines that will increase freedom for the student and yet be comfortable for parents can be helpful.

Returning to School after a Break

Much of college life and most campus services are geared to the just-out-of-high-school 18- to 22-year-old college student. But some 3,650,000 students age 25 or older—1 out of every 3—were enrolled in 2- and 4-year colleges in 1975, and the numbers rise each year. The typical older student is faced not only with the usual problems of academic work, but with a variety of adjustment difficulties, many of which are not addressed by the colleges themselves.

One such difficulty is returning to the self-discipline of study, often after many years out of the classroom. Lack of confidence added to the trauma of sitting in lecture halls filled with bright young men and women can be intimidating. But students past their early twenties can be reassured by recent studies showing that intellectual performance does *not* decline with age. (In some areas, in fact, it improves.) Other studies indicate that over-thirties have fewer academic problems than younger students (Roelfs). Older students, especially in courses like this one, where life experience is an important element, can contribute very tangibly to the group, often raising the academic effort of all (Carnegie Commission).

Returnees to higher education include military veterans, men and women looking for new career opportunities or wanting to move up the career ladder, and retirees seeking stimulation through learning. But a majority are women—often prompted by the consciousness raising of the feminist movement as well as by foreshadowings of loneliness and uselessness when children leave the nest. In addition to readjusting to academic challenges, women must often insert them into already crowded schedules of homemaking, child care, community work, and sometimes a job. Many women have husbands who share home and child-care chores; others are heads of households and must carry all these burdens on their own.

In some colleges, special counseling is made available to returnees. At others, group sessions and even classes are set up to help students deal with their special problems. When a woman confesses that every time she starts to read a book for one of her courses she falls asleep, and finds that many other women have the same problem, she becomes less concerned that "something is wrong with me." With a trained leader, these students can often discover ways of coping with such problems. For example: Read first, do dishes later. Or read sitting up, not in bed. In colleges where special provisions are not made for older students, they can form their own groups with the goal of talking through their needs and winning attention for them.

LOOKING BACK

REVIEWING CONCEPTS IN CHAPTER 2

- Confusion, lack of confidence, and rebelliousness are characteristic of the normal identity crisis, but young adults can emerge from this crisis more "together" than before.
- Identity, finally, is the result of heredity, childhood influences, later influences, and mature decision making; it changes as our lives change.
- Maturity is an ongoing lifelong process; though we strive toward its many components, we cannot expect to exhibit all of them at all times.
- A search for meaning in life—through religion or other channels—is a part of the lives of many; a system of belief, of moral values, can contribute to mental health.
- Stress of many kinds is an important element in life and growth; the anxiety that results from stress signals us that something is wrong, and that we should respond.
- One can respond to stress with defense mechanisms which usually do not solve our problems, or with competent coping which usually does.
- Competent coping begins in infancy, but can be learned at any time of life.

- Coping with college can often be difficult, especially during the initial adjustment period. Specific problems differ for commuting students, older students, and young students living away from home for the first time. All can benefit from learning to balance work and play and to prevent and cope with fatigue.
- Coping with the changing relations with parents can be eased when students recognize the fears and concerns parents have as their children reach maturity.
- As the influence of parents wanes, the influences of their peers become paramount in the lives of college students, helping them grow toward maturity.

3 WHEN MENTAL HEALTH BREAKS DOWN

WHAT'S AHEAD IN CHAPTER 3 Is there agreement on what behavior that varies from the normal represents? What are the major theories that explain mental illness? What is the most common mental illness among Americans? How can you recognize it in yourself or others? When does it need professional treatment? How common is suicide? Can you always tell when a person is going to take his or her own life? How can you handle the person you suspect is going to attempt suicide? Who needs help with problems of mental health? Where can such help be found? Is there one best way to treat mental illness? What approaches are available to mental illness? What approaches are available to mental health professionals and their patients or clients?

When people can no longer cope with life's problems, when they become detached from reality, they are declared to be *mentally ill*. When they behave strangely or differently, they may be called *abnormal*. When they commit senseless crimes, they are often said to be *sick*. Yet there is little agreement on what these terms mean, on whether such behaviors represent mental illness or a variety of mental illnesses, or indeed, on whether they can be called "illnesses" at all.

THEORIES OF MENTAL ILLNESS

In ancient times, irrational behavior was considered the result of demons and evil spirits taking possession of a person. The Greeks,

National Library of Medicine

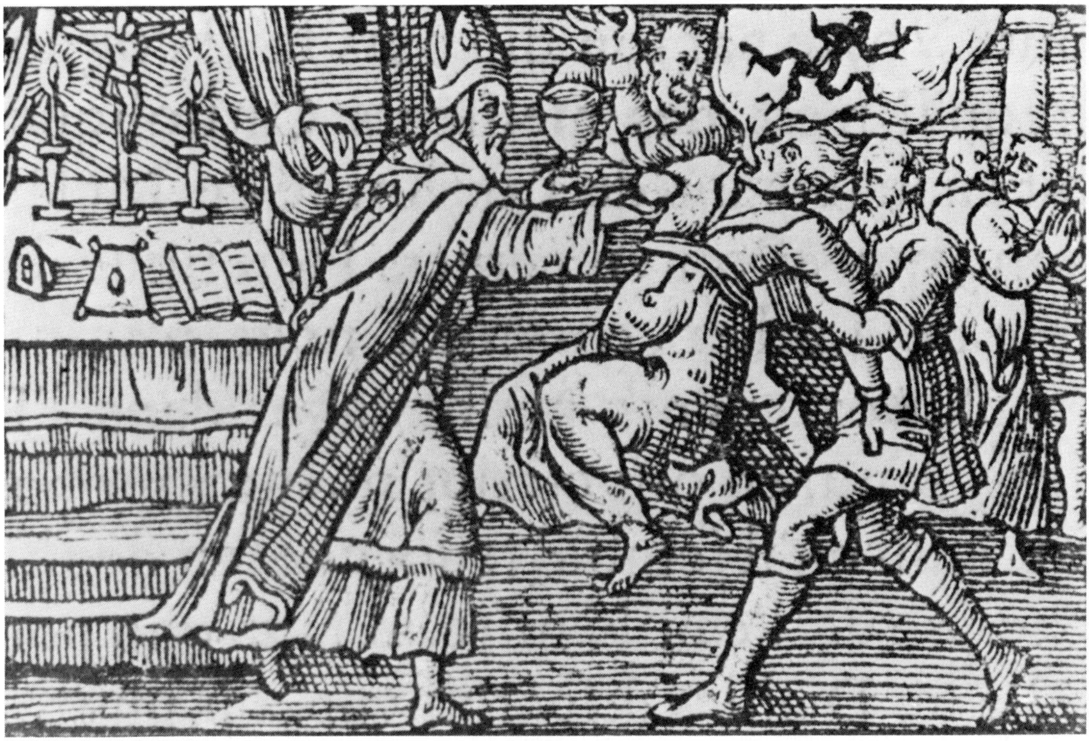

The concept of irrational behavior as sickness rather than possession by evil spirits gained widespread acceptance only in modern times.

on the other hand, looked upon irrational behavior as a physical problem—caused by an imbalance of body fluids called "humors" (an excess of "bad humors" led to depression), or by displacement of an organ. In the highly superstitious Middle Ages, the theory of possession by demons revived. It reached a zenith again in the witch-hunts of Europe and America.

Though the concept of irrational behavior as an "illness" reappeared during the Renaissance, it was not until the end of the nineteenth century and the beginning of the twentieth that the medical model gained wide acceptance and categories of illnesses were devised.

Categorizing Mental Illness

Today, some psychiatrists are again questioning the illness theory. Psychiatrist E. Fuller Torrey suggests that diseases are something we have and behavior is something we do, and that except for a small percentage of people with true brain disease, most people labeled mentally ill are not ill but have "problems of living." He sees an educational, not medical, model for behavior disorders. Individuals who behave irrationally do not need a doctor and medicine, but a tutor and a reeducation program to improve coping skills.

Karl Menninger (*c*), dean of American psychiatrists, has dismissed attempts at diagnos-

Traditional Categories of Mental Illness

Psychoses Psychoses are major mental disorders of organic (physical) and/or emotional (psychological) origin in which there is a departure from normal patterns of thinking, feeling, acting. Commonly characterized by loss of contact with reality, distortion of perception, regressive behavior and attitudes, diminished control of impulses and desires, delusions and hallucinations, and in some cases, chronic and generalized personality deterioration. Examples include:

- *Schizophrenia* No two cases are exactly alike but usually there is intolerable loss of self-respect, self-esteem, and ego, as well as disorganization of personality, distorted and deranged mental processes, and a retreat from reality.
- *Paranoia* In this relatively rare disorder, a person who seems otherwise normal has delusions of persecution ("Everybody is out to get me!") and/or delusions of grandeur ("They want to get me because I'm Napoleon!").
- *Manic-depressive psychosis and the depressive illnesses* These illnesses are extreme manifestations of the "blues." Manic-depressives alternate between periods of extreme "highs" and periods of depression. (See "Depression," page 44.)
- *Organic or structural psychosis* This kind of psychiatric disorder results from a physical disturbance of brain function due to a tumor, infection, or injury—what Torrey would call a "true brain disease."

Psychoneurotic disorders or neuroses These are conditions in which individuals attempt to cover up unresolved conflicts or problems in inappropriate ways. Neuroses are usually less severe than psychoses, with very little loss of contact with reality—though thinking and judgment may be impaired. We all exhibit some symptoms of one or another neurosis at some time in our lives, but unless they persist or recur frequently they need not arouse concern. Unresolved conflicts can be covered up in many neurotic ways:

- *Anxiety reaction* Feeling uneasy and apprehensive out of proportion to daily problems.
- *Conversion reaction* Converting the conflicts to bodily symptoms such as blindness, deafness, and paralysis.
- *Depressive reaction* Being depressed and "blue."
- *Dissociative reaction* Trying to separate ourselves from the conflicts through amnesia, sleepwalking, dream states, multiple personalities.
- *Obsessive compulsive reaction* Being rigid, inflexible, and highly critical of others, and following repeated rituals such as handwashing or arranging a desk in a minutely detailed pattern.
- *Phobic reaction* Transferring emotions from the original object—say a parent—to some unrelated situation or object by showing unrealistic and persistent fear of it. Some common phobias are: *Acrophobia*, fear of heights; *agoraphobia*, fear of the marketplace; *claustrophobia*, fear of closed places; *panophobia*, fear of everything; *xenophobia*, fear of strangers.

Personality disorders These are distorted personalities developed in childhood. Some believe these problems develop because of lack of love, care, and guidance; others suspect they are the result of inborn defects. Affected persons do not usually exhibit the tension, anxiety, and mental and physical symptoms common in neuroses.

TABLE 3.1 Menninger's five levels of dysorganization The ego reacts to stress

FIRST LEVEL	SECOND LEVEL	THIRD LEVEL	FOURTH LEVEL	FIFTH LEVEL
Nervousness Slight failure in coping Increase in aggressive impulses, fear, anger, frustration Tension, sleep problems, grouchiness, irritability, restlessness Mild psychosomatic ills	So-called neuroses Tension-relieving devices to block or repress destructive impulses: withdrawal, blocking out, phobias, recklessness, rituals, compulsions, sexual perversions, personality changes Sense of failure, disappointment, uselessness, joylessness Accident proneness More serious psychosomatic ailments	Loss of control of destructive impulses Chronic mild aggression Sudden explosive violence	So-called psychoses Further ego failure Disruption of thought as well as behavior Loss of contact with reality Depression, mania, delusions, withdrawal from social standards, paranoia, delirium	Total emotional collapse Abandonment of the will to live Often ending in suicide
When underlying cause is relieved, so are symptoms. If stress continues, person may move on to second level.	If underlying tension is not relieved, person may sink to third level.	Further threat to ego; added or continued tension may force person to fourth level.	This is the last line of defense against ego collapse.	

Source: Menninger, Mayman, and Pruyser, pp. 153ff.

tic classification as "sheer verbal Mickey Mouse." Rather than accepting the traditional division of behavior disorders into psychoses and neuroses, Dr. Menninger sees the process as a failure of the individual's coping mechanism to protect self when conflict and anxiety become intolerable. (See Table 3.1.)

Some experiments have also raised questions about the validity of traditional diagnostic categories. In one experiment, for example, three psychiatrists jointly interviewed each of 35 mental patients. They agreed on the overall major disease category in only 46 percent of the cases, and on the specific diagnosis only 26 percent of the time (Ash).

In another rather well-publicized experiment, Dr. D. L. Rosenhan, a Stanford psychologist, arranged for a number of perfectly sane people, mostly graduate students, to seek admission to a dozen different mental hospitals, by telling the admitting psychiatrist that they were hearing voices saying things like, "empty . . . hollow . . . thud." Everything else in their histories was perfectly normal. Yet all were admitted—one as a manic-depressive, the others as schizophrenics. After admission, they behaved in a perfectly normal fashion. Still, they were kept in the hospitals for from 7 to 52 days. Interestingly, many of the "real" patients recognized these admissions as phonies. But the hospital staffs did not. The researchers' conclusions: "Any diagnostic process that lends itself so readily to massive errors of this sort cannot be a very reliable one."

Dr. Harry Milt, whose *Basic Handbook on Mental Illness* has long been a standard in the mental health field, agrees that identification of mental illness is not nearly as precise as diagnosis of pneumonia, tuberculosis, coronary thrombosis, or appendicitis, and that no two cases of mental illness are identical. But he supports the concept of the medical model for explaining behavioral problems because of the very close links between mind and body, and between mental well-being and physical health.

Causes of Mental Illness or Maladaptive Behavior

There is no single cause of mental disorder. Some cases are clearly of physical origin, caused by infections that affect the brain, such as syphilis, meningitis, encephalitis; injuries to the brain; or a tumor growing in or near the brain. Recently, many researchers have begun to see chemical and hormonal imbalances, genetic defects, and possibly, inborn errors of metabolism involved. Some believe that dietary deficiencies, allergic responses, lack of sleep, and drug or alcohol abuse may also be contributory. There is also strong evidence that susceptibility to some forms of mental illness is inherited.

The largest category of mental illnesses, the neuroses, as well as some psychoses, are believed to be entirely psychogenic (*psycho* = mind + *genic* = cause), that is, caused by negative experiences in life, such as: lack of love, of success, of fulfilling human relationships; loss of loved ones; physical or emotional abuse or other trauma. Poorly developed coping skills can also lead to mental breakdown. Some psychiatrists hold that an inherited susceptibility may make certain people more vulnerable to damage from environmental influences. This may be true in many cases of depression.

DEPRESSION

Jennifer sat in her room all day—didn't eat, brush her hair, dress, or eat. She refused to talk to anyone, drowned her sorrows in loud stereo music, and cried a lot. She and her boyfriend had just broken up. By the next day, she was able to drag herself to classes, spoke a few civil words to friends, cried only a little. By the end of two weeks, she was laughing again. Her appetite was back. She was sleeping better and could concentrate on her work.

Jennifer had gone through a mild period of depression, the single most prevalent form of mental disorder in the United States. Dr. Nathan Kline, a pioneer in drug therapy for depression, calls it "the common cold of psychiatric ills." Depression, which can strike anyone at any age, is blamed for a large proportion of suicides and is also sometimes credited with some of the world's great literature, art, and music. Indeed, many prominent persons have suffered extensive bouts of depression. Winston Churchill referred to it as his "black dog." More recently, astronaut Edward "Buzz" Aldrin and U.S. Senator Thomas Eagleton attracted attention when they admitted suffering from depression.

Causes

Few of us have not at some time experienced depression—"the blues"—because of crises in our lives. This is *normal depression.* Like Jennifer's, it usually clears up by itself in a

WHEN TO SEEK HELP

Symptoms of Depression

According to Dr. Frederick Goodwin of the National Institute of Mental Health, one is probably clinically depressed if he or she exhibits:

1 Dysphoric (blue) mood: prominent and persistent feelings of depression, hopelessness, emptiness, etc.
2 Clusters of symptoms, including at least five of the following:
- Appetite disturbance (decrease or increase)
- Sleep disturbance (decrease or increase)
- Loss of energy, fatigue
- Psychomotor slowdown or speedup (agitation)
- Loss of interest in usually pleasurable activities (sex, parties, school, work, sports, etc.)
- Slowed thinking, decreased ability to concentrate or remember
- Self-blame and inappropriate guilt
- Recurrent thoughts of death or suicide

3 Duration of the above for at least two weeks
4 Impaired functioning

The depressed person may also experience such physical symptoms as dry mouth; rapid breathing; unexplained aches and pains; nausea; bowel changes; sweating; cold, clammy, tingly hands and feet; and general hypochondria.

very short time. But an estimated 10 million Americans react to life's problems—most often a loss, disappointment, change, frustration, or threat to identity—with depression deep enough or long-lasting enough to interfere with their functioning. This is *neurotic depression.* Symptoms usually disappear when stress is lifted.

Another 6 to 8 million have medically triggered depression that appears out of the blue, apparently unrelated to life's problems. It may be caused by hereditary factors, hormonal or chemical imbalance, dietary deficiency, or drug or allergic reaction. This *psychotic depression* is more serious and more complex. It is usually divided into two main types: (1) *bipolar depressive disease,* also known as manic-depressive psychosis, in which the individual swings from deep depression to unexplained "highs," during which he or she feels all-powerful and all-wise, and becomes difficult to control; (2) *unipolar depressive disease,* in which the patient has bouts of depression and is severely withdrawn and uncommunicative, or behaves in an extremely agitated fashion.

In all cases of depression—from the mildly neurotic to the psychotic—*there is a very real risk of suicide.* Unexpectedly, the patient may be most susceptible to suicide when the depression begins to lift.

Treatment

One does not have to be a psychiatrist to help a friend shake a case of mild neurotic depression. A shoulder to cry on, a sympathetic ear, a chance to relax and get away, to play tennis or ski, to be successful at something can all help. Even depressed monkeys snap back when they are forced out to play by healthy monkeys. A depressed person may find it

Depression and Humor: Laugh, Clown—Laugh!

In a study of 55 of the top comics in the country, psychiatrist Samuel S. Janus concluded that most comedians are severely depressed, anxious, and fearful. Many experienced severe trauma during childhood. Looking back, they often feel that life has presented them with situations in which they were misunderstood, picked on, or belittled. Their jokes, often voicing deeply felt rage, are aimed at things about which they feel powerless. Humor is their way of coping with depression, of defending against what they see as a hostile and inhumane world. For most, this way of coping appears successful. Dr. Janus describes the comics in his study as "very stable people, good family men" with a divorce rate lower than that in show business as a whole.

difficult to do routine chores, and so help in setting up a regular schedule may be useful, too. If, however, symptoms continue for more than a week or two or interfere with functioning, then professional help as described later in this chapter may be needed. The prognosis is good because depression is generally very responsive to treatment.

SUICIDE AND SELF-DESTRUCTIVE BEHAVIOR

A young woman despondent over a broken engagement hangs herself in her college dorm. A graduate student with no apparent problems hurls himself from an apartment house window. An elderly man, alone and ill,

Thoughts on Manic-Depression

The first time it happened, I was in my twenties. Suddenly I got terribly, terribly depressed. But people just slapped me on the back and said, "Buck up!" You know, "buck up," doesn't help, not when you're sick. It's a good idea when somebody's died, or there's been a divorce or something. But when you're sick . . . you need a doctor.

Then came the more dangerous manic part. It's being terribly happy, terribly up, terribly fast—wild ideas, wild decisions, a lack of censorship inside yourself. You feel you can do anything, you're afraid of nothing. But then you go too far and you're a menace to society and to yourself.

Josh Logan, broadway director, manic-depressive maintained on lithium

It's much easier to live with a man in depression because you're needed. . . . It's the manic period that's difficult. The doctor told me that a man in that state is rather intimidating and I would need great strength to cope with him. I had to be able to actually say, "I don't agree with you." But I wouldn't be drawn into a confrontation. I'd rather lock myself in the bathroom. These arguments don't wear them down, but they do wear you down. It's also important to remember that in a case like my husband's—when the depression is a disease—that you and other members of the family aren't responsible for it. Now I feel so secure—with lithium. It's like insulin for a diabetic, a life saver. His depressions are really gone. His heights are not as high. . . . We aren't on ball-bearing roller skates anymore, but we still skate around quite a bit. And he's no less creative now that he's cured.

Nedda Harrigan Logan, his wife

turns on the gas jets and dies quietly. Suicide, the second most common cause of death among persons 15 to 24, is responsible for 4500 to 5000 deaths in that age group each year and for thousands more in other age groups, especially elderly males. Suicide rates have been rising in the 1970s, particularly among minority males and American Indians (Frederick and Lague).

Three times as many women attempt suicide as men, but three times as many men are successful. Women tend to use less final and less violent methods such as poison or pills, while men are more likely to use guns or explosives. But the use of violent means by women is increasing, and more men are attempting suicide (Faigel).

But the statistics are only the tip of the suicide iceberg; thousands of suicide attempts probably go unreported. One reason is the taboo about suicide—90 percent of college-educated people in one study expressed negative attitudes toward those who commit or attempt suicide (Frederick, *b*). ("If a member of my family did that, I could never forgive them, no matter what!" or "A person who does that is a weak sister. . . . It's a horrible thing.") Other reasons for underreporting include the facts that life insurance policies are not valid in the case of suicide, that religious faiths often deny burial rights, and that the family is embarrassed.

In addition, a large number of suicidal deaths are mistakenly listed as accidents or natural deaths, though they result from the same kind of self-destructive tendency required to aim a pistol at one's head. The person continually taking risks—sky diving, race car driving, or driving recklessly—is often suicidal. So is the man with a lung irritation who will not stop smoking, the woman who knows her liver is deteriorating but will not stop drinking, and the person with chronic illness who refuses to take medication or follow doctor's orders.

Just as some accidents are suicides, some suicides are accidents. The suicide often does not intend to succeed, but rather to manipulate others—to win back the affection of a rejecting lover, get attention from a parent, punish someone. Sometimes the hoped-for rescue does not come and death does. Many adolescent suicides may be in this category, because most teenagers do not want to die (Faigel).

Recognizing the Potential Suicide

Though depressed persons are 500 times more likely to commit suicide than others in the population, many suicides display no apparent signs of depression or other mental disorder before their attempts (Blaine and McArthur). They may, however, share certain common sociological traits. Self-destructive youths, for example, often have little verbal communication with parents and show signs of depression, insomnia, worry, lack of appetite, heavy use of drugs, cigarettes, or alcohol, general inefficiency and a dropoff in

Following a suspected suicide, authorities often do a psychological autopsy—putting together information about the person and the events leading to the death. Often they can conclude for certain whether or not the death was suicide. Sometimes they discover that the victim did not really intend to die—but merely to make a point. That's what happened with a Maryland farmer who had frequent fights with his wife—and controlled her by going to the barn, standing on a barrel, putting a noose around his neck, and threatening to hang himself. She always implored him not to, and peace would return to the family. On one occasion, the barrel had been removed and the farmer used an orange crate instead. The crate collapsed, and before his wife could get to the barn to "talk him down," he was dead.

academic achievement. They may have been rejected or abused by parents and may show a desire to "get even" with them or with others. There may be a history of "accidental" poisoning or other self-destructive behavior. Males may have lost a father through death or divorce or have a father who is too busy for them. Females often have poor relations with their mothers, and have weak and ineffectual fathers (Frederick, *a*).

Though it is true that many who commit suicide never talk about their plans, it is not true that people who talk about suicide never carry out their threats. Any verbalization of suicidal thoughts ("I can't take it any more," or "Everybody would be happier with me out of the way") should be taken seriously. Not everyone who says such things is really contemplating suicide, but if anyone makes such comments frequently or shows other signs of deep depression, chances are that help is needed. If a threat is laughed off, the person may feel a need to carry it through just to prove it was serious.

A friend need not hesitate to ask someone suspected of having self-destructive thoughts whether the suspicion is true. This *does not* put ideas into a person's head. Rather, it is a relief to know that someone is listening and taking you seriously.

Sometimes suicidal intentions are only expressed indirectly. ("I won't be around next semester—you can have all my books," or "If anything happens to me, I want you to take care of Rover.") Many individuals thinking about suicide begin to put their lives in order, check insurance policies, review wills, give away valued possessions, call old friends and reminisce. They may appear serene.

Other warning signs may be less distinct: generalized depression; anger and a wish to get even with others; isolation and withdrawal; a sudden change of mood toward contentedness or nonemotional cool following deep depression (this usually follows the decision to go ahead with suicide); heavy smoking, drinking, or other drug use; "accidental" poisoning; purchase or talk of obtaining poisons, guns, ropes, sleeping pills; and unusually reckless behavior of any sort (Frederick and Lague).

How to Help

Friends or relatives can take a number of constructive steps in the face of a suicide threat: (1) Listen—really listen to the person's problems. (2) Be reassuring and supportive. (3) Avoid leaving the person alone. (4) Get professional help as soon as possible. There are some don'ts, too: (1) Don't try to analyze the person's behavior during the crisis. (2) Don't argue about whether he or she should live or die (there must be only one position—life). (3) Don't assume things will get better by themselves—they don't always.

WHEN HELP IS NEEDED

On Campus

- Tony, an "A" student in high school, seems unable to put things together in the competitive college he attends.
- Angie is in love for the first time, but because of her upbringing and religious values, she does not want her relationship with Greg to include sexual intimacy. She is uncertain of how to keep Greg without yielding.
- Neil is depressed because of a letter from his girlfriend back home breaking off their engagement.
- Kathy, whose mother is critically ill 1000 miles away, feels unable to cope with that worry and schoolwork too.
- Bob, a returning veteran, has suddenly become terrified of crowds, spends most of his time in his room, and sometimes feels as though he'd like to "end it all."
- Marilyn fears she may have to drop out of school because of the difficulty she is having juggling coursework, children, and household chores.

Back from Suicide

A year ago, things were so bad that they couldn't get any worse. But I was convinced they would never get better. I couldn't stand talking to anyone. I couldn't concentrate enough for light reading, let alone schoolwork. I did nothing but sleep, cry, and have headaches. I started to fantacize about killing myself, imagining all the different ways it could be done, wondering which would hurt the least.

That scared me into something my friends had pushed but I'd resisted: counseling. I went through a half-dozen well-intentioned shrinks, psychiatric social workers, psychologists, mental health counselors—until I finally found someone I could relate to.

Now things are great and getting better all the time. I'm discovering real friends and real academic interests, and getting involved in extracurricular activities. Of course, I'm still not doing that much schoolwork—I'm having too much fun.

College junior

Many people believe that counseling or psychotherapy is only for those who are suffering from serious mental illness. They fear it will stigmatize them. The fact is that in a typical college of 5000, only 10 to 25 students will develop serious mental illness while at school. Yet hundreds will seek help each semester for ordinary problems of living. All of the above students would benefit from doing so.

Where students should go for competent counseling depends on the services available at their schools and the types of problems they face. Tony might want to see an academic advisor, a dean, study counselor, or teacher; Neil, a peer counselor or dormitory health aide; Kathy, a chaplain, physician, or psychologist; and Bob, a psychotherapist or psychiatrist. Marilyn might benefit from a self-help group for married or older students. Vocational counselors can help students struggling with career decisions, and almost any sympathetic person can help the young student who is having difficulty adjusting to college.

Only about 10 percent of United States colleges have full mental health services that include staff psychiatrists. However, almost all colleges have some general counseling services—through the dean's office, affiliated counseling services, peer counseling, or the campus health service. Many will also arrange consultation with a psychiatrist or psychologist for seriously disturbed students. Often, however, students will have to seek help off campus.

In the Community

On any given day, 30 of every 100,000 Americans are in acute psychiatric facilities; 30 to 50 are under long-term care in hospitals; and 60 to 100 are receiving extended care outside of hospitals for mental disorders. Approximately 2 in every 100 will get some form of mental health care each year.

Who Can Help?

Very often, *the first line of help* is all that is needed—a friend, a parent, a spouse, a teacher to listen and understand. If problems are not eased, *the second line of help* will be needed—the family doctor, a cleric, a dean, or an advisor. When these people cannot do the job, they will direct the individual to *the third line of help*—the mental health professional (see Table 3.2).

In low-income areas, studies have found, persons with problems turn not to physicians or clergy for help, but to sensitive nonprofessionals—police officers, beauticians,

TABLE 3.2 Who's who in health care Mental health professionals

TITLE	TRAINING*	PROFESSIONAL ORGANIZATIONS*	COMMENTS
Psychiatrist	M.D. plus specialty in psychiatry	American Psychiatric Assoc. American Board of Psychiatry and Neurology	The only therapist allowed to prescribe drugs
Psychologist	Ph.D., Ed.D., M.A., or M.S. in psychology plus internship	American Psychological Assoc. American Board of Examiners in Professional Psychology National Register of Health Service Providers in Psychology	
Psychoanalyst	Psychiatry, psychology, or social work plus training in psychoanalysis	American Examining Board of Psychoanalysts, Inc. American Psychoanalytic Assoc. American Academy of Psychoanalysis	Must have professional background or training
Psychiatric social worker	M.S.W. with special training in psychiatric case work	Academy of Certified Social Workers National Assoc. of Social Workers Registry of Health Care Providers in Clinical Social Work	Counseling, rehabilitation, aftercare
Psychiatric nurse	R.N. with special training in psychiatric nursing		Group therapy and individual therapy under supervision of psychiatrist
Other counselors and therapists	No special training		Be wary!

*Check credentials with local mental health agency or a national registry. Many states require no licensing and do not regulate counseling services. Ask about training and credentials.

barbers, bartenders, school crossing guards, scout leaders, and teenage gang leaders. These people have been dubbed "gatekeepers," because they open or block entry into the mental health system. Their informal, underground "psychiatric" practices have long been condemned by professionals. But recently, their value has been recognized. Some professionals have even begun to train bartenders, police officers, beauticians, etc., to be part of the mental health system, giving them the skills to direct those in need to the proper source of help (Snyder).

Where Is Help Available?

The community mental health center is rapidly overtaking older state services in handling *all* types of care—inpatient, outpatient, day and night care. If there is one in your community, you may want to turn there first. Help may also be found at outpatient psychiatric clinics that are independent or part of a general hospital, at psychiatric hospitals, at family service agencies, and from therapists in private practice. Emergency cases may be referred to crisis centers equipped to handle

Ken Heyman

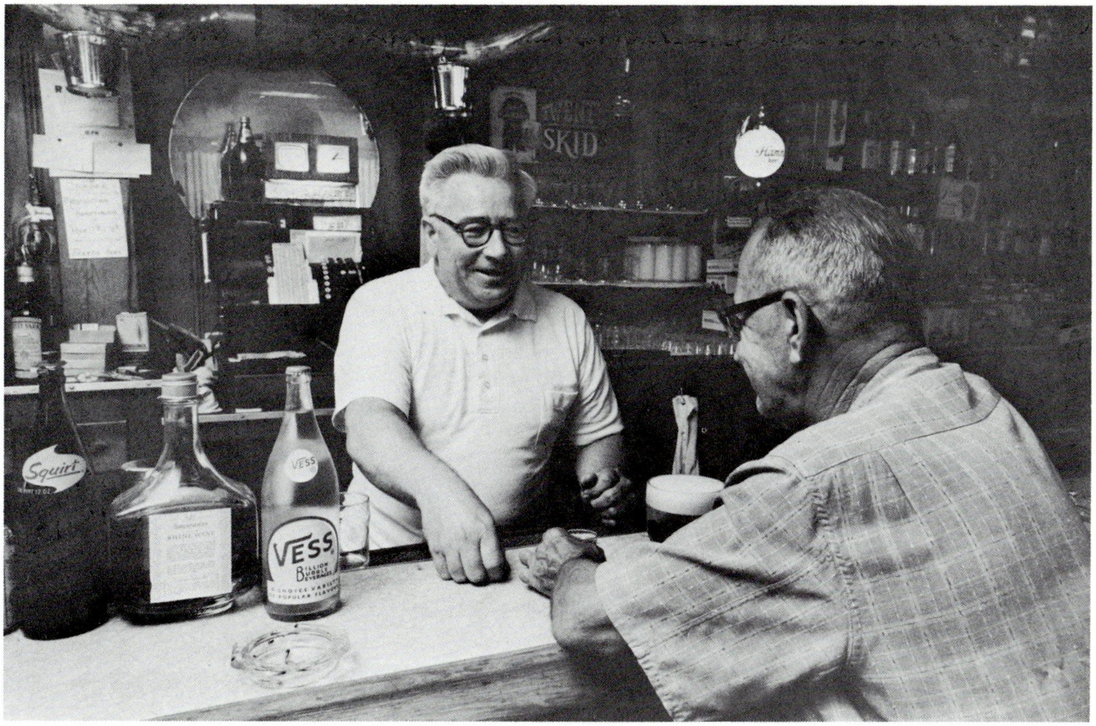

Persons with problems may turn to sympathetic "gatekeepers" who open or block entry into the mental health system.

suicide threats and other can't-wait situations.

New federal policies recognize that institutional stays longer than a year may be self-defeating—making it more difficult for patients to face the realities of the outside world when released. Thus, residential care in a hospital or institution is not likely to be suggested, except for those unable to function at all, or who are dangerous to themselves or others. The trend in residential care is to think small—turning away from "warehousing" in vast mental hospitals toward smaller private hospitals, licensed nursing homes, group homes that simulate family life, halfway houses for those about to return to the community, boarding homes, sheltered care and sheltered workshops, day-care centers for patients who sleep at home, and night care for patients who are able to leave the center to work by day.

New programs have brought renewed life to many former long-term mental patients. But poor follow-up in the community has left some released patients floundering and aimless.

APPROACHES TO TREATMENT

We are a long way from knowing all the answers in the treatment of mental illness. But new approaches and refinements of older treatments offer more hope to the mentally ill than ever before. Many therapists combine treatments, varying them to fit the patient's

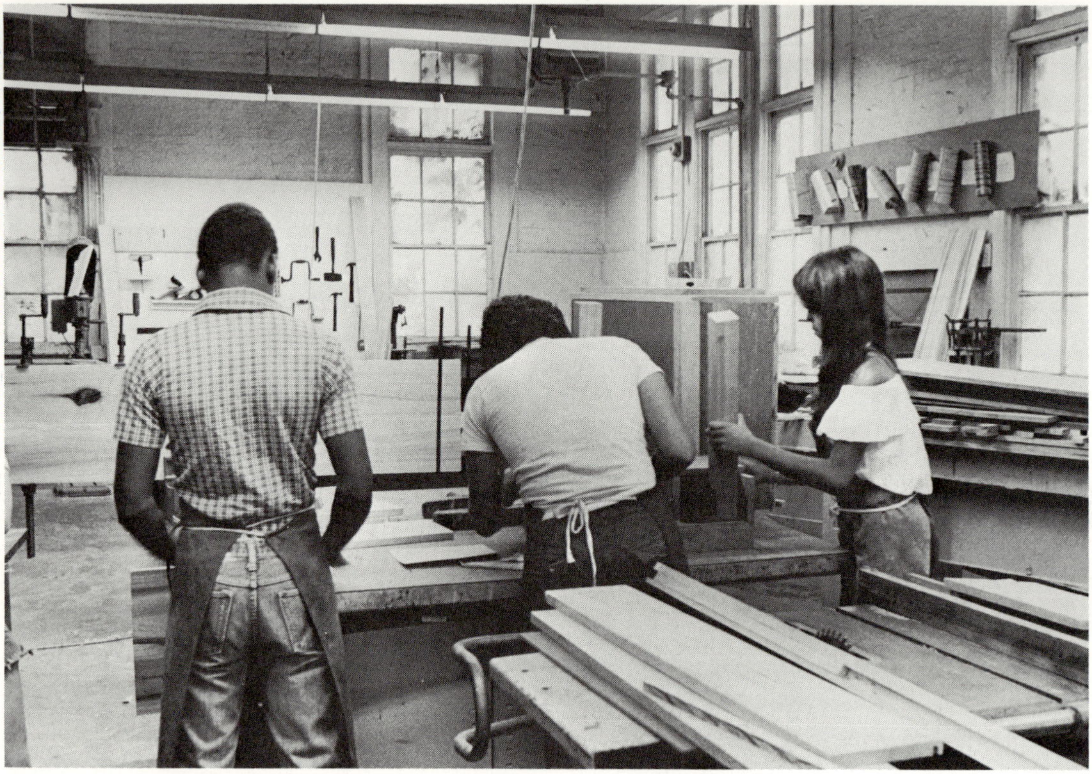

The Hawthorne Cedar Knolls School/Brian Alpert, Keystone

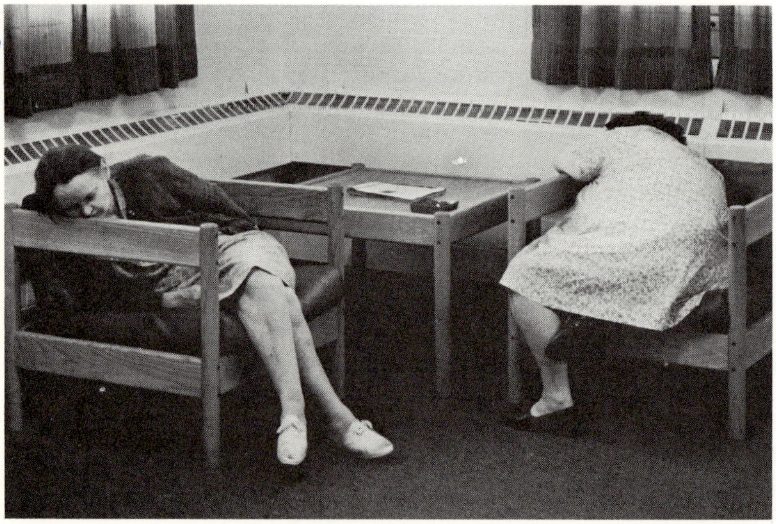

Burk Uzzle/Magnum

Contrasting sharply with the traditional institutions that "warehouse" patients indefinitely, modern mental health facilities offer a wide variety of therapies aimed at returning the patient to the community as soon as possible.

needs. Others depend upon just one or two treatments. Patients who "aren't getting anywhere" with the techniques of one practitioner can try another. Some therapies overlap. The major ones in use today are described below.

Psychotherapies

Psychoanalysis Based on Sigmund Freud's theories, psychoanalysis aims to uncover the origins of patients' problems by probing their pasts through free association and dream analysis. When hidden emotional conflicts responsible for unwanted behavior surface and are recognized by the patients, patients should be able, it is believed, to eliminate the inappropriate behavior. During therapy, patients are expected to transfer their feelings toward parents to the therapist who, unlike the parent, is accepting and nonjudgmental. The emotions forbidden in childhood—hate, hostility, dependency, greed, love—can now be openly expressed. Once expressed, they no longer control the patients who are now free to live in the present, to live a life determined by conscious choice rather than childhood traumas.

Psychoanalytically oriented therapy This kind of therapy also aims to uncover repressed feelings. It does not, however, attempt to completely rebuild the personality. Rather, by breaking the neurotic pattern, it aims to strengthen and reshape personality.

Supportive therapy Supportive therapy, using inspiration, reassurance, persuasion, counseling, and reeducation, is directed toward reinforcing patients' defenses and helping them repress disturbing thoughts and feelings. It is often used with or without drug therapy to tide a person over a traumatic event such as a death or divorce. It may also be useful with patients whose egos (or selves) are too fragile to withstand the deep probing of psychoanalysis, or whose symptoms are not serious enough to warrant deeper therapy. Unlike psychoanalysts, who are usually nondirective, supportive therapists may offer the patient suggestions for action.

Behavior modification This major new therapy is based on the theory that the inappropriate behavior is "learned" and can be "unlearned" with a system of rewards and punishments. A child who always speaks out of turn in class can be conditioned to stop doing so by the teacher's ignoring him instead of scolding. When he raises his hand before speaking, he gets extra praise and commendation. Other unwanted behaviors—smoking, for example—can be erased through punishment or "aversion therapy." Each time the unwanted behavior occurs, an electric shock is administered, permanently associating the formerly pleasant activity with pain. Wanted behaviors an individual does not have—assertiveness or social ease—can be taught, too, via reward.

Although behavior modification was first greeted with distrust and criticism by the psychiatric community—as making mice of men (and women)—it has recently gained wide support as a useful therapeutic tool.

Reality therapy Reality therapy, developed by William Glasser, takes a position contrary to traditional psychoanalytic theory. It postulates that neurotic behavior is caused by the inability to fulfill the two essential needs: to love and be loved, and to feel worthwhile to oneself and others. Therapy is based on intense personal involvement, facing reality, rejecting irresponsible behavior, and learning better ways. Unlike psychoanalytic therapy, the aim is not to gain insight or to lower the high goals of the superego or conscience, but to increase accomplishment to meet these goals.

This is achieved through the patient's accepting responsibility for his or her own behavior. Neither a difficult childhood (it cannot be changed) nor "mental illness" (there is no such thing) is an acceptable excuse for irresponsible or irrational behavior. The therapist first develops a strong relationship with the patient and then begins to reject the person's grossly irresponsible behavior—without rejecting the person.

Transactional analysis TA is based on recent research that has turned up evidence that all our past experiences are stored, word for word, feeling for feeling, in our brains. Probes of the brain during surgery have "brought back" exact feelings and dialogues. A related word, a sound, a sight, or a smell can also bring them back. We hear a song and feel inexplicably happy or sad. We hear a name and become furious.

TA assumes that each event or transaction of the past affects us today. It categorizes external events recorded before age 5, dominated primarily by parents, as *Parent* self; internal reactions to such events, the feelings we had as children, as *Child* self; and data acquired, thought about, and tested from about 10 months of age onward, as *Adult* self. TA aims to make us use our Adult (our rational selves) to control our Parent (the things we learned automatically in childhood and should rethink) and our Child (the part of us that reacts with feelings but no thought). The goal is for each of us to feel OK and to feel that others are OK, too (T. Harris).

Group therapy Tried experimentally in the 1920s and 1930s, this approach did not become popular until after World War II, when large numbers of returning GIs in need of psychiatric treatment overwhelmed mental health facilities. In group therapy, one therapist could serve many patients. For some, group therapy is more successful than one-to-one treatment. For others, it is most effective when combined with traditional therapy. Dr. Harry Milt describes the dynamics of group therapy this way:

> Fears are expressed, strong emotions are voiced, hostilities spill out, aggressive or passive or negativistic roles are assumed. Slowly, change takes place. New facets of the personality of each patient come out—less defensive, less fearful, more protective of each other, more concerned about the therapist, about the group . . . anxieties and depressive states are lessened, compulsive acts become less fixed, phobias lose their hold. (p. 81)

The success of group therapy depends primarily upon the skill and sensitivity of the group leader and on the group's composition. A group of only silent types will get nowhere. Insensitive or explosive persons can destroy a group. The overly sensitive may break down under criticism or be unduly upset by the ills of others.

Group therapy is not a game. It is serious treatment. It differs from sensitivity and encounter sessions, which are aimed at "well" people who want to enrich their lives.

Self-help groups Applying principles similar to those of Alcoholics Anonymous, self-help groups for psychiatric patients serve not to replace psychiatric help, but to supplement it. In Recovery, Inc., the largest such organization, small groups led by trained former mental patients, jointly strive to find better mental health through "will power" and other principles laid down by the founder, the late Dr. Abraham A. Low. Self-help groups can help patients return to normal lives after illness and lessen pressure on overloaded psychiatric professionals.

Family therapy Family therapists view an emotionally disturbed individual as part of a psychiatrically sick family. Their goal is to treat the entire family and its relationships. It may be useful in steadying a shaky marriage. In some forms, the therapist has two or more family members go through a series of negotiations, with each trying to change the other. Another variation seeks to manipulate the family's environment to reduce stress. A job or school may be changed, an interfering relative moved to other quarters.

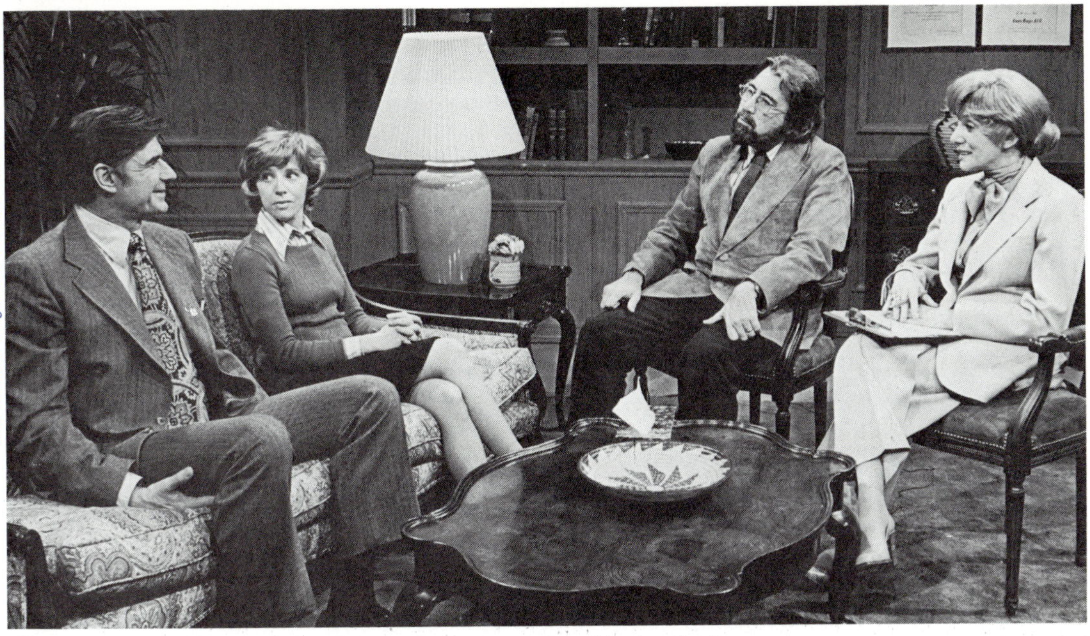

Drs. Laura J. Singer and Richard Robertiello/Metromedia

Co-therapy is just one of a variety of approaches used in family therapy.

Physical Therapies

Drug therapy This is the most widely used physical therapy for mental disorders. The psychotherapeutic drugs most frequently used are tranquilizers which calm the patient, psychic energizers or antidepressants which bring them out of depression, and lithium carbonate, which has been successful in treating the manic phase of manic-depressive psychosis. Exactly how these drugs work is uncertain, but they are believed to affect brain chemistry.

Drug therapy has brought about great changes in the care of mental patients—often replacing the straitjacket and other restraints for the aggressive or violent patient, bringing withdrawn patients to a level of awareness that allows them to be reached by therapists, and helping outpatients to function in the community during treatment. Some therapists warn that drugs should not be used as a crutch, but only as a tool to draw the patient into a treatable state. They prefer to take over from that point with psychotherapy. (For a discussion of the misuse and abuse of psychotherapeutic drugs, see Chapter 15.)

Convulsive therapy Used less frequently since the advent of drug therapy, this treatment for deep depression creates mild convulsions in the patient. The convulsions, believed to restore chemical balance to the brain, can be produced by: (1) electroconvulsive shock (ECT), popularly known as shock treatment, in which mild electric current is applied to the scalp of an anesthetized patient; (2) inhalation of an etherlike gas; (3) injection of a chemical convulsive agent. Relief of symptoms usually occurs after 6 to 8 treatments. Gaps in memory—usually temporary—are often a side effect of ECT.

Psychosurgery or lobotomy Seldom used today, this surgical removal, severing, or destruction of brain tissue with the intent of altering behavior is highly controversial. Though the concept that lobotomy transforms a patient into a "vegetable" is untrue, most patients do lose some mental capacity and some suffer serious memory deficiencies. Psychosurgery is not always effective in relieving psychosis, though violent behavior is often reduced. Today it is generally used only when all else fails.

LOOKING BACK

REVIEWING CONCEPTS IN CHAPTER 3

- Irrational or maladaptive behavior and detachment from reality have, through the ages, been attributed to many causes. Even today, professionals do not all agree about the mechanisms of mental breakdown.
- Mental illness can be caused by physical damage to the brain, by genetic defect or inherited susceptibility, by influences during childhood, or by the inability to cope with stress at any time in life; possibly by chemical changes in the body, dietary deficiency, or allergic response as well.
- Depression is the common cold of mental disorders. It can be reactive (a reaction to loss, frustration, disappointment in life) or it can be endogenous (caused by some internal physical mechanism).
- We all experience normal depression at some time in our lives, and it usually cures itself—often with a little help from friends. More serious depression may require psychotherapy and/or drug treatment.
- Suicide is a major killer of young people, and is probably underreported. Suicide threats and hints should be taken seriously; those contemplating suicide can be helped, and can build normal lives thereafter.
- Help for the mentally disturbed is available on several levels—ranging from friends and family for minor illnesses to psychiatric professionals for serious ones.
- Most treatment today has moved out of institutions to outpatient care—except when the patient is a danger to self or others.
- Approaches to treatment may vary widely; all have some success, but none are 100 percent successful. Treatment should be tailored to the individual, to the type of illness, and to the therapist. Good therapist-patient relationships are essential.

II

II

PREVENTION: STAYING WELL

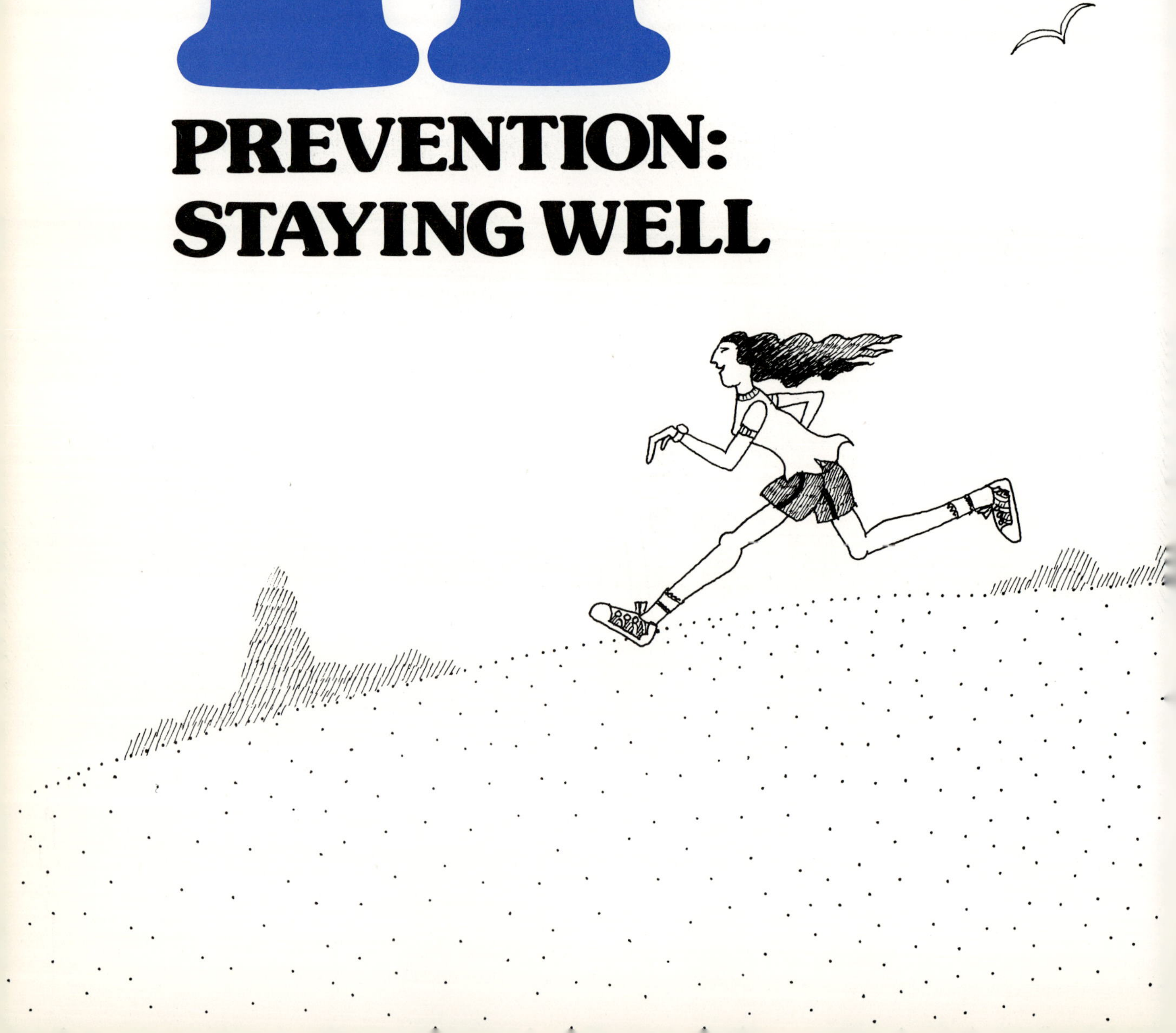

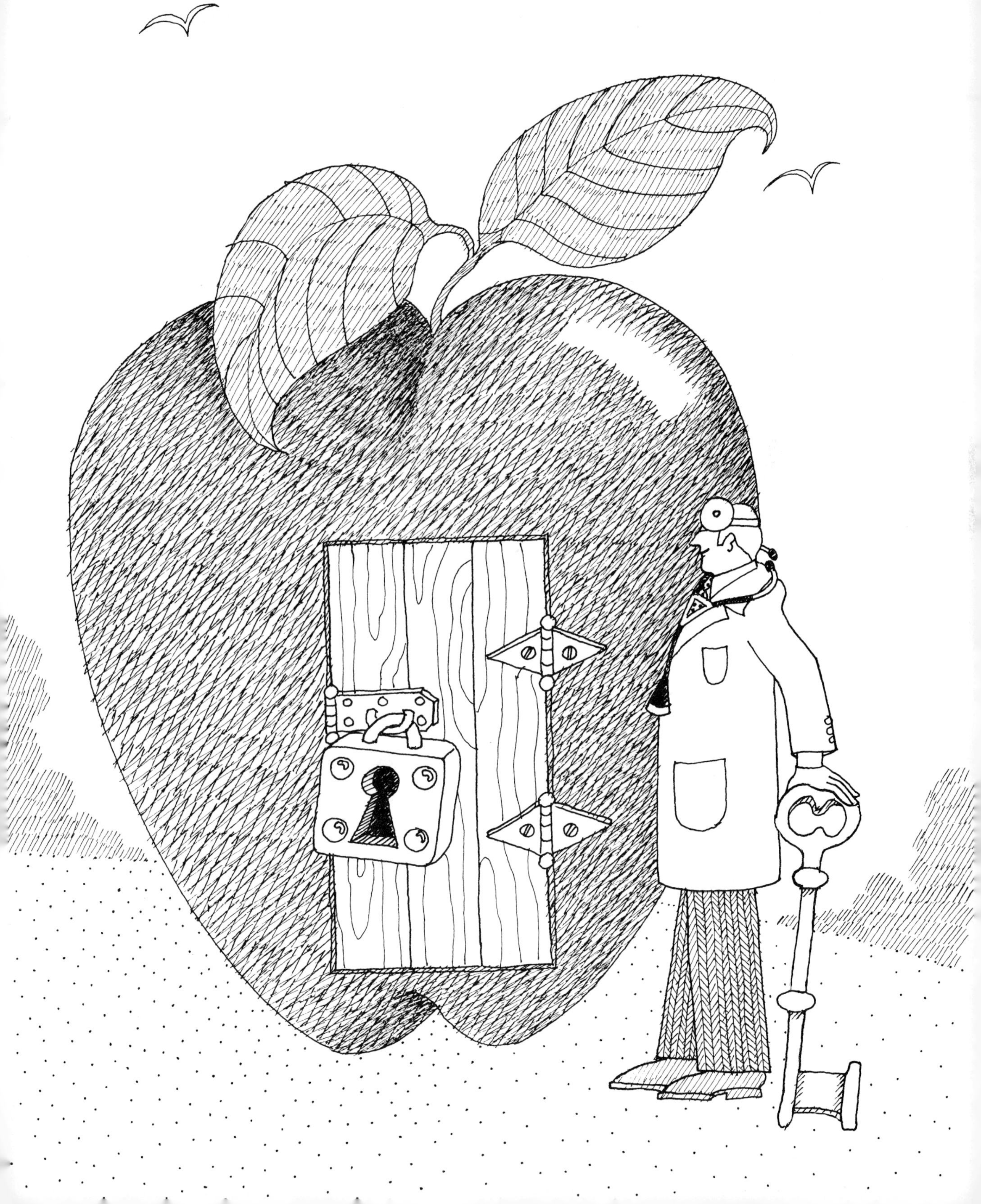

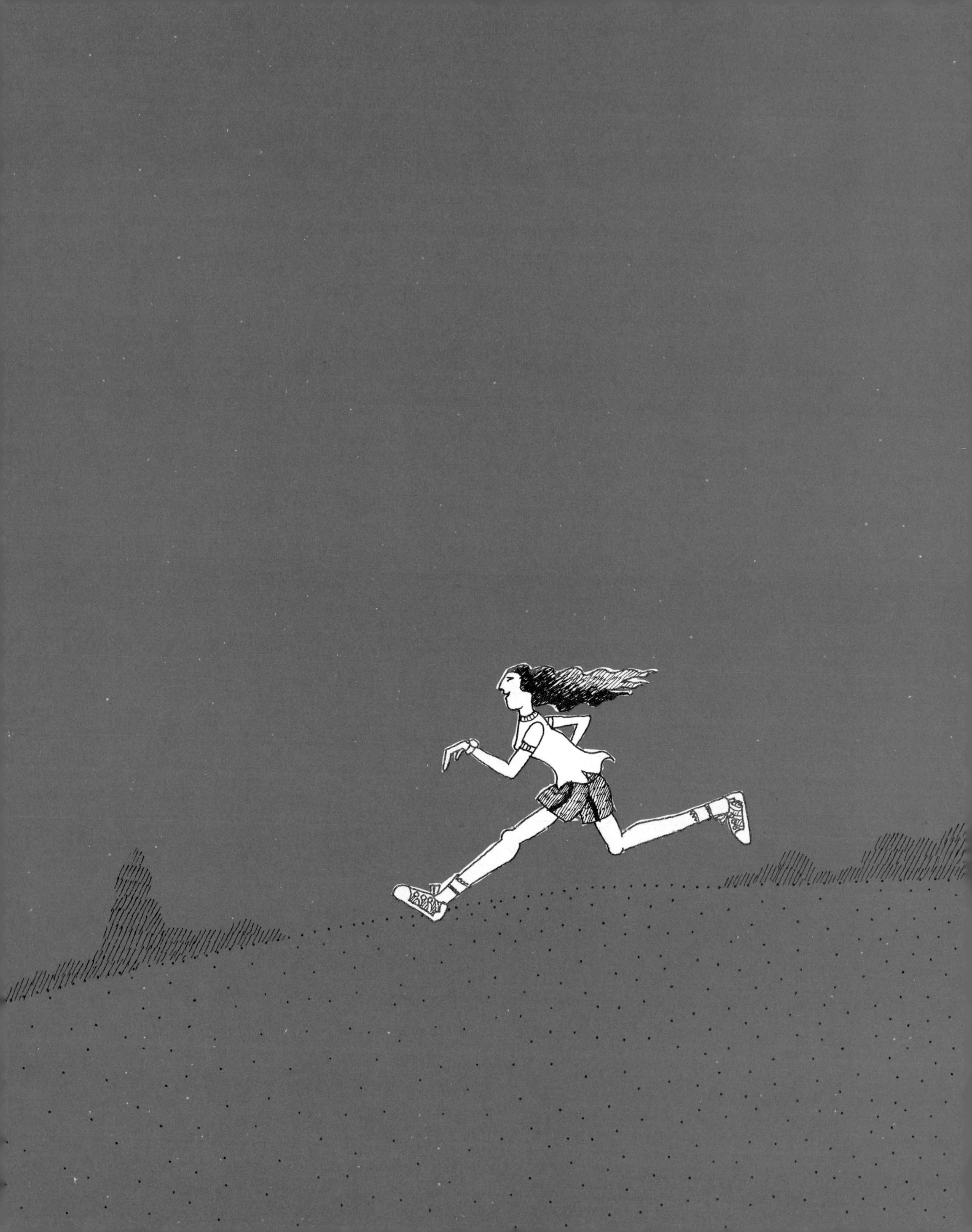

4

YOU AND YOUR PHYSICIAN—PARTNERS IN PREVENTION

WHAT'S AHEAD IN CHAPTER 4 What is the role of prevention in modern health care? How can patients develop good patient-physician partnerships? How can they get the most out of these relationships? Is the physician solely responsible for medical record keeping? Does a regular health checkup pretty much guarantee good health? What constitutes a good physical examination? What are the ways in which our bodies speak to us? How can understanding our bodies' messages help us to better health? What part do physical activity and rest play in building and maintaining good health? What kinds of exercise most benefit heart and circulatory system? How can a life-long exercise program be developed? What is the result of loss of sleep? How much sleep does the average person need and what factors may disturb sleep? Can drugs improve sleep for the sleepless?

When Sister Elizabeth Kenny, an Australian nurse, devised a physical therapy approach to treating the victims of infantile paralysis (polio), hope dawned for thousands of children crippled by the disease. However, when Dr. Jonas Salk later perfected a vaccine to prevent polio, it meant that children would not have to be crippled at all. Cures and treatments are important elements of medicine, but the ultimate goal is prevention.

Folk wisdom has long recognized that a gram of prevention is worth a kilogram of cure. In fact, the ancient Chinese wisely paid doctors to keep them healthy. In biblical

Quarantine—separating those with infectious disease from others to prevent disease spread—is an old preventive measure:

> The Queen commands that the superintendent and a surgeon appointed by the authorities examine every Saturday all the whores in the house of prostitution. And if one is found who has contracted a disease from coitus, she shall be separated from the rest and live apart, in order that she may not distribute her favors, and may thus be prevented from conveying the disease to the youth.
>
> From a public health law to prevent the spread of venereal disease in Avignon, France (1347)

times, there were modest beginnings toward the kind of preventive health measures we recognize as important today.

Over the next 3000 years, preventive medicine made slow, sometimes unsteady progress. Not until the eighteenth century, however, were giant preventive strides taken:

- Edward Jenner's successful vaccinations against smallpox, which led to virtual elimination of the disease and, eventually, to vaccination against many other dreaded ills
- James Lind's recognition that scurvy could be prevented by eating of citrus fruits, which led to understanding and prevention of other deficiency diseases
- Ignaz Philipp Semmelweiss' observation that washing hands before delivering pregnant women could prevent deadly childbed fever, which dramatically reduced deaths, first in childbirth and later in surgery
- Louis Pasteur's work on the germ theory of disease and the development of procedures for pasteurizing milk which wiped out the once common milk-borne diseases
- Public health measures, pioneered by people like Walter Reed, which aimed at eliminating disease-carrying populations of rodents, flies and other insects
- The purification of water systems

Today techniques for the prevention of disease have multiplied tremendously. Yet the death and disability rates from preventable illnesses and injury—as can be seen in Table 4.1—continue to be high. The reasons, as discussed in Chapter 1, are many. The solutions, for the most part, lie in the hands of individuals who work in partnership with their physicians and other health care professionals.

THE PATIENT-PHYSICIAN PARTNERSHIP

Lay people are sometimes passive to an extreme—like the woman Dr. A. Russell Lee used to tell about. She had, as he spun the story, telephoned a doctor to hurry out and visit her long invalided husband, Henry. "He's taken a turn for the worse," she reported urgently. "Can you come right out and see him?"

The doctor drove out immediately, was ushered into Henry's presence, found him flat on his back and apparently no longer breathing. He felt his pulse, found none, and said sadly to the new widow, "You're right, Sarah. Henry took a turn for the worse alright. He's dead." At which Henry sat bolt upright in bed and exclaimed in dismay, "I am not!" His wife pushed him back onto the pillow. "Lie down on that bed, Henry," she exclaimed. "The doctor knows best!"

Sehnert and Eisenberg, p. 108

The Activated Patient

Few of us are as thoroughly intimidated by the physician as the caricatured Sarah, but the picture of the passive patient is a familiar one. Until recently, there has been an "almost universally held faith and unquestioning trust in the wisdom of the doctor . . . the 'medical mystique'" (Belsky and Gross, p. 17). But things are changing. Many people are coming

TABLE 4.1 Leading causes of death (1976) and means of prevention

RANK	CAUSE OF DEATH	NUMBER OF DEATHS (DEATHS PER 100,000 POPULATION)	PREVENTIVE MEASURES
1	Diseases of the heart	759,550 (353.9)	Reduction of risk factors: smoking, high blood pressure, high cholesterol intake, inactivity, stress, etc. (Chap. 10)
2	Malignant neoplasms (cancers including those of lung, breast, skin, digestive tract)	374,780 (174.6)	Cessation of smoking; reduction of air pollution and of carcinogens in food, air, water; avoidance of excess exposure to hot sun and unnecessary x-rays; adequate fiber in diet and low fat intake; early detection and cancer screening; self-examination (Chap. 10)
3	Cerebrovascular disease (stroke)	189,100 (88.1)	Control of high blood pressure; screening programs (Chap. 10)
4	Accidents	100,430 (46.8)	Use of seat belts; avoidance of driving under influence of alcohol or drugs or with an intoxicated driver; reduction of home and job risks; installation of fire protection and escape equipment (Chap. 11)
	Motor vehicle	45,800 (21.3)	
	Other	54,630 (25.5)	
5	Influenza and pneumonia	62,980 (29.3)	Immunization when available; good care of respiratory illnesses to prevent complications; reduction of air pollution, smoking, other irritants (Chap. 9)
6	Diabetes	35,090 (16.3)	Reduction in use of sugar and in obesity; treatment of those affected (Chap. 9)
7	Cirrhosis of liver	31,130 (14.5)	Avoidance of heavy alcohol consumption (Chap. 16)
8	Arteriosclerosis	28,760 (13.4)	Reduction in consumption of animal and other saturated fats; exercise; cessation of smoking; reduction of other heart risk factors (Chap. 10)
9	Mortality in early infancy	24,870 (11.6)	Improved prenatal care and diet; avoidance of x-rays and drugs during pregnancy; genetic counseling; prenatal (Tay Sachs, Rh, Downs) and postnatal (PKU) testing; improved newborn care and treatment (Chap. 23)
10	Bronchitis, emphysema, asthma	23,840 (11.1)	Cessation of smoking; reduction of air pollution and of on-the-job lung irritants (Chaps. 9, 17)
11	Suicide	25,200 (11.7)	Improvement of coping techniques; better mental health care and treatment; early recognition and treatment of potential suicide victims; more opportunities for success and satisfaction for individuals (Chaps. 2, 3)

Source: Developed from data in *Vital Statistics of the United States,* U.S. National Center for Health Statistics.

HEALTH CONSUMER TIPS

Questioning the Physician*

1 What is the diagnosis? ______
2 What is the cause and how can I prevent it from happening again? ______
3 Are there any helpful patient education materials on this condition? ______
4 Are there any medicines I should be taking? ______
5 Are there any special side effects or instructions in reference to this medicine? ______
6 Will a return visit be necessary? ______
7 Any treatments I need to follow at home? ______
8 Any limitation on my activities? ______
9 Any precautions? ______
10 Shall I call for lab reports? ______
11 Am I to report back to the doctor by phone? ______

*Adapted from Sehnert and Eisenberg.

to view physicians not as gods, but merely as experts in a discipline that is a long way from knowing all the answers. They recognize that physicians are human and are susceptible, as we all are, to error. They are switching from the authoritarian parent–docile child relationship to a patient-physician partnership.

Activated patients who have a nagging suspicion that their physician is wrong—that something has been missed, or that the suggested surgery or prescribed drug is not needed—do not obediently follow doctor's orders despite their misgivings. Nor do they ignore the doctor's recommendations. Instead, interested in making informed health decisions, they question the physician, communicating their doubts and fears. If the question is a major one, involving surgery, for example, they request a consultation with a specialist, or another physician. Most doctors are willing to invite a second opinion.

If attempts at communicating appear to fail, if requests for explanations of illness or drug side effects or alternative treatments meet repeated resistance or disinterest, if there is a lack of trust in the physician, activated patients look for a new doctor. A one-sided partnership is difficult to maintain. But patients who switch from doctor to doctor, trying to find one willing to follow *their* orders, do not develop a partnership either, and are not likely to get good medical care.

Self-Care

Many health care authorities believe that patients can go beyond participating in health decision making, that they can be trained in many minor medical procedures including observation and reporting of symptoms, measurement of vital signs, record keeping, and treatment of the 70 percent of illnesses that may not require a physician's attention. Allowing patients to perform medical procedures has many precedents: self-administration of insulin by diabetics, even juveniles; operation of complex dialysis machines by kidney patients and their families; and blood pressure monitoring by patients with hypertension. This approach is seen by many as the only practical solution to both spiraling medical costs and shortages of health care personnel. To this end, a small but growing number of physicians, hospitals, schools, and medical groups are training patients in basic skills. *Alive and Well*, through self-care sidebars, will attempt to do likewise.

Health Record Keeping

A student traveling in Europe collapsed while strolling along Rome's Via Veneto. Police, who found pills in his knapsack, assumed he was just another drug addict who had taken an overdose. Fortunately, hospital personnel, searching his belongings for further clues, came up with a little booklet containing the youth's complete medical history. He was a diabetic who had slipped off his diet when confronted with the rich pastries in a Via Veneto cafe, and gone into a coma. If he had not had a Medical Passport[1] in his pocket he might have died.

Many diabetics, epileptics, and others with chronic illnesses or allergies wear Medic-Alert bracelets or pendants. But the Medical Passport, a complete personal medical record, is recommended for everyone. (A variation can be found in the Appendix.) Keeping one's own health records is a new concept to most people. For so long we have left this task to the physician or other professional. Yet the benefits of keeping your own health records are many: (1) Vital information is handy for filling out medical forms, in an emergency when neither patient nor family can remember such details as blood type or last tetanus booster, or when you are far from home or your physician is away; (2) x-ray dosage can be monitored and unnecessary repeats avoided; (3) tests do not have to be repeated each time you move or change doctors; (4) care of the several physicians most of us see can be coordinated. The passport also lists such useful information as eyeglass prescriptions, health insurance number, and name and phone number of family doctor.

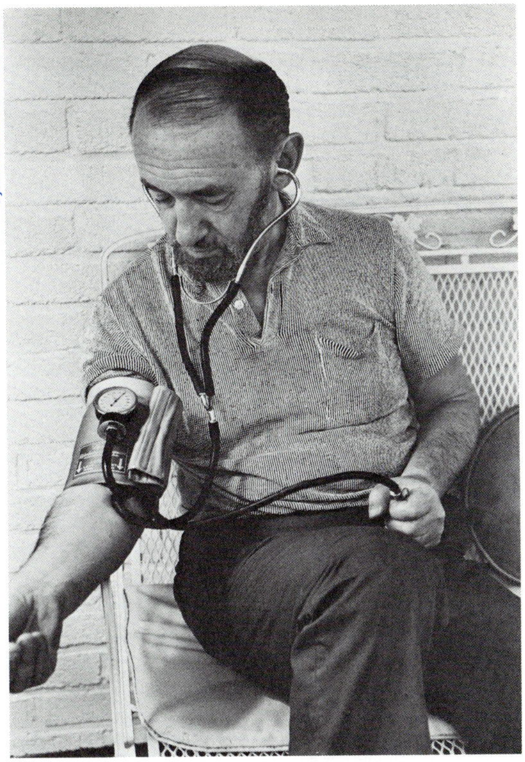

Sybil Shelton/Monkmeyer

The patient as a partner in health care: laypersons can become more involved in their own health care, learning simple procedures and working in active cooperation with their physicians.

The Activated Student-Patient

Campus health services, once limited to infirmary facilities for coughs and quarantines, now often offer advice on health maintenance and preventive medicine, and counseling in such once-taboo areas as abortion, VD (venereal disease), contraception, drug abuse, and mental health. Confidentiality between students and medical staff is legally protected so that students can feel free to "open up."

At some schools, students are very much involved in health care—serving on advisory committees, acting as health and sexuality counselors, and otherwise contributing as activated consumers of health care. Health facilities on college campuses range from nonexistent to elaborate medical centers. It is a good idea for students to find out exactly what services are available—before the first fever or sprained ankle.

[1]Available from Medical Passport Foundation (nonprofit), P.O. Box 820, Deland, FL 32720.

TABLE 4.2 Most serious threats to the lives of young adults (15- to 24-year-olds)

FEMALES				MALES			
WHITE	RATE* (*n*)	OTHER	RATE* (*n*)	WHITE	RATE* (*n*)	OTHER	RATE* (*n*)
Accidents	26.4 (4517)	Accidents	19.2 (585)	Accidents	97.1 (16,986)	Accidents	76.0 (2228)
Cancer	5.2 (885)	Homicide	17.8 (518)	Suicide	19.2 (3354)	Homicide	70.2 (2057)
Suicide	4.9 (839)	Cancer	4.8 (146)	Homicide	10.6 (1850)	Suicide	14.7 (432)
Homicide	3.6 (613)	Heart diseases	4.4 (134)	Cancer	8.0 (1402)	Cancer	7.7 (226)
Heart diseases	1.4 (248)	Suicide	4.0 (122)	Heart diseases	2.8 (489)	Heart diseases	6.9 (201)
Inborn defects	1.2 (203)	Influenza, pneumonia	2.5 (75)	Inborn defects	1.6 (274)	Influenza, pneumonia	2.7 (79)
Influenza, pneumonia	1.2 (200)	Cerebro-vascular	1.9 (57)	Influenza, pneumonia	1.5 (257)	Cerebro-vascular	2.5 (74)
Cerebro-vascular	1.0 (168)	Pregnancy†	1.8 (55)	Cerebro-vascular	1.2 (207)	Inborn defects	1.9 (55)
Pregnancy†	0.5 (82)	Inborn defects	1.2 (36)	Benign tumors	0.3 (55)	Anemias	1.6 (48)
Diabetes	0.4 (64)	Anemias	0.9 (28)	Diabetes	0.3 (55)	Cirrhosis of liver	1.1 (31)
		Cirrhosis of liver	0.9 (28)				

*Rate per 100,000.
†Complications of pregnancy, childbirth, and recovery from childbirth.
Source: National Center for Health Statistics, 1976.

THE PERIODIC MEDICAL EXAMINATION

A middle-aged man has his annual checkup at his doctor's office and is pronounced fit. He goes home reassured. That night, he suffers a heart attack.

Such occurrences are not uncommon. A checkup is not a blanket one-year insurance policy guaranteeing good health. It is only a small part of a health maintenance and disease prevention program. Medical opinion is divided on the value of the periodic physical examination. Some physicians believe that the checkup is unnecessary, that it is more practical for the patient to see the physician when a specific complaint surfaces. They point out that few illnesses are discovered in relation to the cost of health screenings, that some of these cases cannot be treated or cured anyway, and that when treatment is possible, it is often not carried out.

Most health care professionals, however, maintain that, despite flaws, checkups are valuable because: (1) they help the physician detect conditions (cancer or high blood pressure, for example) that can be best controlled or cured in the earliest presymptom stages; (2) they establish baselines (readings of blood pressure, blood chemistry, and so on, that are normal for each individual), variations in which at a later date might be indications of trouble; (3) they allow patients to unburden themselves by discussing nagging problems and give the physician an opportunity to reassure, to guide, to educate; and (4) they strengthen the ongoing doctor-patient relationship.

Perhaps the key to evaluating the worth of the periodic physical is the quality of the examination itself. If an overweight 25-year-old smoker is put through a battery of tests, told the results are normal, and asked to return next year, he might as well have saved his money. If, however, the physician takes the time to discuss the importance of weight loss and of kicking the smoking habit, prescribes programs for accomplishing both, and arranges a follow-up visit to give the patient needed support, then the checkup fee was well spent.

How often? Some physicians prefer to see their patients at least once a year, but do a full series of tests less often. Others recommend a full examination every other year until age 50, annually thereafter. Dr. Keith Sehnert, active in the promotion of patient self-care, recommends full-scale checkups every five years until age 40, every three years from 40 to 50, every two years between 50 and 60, and annually from then on. Those patients with known medical problems, those on any regular medication (including birth control pills), and those whose family histories indicate high risk for a particular disease should see their physicians more often.

Where? You can get a checkup at your doctor's office; at a major medical center such as the Lahey or Mayo Clinics; at a preventive care center such as New York's Preventive Medicine Institute–Strang Clinic; at a health maintenance organization, if you are a member; or in a few instances, at your college health service. Ideally, the examinations should take place at the same facility each time to assure continuity. And all reports should be forwarded to your own family physician for further evaluation and consultation.

Preventive Medicine Institute/Strang Clinic

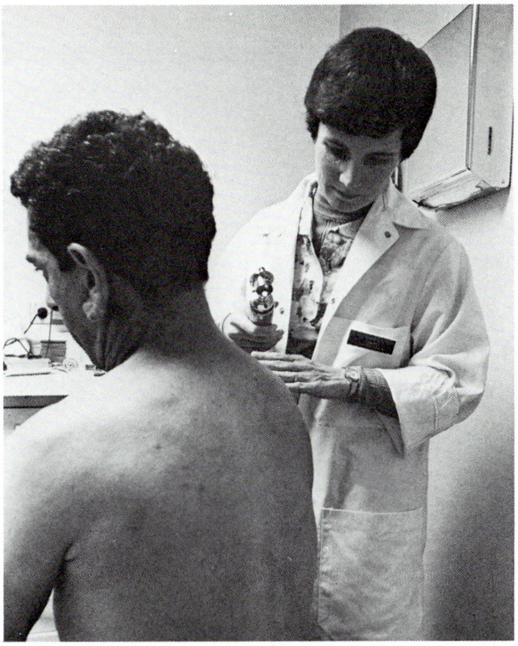

The periodic medical examination is only a small part of a health maintenance and disease protection program. Without follow-up changes in lifestyle the examination may be worthless.

What should a health checkup include? The exact agenda may vary depending on such factors as sex, age, race, family history, chronic conditions, health habits, and the physician's own convictions. But, in general, most checkups include the following basics:

- *A health history* Some physicians believe the health history is *the most important* part of any exam. Its questions—about previous illnesses, health of close relatives, known allergies and sensitivities, and emotional or physical problems one might not think to mention to the doctor—can often tell the physician more than any number of expensive tests.
- *The physical exam* The examiner—the doctor or an assistant—checks the patient from scalp to sole for abnormalities, ob-

WHEN TO SEEK HELP

Between Checkups

Consult a physician or stop in at the school health service, if you experience the symptoms listed below.*

1 Any of the following, not explained by a known illness or condition, that is not "normal" for you:

- Bleeding (other than menstrual) from any body opening
- Blood in urine, bowel movement (black or red), vomit, or coughed-up material
- Dizziness, blackouts, falling, fainting
- Numbness, paralysis, extreme weakness, tingling
- Convulsions
- Bowel changes—diarrhea, constipation
- Very high or very low fever
- Difficulty with breathing, urination, hearing, seeing, speaking, swallowing, digestion
- Blueness or yellowness of skin
- Unexplained black and blue marks or red streaks on skin
- Personality changes
- Red ear drum

2 Any of the following that is severe, prolonged, or recurrent:

- Sore throat, hoarseness, cough
- Vomiting
- Pain

3 Any of the following that is sudden:

- Severe pain
- Rapid, irregular, or very slow pulse

4 Any of the cancer warning symptoms described in Chapters 6 and 10.

*See also *When to Seek Help* sidebars for mental, dental, and other problems, listed in the Index.

serving such indicators of health as posture, walk, speech, general appearance, and behavior; examining eyes, ears, mouth and teeth, throat and nose; checking for masses, swellings or tenderness in the neck, abdomen, groin, and armpits; inspecting the condition of genitals and breasts; looking for any abnormal markings or lesions on the skin; observing the mobility and general health of arms and legs, hands and feet; checking for neurological problems with such tests as the familiar hammer-on-the-knee reflex test. Vital measurements are taken—height, weight, blood pressure, pulse, possibly temperature and respiration—and lungs and heart checked with a stethoscope. Checkups should include internal rectal examination with a proctoscope for persons over 40, vaginal examinations for women, and prostate examinations for men.

- *Diagnostic tests* The list of available diagnostic tests grows daily, but few people undergo even a small fraction of them (see Table 4.3). Most general checkups include basic blood and urine analyses, possible chest x-ray (particularly for smokers), and electrocardiogram (ECG or EKG) to measure heart activity in those over 40. A stress ECG (discussed on page 82) is highly recommended by the American Heart Association. Additional tests will be ordered for those who have particular complaints (digestive problems or headaches, for example) and for those who live or work in hazardous environments.
- *Consultation* Without a consultation to discuss findings and receive follow-up care instructions, even the best of examinations is worthless. Patients can use this visit to ask questions about anything in the checkup that was not understood, or to tell the physician about lingering concerns.

HEALTH CONSUMER TIP
X-Ray Safety

X-ray and fluoroscopic* examinations are extremely valuable in diagnosing a wide variety of ailments from broken bones and dental disease to tumors and pneumonia. But radiation from x-rays is known to cause cancer at high or repeated doses; it can also cause genetic damage in unborn children. Just how much x-ray radiation is hazardous, however, is the subject of wide disagreement. A few experts suggest that it is harmful at almost any level; others maintain that ordinary use is harmless; most suggest weighing risk against benefits in each case. While the debate goes on, consumers can protect themselves by using the following x-ray guidelines:

- The potential benefits of an x-ray exam should outweigh the potential risks.
- X-rays should be used only when other, safer diagnostic tools are not available.
- Routine x-ray examinations should be avoided except for: chest x-rays for heavy smokers or those who show positive TB tests; mammography for women over 50 or those over 35 with a personal or family history of breast cancer. Otherwise x-ray should be used only when something in the physical exam or personal history indicates the need for further investigation.
- X-rays should be administered to a woman who is or might be pregnant only when absolutely necessary and when no other procedure can be substituted. If possible, the exam is best postponed until after the third month of pregnancy, and the uterus shielded with a lead apron.
- X-rays should not be retaken when previous ones are available. You can have them transferred from one doctor to another.
- X-rays should be administered in a facility regularly licensed or inspected by a state or other agency. Equipment should be up-to-date, in good condition, and operated by well-trained, conscientious technicians under the supervision of a full time radiologist.
- X-ray beams should, when possible, be adjusted so only the necessary area is exposed; other areas, particularly reproductive organs, should be shielded with a lead apron.
- The patient should follow orders precisely. Otherwise, pictures might be ruined and need to be retaken, increasing exposure.

*Fluoroscopic examination allows for immediate viewing of internal organs in motion.

TABLE 4.3 Common diagnostic and screening tests

TEST	DESCRIPTION	DISEASE(S) DIAGNOSED	INDICATIONS FOR USE
		BLOOD TESTS	
Complete blood count (CBC), or computerized analysis	Count and examination of white blood cells, red blood cells, hemoglobin, etc.	Anemias, leukemias, infections, mononucleosis, internal bleeding	Screening*; fatigue, unexplained fever or illness
Sed(imentation) rate	Measures rate at which red blood cells settle	Can rule out infection and several other disorders	Screening*; unexplained illness
Lipid tests	Measures levels of cholesterol, triglycerides, VLDL, HDL, LDL	Potential heart disease	Screening*; chest pain; other symptoms of heart problems
Glucose and glucose tolerance	Measures levels of glucose (sugar)	Diabetes, other metabolic disorders	Screening* when symptoms of diabetes appear
Bilirubin	Measures bilirubin levels	Liver and blood diseases	Screening*; jaundice (yellowing)
BUN, uric acid	Urea-nitrogen tests	Kidney malfunctions	Screening*; urinary irregularities
Prothrombin, coagulation rate, platelet	Tests of blood clotting time	Bleeding disorders	Hemorrhaging; blood clots; surgery
VDRL	Veneral disease research lab screening	Syphilis	Screening*; exposure to syphilis; marriage; pregnancy
Wasserman	Antibody test for VD	Syphilis	Screening*; exposure to syphilis; marriage; pregnancy
T_3, T_4, PBI (protein-bound iodine)	Tests for thyroid function	Thyroid disorders	Symptoms of thyroid malfunction
		URINE ANALYSIS	
Glucose test		Diabetes, hypoglycemia	Screening*; symptoms of diabetes, hypoglycemia
Hormone test		Metabolic, endocrine disorders	Symptoms of hormone excess or deficiency
Microscopic exam for blood, microbes		Kidney, bladder, gall bladder disorders	Symptoms of urinary tract problems
		X-RAYS	
Bone x-ray		Fractures, tumors, abnormalities	Suspected fractures, tumors, abnormalities
Chest x-ray		Pneumonia, emphysema, cancer of lung, heart disorders, lung disorders, TB	Cough; screening* for heavy smokers; chest discomfort
GI series	X-ray of digestive tract	Digestive disorders, obstructions (e.g., ulcers, tumors)	Chronic indigestion, diarrhea, constipation, other digestive disturbances

*Tests used to screen for nonsymptomatic or early stage disease in healthy persons.

TEST	DESCRIPTION	DISEASE(S) DIAGNOSED	INDICATIONS FOR USE
		X-RAYS	
Mammography	Breast x-ray	Cancer of breast	Screening* in women over 50, or at high risk of breast cancer
Scanners (CAT, EMI, ACTA)	Flat crosswise views of internal organs	Can help diagnose tumors, blood clots, hemorrhages, etc., especially in brain	Symptoms of brain damage or other internal disorder *Note:* Very expensive; low radiation levels; safer than angiography
		CYTOLOGY, CULTURES	
Pap smear	Microscopic exam of secretions of uterine cervix	Cervical, uterine cancer or abnormalities	Screening* in women; abnormal bleeding or discharge from vagina
Sputum test	Microscopic exam of sputum	Respiratory diseases (cancer, pneumonia)	Screening* in smokers; symptoms of respiratory disease (cough, etc.)
Throat smear	Swab of throat to examine mucus	Strep throat (indicates need for antibiotic therapy)	Severe sore throat, usually with fever; possible carrier status
Stool exam	Tests for hidden blood, other abnormalities	Cancer of digestive tract; parasites	Screening* especially when digestive disturbance present
Gonorrhea culture	Culture of genital secretions to determine presence of gonorrhea	Gonorrhea	Costly and time-consuming, but can turn up nonsymptomatic cases
		OTHER TESTS	
Ultrasound	Use of echoes from high-frequency waves to examine internal organs; especially soft tissue	Eye, abdominal, lymph node problems; also used to determine fetal position and abnormalities of fetus in utero	Possible deformity of fetus; abnormal position of fetus; symptoms of diseases of various body organs *Note:* Safer than x-rays
Thermograph	Use of heat sensor to discover abnormalities	Breast cancer	Screening* in women over 50 or in high-risk categories
BMR	Oxygen test of basal metabolism	Thyroid malfunction (test less used today)	Symptoms of thyroid malfunction
Tonometry	Measures eyeball tension	Glaucoma	Eye pain or discomfort; screening* in older persons
Spirometry	Measures respiratory capacity	Emphysema, other respiratory disorders	Screening* especially in smokers

LISTENING WHEN THE BODY SPEAKS

Rarely does something go wrong, either physically or psychologically, without our bodies giving us fair warning. Some warnings are loud and clear—pain or bleeding. Others are more subtle—fatigue, loss of appetite. Still others can only be detected by means of medical instruments—fever, high blood pressure, abnormal heart beat—or upon examination—breast lumps, mouth sores. Learning how to recognize these symptoms, what they mean, and how to measure and report them is an important part of preventive medicine for the activated patient-partner.

General Warning Signs

Pain The symptom that most often brings people to seek medical treatment, pain is an important warning. Though its mechanisms are not fully understood, it can be divided into three types: (1) *psychogenic pain*—pain of psychological origin, felt by the patient, but for which no physical causes can be found; (2) *trauma pain*—pain resulting from injury; and (3) *organic pain*—pain caused by an actual lesion or obstruction somewhere in the body, such as a tumor pressing on an organ. In all cases, the pain is transmitted to the brain by the nerves. If the nerves are severed, there is no pain, no feeling at all.

Individual pain thresholds vary. Some persons are incapacitated by minor pain; others can tolerate large amounts. Women are said to be able to endure more pain than men. Use of painkillers like aspirin from childhood on to "cover up" pain often reduces our ability to cope with common pain. Fortunately, no matter how bad a pain is, when it is gone, it becomes difficult to remember (Hackett, *d*).

It has been said that God created pain for an important purpose—warning—and then forgot about it (Hackett, *d*). When pain continues, it serves no purpose. Recent studies indicate that the body manufactures a pain-

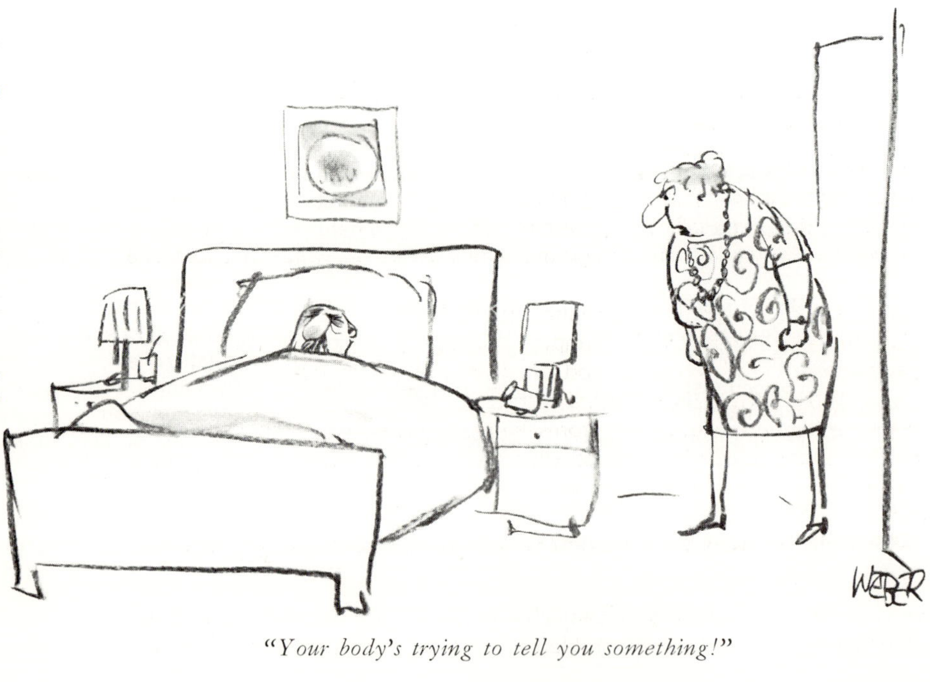

"Your body's trying to tell you something!"

SELF-CARE

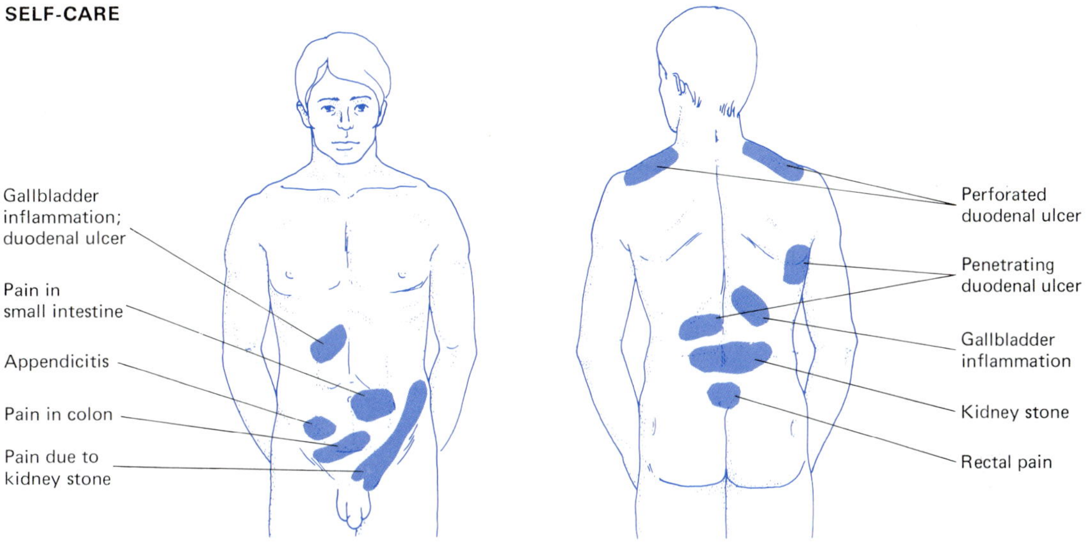

FIGURE 4.1 Common pain sites. Pain is often referred to parts of the body not directly involved in the disease or disorder causing the pain. [*After Sehnert and Eisenberg, p. G117.*]

HEALTH CONSUMER TIP

Reporting Symptoms to the Physician

Patient-partners can help the physician with the diagnosis by being prepared to answer the following questions about symptoms, particularly pain:

- *Intensity* How severe is the symptom?
- *Duration* How long does it last? (Time it, if you can.)
- *Pattern* Is it constant, rising and falling, or intermittent?
- *Location* Be specific, even mark it with a magic marker if it is pain that comes and goes (see Figure 4.1).
- *Radiation* How far does it spread from its central location? (See Figure 4.1.)
- *Quality* Is pain throbbing, stabbing, dull, crampy; is a cough dry or productive?
- *What influences the symptoms* What (a food or activity) seems to induce them? What makes them worse? What relieves them (rest, a certain position)?
- *Related symptoms* Are there any other symptoms that appear to be associated with the one that has brought you to the doctor (tenderness, swelling, cough, dizziness, or double vision along with the headache, or rectal pain along with the bleeding)? Or any recent injury that might be related?
- *Recurrence* What is the history of the symptom? How frequently has it recurred? When did it appear before?

It is also important to tell the physician about any chronic illness, medications or other drugs taken. Keeping a written record of symptoms, problems, and questions makes reporting easier.

WHEN TO SEEK HELP

Headache

Headache, or pain in the head, is one of nature's most common warning signals. When it results from the tensing of muscles in the back of the neck, reducing the supply of blood and the oxygen it carries to the brain, it is saying slow down, ease up, you are too uptight. Headache can also be saying you are partying or drinking too much, not sleeping enough, tired or hungry, or breathing noxious fumes. Sometimes headache signals physical illness—sinusitis, fever, dental problems. Certain headaches say see the doctor immediately:

- An almost constant headache that follows an injury to the head—immediately, weeks, or even months later
- A persistent headache that is accompanied by neurological disturbance of vision, hearing, coordination, speech, confusion, or lapses of consciousness
- A headache that is associated with convulsions, psychological changes, fainting, or paralysis
- A headache that is sudden and severe, especially if accompanied by nausea, vomiting, or diarrhea
- A headache that is daily or frequent or interferes with functioning

Rest, quiet, fresh air, sleep, food, or relaxation exercises may relieve headaches. Aspirin (as directed) may help until a doctor is seen. But regular use of painkillers for headaches can mask a serious condition and should be avoided.

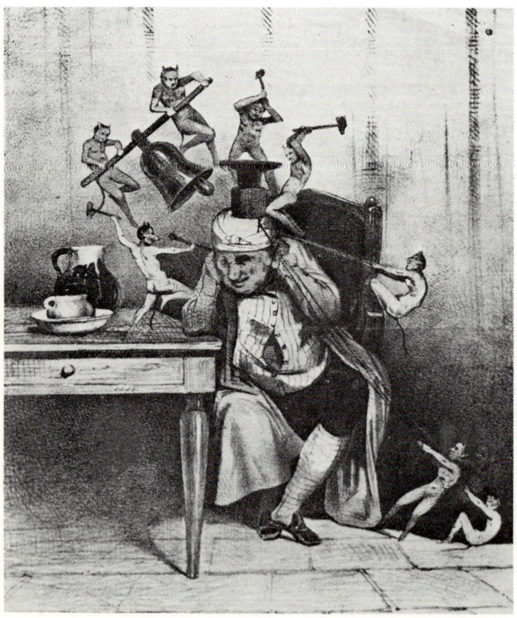

Daumier/Culver Pictures

killer of its own—endorphine—which is more powerful than morphine. Learning how to stimulate it would be a major breakthrough in pain treatment. To help patients with chronic pain that does not respond to treatment of the underlying cause, special pain clinics now use a variety of approaches: hypnosis, electrical stimulation, severing of nerves, injection of nerve blocks, acupuncture, physical therapy, heat and cold therapies, drugs, and such psychological approaches as behavior modification, biofeedback, counseling, and psychotherapy. In most cases, some degree of pain relief is achieved.

Other general warning signs These include the following:

- *Blood* in sputum, in urine, in feces; frequent nosebleeds; bleeding gums; and vaginal bleeding

SELF-CARE

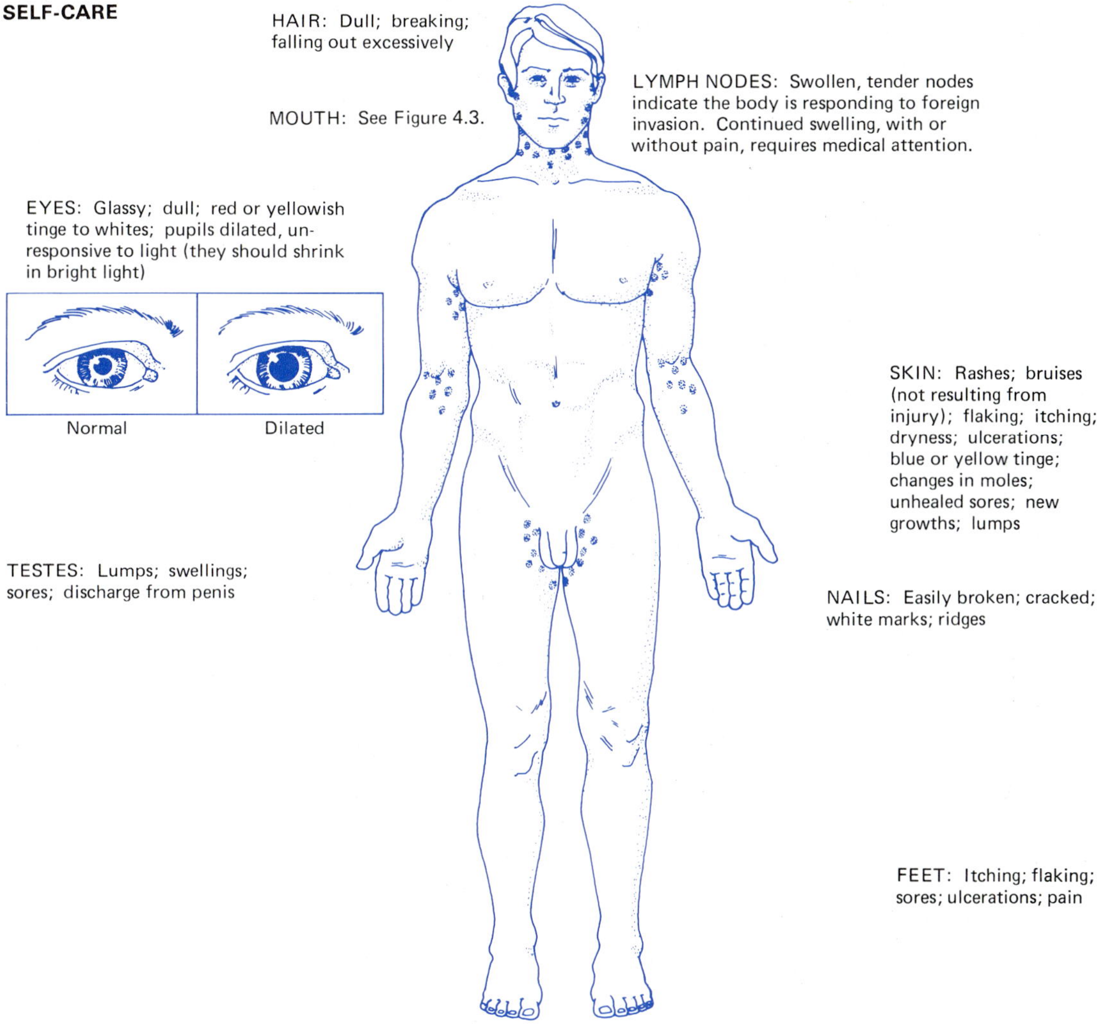

FIGURE 4.2 Self-examination. Get to know your body when it is healthy, so that you can recognize when it is not. For example, the average individual has 40 noncancerous (benign) skin markings or tumors—moles, "freckles," "beauty marks," skin tags, warts, and the like. Become familiar with yours, their sizes, colors, locations. Use a full-length mirror and check for changes every three to six months. Look, too, for any of the possible signs of illness shown above. If any are noted, a physician should be consulted. For female breast examination, see Figure 4.4.

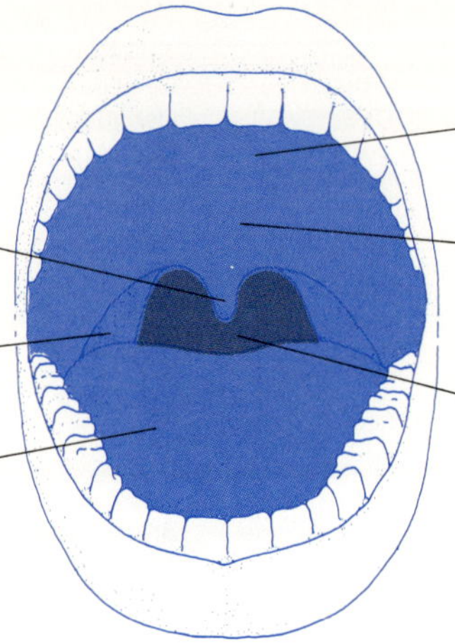

FIGURE 4.3 Self-examination of mouth and throat. For a good view of the throat, the handle of a spoon can be used to depress the tongue while the patient says "ah." A penlight can provide enough light. A reddened throat with patches of yellow or white exudate (mucus), possibly giving a "cobblestoned" appearance, may indicate strep throat (a bacterial infection of throat or tonsils). A throat culture can confirm the diagnosis. The mouth should also be examined periodically for the dental problems and oral cancer warning signals listed on page 143.

- *Fatigue*; *loss of appetite*
- *Unexplained itching*
- Suddenly *increased appetite or thirst*
- *Swelling*, which can indicate infection (pain, heat, redness), bleeding under the skin (if there is a black-and-blue bruise), internal bleeding, or accumulation of fluid (edema, which can be a sign of heart failure or other circulatory difficulties).

Discovering Body Signals through Self-Examination

Some 1800 years ago, Plutarch noted, "The man . . . is but a blind and deaf tenant in his own body, who gets his knowledge [of his own health] . . . from another, and must inquire of his physician whether his health is better in Summer or Winter, whether he can more easily tolerate liquid or solid foods, and whether his pulse is naturally fast or slow." Plutarch was probably among the first to recommend self-examination. Today most physicians recommend it, particularly as a way of detecting early cancer. Figures 4.2, 4.3, and 4.4 show how and when basic home examinations can be performed.

Warning Signals that Need to Be Measured

Calling the physician and saying, "I think I have a fever," or "I seem to be losing weight no matter what I eat," is not much help. The doctor needs to know fever readings or the amount of weight lost in a specific time period. It helps for patient-partners to be able to take basic physical measurements, and to be familiar with the baseline figures that are normal for them.

Body temperature The healthy body usually maintains temperature within a narrow range—averaging between 97.7° (36.2°C) before getting up in the morning and 99.6° (37.6°C) at its late afternoon peak—no matter what the environmental temperature may be. Figure 4.5 shows how to measure temperature.

Many factors affect body temperatures: thyroid malfunction, ovulation in women, time of day, exercise, and emotional upset. When body temperature rises above 100° (37.8°C), it is a signal that the body is responding to an infection or other abnormality, trying to overcome the germs with heat, and stimulating the body's defenses. Fever serves a useful purpose, and adults with slight fevers usually require no treatment. But high fever can be damaging to body cells—especially in the brain—and is particularly dangerous in ba-

SELF-CARE

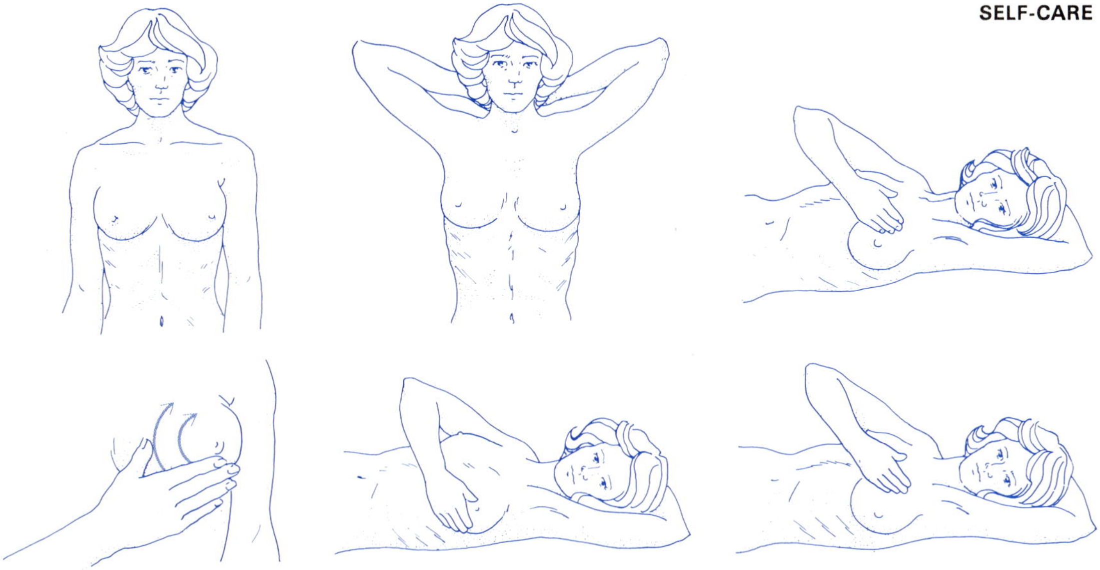

FIGURE 4.4 Self-examination of the breast should be performed monthly following the menstrual period. Women past menopause should perform the examination on the first day of each month.

1 Sit or stand in front of your mirror, with arms relaxed at your sides, and look for any changes in size, shape, or contour of your breasts. Look for puckering or dimpling of the skin or changes on the surface of the nipples. Gently press each nipple to see if any discharge is present.

2 Raise both arms over your head and look for the same things.

3 Lie down, pillow or bath towel under your left shoulder and left hand under your head. With the fingers of your right hand held together flat, examine your left breast this way:

a Imagine your breast divided into four areas like a clock: 12:00, 3:00, 6:00, and 9:00. Starting at 12:00 (and pushing down gently until you can feel the chest muscle underneath), move your fingers clockwise from 12:00 to 3:00 and on around in a small circle. Then move your hand up 2 inches and make another circle in the same way; then move up another 2 inches and repeat until entire breast is examined. If you notice a lump at any point, note its position on the "clock" so that you can report it exactly to the physician. (At the inner area of the breast, you may feel a ridge of firm tissue; this is normal.)

b Finally, bring left hand down to side and examine upper breast out to and including the armpits.

4 Repeat the same procedure on your right breast, using your left hand.

REPORT ANY UNUSUAL LUMPS, DIMPLES, OR OTHER CHANGES TO YOUR DOCTOR IMMEDIATELY. BUT DON'T PANIC—MOST CHANGES TURN OUT NOT TO BE CANCER.

SELF-CARE

FAHRENHEIT (°F) CELSIUS (°C)

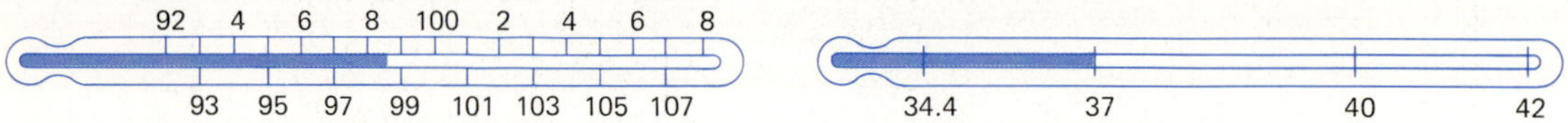

On a Fahrenheit thermometer the long line immediately to the left of the end of the mercury column is the full degree. Each small line represents 0.2 degree. Thus the thermometer above reads 98.6°F.

A Celsius thermometer is read in the same way, but on a scale of 34.4 to 42.0°C.

ORAL READINGS	°F	°C
Normal	98.6°	37.0°
Mild fever	99-100°	37.2-37.8°
Moderate	101-104°	38.3-40°
High fever	104° plus	40° plus

Baseline or normal temperature varies from person to person. One degree above this baseline indicates a mild fever.

FIGURE 4.5 Measuring body temperature.

1 Disinfect the thermometer with alcohol; rinse it with cold water.

2 Holding plain end, shake thermometer down until mercury drops below 96°F or 35.5°C. (Use a wrist motion; practice over a bed or couch.)

3 Place thermometer in patient's mouth, under the tongue. The lips should be kept closed around the thermometer, and the patient should breathe through the nose.

4 After 3 minutes, remove the thermometer and rotate it in good light until you see the flat ribbon indicating body temperature. Read as shown in the drawing.

5 Wash the thermometer with soap and *cold* water, rinse, and store it carefully, away from heat.

Note: Do not take temperature for 15 minutes after the patient has had something hot or cold to eat or drink.

Rectal readings, which are about 1° higher than oral readings, are preferred for young children or when nasal congestion forces the patient to breathe through the mouth. The thermometer, preferably with round bulb tip, is lubricated with petroleum jelly or oil and inserted about 1 inch into rectum.

bies and young children whose temperature-regulating mechanisms are not well developed. Since death usually occurs at about 107.6° (42°C), it is important to treat high fevers immediately.

Heartbeat or pulse Heartbeat, or pulse, can be influenced by blood pressure, body temperature (10 beats per minute increase for each degree of temperature rise), excitement, exercise, or illness. The average rate is considered to be 72 beats per minute, though the normal range, depending in part on physical conditioning and size, can be anywhere from 54 to 80 in adults (slightly higher in females than in males). In children, the rate is much higher: 82 to 180. Very rapid heartbeat is best measured with a stethoscope, but ordinary variations can be detected as shown in Figure 4.6, by taking the pulse. It is important, too, to note whether the pulse is irregular or weak, and whether it is skipping a beat.

Respiration The healthy adult takes about

SELF-CARE

Treating Fevers—Low and High

1 *If fever is very high:*
- Give cool drinks if patient is awake.
- Loosen or remove clothing.
- Apply icy wet towels or sponge with cold water or bathe in cold water.
- Administer aspirin as directed on the bottle.

2 *If fever is very low:*
- Give hot drinks if patient is awake.
- Cover with blankets, sweaters, etc.

3 In either case, call a physician or take the patient to an emergency room, clinic, or infirmary.

18 to 20 breaths per minute, children more—though there are variations. Respiration slows during sleep, speeds up during exercise. But very slow or very rapid respiration at rest can indicate illness, often lung disease. Respiration rate can be measured by placing one's hand on the patient's chest—ring finger on collarbone, thumb a few ribs lower—and counting the number of rises of the chest in 60 seconds. Sometimes this can be done visually, simply by watching the chest rise and fall.

Blood pressure High blood pressure can be a disease in itself, or can signal another disease (see Chapter 10). Sehnert has compared measuring the pressure of the blood as it flows through the arteries to listening to the flow of water through a hose. When the hose is kinked shut (which is analogous to tightening the blood pressure cuff and stopping the blood flow), water stops flowing and there is no sound. When the kink is loosened (opening the valve and letting blood flow again), there is a turbulent sound as water rushes into the hose once more. The readings as the swirling sound begins (systolic pressure) and as the flow smooths and the noise disappears (diastolic pressure) constitute the blood pressure reading. Figure 4.7 shows how to measure blood pressure.

EXERCISE: PREVENTION IN ACTION

Keen observer-author Plutarch recognized the value of exercise as preventive medicine when he declared that: "Health is not to be purchased by idleness and inactivity. . . . The man who thinks to conserve his health by uselessness and ease does not differ from him who guards his eyes by not seeing, and his voice by not speaking."

Today's medical community agrees that inactivity can be hazardous to health. During the presidency of John F. Kennedy, great concern arose over the fact that we had become a nation of sedentary spectators, most of whom regularly neglected exercise. A campaign, led by the President, was launched to develop physical fitness programs. Nearly 20 years later, most Americans would still rather ride than walk, watch the game of the week than play in one themselves. They empathize with the late educator Robert Maynard Hutchins who once declared, "Whenever I feel the urge to exercise, I lie down until it goes away." But millions have joined the pursuit of fitness—through jogging, tennis, squash, swimming, bicycling, and so on.

Dividends of Regular Exercise

Exercise, as an integral part of one's lifestyle,

affects health directly and indirectly in a variety of ways. It may lower blood pressure (or raise it when it is too sluggish), enhance sleep quality (while making the exerciser more alert overall), improve circulation and digestion, ease constipation (by toning abdominal muscles), and even, by relieving tensions, help to prevent ulcers and other psychosomatic disorders. In addition, it can increase strength, endurance, speed, and agility, and can improve coordination, flexibility, accuracy, balance, steadiness, timing, rhythm, and reaction time. Many people exercise to enhance general fitness, to maintain or lose weight, to achieve better appearance, to gain a feeling of well-being, and of course, for enjoyment. Exercise can also be helpful in restoring function in those disabled by injury, illness, or birth defect.

Regular exercisers also report increased vigor, more interest in and stamina for sex—at all ages—and what has been called "the exercise high." Adrenalinelike products called *catecholamines* secreted during strenuous exercise have a stimulating effect on mind and body, helping to create a lift and a feeling of well-being that is physiological as well as psychological. Studies have shown exercise to be helpful in elevating the mood and attitudes of depressed patients.

The most important reason for exercising, however, may be to improve cardiovascular (*cardio* = heart + *vascular* = blood vessel) or

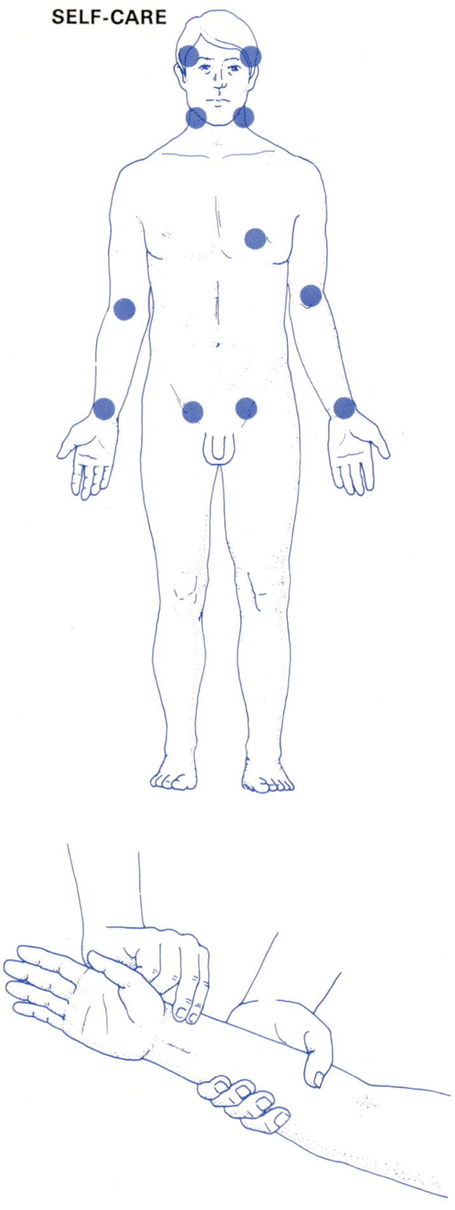

FIGURE 4.6 Measuring heart rate.

Taking pulse during rest: The pulse can be counted at any one of the starred pulse points, although wrist and neck are most often used. Using index and middle fingers, seek the pulse point—on the wrist, for example, on a line up from the thumb. When you have it, count the number of beats in a 15-second interval and multiply by 4. The result is the pulse beat or heart rate (e.g., 18 × 4 = 72).

Taking pulse during exercise: Because the pulse slows down very rapidly after exercise, it must be counted *immediately* when exercise is stopped in order to get the pulse beat during activity. Count for only 10 seconds and multiply by 6 to get a full minute's count.

SELF-CARE

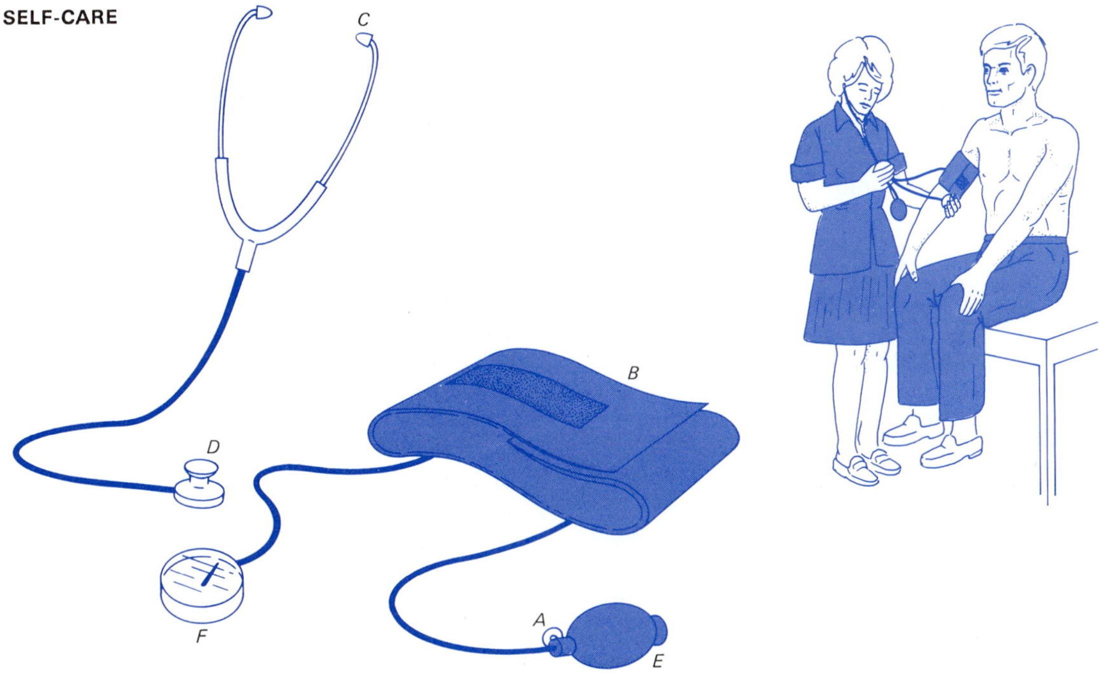

FIGURE 4.7 Measuring blood pressure.

1 Loosen the valve (*A*) and press air out of the blood pressure cuff (*B*).

2 Wind cuff around upper arm of patient as shown, about an inch above the bend in the arm.

3 Put ear pieces (*C*) of stethoscope in your ears, facing them forward.

4 Find pulse beat in arm below cuff with fingers. Place listening piece (*D*) over the pulse.

5 Close valve (*A*) and squeeze pump (*E*) to inflate cuff. Inflate up to about 180 on the gauge (*F*). Immediately loosen valve slightly, allowing air to escape gradually. Watch gauge. The point at which you begin to hear the pulse beat is the *systolic pressure*. The point at which the pulse beat disappears is the *diastolic pressure*. The pressure is recorded as systolic/diastolic, e.g., 120/70.

cardiorespiratory (*respire* = to breathe) fitness, known as CRF.

If you have ever bounded up three or four flights of stairs or run several blocks to make a class on time, and found your heart pounding, your lungs gasping for air, you know what happens when a cardiorespiratory system is not functioning at peak effectiveness. A well-conditioned system efficiently delivers oxygen to the muscles and other parts of the body; it also burns oxygen more efficiently. Thus, under sustained physical stress, when more oxygen is needed, the system easily meets that need. When our bodies are out of condition, our hearts must work harder to push more blood to feed more oxygen to our muscles—and so they beat more rapidly.

Regular vigorous exercise improves CRF

and apparently reduces the risk of death from heart attack. In one 22-year study of longshoremen, researchers found that a regular pattern of hard physical labor nearly halved the risk of heart attack (Paffenbarger et al.). Another study indicated that the more strenuous the exercise (running instead of walking), the greater the protection against heart disease.

Planning an Exercise Program

Anyone accustomed to a sedentary existence should have a medical checkup before beginning an exercise program (Zohman)—especially if he or she smokes; is more than 20 pounds overweight; or has had heart trouble, pains in the chest, irregular heartbeats, or palpitations, or an abnormal ECG reading. This applies, too, to anyone who has a chronic illness (diabetes, high blood pressure, asthma, etc); anyone who has experienced cramps or aches and pains in joints or muscles, emphysema, or shortness of breath; anyone whose immediate relatives have had heart trouble before age 60; and anyone over 30 who is just plain out of shape. Those under 30 who have had a checkup with normal findings within the last year can begin exercise without another visit (Cooper).

Ideally, the examination—especially for over-forties—should include a stress ECG. In this stress test, the subject handles gradually increasing work loads on a stationary bicycle or treadmill while connected to equipment that measures cardiovascular capacity and oxygen consumption. A cardiologist (heart specialist) carefully monitors the patient during the entire test, and stops it when 85 percent of capacity is reached, or when an abnormal reading flags a warning. The test may show up abnormalities such as narrowing blood vessels to the heart that an ordinary prone ECG would miss. It's like testing a car on the road instead of on the showroom floor. On the basis of the results, the physician can write a personalized exercise prescription for the patient. (See Figure 4.8.)

What kind of exercise? Not all exercise will increase CRF. Lifting weights, many kinds of calisthenics, isometrics, sprinting, and tennis doubles are among those that do *not*, because they fail to bring the heart rate up to a training point and keep it there for a suitable period. Good CRF exercises are both aerobic and isotonic. (See Figure 4.9.)

The exercise level aimed for is one that is neither too mild nor so strenuous that it causes excessive fatigue or aches and pains. The goal is to bring exercisers to a target zone somewhere between 70 and 85 percent of their individual *maximal aerobic power*—the exhaustion point at which, no matter how hard they try, the heart and lungs cannot deliver any more oxygen to the tissues or remove the waste products from them fast

HEALTH CONSUMER TIPS

Beware Instant Fitness Promises

Fitness can be developed only if the individual is committed to aerobic exercise or activity over an extended period of time. Promises of instant fitness—at a spa or health club or through the use of weights or other gadgets—are highly suspect, especially when they are associated with high-cost contracts. Such products or programs (and any contracts that must be signed) should be checked with a local Better Business Bureau or Consumer Fraud unit and possibly with your physician or other health care professional before you make a purchase or sign a contract.

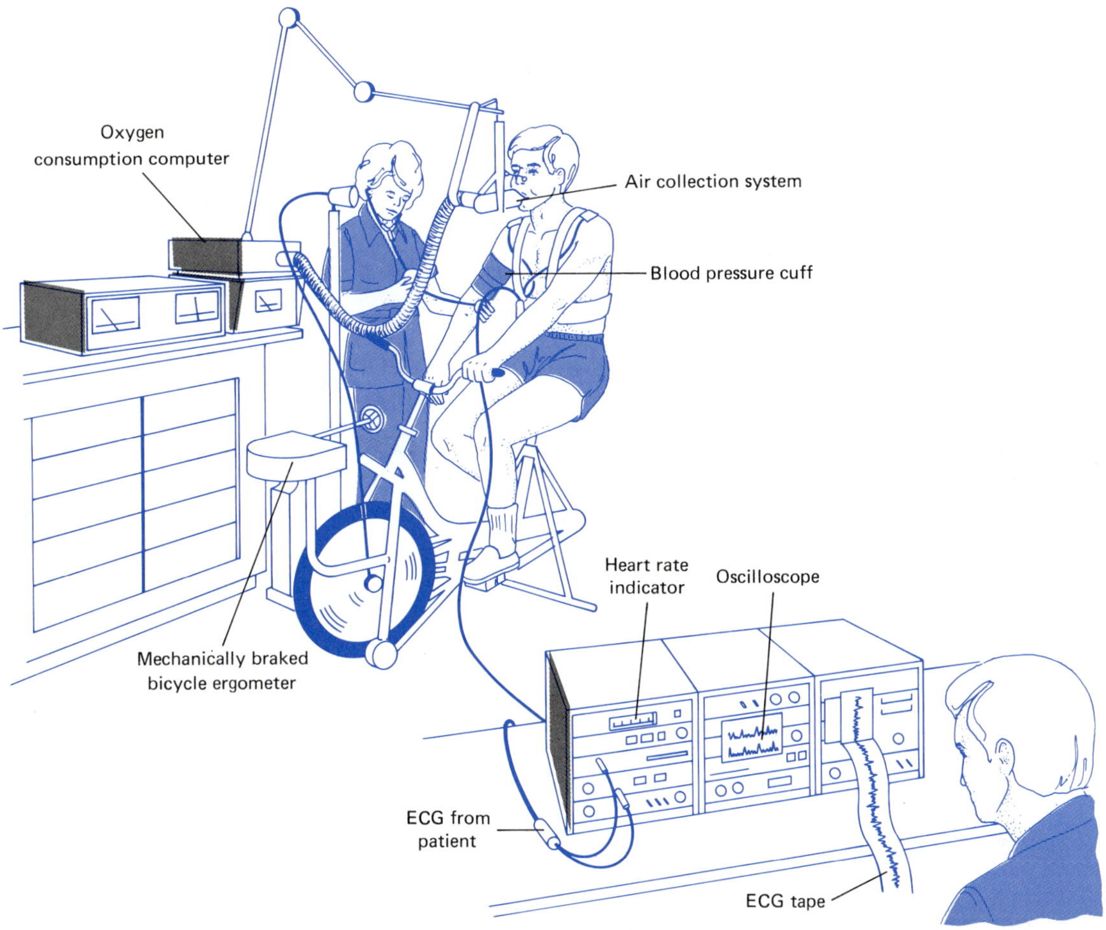

FIGURE 4.8 This exercise stress test evaluates the condition of the cardiorespiratory system while an individual is in motion. Such examinations have turned up many instances of impaired heart function in persons who had appeared perfectly normal. [*Adapted from Lenore R. Zohman,* Exercise Your Way to Fitness and Heart Health, ©*CPC International, Englewood Cliffs, N.J. Single copies available gratis from Mazola Health Book, Box 307, Dept. 2D, Coventry, Conn. 06238.*]

enough. In most normal individuals, at about this time, as the oxygen transportation system is breaking down, the heart reaches its top beating capacity, known as the *maximal attainable heart rate*. Because heart rate is easy to determine by taking the pulse, most exercise programs are based on heart rate rather than aerobic power. Figure 4.10 shows maximal average heart rates for adults, and the target zone for exercise. Figure 4.6 shows how to take the pulse.

Exercise that brings the heartbeat, or pulse, into the target zone for 20 to 30 minutes at each workout will create a *training effect*. If

ISOTONIC EXERCISES

Dynamic exercises that are rhythmic and repetitive, and involve motion. They result in rhythmic tensing and relaxing of muscles and thus in improved blood circulation. They can be aerobic or anaerobic.

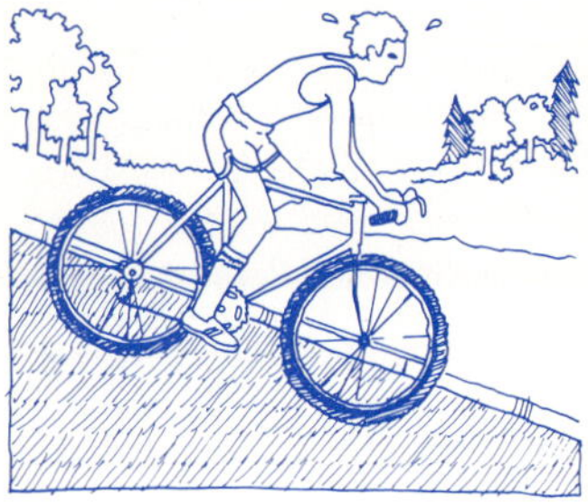

AEROBIC

Exercise that steadily supplies enough oxygen to exercising muscles for as long as the exercise continues: for example, bicycling, jogging, walking. They allow the rider or jogger to attain a balance between the oxygen needed and the oxygen getting through to the lungs and the cardiovascular system. Any isotonic exercise that can be continued for more than 2 minutes is probably aerobic.

ANAEROBIC

An exercise that cannot be kept up at a sustained rate because the body cannot continue to supply oxygen at so high a rate. Sprinting is an example of anaerobic activity.

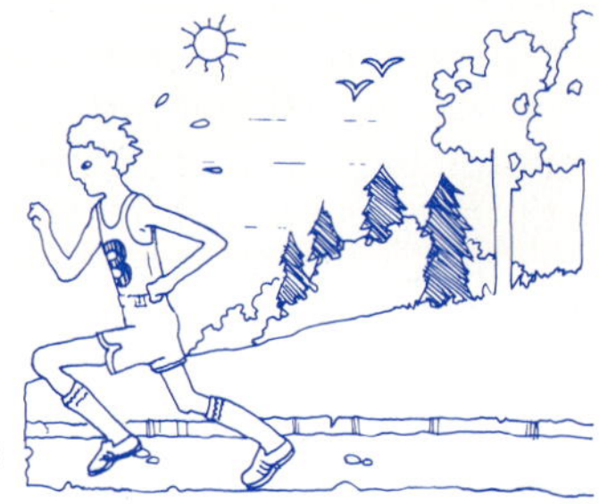

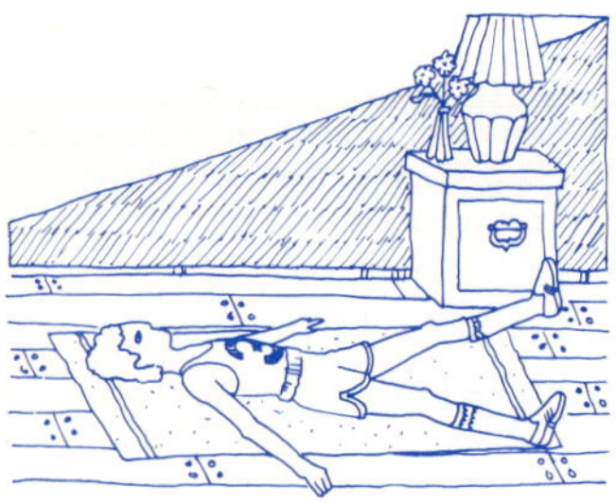

CALISTHENICS

Depending on how they are done, these can be isotonic or isometric, aerobic or anaerobic. When the body is kept constantly in motion (resistance followed by movement), the exercise is isotonic; when the body is in holding position, the exercise is isometric. Some calisthenics aid CRF, others do not significantly do so.

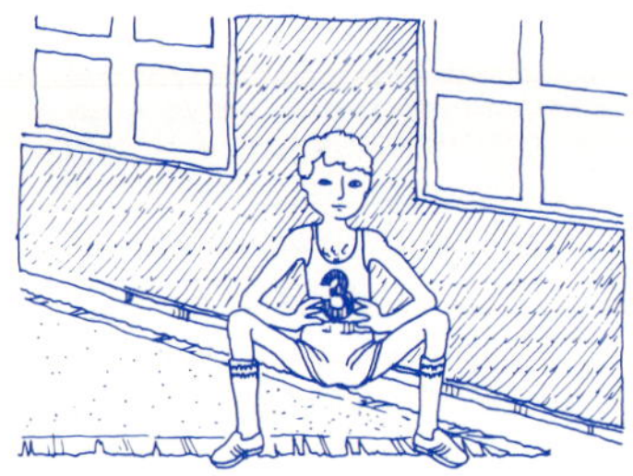

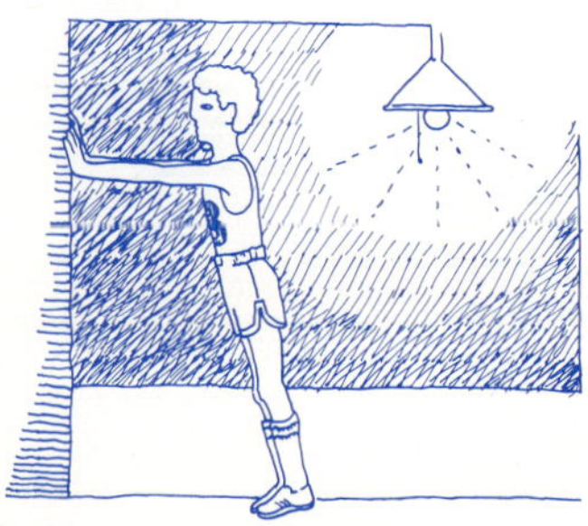

ISOMETRIC EXERCISES

A static form of exercise with little or no movement– such as lifting an unliftable object, pushing against a wall or a weight, squeezing hands together, carrying a heavy suitcase. These increase muscle power and strength, do not aid in developing CRF, and can be dangerous for heart patients. They can cause muscles being strengthened to shorten and tense up, squeezing blood vessels and decreasing blood flow through the heart.

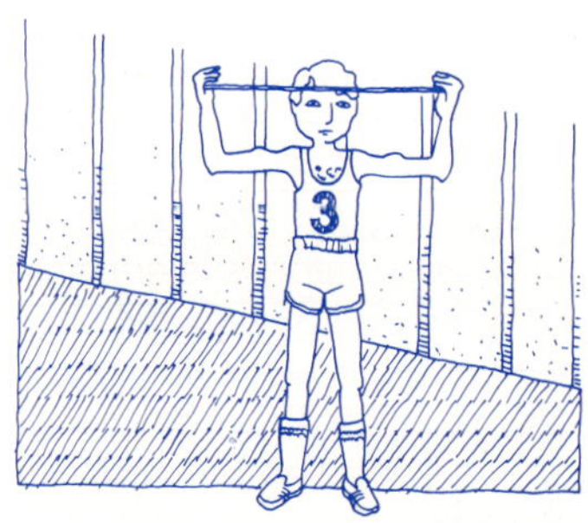

FIGURE 4.9

such exercise is done at least three times a week and continued over a long period, cardiorespiratory fitness will be improved.

Approaching the exercise Heidi and Susan, roommates at a state college, decided to begin exercise programs. Enthusiastic Heidi couldn't wait to begin. The next day was cold and damp, but she was out on the track determined to run 2 miles—and, to everyone's surprise, she did. But it took her 20 minutes to limp home exhausted, cold, wet, and discouraged. She spent a lot of time thereafter talking about exercise, but none in carrying it out.

Susan was a more patient sort. Just a couple of laps the first day. A little further the next. When the weather was cold and damp, she used a jump rope or the indoor track. On nice days, she jogged through the woods, or around the campus with a friend, rather than endure the monotony of the track. Susan was still exercising at semester's end, and she continued her program at home for the summer. She had built pleasure, not pain, into her exercise program. And she kept in mind her short- and long-term rewards: a better figure, more stamina, better health, and possibly longer life.

Integrating exercise into your life Some busy people build physical activity into their daily schedules. They walk up stairs rather than use the elevator; get off the bus a stop or two early and walk the rest of the way to school or job; scrub floors instead of mop-

FIGURE 4.10 The exercise training pattern for young adults. More strenuous exercise—e.g., jumping rope, hard running—requires less time in the target zone. The maximum heart rate holds for only two-thirds of the population. The figure is based on a hypothetical maximum of 200 beats per minute. [*Adapted from Lenore R. Zohman,* Exercise Your Way to Fitness and Heart Health, *©CPC International, Englewood Cliffs, N.J. Single copies available gratis from Mazola Health Book, Box 307, Dept. 2D, Coventry, Conn. 06238.*]

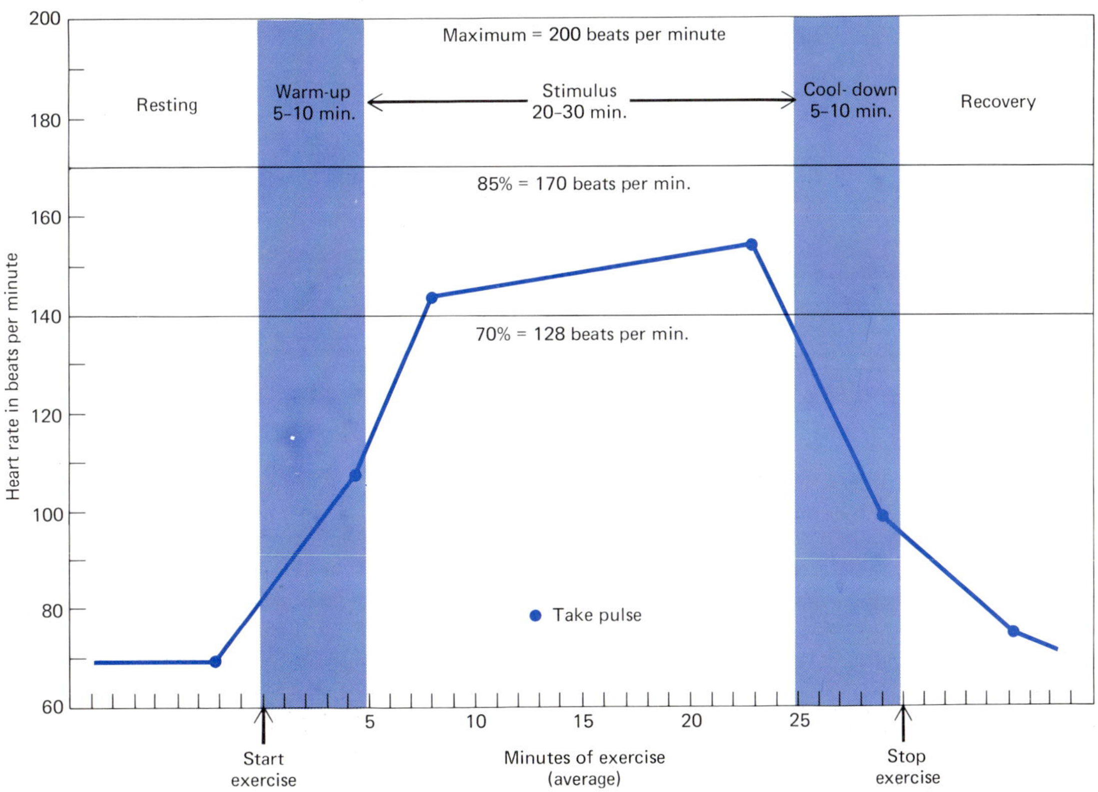

SELF-CARE

Exercise Tips

1 Select activities you enjoy (see chart for choices), and do them with someone else if you like.
2 Start off *very* slowly. If fatigue or other symptoms such as cramps, aches and pains, or breathlessness appear, go into a cool-down period and then stop. (If there is chest pain or discomfort, stop immediately.) Increase exercise gradually—an extra block of running, 10 more rope skips, or $^1/_{10}$ mile more on the stationary bike, for example.
3 Start each session with a warm-up and end with a cool-down period. These are very important. Warm-up (walking or very slow bicycling, for example) assures that the heart and circulation will not be taxed suddenly. It also helps avoid joint and muscle injury and soreness. The cool-down is equally important. An abrupt stop in exercise may trap blood in muscles which have stopped moving, cutting the supply of blood circulating back to brain, heart, or intestines. Dizziness, faintness, extra heartbeats, or nausea may result.
4 Reach your target zone (see Figure 4.10) and stay there for 5 minutes at first. Work up to a goal of a minimum of 20 minutes on target. Take your pulse as shown in Figure 4.6 at the appropriate moments. Or follow a point system such as the one developed by Dr. Kenneth Cooper and described in his book, *The New Aerobics.*
5 Exercise at regular times, at least three times weekly. Don't miss more than two days between workouts or you will slip backward.
6 Remember that poor health habits—lack of rest, poor diet, smoking, or use of drugs, for example—can sabotage an exercise program.

ping them: use people-powered rather than electrically powered tools.

SLEEP—ANOTHER FACET OF PREVENTION

Sleep, important to well-being, is an essential part of any prevention program. What happens when humans are deprived of sleep?

> In January 1959, under medical supervision, a 32-year-old disc jockey named Peter Tripp undertook to stay awake for 200 hours in a Times Square booth for the March of Dimes. After two days and two nights, Tripp began to report hallucinations—finding "cobwebs" in his shoes, for example. At 100 hours, simple mental tests were torture for him. He had trouble remembering, and saw the tweed suit of one scientist as a suit of "furry worms."
>
> After 120 hours, scientists saw the spectacle of a suave New York radio entertainer trying vainly to find his way through the alphabet, "like a blind animal trying to feel his way through a maze."
>
> By 170 hours, Tripp was no longer sure he was himself. He seemed awake, but his brain wave patterns resembled those of sleep. In his psychotic delusions, he was convinced his doctors were conspiring to send him to jail. On the last morning of his 8-day, 16-hour wakathon, Tripp stripped to the shorts for an examination by Dr. Harold Wolff of Cornell. Suddenly, gazing up at the doctor, Tripp came to the macabre conclusion that the doctor was an undertaker about to bury him alive. He broke for the door and dashed down the corridor with doctors in hot pursuit. Nightmare illusions and reality had merged. Only with great difficulty was Tripp persuaded to make a final appearance in the glass-windowed broadcast booth in Times Square—after which he slept for 13 hours. (Adapted from Luce, *b*)

Sample Exercise Program

1 *Five-minute warm-up* Include such activities as stretching of arms and legs followed by toe touching, pushups and sit-ups, rapid walking, then slow jogging or biking.

2 *Selected conditioning exercises**

- Walking (3 miles per hour or more)
- Jogging (5 miles per hour or more)
- Running (5.5 miles per hour or more)
- Bicycling (6 miles per hour or more)
- Swimming
- Stationary running (in place)
- Stationary bicycling
- Running up and down stairs
- Basketball
- Jumping rope
- Cross-country skiing
- Heavy housework (washing windows, mopping floors, vacuuming for at least 20 to 30 minutes)
- Heavy chores (chopping wood, digging steadily for at least 20 to 30 minutes)
- Tennis *singles*, handball, squash, table tennis, volley ball, badminton (only when skilled, vigorous, continuous play with player always on the move)

3 *Five-minute cool-down* Walking or very slow jogging or bicycling until pulse drops down to about 100 to 108 beats per minute.

*The more strenuous the exercise, the less time needed to complete a period of conditioning exercise. Jumping rope requires less than the average 20 minutes in the target zone; walking rapidly requires more. Bicycling at 12 miles per hour requires less time; at 6 miles per hour more. Slow walking (3 miles per hour) requires an hour or more for any conditioning to take place. All exercises must be continuous for training effect to take place.

The following exercises do *not* provide a training effect: water skiing, weight lifting, tennis doubles, golf (unless one reaches target zone by pulling cart and carrying clubs), most calisthenics, paddleball, light housework, strolling (under 3 miles per hour), bowling, downhill skiing, universal gym exercises, isometrics.

Some sleep deprivation experiments have not resulted in such extremes of psychotic behavior. A 17-year-old high school boy went through an 11-day experiment with only occasional hallucinations, fragmented speech and thought, blurred vision, and some involuntary movements. Researchers have suggested that age and differences in general stability probably accounted for the young man's easier time (Luce, *b*).

Most people can recall feeling "too tired to think," or grumpy and unpleasant, possibly even experiencing visual illusions following a night or two of sleepless cramming for exams. The most difficult hours are usually those during which we would ordinarily be sleeping. Performance and general condition improve during the usual waking hours. Evidently, sleep or no sleep, our bodies are following some preset internal clock.

The Biological Clock

Night follows day. Seasons change. Tides ebb and flow. The morning glory opens its scented blossoms each morning, closes them each night. Birds migrate at the same season every year. The world has rhythm, and human beings are part of the orchestra. Monthly patterns are most familiar in the female's menstrual cycle, but researchers have discovered that men, too, undergo monthly changes—including a weight change of 1 or 2 pounds, and variations in urinary hormones. Other patterns, both longer and shorter than a month, have also been recognized in humans. Understanding these patterns can illuminate many aspects of human variability—in symptoms of illness (suicides peak in May and arteriosclerosis around January in temperate climates), in response to treatment, in learning and job performance (B. S. Brown).

Circadian cycles The most studied of human cycles is the circadian (*circa* = around + *dia* = day) or 24-hour cycle, and this is the cycle most relevant to a discussion of sleep. All creatures—from the massive elephant to the delicate butterfly—suspend activity for a prolonged rest once in every 24-hour period (Luce, *a*).

Humans and primates differ from most other animals in that their 24-hour cycles are *diurnal*—they are awake during the day and asleep at night. Some people manage to alter this pattern because they work nights. Others—"night people"—just naturally prefer a night cycle.

Though the 24-hour circadian cycle is difficult to alter, it can be reset, if one relocates from Honolulu to Chicago, for example. But it takes time. Following arrival in Chicago, body time is out of phase with clock time in what is known as "jet lag." Fatigue, hunger, and readiness for activity are experienced on the old schedule. By the end of two weeks, the traveler feels adjusted, but tests indicate that internal body functions have not yet switched over completely (Luce, *a*).

Sleep cycles The period of sleep, research has shown, is not a single state of being, but a series of cycles. During a typical night's sleep, we go through a sequence of the stages shown in Table 4.4 approximately every 90 minutes, starting with stage I (near wakefulness), moving down to stage IV (deep sleep), and back up to REM (rapid eye movement, when most dreaming takes place) sleep. There is more stage IV early in the evening, more REM toward morning.

Persons entirely deprived of sleep appear to make up for it by very long periods of stage IV sleep. Subjects denied stage IV sleep for a few nights in experimental situations begin to complain of bodily malaise, apathy, and depression. Those deprived of REM sleep report irritability and sometimes anxiety; at times, they appear to be truly disturbed (Dement).

The Need for Sleep

Sleep, like most other human functions, is an individual matter. Some people do not feel rested unless they have had 12 hours of sleep. Others—usually very efficient sleepers who

HEALTH CONSUMER TIPS

Biorhythms

Though the existence of biological rhythms in all living things is well substantiated, there is presently no scientific support for the belief that "biorhythms," based on date of birth, control our physical, emotional, and intellectual ups and downs. Nevertheless, computerized biorhythm charts or kits for home preparation are sold by several firms reportedly taking in large sums of money in the enterprise. Anyone who invests in a personal biorhythm chart should do so with the awareness that the concept is an entertaining but hardly scientific gimmick—and that warnings about "bad days" can become self-fulfilling prophecies.

TABLE 4.4 Stages of sleep

DROWSINESS	STAGE I	STAGE II	STAGE III	STAGE IV	REM
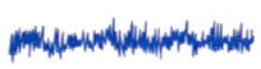	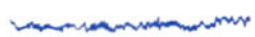	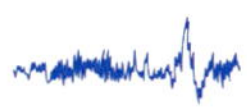	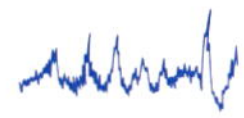	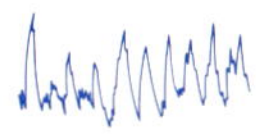	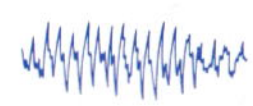
Body temperature declining	Respiration more even; pulse slowing; body muscles relaxing	Eyes may roll slowly; slowdown continues	Respiration even; pulse slows further; blood pressure and temperature continue to drop; muscles very relaxed	Respiration slow and even; pulse, temperature continue to drop; growth hormone at peak	Pulse, blood pressure, respiration wildly variable; temperature drops
Images float in dreamlike fragments	Some unstructured, fragmentary, thoughtlike dreaming possible				Period of vivid dreams, rapid eye movements
Serene state devoid of deliberate thought; easily disrupted	Light sleep; subject easily awakened by noise or spoken word	Sound sleep, yet easily broken (subject, awakened, might feel he or she had been thinking or in reverie)	Loud noise or soft calling of name can awaken subject	Oblivious sleep; subject hard to awaken, but loud sound or calling of name will cause slow awakening	Subject hard to awaken
	Myclonia (feeling of falling or floating, ending in jerking; awakening) may occur			Sleepwalking, talking, bedwetting, and night terrors may occur	Penile erections in males; change in female erectile tissue; ulcers, migraine may flair; heart attacks may occur

have very little stage I and II sleep and a great deal of REM and stage IV—do very well on 4 hours. There have been some poorly documented claims that humans can exist without sleep of any kind. All sleep deprivation studies made in the United States, however, indicate that sleep is as essential as food and drink if we are to function effectively. Still, scientists do not agree on why we need sleep, or what it does for us.

Sleep needs change with age, illness, pregnancy, mood, or stress. Sometimes the

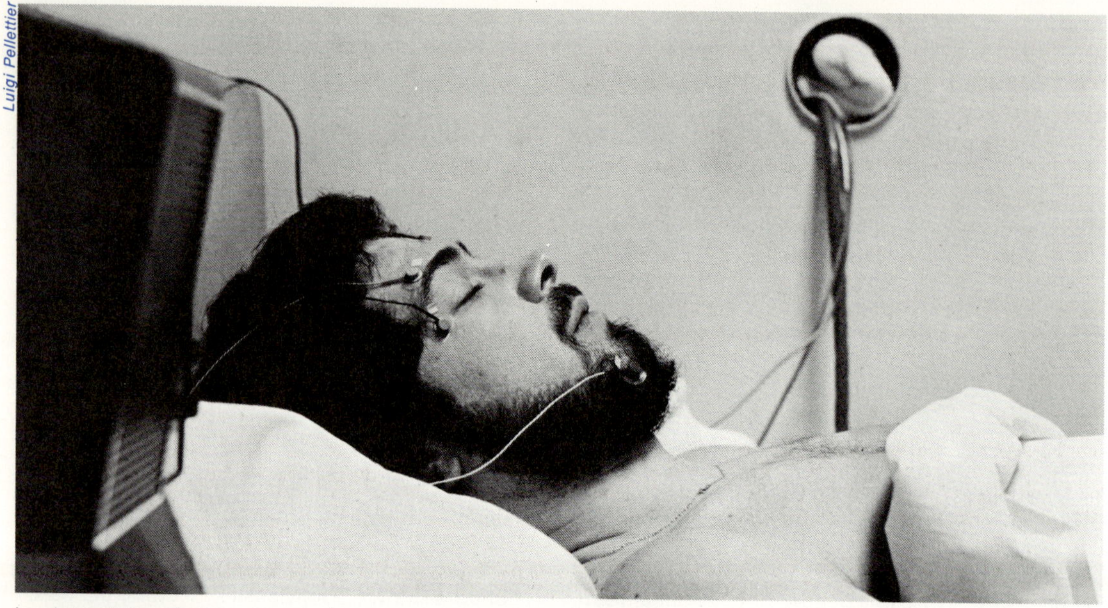
Luigi Pelletier

In sleep laboratories, researchers study the stages of sleep and the effects of sleep deprivation.

changes are inexplicable. A 23-year-old graduate student, accustomed to sleeping 6 to 8 hours a night, awoke at 2 A.M. after 4 hours of sleep and was unable to go back to sleep. The next night, the same thing happened. Unwilling to just lie in the dark and do nothing, he lit a candle and returned to his studies. This 4-hour pattern continued for the rest of his life of 80 years, during which he became an internationally known scholar (Dement).

Generally, sleep requirements decrease with age. Average time for newborn infants is 16 hours, for 16-year-olds 10½ hours, and for graduate students 8 hours. Elderly people often manage on 6 hours, but they need additional rest periods. Deprived of sleep for one or several nights, we generally make it up by sleeping longer at the first opportunity (Dement).

Sleep Problems

Most people experience an occasional sleepless night, but for an estimated 20 million Americans, every night is sleepless. Some have difficulty falling asleep, others awaken frequently during the night, still others awaken early in the morning. Their problem is called *insomnia* (*somnia* = sleep). There are several types of insomnia.

Pseudoinsomnia (*Pseudo* = false.) A good many insomniacs, when tested in a sleep lab, turn out to be sleeping normally—often a full eight hours or more. In at least one case, the subject slept, but dreamed he was awake. Other cases of pseudoinsomnia are not as easily explained (Scarf).

True insomnia Genuine insomnia has many causes including: (1) external stimulation—noise, lights, etc.; (2) uncomfortable surroundings—lumpy mattress, heat, cold; (3) genetic or neurological disorder or illness; (4) mild aches and pains not noticed during the day; (5) indigestion; (6) muscular twitches (the feeling of falling) felt in early sleep; and (7) worry and stress.

Sleep apnea (*a* = without + *pnea* = breath.) Breathing lapses can also disturb sleep. When persons suffering from these lapses fall asleep, their brain breathing centers turn off. After 60 to 100 seconds, their bodies hungry for air, they awaken. This pattern can be repeated throughout the night. Those who are aware of the awakenings consider themselves insomniacs. Those who do not notice them complain of unexplained tiredness and a need to sleep during the day. Because of this need, they are called *hypersomniacs* (*hyper* = over).

Drug-induced insomnia It is well known that stimulants like amphetamines and caffeine can cause sleeplessness. Less recognized is the fact that "sleeping pills," too, can lead to insomnia (Dement). The depressant drugs used in prescription sleeping aids do aid sleep—for a few nights. Then two things happen: (1) the body becomes adjusted to the dose and more is needed for the drug to be effective, and (2) sleep patterns become disturbed because the drug depresses REM sleep and often stages III and IV as well. This often leads to self-prescribed increases in dosage and then drug dependency. Use of the drugs disturbs sleep, but abrupt withdrawal brings on nightmares and other withdrawal symptoms. Dr. Anthony Kales of Penn State Medical School Sleep Research and Treatment Facility suggests that the only safe course is gradual reduction of the dosage *under medical supervision* until withdrawal is accomplished. (For more on the effects of depressants, see Chapter 15.)

Idiopathic insomnia Many cases of insomnia are labeled *idiopathic*, of no known cause.

Narcolepsy Once thought to be a rare condition, this sudden, overwhelming, irresistible sleepiness is now believed to affect as many as 100,000 Americans, with many times that number marginally narcoleptic. Alert most of the day, narcoleptics can fall asleep driving a car, talking on the telephone, or making love. They should be under the care of a physician familiar with the condition and should, if

SELF-CARE

Combating Insomnia

- Exercise strenuously during the day—but not before bedtime. Yoga, meditation, or biofeedback may also be helpful.
- Find your natural rhythm. You'll sleep best when body temperature drops.
- Make a routine of going to bed; ritual helps. Take a warm bath, read a soothing book, watch TV, relax, put aside problems.
- Have warm milk or a protein snack before bed. Avoid sugary snacks, coffee, tea, colas, chocolate—they can keep you awake.
- Keep covers off your head. Covering up cuts down on oxygen and increases carbon monoxide, causing headaches and even abnormal heart rhythms.
- Not sleeping may be a habit. Change surroundings and other conditions to encourage sleep.
- Don't just lie there tossing; read, sew, write a paper.
- Resort to pills only under a physician's directions. Nonprescription sleep aids have not been proven effective and can, if abused, lead to psychological problems.
- Reduce time in bed. You may be sleeping too much.
- If worry is keeping you from sleep, try to solve the underlying problems causing the worry.
- If you can't sleep, don't worry. Anxiety makes sleeplessness worse, and loss of sleep won't do any real harm. If sleeplessness continues, see your physician.

necessary, take prescribed medication to prevent attacks of sleep when driving or operating machinery.

Dyssomnia This broad category of sleep disorders occurring during the oblivion of stage IV sleep includes somnambulism (*somni* = sleep + *ambulare* = walk), night terrors, and bed-wetting. These problems are found most often in children, but occur in adults as well. (One of every 100 men in the U.S. Army has been found to suffer from nocturnal enuresis, or bed-wetting.) Sleepwalking and night terrors are completely forgotten by morning, and treatment is often not advised. The problem usually disappears by itself. Safety precautions—locked windows and doors, etc.—are, of course, necessary to protect the sleepwalker.

LOOKING BACK

REVIEWING CONCEPTS IN CHAPTER 4

- Preventive health practices are the most important elements in modern health care.
- The periodic physical exam is only a small part of prevention, and unless it influences the individual's lifestyle it may be next to worthless.
- Physicians are fallible, and activated patients recognize this in establishing a doctor-patient relationship. They follow doctors' orders, but not until they have questioned anything they do not understand.
- Patients can learn to keep their own health records, and have a right to see those the physician keeps for them.
- Our bodies speak to us in many ways. Learning to listen to and understand body language makes a patient a more effective health consumer and contributes to disease prevention.
- Both regular physical activity and adequate sleep are necessary for optimal physical and mental health as well as for disease prevention. In addition, aerobic exercises improve cardiorespiratory fitness.
- The most successful exercise programs are those that build in pleasure, are easy to keep up with, fit one's lifestyle, and are tailored to individual special needs.
- When humans are deprived of sleep for long periods, their performance level slips—both physically and mentally; they may also exhibit symptoms of mental illness.
- Sleep and many other functions are linked to our inner biological clocks. Sleep needs vary from person to person and even out over a period of time.
- Sleep can be disturbed by noisy or distracting surroundings, poor physical and mental states, drugs, breathing difficulties, and causes unknown.

5

NUTRITION: ARE WE WHAT WE EAT?

WHAT'S AHEAD IN CHAPTER 5 What influences food choice? How do decisions about what to eat in our modern society differ from those made by more primitive peoples? How does nutrition influence health? What is malnutrition? How common is it in this country? What is overnutrition? What are the nutrients that our bodies require? What factors may influence individual requirements? How are recommended dietary allowances (RDAs) of the various nutrients best used by the average person? How can you best assure that you are getting an adequate amount of all the nutrients? What are empty calories? What are the dangers of fad diets? Does the promise "100 percent natural" guarantee the consumer either nutritive value or food safety? How is a weighing of risk versus benefit used in determining the appropriateness of using a particular food additive? In what ways may the handling, storage, and preparation of food be a threat to health? How serious a menace is overweight in the United States today? What is the *only* way to take off weight? How do overweights and normal weights differ in eating habits and physical activities? What kind of changes will help a person to attain and to maintain desired weight? When may drastic action be necessary for the overweight? Who should make the decision to take such steps?

Three or more times a day, more than 1000 times a year, we make decisions that can cause or prevent disease,[1] influence our ability to learn and to respond to physical and emotional stress, and affect the health of our children and our children's children. We make these decisions every time we eat. According to noted nutritionist Jean Mayer, we have failed to increase the lifespan of the adult American not because of lack of effort and money, but because we have often not made these decisions wisely. Suggests Mayer (c), we have neglected the best and easiest kind of preventive medicine: good nutrition.

WHY WE EAT AS WE DO

- *Breakfast A* A cup of black coffee and half an orange.
- *Breakfast B* Whole wheat toast, orange juice, bran cereal or oatmeal, and tea—no eggs because of cholesterol.
- *Breakfast C* Cantaloupe, two fertile eggs, a heaping bowl of cottage cheese, and a large glass of raw milk.
- *Breakfast D* A 4-ounce serving of broiled chicken, half a slice of rye bread with margarine, and a glass of milk.
- *Breakfast E* Bran flakes, corn flakes, and a high-protein cereal with low-fat milk, blueberries, half a slice of rye toast, and two cups of black coffee.

How would you evaluate these breakfasts? Do you think that the people who selected them know much about nutrition? Actually, all five breakfasts were chosen and eaten by prominent nutritionists.[2] They run the gamut from conservative establishment to radical antiestablishment, and they give us an inkling of the wide differences and preferences existing in the nutritional arena.

[1]Including 6 of the 10 leading causes of death: heart disease, some cancers, stroke, diabetes, arteriosclerosis, and cirrhosis.

[2]Breakfast A was chosen by Dr. George Watson, biochemist at California's Lancaster Institute; breakfast B, by Dr. Jean Mayer, leading nutritionist and educator; breakfast C, by the late Adelle Davis, author and nutritionist with an antiestablishment reputation; breakfast D, by Dr. Carleton Fredericks, author and lecturer with an antiestablishment attitude who teaches at the university level; and breakfast E, by Dr. Frederick Stare, Harvard nutritionist-author and frequent food industry advocate (Curley; Blinn).

For many reasons, these differences of opinion are not surprising: (1) nutrition is an infant field in which few absolute rules have yet been laid down; (2) new concepts in nutrition are often proposed before old ones filter down to American tables; (3) the field attracts untrained self-proclaimed experts serving a mixed salad of fact, fad, and fantasy, as well as serious scientists; (4) nutrition is inescapably influenced by a multibillion dollar food industry, and by individual lifestyles and backgrounds. Evidence suggests that even if scientists could draw up the perfect diet, most people would not eat it (Yudkin).

Factors that Affect Food Selection

Food choice is governed not just by a list of do's and don'ts, but by our family and ethnic background, the part of the country or the world we come from and live in, our moods, and how much time we have to eat. It is colored, too, by the weather (hot oatmeal in July?), by food allergies and sensitivities (millions of adults, particularly of African or Asian origin, cannot drink milk), where we are eating, our economic circumstances, and how we are feeling about life in general.

In recent years, food choice has been influenced by the development of "convenience foods" and by the advertising media. On a typical Saturday for example, children watching one station in Boston between 7 A.M. and 2 P.M. saw 67 commercials urging them to eat or drink highly sweetened products (Charren and Sarson). The Federal Trade Commission (FTC) has proposed a ban on *all* advertising directed to young children.

A Historical Perspective

Our earliest humanlike ancestors, anthropologists believe, were herbivorous—eating herbs, berries and nuts, and leaves. When the world entered a 12-million-year drought and supplies of vegetarian foods dwindled, our primate ancestors became hunters to supplement the slim pickings. Their diets then became rich in protein, moderately rich in fats, and rather poor in carbohydrates, for which fruits were their chief source. About 10,000 years ago, with the discovery that seeds could be planted and crops harvested, agriculture was born. Farming was easier and less hazardous than hunting and higher in yield. Grains—bread, rice, tortillas, pitas, kashas, etc.—therefore became the staple food for much of the world and diets became richer in carbohydrates, mostly starches, and poorer in both proteins and fats.

The next major change in food habits came with industrialization. With foods refined and processed in factories, instead of eaten as grown, the link between palatability (or taste) and nutrition (or healthfulness) broke down. No longer did craving something sweet mean wanting a piece of fruit full of vitamins and minerals. It could mean wanting a soft drink, hard candy, or ice pops containing no nourishment at all. In 1900, 40 percent of our calories came from fruits, vegetables, and grains, mostly fresh; today only 20 percent of our calories are from these sources. Calories often come from "nonfoods." In 1975, Americans consumed an average of 295 cans of soda each (Senate Select Committee).

In thinking about diet today, then, it is no longer possible to rely solely on what pleases our palates. We need to know something about what it is in foods that pleases our bodies and the cells that compose them.

NUTRITIONAL NEEDS

Our bodies function as chemical factories, producing, storing, burning, releasing, and excreting the huge numbers and varieties of substances needed to keep us healthy. Many of the chemicals required for these processes are produced within the body. Others must be taken in as raw materials—from food.

By trial and error, scientists have compiled a list of many of these essential chemicals or nutrients. But though diets made up of known nutrients from this list may maintain health, scientists are aware that the current list of nutritional needs is incomplete. A varied diet assures that we will get needed nutrients—known and unknown. Known nutritional needs include: calories and the proteins, carbohydrates, and fats that provide them, dietary fiber, water, vitamins, and minerals.

> Whatsoever was the father of a disease,
> an ill diet was the mother.
> Old proverb

Calories—Source of Energy

Though it sometimes seems that the calorie is U.S. Public Enemy Number 1, the fact remains that we cannot live without the much-maligned, much-counted, much misunderstood calorie. A calorie is the amount of heat energy required to raise the temperature of 1 kg of water 1°C. Calories provide the energy to operate that chemical plant, our body, and the fuel for all our physical and mental activities. The various kinds of caloric energy—five slices of bread, an hour of walking at moderate speed, an ounce of body fat, for example—are roughly equivalent in quantities of energy.

Calories in the diet come from three major sources: fats (an average of 9 calories per gram) and proteins and carbohydrates (averaging 4 calories per gram). Alcohol, not considered a nutrient, contains 7.1 calories per gram. The marriage of science to weight watching has given birth in recent years to charts that tell us the *approximate* calorie count of just about any food, from corn bread to caviar (see Table 5.9). Charts have been developed, too, to suggest calorie requirements for individuals, but again, these are approximations, varying from person to person (see Table 5.1).

Protein

The name "protein" from the Greek *proteios*, or primary, is well chosen, for protein is of

TABLE 5.1 Recommended daily dietary allowances of calories and protein*

	AGE, years	WEIGHT kg	WEIGHT lb	HEIGHT cm	HEIGHT in	ENERGY, kcal	PROTEIN, g
				MALES			
	15–18	61	134	172	69	3000	54
	19–22	67	147	172	69	3000	54
	23–50	70	154	172	69	2700	56
	51+	70	154	172	69	2400	56
				FEMALES			
	15–18	54	119	162	65	2100	48
	19–22	58	128	162	65	2100	46
	23–50	58	128	162	65	2000	46
	51+	58	128	162	65	1800	46
Pregnant						+300	+30
Lactating						+500	+20

*The allowances are intended to provide for individual variations among most normal persons as they live in the United States under usual environmental stresses. Diets should be based on a variety of common foods in order to provide other nutrients for which human requirements have been less well defined.
Source: RDA.

primary importance to all living things. It is used in repairing, rebuilding, and replacing cells. It is produced in the body using protein building blocks called *amino acids*, some of which are synthesized (produced) in the body, others of which must come from the foods we eat (essential amino acids). For the body to function well, we need all the amino acids in the proper proportions. If one is missing, like a hockey team with one player in the penalty box, the team carries on, but less ably. If all, or almost all, amino acids are missing from the diet, the game of life grinds to a halt.

Total protein starvation and protein-calorie malnutrition are common in many underdeveloped countries, but in regions of plenty like the United States, people are more likely to suffer from an imbalance of the essential amino acids. This type of imbalance can be avoided by choosing protein foods from a wide variety of sources. Animal proteins (such as meat, eggs, poultry, fish, milk, and cheese) tend to be complete sources of amino acids, while vegetable proteins (such as beans, peas, grains, and nuts) are not.

Carbohydrates

Carbohydrates—starches and sugars—are the single highest source of calories in the American diet, providing 46 percent of typical calorie intake. Converted to glucose (blood sugar) by the digestive process, carbohydrates are the main source of energy for the human body—essential for muscular activity, nervous system functioning, and the maintenance of body temperature.

If the level of glucose in the blood climbs too high, hormones—primarily insulin produced by the pancreas—are released to convert the excess into glycogen for storage in the muscles and liver. When glycogen storage reaches capacity, excess glucose is stored as fat. Should blood-sugar levels drop, glucose is released and reconverted into readily usable glucose. When glycogen stores are exhausted, body reserves of fat are called upon for energy. Should these be depleted, the body is forced to a dangerous last resort—withdrawing protein from the cells for use as energy. In some persons, the blood-sugar-regulating mechanisms go haywire. Then blood-sugar levels become very high as in diabetes (*hyper*glycemia) or very low (*hypo*glycemia). (See Chapter 9.)

Carbohydrates, often an inexpensive source of calories, abound in such foods as bread and other baked goods, cereals, rice, noodles and macaroni, most vegetables and fruits, jams and jellies, candy and soft drinks, honey, maple syrup, and table sugar. High carbohydrate intakes require an accompanying high intake of the B vitamins. In nature, such staple carbohydrates as whole grain breads and cereals are high in the essential B vitamins. Processing, however, removes the B vitamins and a diet of unenriched, refined carbohydrates could lead to a B vitamin deficiency.

Sugar: A special note As late as the eighteenth century, you needed a key to get into the locked sugar boxes of the rich. Not until the mid-eighteenth century, when mass production and the discovery that sugar could be refined from beets brought costs down rapidly, did sugar cease to be a luxury item. A rapid rise in its consumption followed. More recently, sugar has appeared unexpectedly in a

TABLE 5.2 Processed sugar in everyday foods*

FOOD	SERVING SIZE	TEASPOONS OF SUGAR
Candy bars	1 ounce	5
Brownies	2 × 2 × ¾ inches	3
Ice cream	½ cup	5–6
Apple pie	1/6 of pie	12
Ginger ale	6 ounces	3⅓
Cola	6 ounces	4½
Jam	1 tablespoon	3
"Natural" cereal	¼ cup (1 ounce)	2
Cocoa Krispies	¾ cup (1 ounce)	3
Special K	1¼ cups (1 ounce)	0.6
Captain Crunch	¾ cup (1 ounce)	3
Wheat Chex	⅔ cup (1 ounce)	0.4
Jello	½ cup	5
Peaches, canned, heavy syrup	½ cup	4
Tang breakfast drink	½ cup	4
Hi-C orange drink	¾ cup	5
Coffee-Mate nondairy creamer	1 teaspoon	0.65
Wishbone Russian dressing	1 tablespoon	1
Hamburger Helper	¼ cup	3
Ketchup	4 teaspoon	1
Shake 'n Bake Barbecue	¼ cup	6

*Read labels. Sugar is also found in bread, spaghetti sauce, peanut butter, prepared dinners, boullion cubes, soups, vegetables, crackers, yogurts, and hundreds of other products. It is the major ingredient (first on the label) in Shake 'n Bake Barbecue Style, Tang, General Food Cafe Vienna, Ovaltine, Carnation Breakfast Bars, and La Choy's Sukyaki Sauce Mix.

Source: "Science in the Public Interest"; *Consumer Reports,* March 1978, pp. 136–142; Jim Wright, p. 31.

variety of ready-to-eat convenience foods—everything from salad dressings to corned beef hash.

Though sugar provides fuel to be burned for energy when needed—as do starches, proteins, and fats—nutrition experts find no evidence justifying sugar industry claims that sugar somehow gives "extra" energy. Sugar may provide an energy spurt by elevating blood-sugar levels more quickly than other calorie sources; but the levels then drop more quickly, leaving the individual hungry and tired. While protein raises blood-sugar levels more slowly, it keeps them up for a longer period.

Is sugar "good food," as the sugar industry claims? Or is it the cause of many of humankind's ills, as some scientists assert? Says Jean Mayer: "I can find nothing good, nutritionally, to say about sugar. The calories are present, but the nutrients are not. And the difference between a good and bad diet is how much of the nutrients you get with the calories" (*d*, p. 196). A diet high in the empty calories of sugar will inevitably either be deficient in necessary nutrients or contain an excess of calories, or both.[3]

Some scientists have suggested that the dangers of sugar go beyond empty calories. Dr. John Yudkin, British physician, biochemist, and professor of nutrition, points to evidence that associates sugar with:

1 *An increase in dental decay* This is well accepted (see page 133).
2 *An increase in heart disease, hardening of the arteries, and increases of certain fats in the blood* This theory is not yet substantiated.
3 *Diabetes* Heavy sugar intake may be responsible for fouling up the metabolic system, causing a breakdown in insulin production, particularly in adults with a family history of the disease.[4]
4 *Hypoglycemia* Heavy intake may cause *low* blood sugar, though proof is lacking.
5 *Acceleration of the lifespan* There is an unproved theory that sugar may be responsible for earlier maturation in affluent countries, and by accelerating the life cycle may in the end shorten it.

Other researchers have suggested links between sugar and high blood pressure, gout, digestive problems, susceptibility to infection, nearsightedness, mental disturbances, skin disorders, cancer, and hyperactivity in children. Much more research is needed before the role of sugar in these ailments can be proved or disproved.

In the meantime, since many nutritionists agree that we do not need sugar in our diets, cutting down on refined sweets may be wise (Briggs). Many authorities suggest that the best way to break the "sweet tooth" habit—the more we eat, the more we want—is to stop it before it begins, in childhood, by eliminating added sugar in infant formulas, baby foods, and treats.

Fats

Like carbohydrates, fats are primarily an energy source, though some fats contain significant quantities of vitamins and/or provide essential fatty acids. Fats also make food tastier, delay the emptying of the stomach (giving a stick-to-the-ribs feeling), make up part of the structure of the cells, cushion vital organs with fat pads, and allow the use of protein for body building.

Dietary fats are generally classified as: (1) *Saturated*, those saturated with hydrogen.

[3]Brown sugar, raw sugar, and honey have only a trace of vitamins and minerals and are barely more nutritious than "white" sugar.

[4]An Israeli study at Hadassah Hospital found that immigrant Yemenite Jews arrived in Israel without any signs of diabetes. After 20 years on the high-sugar Israeli diet, the rate of diabetes among their descendants had risen to the 3 to 5 percent common in Israel (Ahron Cohen).

They are chemically inactive, and are used by the body as sources of energy, and as carriers of fat-soluble vitamins. They include chicken fat, lard, butter, hardened (hydrogenated) vegetable fats, and coconut oil. (2) *Polyunsaturated*, chemically active and important in many body processes. They supply essential fatty acids which are as necessary as vitamins and minerals. They include many liquid vegetable oils, such as corn, soybean, and safflower oils. (3) *Monounsaturated*, containing some hydrogen and thus only partially saturated. They include peanut and olive oils.

Cholesterol, more like a wax in consistency than ordinary fat, is manufactured by the body in needed amounts. When cholesterol is taken in the diet, manufacture slows down—but not enough to compensate for the added intake. Thus large dietary intakes may lead to increased levels in the blood, a condition linked to the development of cardiovascular (heart and blood vessel) diseases and possibly to some cancers. Many nutritionists and physicians recommend a *prudent diet*, one that is low in cholesterol and in saturated fats. (See Chapter 10.)

Dietary Fiber

In 1932, a well-known physician wrote that the "fad for . . . rabbit food" was responsible for much of the indigestion prevalent and was "worth $300 a month to any good stomach specialist."

Today, most nutrition experts have a somewhat different view. "Rabbit food"—known scientifically as dietary fiber—is the material that surrounds the cell walls of plants, providing both support and protection. In the form of bran, it has long been promoted by cereal manufacturers as a natural laxative. Indeed, increased fiber in diet often does relieve constipation.

It may do more. Recent large-scale studies have shown that primitive peoples with very high intakes of dietary fiber have very little heart disease and colon cancer. When they move to "civilized" areas where low-fiber foods such as meats, dairy products, and refined carbohydrates (white bread, smooth cereals, sugar) are mainstays, they fall victim to these diseases (Burkitt).

Preliminary evidence has also shown dietary fiber to be related to other digestive tract diseases (diverticulosis, gallbladder disease, appendicitis), other heart and blood vessel conditions (atherosclerosis, hemorrhoids), and metabolic disorders such as obesity and diabetes. Studies are underway to substantiate these reports. In the meantime, anyone wishing to switch to a high-fiber diet should do so gradually to avoid intestinal irritation. Table 5.3 shows the true fiber content, as determined by new analytic methods, compared with the old crude fiber content, of some common foods.

Water

Water ranks second only to oxygen on the list of things essential to life. About one-half to three-quarters of the human body is made up of water. A person can live for days or even weeks without food, but only a few days without water. Water assists in forming the building blocks for cells, and is a part of most of them; it is the environment in which cells live; it is the main constituent of body fluids, secretions, excretions; it carries nutrients and waste materials; it is involved in digestion and regulation of body temperature through perspiration and respiration.

Only a small part of the water necessary for these many functions is obtained directly from the kitchen faucet. Most of it comes from other beverages (coffee, tea, juice, milk, soft drinks) and from soups, fruits, and vegetables. A small amount is produced by the body as the end product of the burning of food for energy.

We require additional quantities of water in hot weather when perspiration is profuse, in dry weather when mucous membranes lose more water, when we are on high-protein

TABLE 5.3 True fiber content of some foods

FOOD ITEM	TRUE FIBER*	CRUDE FIBER*
BREADS		
White	2.72	0.2
Whole wheat	8.50	1.6
BREAKFAST CEREALS		
All-bran	26.7	7.8
Cornflakes	11.0	0.7
Grape Nuts	7.0	N.A.†
Rice Krispies	4.47	N.A.†
Puffed Wheat	15.41	2.0
Sugar Puffs	6.08	0.9
Shredded Wheat	12.26	2.3
Special K	5.45	N.A.†
VEGETABLES		
Broccoli tops, boiled	4.10	1.5
Brussel sprouts, boiled	2.86	1.6
Cabbage, boiled	2.83	0.5
Cauliflower, boiled	1.80	1.0
Lettuce, raw	1.53	0.6
Onions, raw	2.10	0.6
Carrots, boiled	3.70	1.0
Turnips, raw	2.20	0.9
Baked beans, canned	7.27	N.A.†
Peas, canned	6.28	2.3
Potatoes, french fried	3.20	1.0
Tomatoes, fresh	1.40	0.5
Tomatoes, canned	0.85	0.4
Sweet corn, cooked	4.74	0.7
FRUITS		
Apples, without skin	1.42	0.6
Apples, with skin	N.A.†	1.0
Bananas	1.75	0.5
Grapefruit, canned	0.44	0.2
Peaches, with skin	2.28	0.6
Plums, with skin	1.52	0.4
Strawberries, raw	2.12	1.3
NUTS		
Brazil	7.73	3.1
Peanuts	9.30	1.9
Peanut butter	7.55	1.9

*Number of grams of fiber per 100 grams of edible food.
†Not available.
Sources: United States Department of Agriculture; and David Southgate, researcher, Medical Research Council, Cambridge, England.

diets, during breast feeding, and during periods of strenuous physical activity. Water deprivation during physical exertion can lead to serious acute illness, permanent health damage, or even death from heat exhaustion. An educational program informing athletes and their coaches that water lost through sweating must be replaced at regular intervals is credited with considerably reducing the death rate from heat stroke on athletic fields.

Vitamins

Even ancient peoples recognized the relationships between some foods and health. But it was not until this century that the minute substances in food that kept us healthy were clearly identified and grouped. In 1912, Casimir Funk named these substances "vitamines" (*vita* = life + *amine* = class of chemical compound to which it was believed vitamins belonged). Today, it is known that vitamins are not all amines, but are chemically diverse. They are usually arbitrarily classified into two groups: (1) *fat-soluble vitamins* (those found most often in food fats), which include vitamins A, D, E, and K, and (2) *water-soluble vitamins*, which include all the others.

Vitamins play a dynamic, constantly active role as catalysts in body processes such as the release of energy from foods, growth of body tissues, and proper functioning of nerves and muscles. The quantities of vitamins needed to accomplish this vital work are miniscule. Indeed, an entire day's supply can be packed into a small capsule, but a well-chosen assortment of foods is a better and tastier way to meet these needs. (See Table 5.4.)

A variety of preliminary studies suggest that individual vitamins—particularly C and

National aspirations affect the nutritional standards set in each nation. A report of the Ministry of Health and Welfare on Nutrition in Japan, for example, said that the aim in Japan is "to become one of the healthy, able-bodied and able-minded peoples of the world and in a well-grown size, too . . . we are not satisfied to be in the present physiques, which are, compared to many other nations, rather dwarfish." (*Nutrition in Japan, 1960*)

E—may be of value in treating or preventing a number of disorders not caused by deficiency of the vitamin in question. The best known of these claims is the assertion that vitamin C can prevent, cure, or at least minimize a cold. This assertion is discussed on page 210.

It is not likely that further study will show that vitamins can work all manner of miracles. What is likely is that some off these "miracles" will prove to be—as did the citrus cure for scurvy—good sound science. Others will be discarded as faddist fantasies.

Meanwhile, it is wise to be wary of heavy self-dosing of vitamins. Massive doses of some vitamins—particularly A and D over long periods—can cause hypervitaminosis and serious illness. On occasion, illness can occur from even a single massive dose of a vitamin. Arctic explorers, for example, who ate large quantities of polar bear liver rich in vitamin A became very ill.

Minerals

More than 60 inorganic (nonliving) elements have been found to be components of living organisms. Many of these are essential in human nutrition. Calcium, phosphorus, magnesium, potassium, sodium, and chloride—the major or macro minerals—are needed by the body in amounts of 100 milligrams or more. Trace elements, such as iron, iodine, copper, manganese, fluorine, chromium, and zinc (which appears to be valuable in a wide range of disorders), are needed in small, nearly infinitesimal amounts. It is expected that as study techniques improve, other elements, such as nickel, tin, vanadium, and silicon, will be found to play vital roles in the physiological processes.

Mixed diets of well-chosen foods that include the recommended amounts of animal protein usually contain most of the known needed minerals and trace elements in sufficient quantity for good health. Fluorine (present in some water systems, absent in others) and iodine (usually short in regions away from saltwater seas) are exceptions, and diets may need to be supplemented with these. Women in their child-bearing years may also need iron supplements. Overdoses of some minerals, including iron and fluorine, are possible.

Sodium chloride is historically treasured (the word salary comes from the Latin *salarium*, or "salt money" paid to Roman soldiers), tasteful, and innocent-looking. But salt can be as much danger as delight. Of course, the body needs salt, nature's artful blend of sodium and chloride, to keep body fluids in balance. Various authorities recommend a daily intake of from 1 to 5 grams at normal temperatures and work loads, more at high temperatures and work levels. Yet the usual American adult takes in 6 to 10 grams daily (RDA), not only in pretzels and potato chips, but hidden in a wide variety of foods from cakes and cookies to bouillon cubes that are almost half salt.

This high salt intake may be responsible in part for the wide incidence of high blood pressure in the United States (see Chapter 10) and for some kidney problems. It is possible to cut down on salt by limiting the use of ready-to-eat foods, using spices, herbs, and lemon juice in place of salt, increasing fluid intake to flush excess salt from the system, reducing intake of fluid and salt-retaining carbohydrates, and taking the salt shaker off the table.

TABLE 5.4 Vitamins

VITAMIN	REASONS FOR	EFFECTS	SOURCES
		FAT-SOLUBLE VITAMINS*	
A (retinol), 5000 IU†	New cell growth; healthy skin, bones, other tissue; night and color vision	*Too little:* Night blindness; blindness; dry skin susceptible to infection; poor bone, tooth development. *Too much:* Headaches, nausea, irritability; peeling skin, hair loss, bone pain, enlarged liver and spleen; retarded growth in children; menstrual problems; death.	Liver, fortified margarine, eggs, butter, whole milk, fortified skim milk; green and yellow vegetables (as carotene, converted to vitamin A by the body)
D (calciferol), 400 IU†	Absorption and utilization of calcium and phosphorus; protein metabolism	*Too little:* Rickets in children (skeletal deformities); osteomalacia in adults (soft bones). *Too much:* Nausea, weight loss, weakness, frequent urination; hypertension, kidney damage, calcium deposits in soft tissue; death.	Direct exposure of skin to sunlight; fortified milk, fish-liver oils, fatty fish (salmon, tuna), egg yolk
E (tocopherols), 30 IU†	Prevention of oxygen from destroying such substances as vitamin A (antioxidant)	*Too little:* None known in adults; rare anemia in premature infants. *Too much:* None certain.	Vegetable oils, beans, eggs, whole grains, wheat germ, liver, green leafy vegetables, almonds, margarine
K	Clotting of blood	*Too little:* Bleeding, liver damage. *Too much:* None known in adults; synthetic form causes jaundice in newborns.	Produced in intestines; lettuce, spinach, kale, cabbage, liver, cauliflower, egg yolk
		WATER-SOLUBLE VITAMINS‡	
C (ascorbic acid), 60 mg†	Growth; tissue repair; wound healing; tooth, bone, hemoglobin repair; various metabolic processes	*Too little:* Scurvy (weakness, bleeding, weight loss, anemia, weakened capillary walls). *Too much:* Possibly destruction of B_{12} or increased risk of kidney stones.	Citrus fruits, tomatoes, cantaloupe, strawberries, peppers, green leafy vegetables, fresh potatoes, other melons and berries
B_1 (thiamine), 1.5 mg†	Carbohydrate metabolism; growth; fertility; nerve tissue function	*Too little:* Beri-beri (dysfunction of nervous system); loss of appetite, retarded growth, nausea, heart problems, leg pain, spastic colon. *Too much:* None known.	Whole grain flours and cereals, peas, nuts, seeds, soybeans, pork, organ meats, enriched flours and cereals

*Stored in the body; we are not dependent on daily supply. Toxicity can build up.
†RDA for adults and children over 4 years of age.
‡Not stored in body; supply needed daily. Large doses may act as drugs.
Sources: Jean Mayer, *d,* pp. 260 ff; "A Primer on Vitamins," U.S. Department of Health, Education, and Welfare.

VITAMIN	REASONS FOR	EFFECTS	SOURCES
B_2 (riboflavin), 0.6 mg†	Metabolism of carbohydrates, protein, fat	*Too little:* Lip sores and cracks; sore mouth; itching, burning eyes; sensitivity to light. *Too much:* None known.	Leafy vegetables, whole-grain and enriched flours and cereals, liver, cheese, lean meat, eggs, milk, beans and peas
Niacin (B_5, PP), 20 mg†	Healthy tissue cells	*Too little:* Pellagra (rough skin, mouth sores, diarrhea, mental disorders). *Too much:* Flushing of skin; sometimes jaundice.	Liver, lean meat, peas, beans, whole grains, fish, poultry, nuts, seeds, wheat germ
Pantothenic acid 10 mg†	Growth, metabolism; many body processes	*Too little:* Headache, fatigue, nausea, cramps, poor coordination, personality changes, tingling hands and feet. *Too much:* None known.	Liver, eggs, white potatoes, sweet potatoes, peas, wheat germ, bran; widely found except in highly processed foods
Folic acid (folacin), 0.4 mg†	Cell health; metabolism; production of red blood cells	*Too little:* Type of anemia; intestinal distress; smooth, red tongue. *Too much:* None known.	Liver, green leafy vegetables, fresh oranges, nuts, navy beans, whole wheat products
B_6 (pyridoxine), 2 mg†	Growth; maintenance of body functions; protein metabolism	*Too little:* Irritation around eyes, mouth; sore mouth, smooth red tongue; weight loss; dizziness and other nervous disturbances; nausea. *Too much:* None known.	Liver, whole grains, potatoes, red meat, green vegetables, yellow corn, wheat germ, bran, fish, seeds, beans
B_{12} (cyanocobalamin), 6 mcg†	Cell function; development of red blood cells; nervous system; intestines	*Too little:* Pernicious anemia; degeneration of spinal cord; sore tongue, weakness, weight loss; back pain, mental and nervous changes. *Too much:* None known.	Primarily animal foods: liver, meats, poultry, fish, eggs, dairy products
Biotin, 0.3 mg†	Metabolism of carbohydrates, fat, protein	*Too little:* (Occurs only when too many raw egg whites eaten over long period.) Skin problems, nausea, anemia, depression, insomnia, muscle pain. *Too much:* None known.	Widely found, especially in egg yolk, meat, milk, nuts, mushrooms

DIET PLANNING: GETTING IT ALL TOGETHER

By now, you may have concluded that you need a slide rule, a pocket calculator, a scale, and 90 minutes a day to plan a proper diet. You don't. Recommended dietary allowances are not meant to be used that way. They are a useful guide for those planning production and distribution of foodstuffs, mass feeding, or food rationing programs, or as a base for nutrition therapy. But individuals should view them only as a spot along the spectrum between deficiency and overdose, calculated to be about the right amount for the "reference" (or average) man, woman, or child.

TABLE 5.5 Minerals essential to good health

MINERAL	REASONS FOR NEED	PART OF*	EFFECTS	SOURCES
		MACROMINERALS†		
Calcium, 800 mg‡	Strong bones and teeth; muscle contractions; normal heart rhythm; blood clotting; transmission of nerve impulses; enzyme activity	Bones and teeth	*Too little:* Rickets (stunted growth, skeletal malformation) in children; loss of minerals, softening bones, in adults. *Too much:* May be related to calcium deposits in soft tissue.	Milk and hard cheeses, green leafy vegetables, canned sardines, salmon with bones, soft cheeses, dried beans and peas, shellfish
Phosphorus, 800 mg‡	Strong bones and teeth; enzyme activity; metabolism	Bones and teeth	*Too little:* (Rare with normal diet.) Weakness, bone pain, loss of minerals from bones, poor growth. *Too much:* Imbalance with calcium.	Organ meats, meat, fish, poultry, eggs; also dairy products, nuts, beans, and peas
Magnesium: 300 mg (females),‡ 350 mg (males)	Metabolism; enzyme activity; body temperature regulation; nerve and muscle contraction; protein synthesis	Soft tissue; bones	*Too little:* (Rare except in alcoholics or those on diet limited to a few highly processed foods) weakness, tremors, delirium and depression, and other nervous disorders. *Too much:* None known.	Whole grains, nuts, beans, spinach. (Processing may destroy much magnesium.)
Sodium (Need varies with work, weather, health, etc.)	Regulation of water balance; muscle contractions; nerve irritability	Fluid outside cells	*Too little:* (Rare) nausea, diarrhea, abdominal and muscle cramps. *Too much:* Probably related to high blood pressure.	Salt, salted foods, MSG, soy sauce, baking powder, cheese, milk, shellfish, fish, meat, poultry, eggs, most prepared foods
Potassium, 2.5 gm‡	Water balance; muscle contractions; nerve functioning; heart rhythm; protein synthesis; glucose formation	Fluid inside cells	*Too little:* Muscle weakness, nausea, rapid heart beat, heart failure, loss of glycogen. *Too much:* None known.	Dried fruit, cantaloupe, bananas, oranges, tomatoes, raw vegetables, soybeans, some fish, meats, poultry.
Chloride (Need varies with work, weather, health, etc.)	Water balance; formation of gastric juices; digestive processes	Fluid outside cells	*Too little:* Vomiting, diarrhea. *Too much:* None known.	Salt (sodium chloride) (Alternate source may be needed when salt intake is limited.)

*Much is yet unknown about function of minerals in humans; many work together, are interrelated. These elements are important constitutents of cells, body fluids, and enzymes.
†Needed in amounts of 100 mg or more per day.
‡Daily RDA for typical adult between 19 and 22 years old.
§Needed in small, sometimes almost infinitesimal, amounts.
¶Not enough is known about these elements for an RDA to be set.
Sources: Burton, pp. 127 ff.; Mayer, *b,* pp. 265 ff.; RDA, pp. 82 ff.

MINERAL	REASONS FOR NEED	PART OF*	EFFECTS	SOURCES
		TRACE MINERALS§		
Iron: 18 mg (females),‡ 10 mg (males)‡	Transfer and transport of oxygen	Hemoglobin in blood; myoglobin in muscle, cell protoplasm, and nuclei; many enzymes	*Too little:* Anemia; cell damage. *Too much:* Gray skin color; heart, liver damage; diabetes	Liver, eggs, lean meats, dried fruits, dried beans and peas, whole grains, green leafy vegetables
Iodine: 100 μg (females),‡ 140 μg (males)‡	Thyroid function	Thyroid hormone	*Too little:* Cretinism in infants born of mothers deprived of iodine; goiter. *Too much:* Over long periods, may depress thyroid activity.	Iodized salt; seafood; vegetables grown near sea in iodine-rich soil; dairy products and eggs of animals with rich iodine ration
Copper, 2 mg‡	Formation of red blood cells, nerve walls, and connective tissue; glucose metabolism	Brain, liver, heart, kidneys	*Too little:* None known in adults; anemia in some infants fed *only* cows milk. *Too much:* Rare.	Organ meats, some shellfish, nuts, dried beans and peas, mushrooms, cocoa
Manganese¶	Synthesis of carbohydrates, fats, cholesterol; use of glucose and fats; muscle contractions; bone and pancreas development	Many enzymes	*Too little:* None known in humans. *Too much:* None known.	Most foods, plant and animal, especially whole grains, beans and peas, and nuts
Zinc, 15 mg‡	Digestion, protein metabolism, synthesis of nucleic acids	Insulin and enzymes	*Too little:* (Rare in U.S.) retarded growth and sexual development; anemia, poor wound healing. *Too much:* Nausea, vomiting, diarrhea, fever.	Wheat germ, bran, yeast, whole grains, peas, nuts, lean meats, fish, poultry
Fluorine¶	Decay-resistant teeth; possibly strong bones	Teeth	*Too little:* Tooth decay in children; possibly osteoporosis in adults. *Too much:* Mottled, deformed teeth.	Water, naturally or artificially fluoridated; some foods prepared with fluoridated water
Chromium¶	Metabolism; synthesis of fatty acids and cholesterol; improves insulin efficiency	Skin, fat, adrenals, brain, muscle	*Too little;* Possibly impaired insulin metabolism leading to poor utilization of glucose. *Too much:* None known.	Whole grains, brewer's yeast, meats, corn oil

SELF-CARE

Eating for Good Health

1 Individualize your diet. Consider your size and the level of your physical activity in figuring caloric and other nutritional needs (see Table 5.1) as well as any special diets prescribed by your physician—diabetic, high-protein, low-fat, or whatever.

2 Eat a varied diet—the key to good nutrition. No one perfect food or combination of foods contains all the essential nutrients. Steady meat-and-potatoes or cottage-cheese-and-fruit diets may be deficient in several nutrients. The same is true of diets that rely heavily upon convenience and artificial foods, often enriched with major vitamins and minerals but lacking the trace elements vital to life. Variety also protects us from heávy doses of potential hazards—such as nitrates from bacon every morning and hot dogs every noon.

3 Reduce your intake of the empty calories of sugar in soft drinks, candy, cake, and so on, and of the nearly empty calories in a variety of deceptive nonfoods such as "fruit" drinks, nondairy creamers, and "milk" chocolate. Reduce, too, your intake of processed foods, which are often lower in nutrients and higher in additives than fresh foods.

4 Include in your daily diet the basic foods shown in Table 5.6.

5 If you cook for yourself or others, learn which cooking and storing methods preserve nutritive value best. For example, vegetables retain most of their nutritive value when cooked by the waterless method or in a pressure cooker, or when steamed or stir-fried.

6 If you eat on the run a lot or miss meals, or if you find that the dining hall serves one of the same two or three soggy overcooked vegetables every night, or if you are counting calories, you might consider taking a multiple vitamin and mineral capsule containing the RDAs, and extra iron if you are female. However, it's a mistake to believe that a capsule can be a permanent substitute for good diet. Capsules are intended to supplement good nutrition, not replace it.

Your needs, though somewhere along the same spectrum, will vary according to size, genetic makeup, environment, diet patterns, severity and nature of stress, age, sex, rate of growth, and personal and group aspirations.

The best way to assure a well-balanced diet is to eat a wide variety of foods and to keep in mind the tips in the self-care sidebar shown above.

Tight-Budget Diet

Though food costs have soared, wise decision making makes it possible to combine nutrition and tasty meals at low cost. In most cases, this means avoiding ready-prepared foods, buying foods in season, planning meals around specials or sale items, and selecting foods that have the best cost-nutrient ratio.

One of the best ways of combining low cost with high nutrition is to use vegetable proteins, which are incomplete in themselves, at the same meal with small amounts of animal protein. For example: baked beans with bits of pork; macaroni and cheese; tuna and noodles; lasagna or eggplant parmigiana; chili con carne; Hoppin' John (black-eyed peas, rice, and ham hocks); frijoles refritos (dried kidney or pinto beans cooked and mashed with bits of meat added); cottage cheese and noodles; lentil soup and frankfurters.

Athletic Diets

Over the centuries, a variety of special super-

TABLE 5.6 Daily diet plan

At each meal or at least three times a day:

- A serving of protein food—meat, fish, poultry, cheese, eggs, dried beans, peas, lentils, peanut butter, or combinations such as whole grain cereal and milk.* Alternate beef and pork with fish and poultry Adult males should limit egg intake to three per week.
- One or more servings of a grain food (whole grain preferred, but unbleached and/or enriched also acceptable)—cereal, bread, macaroni, rice (four or five servings per day).
- One or more fruits or vegetables (four per day). One each day should be a dark green or deep yellow vegetable; one or two should be raw. Fresh in season; frozen (retains more nutrients) or canned out of season.
- One or more cups of a beverage—milk, juice, water, tea, coffee (4 to 8 cups per day).

At two meals:

- A milk food—cheese, milk (preferably skim), yogurt.† Occasionally, ice cream. (Butter, cream, and cream cheese do not count as milk foods.)

Some time during the day:

- A citrus fruit or juice, or tomato juice or other food high in vitamin C. (Cooking damages vitamin C content.)
- An unsaturated oil, possibly in salad dressing.
- Iodized salt (unless it worsens acne); but use salt sparingly.
- Butter or margarine as desired and within energy requirement.
- Food high in fiber.

*Minimum serving: 2 ounces meat or fish or equivalent; 3 ounces during pregnancy.
†The equivalent of 4 cups milk per day during pregnancy, two cups for other adults.

diets, featuring everything from royal jelly and honey to huge quantities of meat, sugar, or fat, have been devised for athletes. But current scientific knowledge indicates that the best diet for the physically active is a normal one as recommended in Table 5.6 (Mayer, *b*; Nelson). Calories may need to be increased to meet extra energy needs, but proportions of protein, fat, and carbohydrates should remain about the same: 15, 30 to 35, and 50 to 55 percent, respectively.

Athletes should keep in mind: (1) Increased food intake of any kind will *not* build muscle mass—only exercise can do that. (2) Carbohydrate loading (eating a low-carbohydrate diet when exercising strenously and a high-carbohydrate diet when exercising lightly) may increase endurance, but can be hazardous. (3) Starvation or semistarvation in order to make a particular weight is not only dangerous, but lowers performance. (4) Quick-weight-gain programs, likewise, can be perilous. (5) There is no evidence that vitamin, mineral, or protein supplementation improves performance, and excessive doses may, in some cases, be toxic. There is, however, some indication of an increased need for B vitamins in very active persons. This can be met by ensuring that the extra calories consumed come from highly nutritious foods (Mayer, *b*).

Vegetarian Diet

Millions of people throughout the world have long subsisted on vegetarian diets, out of necessity. Recently, many Americans have adopted such diets, out of choice. Their reasons may be religious, humanitarian, financial, or even the belief that a vegetarian lifestyle leads to less aggressiveness. (The fact that Hitler was a vegetarian tends to undermine this last reason.) Perhaps the most popular justification is political-ecological: the belief that it is wrong to devour an 8-ounce steak that has taken 4 pounds of grain to produce, when that grain could sustain a starving child for nearly a week.

Vegetarians, all of whom exclude meat in their diets, fall into several groups: *strict vegetarians*, who do not eat any foods of animal origin, not even eggs and dairy products; *ovolactovegetarians*, who include eggs and dairy foods in their diets; and *lactovegetarians*, who use dairy products. In addition, people who avoid red meats but will eat fish and poultry are sometimes classified as vegetarians.

Adequate protein can be assured even in a strict vegetarian diet by combining vegetable proteins so as to provide a complete selection of the essential amino acids. The recommended guide to complete protein is to combine legumes (such as beans, peas, or peanuts) with cereals (such as rice, barley, wheat) at each meal—though not necessarily in the same dish. It is difficult, however, for young children to receive adequate protein without milk in their diets.

Studies have shown that the health of vegetarians is, in general, normal. Strict vegetarians are likely to suffer from deficiencies in vitamin B_{12}, calcium, vitamin D, and possibly riboflavin and iodine, but vitamin supplements can fill those gaps (Raper and Hill). Vegetarians appear to have some advantages over meat eaters: they are less likely to be overweight, and they eat a diet high in bulk and low in cholesterol—which should be beneficial in the long run.

A sample vegetarian diet might include:

- *Breakfast* An orange, bulgur wheat with brewers yeast, toasted wheat-soy bread spread with honey
- *Mid-morning snack* Shelled almonds
- *Lunch* Split pea soup, a peanut butter sandwich on whole wheat bread with honey, a salad of fruits and sunflower seeds on lettuce
- *Afternoon snack* Fruit
- *Dinner* Soybeans, brown rice fried with chestnuts and sesame seeds, a green vegetable, and a fruit
- *Evening snack* Raisins

Fad Diets

Dr. Jean Mayer (*b*) suggests three ways in which fad diets are dangerous: (1) *Nutritionally*: Most are based on an imbalance of nutrients (often just one or two "near magic" foods). (2) *Financially*: The costs of specially promoted diet foods are often much higher than the cost of a normal diet. (3) *Intellectually*: Such diets weaken confidence in "organized" medicine and "official" nutrition, leading patients to turn to faddism or quackery instead of seeking needed medical advice.

Zen macrobiotic diets are among the most dangerous. The AMA Council on Foods and Nutrition has condemned the most extreme of these diets (level 7) as a threat to human health. Composed almost entirely of cereals, it can lead to scurvy, anemia, protein and calcium deficiencies, emaciation and general malnutrition, and death from loss of kidney function due to restricted fluid intake.

The Food Consumer

- Government inspectors examining cans of "organic vegetables" find they are ordinary commercial brands with the original labels replaced and considerably higher prices added.
- The sugar industry, disturbed by poor public relations, finances an advertising campaign that says sugar not only tastes good, but is good for you. The campaign is later discontinued at government insistence.
- Vitamin C tablets labeled "100 percent natural" are discovered to contain synthetic vitamin C.
- A synthetic orange drink is claimed to be "more like fresh" than frozen, though it contains water and sugar, while the frozen product is pure juice.

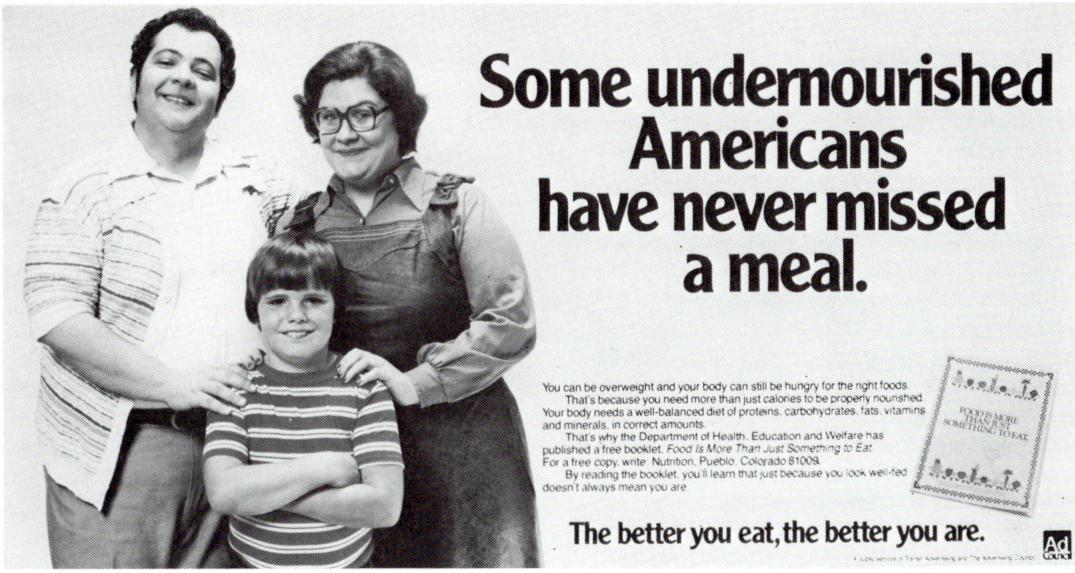

The Advertising Council

Although we usually associate poor nutrition with underdeveloped countries, it is an American problem.

Whether the purveyor is a small health food store owner or a multi-million-dollar food processor, the goal of those in the food industry is to make a profit, not to make consumers healthier. Nor is their advertising meant to educate. Its only aim is to sell products (Hovel). Thus health-conscious consumers must be wary. They must look beyond the come-ons and the razzle-dazzle rhetoric, and carefully evaluate for themselves the quality of the foods they buy.

New labeling laws, requiring foods making nutritional claims to list approximate nutritive content will be of great help to consumers. So can knowing how to interpret lists of ingredients. Although the quantity of ingredients (how much chicken in chicken chop suey?) is still not required on the label, the ingredients are listed in order of quantity. (See Figure 5.1.) When real foods are listed low in order, and chemicals or substances empty of nutritive value (water, sugar, salt) high, the foods are likely to be lacking in trace elements and other nutrients, even if some major vitamins and minerals are added.

MALNUTRITION

For many reasons—including lack of money, education, interest—many people do not succeed at putting together nutritious meals. Although malnutrition is something we usually think of in connection with underdeveloped countries, it is an American problem as well.

The Gould Medical Dictionary describes malnutrition (*mal* = bad) as "defective nutrition." There are two basic types: *undernutrition*, in which an individual lacks one or more nutrients to the extent that specific symptoms or conditions appear; and *overnutrition*, in which an excessive intake of certain nutrients leads to obesity and a variety of illnesses.

Undernutrition

The most severe forms of malnutrition—dramatically evident in starving children with matchstick legs, swollen bellies, and pleading eyes—results from a prolonged and extensive shortage of protein and/or calories due to lengthy or lifetime starvation. Persons suffer-

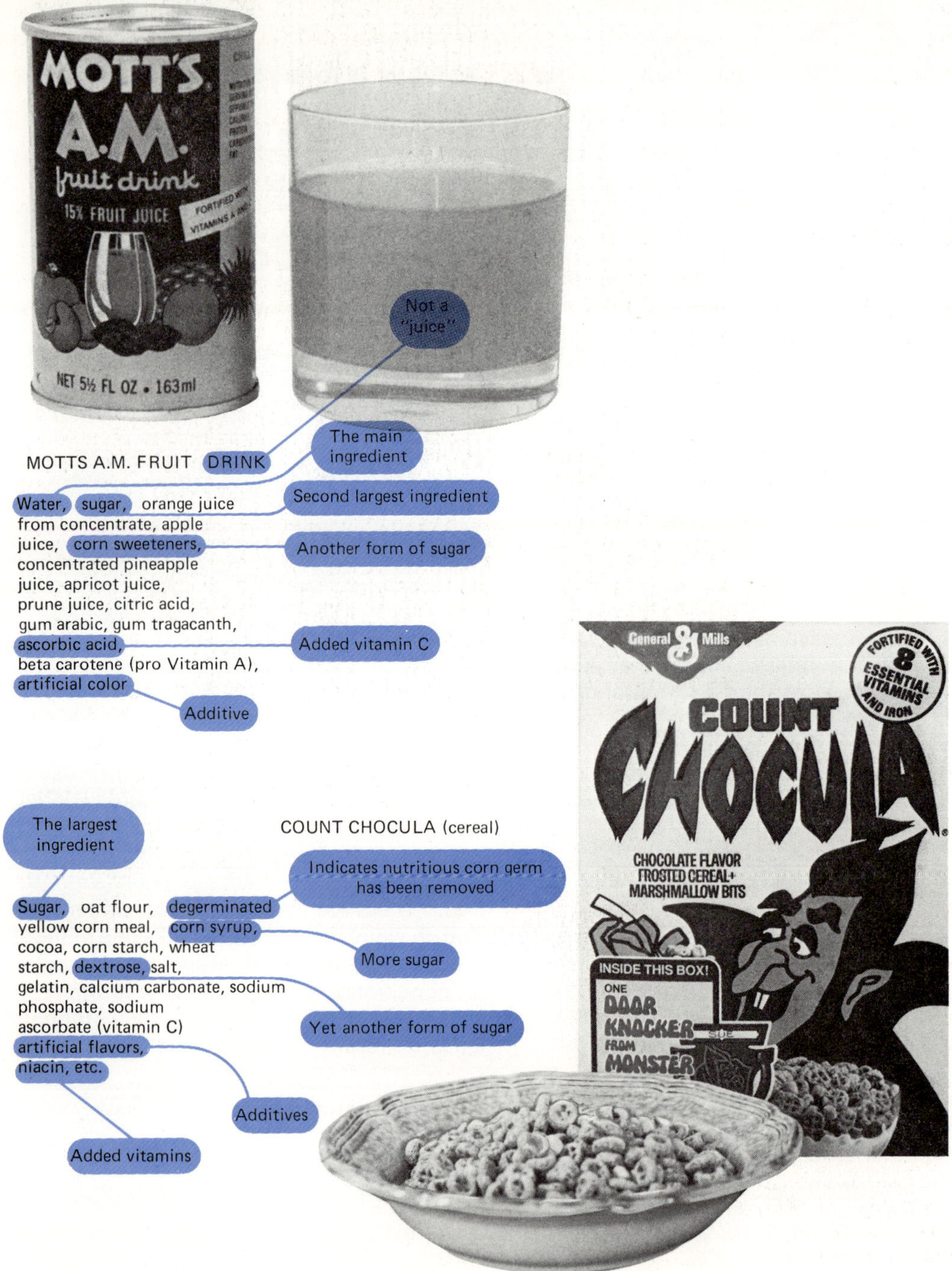

FIGURE 5.1 What food labels tell you.

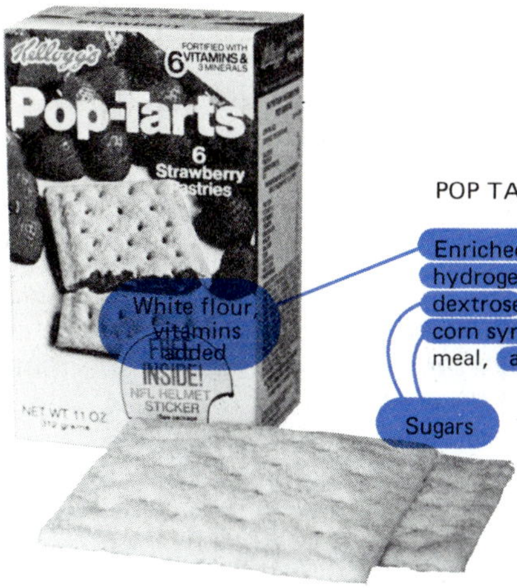

POP TARTS

Enriched wheat flour, partially hydrogenated vegetable oil, dextrose, strawberry preserves, corn syrup, sugar, whey, cracker-meal, apple preserves

White flour, vitamins added

Better for "prudent diet" than hydrogenated shortenings or animal fats, not as good as liquid vegetable oils

Sugars

Contain additional sugar

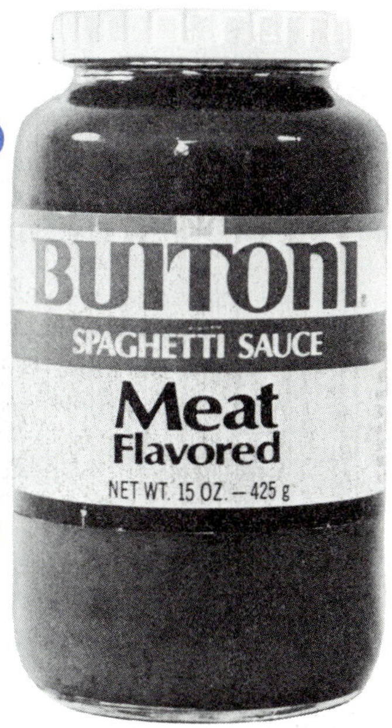

Contains less meat than "meat sauce"

BUITONI MEAT-FLAVORED SAUCE

An empty filler

Tomatoes, onions, vegetable oil, modified food starch, salt, beef, textured vegetable protein, carrots, sugar, celery, spices, natural coloring, natural etc.

Good for "prudent diet"

More salt than beef

Hidden sugar

Not meat, but a nutritious form of protein

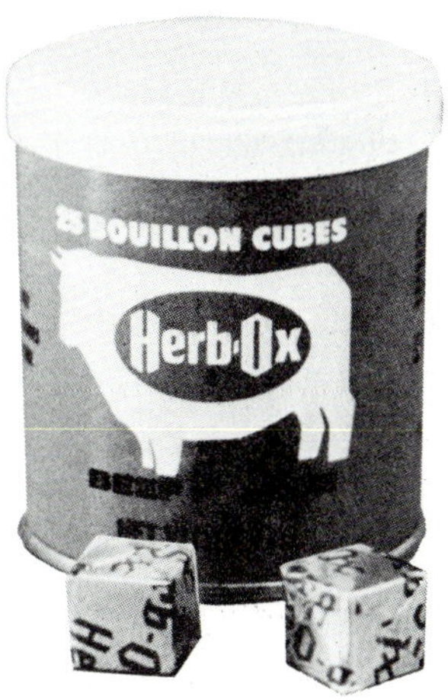

BEEF-FLAVOR BROTH (bouillon cubes)

Salt, monosodium glutamate, onions, potato starch, sugar, vegetable fat, caramel, beef fat, spices

Many bouillon cubes are more than half salt/sodium. Avoid on low-salt diet

Again, unexpected sugar

Diet for a Hungry World

Many experts suggest that reductions in the consumption in the United States of beef and grain alcohol (scotch, rye, etc.) would free grain for millions who are hungry. A 10 percent decrease in beef intake in the United States, it is estimated, could feed 60 million grain eaters for a year. A reduction in the number of pets kept and fed by Americans could also free millions of tons of usable grain.

ing from protein-calorie malnutrition (PCM) usually are deficient in all, or almost all, nutrients. If starvation continues long enough, death results. The symptoms of PCM are obvious, but the kinds of undernutrition more common In the United States often go unnoticed. They can, nevertheless, be devastating.

Inadequate nutrition is found in every group in the population, but is most prevalent among the poor, adolescents, women during their childbearing years, the elderly, Indians and Eskimos, and people with chronic or acute illness or conditions (such as alcoholism or drug abuse) that make extra demands on the body or interfere with the body's use of nutrients.

The effects of malnutrition vary depending upon the stage of life and the nutrients lacking (Read). A child malnourished prenatally (*pre* = before + *natal* = birth) may be born with one or more birth defects, or may even be stillborn. If malnutrition is great during the first two years of life, when brain growth and development are at their peak, there is apt to be mental retardation. Inadequate nutrition in childhood can lead to physical as well as intellectual retardation and possible damage to the body's defenses against disease (Ferguson). During adolescence, it can interfere with or even completely halt the normal growth spurt. In the elderly, malnutrition can lead to excess bone loss and frequent bone fractures, and to early senility. Shortages of specific nutrients can lead to deficiency diseases at any time of life. (See Tables 5.4 and 5.5.)

Without proper nourishment prenatally and in infancy, children of the poor have little chance of absorbing the kinds of education and then getting the kinds of jobs that will enable them to break out of the vicious cycle of poverty. It was recognition of this that led to the federal WIC (women, infants, children) supplemental feeding program, under which pregnant and nursing mothers are given vouchers for specific nutritious foods for themselves and their infants. Supporters of such food programs point out that the programs are economically sound. It has been

Nothing New Under the Sun

In those days again, it was lack of food that drove fainting bodies to death; now contrariwise it is the abundance that overwhelms them.

No modern comment this—written by Lucretius about 2000 years ago

[King Edward IV] by intemperance in his diet, in some sort digged his grave with his own teeth.

Church History, Thomas Fuller (1608–1661)

estimated that $1 in supplemental food can save $6000 or more in later medical costs. Many authorities also believe that food funding can help to reduce later costs of law enforcement, courts, prison systems, and welfare payments.

Overnutrition

A pattern of overfeeding and overeating in the United States apparently begins in infancy and continues throughout life. Overeating, while not as immediately hazardous as undereating, can lead to all the problems of obesity, discussed later in this chapter, and to premature death. It has been aptly pointed out, "The thin rats bury the fat rats." Recent history supports this position. During World War II, the bad news included shortages of meat, sugar, and butter; the good news was a striking reduction in certain diseases, particularly those of the heart.

IS EATING HAZARDOUS TO HEALTH?

It sometimes seems that all our foodstuffs should carry a warning much as cigarette packages do. There is mercury in tuna fish, cholesterol in eggs; botulism can form in a can of improperly processed soup; deadly bacteria multiply in macaroni salad that has not been refrigerated; there can be insecticides on fruit; there is caffeine in coffee and too much salt on potato chips. Considering the poisons that occur naturally in food, that are added to foods, that develop in foods through mishandling, and that are absorbed by foods from pollutants in air, soil, and water, it is easy to wonder: Is there anything safe to eat?

Since most Americans live into their seventies, we can assume that either we are very tough people, or the food we eat is not as hazardous as critics would have us believe. On the other hand, since more and more scientists are becoming convinced that many of our ills are environmentally caused—often by our food—we cannot consider food totally safe either. To add to the confusion, we cannot easily distinguish the safe from the unsafe.

Natural versus Chemical

Some persons have assumed that the way to judge the safety of foods is to categorize them as "natural" and thus safe, or "chemical" and thus automatically hazardous. Let's look at that argument.

Natural foods In spite of the reassuring sound of the word "natural," many completely natural foods present hazards. Butter and eggs have been implicated in heart disease, sugar in tooth decay and more, and spinach, with its high levels of natural nitrates, in infant illness. Even half a strip of licorice a day can cause serious indisposition. Natural milk, salt, and liver in excess can cause illness. A few natural foods are poisonous in any dose—some varieties of mushrooms and raw soybeans, for example. Many natural foods, including wheat, eggs, chocolate, milk, and strawberries, cause allergic reactions in sensitive individuals. Still others, such as cheeses, can cause a toxic reaction in combination with certain drugs. Aflatoxin, produced by a mold that sometimes grows on peanuts, grains, or sweet potatoes, is "natural," but it also causes cancer of the liver, and in fact, is one of the most potent liver cancer-causing substances known. Clearly, "natural" is not synonymous with "safe." Nor does it mean "nutritious": coffee is natural but devoid of food value.

Chemicals Everything we eat has a chemical composition. Phenyl-ethyl-benzyl-hexyl-isioamyl-butyl alcohols mixed with (among other things) caffeine, tannin, geraniol, and essential oils, for example, make up a cup of tea. Acetone, acetaldehyde, methyl butrate,

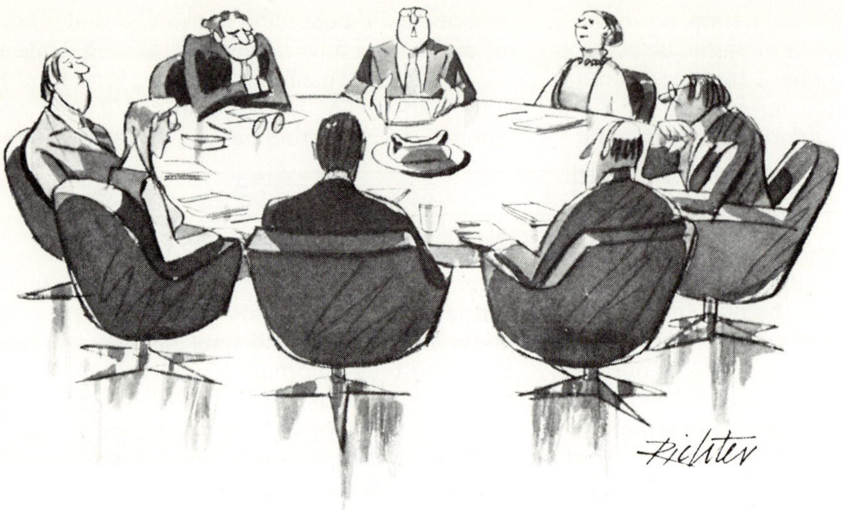

"Granted the public has a right to know what's in a hot dog, but does the public really want to know what's in a hot dog?"

ethyl caproate, hexyl acetate, methanol, acrolein, and crotmaldehyde are in strawberries. Chemicals can be good for humans, as ascorbic acid (vitamin C) is, or bad, as arsenic is. They can be extracted from natural sources (sodium caseinate from milk, lecithin from soybeans) or synthesized in the factory from a wide variety of organic and inorganic materials. Some of these materials, such as coal tars, have long been suspected of being cancer-causing. Others have been used for many years with no apparent ill effects. Some, including nitrites and nitrates, are apparently both helpful and harmful (see page 116). As you can see, it is not easy to put either a safe or an unsafe label on chemicals.

Food additives Additives in commercial food products are used for a variety of reasons: to add vitamins or other nutrients, to improve taste (flavor enhancers), to prevent spoilage (antioxidants), to improve texture (emulsifiers), to control acidity and alkalinity (neutralizers), to color, to sweeten artificially, to keep liquids from clouding, to keep marshmallows moist, to prevent caking, to preserve color, to help in foaming such things as whipped topping. There are also "natural" spices and flavorings added, such as salt, sugar, pepper, and cinnamon, and there are indirect "additives" that originate in wrappings, machinery, and the like. Some additives are more necessary than others. A few manufacturers have successfully eliminated additives from their products entirely.

Additive effects may show up immediately—as when a sensitive person eating food containing monosodium glutamate (MSG) gets a headache or other symptoms characteristic of the "Chinese restaurant syndrome," so named because MSG is heavily used in Chinese cooking. Or they can show up after many years of regular consumption—as may happen with those suspected of causing cancer.

The Role of the FDA

Consumer advocates and some health authorities have criticized the Food and Drug Administration (FDA) for not doing its job of protecting citizens against dangerous foods

Evaluating Additives

Factors considered in evaluating risk versus benefit include:

- Hazard to the consumer
- Consumer needs and wishes
- Requirements of food supply and public health
- Needs of the food producer and processor
- Economic factors
- Availability of methods and mechanisms for regulatory control
- Threat to the adequacy, wholesomeness, or availability of the food supply in the absence of protection afforded by the additive

or food ingredients. Other scientists accuse the FDA of being overprotective, citing the agency's efforts to limit over-the-counter sale of vitamins or its refusal to license reportedly effective European drugs for use here until they undergo United States testing.

How can reputable scientists—at least those not under economic pressures—be at such odds? There are many reasons:

- Additives are only a small number of the some 200,000 new chemicals appearing in the scientific literature each year, an estimated 2000 of which will have an impact on human life. Testing them is difficult, expensive, and sometimes inconclusive or inaccurate.[5]
- Animal tests give scientists only an approximation of the effect a particular substance might have on humans, and yet human testing is often impossible. "Safe" human doses are set at 1/100 the safe dose for test animals.
- Many ill effects of a serious nature develop in only 1 in 100 or 1 in 1000 subjects, and so studies on 30 or 40 animals may not show up a single such effect. But the high cost of testing often prohibits larger studies.

[5]The new Ames test, and similar rapid test procedures, allows screening of new chemicals, and sifting out of those potentially hazardous. The Ames test is done on a special strain of salmonella. If the test chemical causes changes in the hereditary material of the salmonella, it is almost certainly both cancer-causing and birth-defect-causing.

- Many substances used for years with no ill effects have been classified "Generally Recognized as Safe" (GRAS). But concern among consumers about the safety of some of these substances—never subjected to safety testing—prompted a review of the GRAS list.
- Every substance—water, oxygen, vitamins, as well as additives—is toxic at some levels. Thus, scientists cannot say that a particular substance is "safe"—only that "at the concentrations used, it is highly unlikely that this additive does any harm."

There is an exception to the "safe dose" concept. Under the Delaney amendment to the Federal Food, Drug and Cosmetic Act, no food additive is permitted if any dose "is found to induce cancer . . . in man or animal." It was this law that led to the banning of cyclamates and saccharine. Some scientists believe that the law is too limiting, that it does not allow scientific discretion in evaluating cancer-causing effects. Other scientists, however, approve the "zero tolerance" of the law and believe it should, in fact, be expanded to include any substances that at any level cause birth defects.

Because no substance can be declared totally safe, decisions related to food additives are made on the basis of risk versus benefit. For example, the FDA has decided that the addition of enriching nutrients to white bread is important to the general

Some Major Food Controversies

- *Sodium nitrates and sodium nitrites* in bacon, frankfurters, salami, lox, and other smoked foods may be converted into cancer-causing nitrosamines when combined with amines, which are found in many foods, beverages, and drugs. The FDA and industry insist the chemicals must be used to prevent the development of deadly botulism toxins in foods. Consumer advocates suggest that they are not necessary in an age of freezers and refrigerators, and that their main use is to give meat a red color. Permissible levels of nitrates and nitrites have recently been lowered.
- *Red dye No. 2* was used as a red coloring in more than 30 kinds of food products, ranging from ice cream to packaged meats, until 1976, when studies were interpreted by the FDA as indicating that the dye causes cancer in animals. The dye was then banned and replaced in many products by red dye No. 40—about which safety questions were immediately raised, although studies to date have not shown tumor-causing activity.
- *Additives and hyperactivity in children* became an issue when pediatric allergist Benjamin Feingold put forth a theory that hyperactivity and learning disability in children can often be traced to food additives. The theory is as yet unconfirmed.
- *Contaminants in fish* from toxic industrial wastes dumped into waterways have raised questions about the safety of this fish for human consumption. PCBs (polychlorinated biphenyls), for example, have been found in many United States rivers and lakes. This chemical has been found to cause liver cancers and reproductive failures in test animals and a variety of symptoms in workers exposed to it. Environmentalists are urging that use of the chemical be banned or greatly curtailed, and that permissible levels in fish be lowered to protect consumers.
- *Cyclamates and saccharin:* Is either safe? Neither? Both? Cyclamates were banned in 1969 on the basis of a small study that found that at extremely high doses they cause bladder cancer in animals. Further study did not confirm the results. Still, in 1976, after examining a vast amount of evidence, a scientific panel was only 95 percent convinced of cyclamate safety. Because of this nagging doubt, the FDA turned down requests to reinstate use of cyclamates. In 1977, saccharin, long used and believed safe, was banned on the basis of a Canadian study similar to the one that doomed cyclamates. The move brought applause from environmentalists and some scientists who support the theory "better safe than sorry." It raised concern among others in the medical community, however, who feared the ban would lead to a rise in sugar consumption and thus in obesity. They reasoned that the resultant risk of increased deaths from heart and related diseases far outweighed the possible risk of cancer from the use of saccharin. Because of medical and public outcry, the ban was not imposed. Instead this warning label was mandated: "Use of this product may be hazardous to your health. This product contains saccharin which has been determined to cause cancer in laboratory animals."

health, and worth the slight risk to a small number of individuals of overdose of the vitamins and minerals involved. On the other hand, after long study and much public discussion, the idea of adding iron to bread was vetoed even though it would benefit pregnant women and children. The reason for this decision was the potential risk to persons suffering from iron storage disorders—Parkinson's, thalassemia, sickle cell, and others.

Tainted or Dirty Foods

From a public health standpoint, the germs that contaminate our food may be a more

Preventing Food Contamination in the Kitchen

Careless handling of food can cause the microorganisms present in all unsterilized foodstuffs to multiply or can add new germs. To avoid such contamination:

1 Wash hands with soap and water before touching food and after handling raw meat, poultry, or eggs (they harbor germs).
2 Do not handle food if you have an open cut, a cold, or any other infection.
3 Use a fresh, clean spoon for tasting and serving food.
4 Keep hot foods *hot* and cold foods *cold* (see Figure 5.5). Refrigerate foods that will not be served or cooked immediately.
5 If the odor or color of any food is poor or questionable, get rid of it. It may be dangerous. *If in doubt, throw it out.* Discard, too, cans that are swollen or leaking.
6 Defrost meats and poultry in the refrigerator or under running water rather than at room temperature. Cook them completely. Never stuff them until they are ready to go into the oven; and cook stuffing to at least 165°F.
7 Clean all dishes, utensils, and work surfaces thoroughly with soap or detergent and water after each use, giving special attention to dirt-harboring cracks and corners.
8 Refreeze only those foods that are still cold or contain ice crystals and have been held no longer than one or two days in the refrigerator since thawing. *Do not* refreeze ice cream, or any food that is either off color or has a bad odor.

present danger than the pesticides and chemicals in our diet. Food poisoning, according to Dr. Richard L. Doutt, of the University of California's Division of Biological Control, is not just a threat as chemical pesticides are; it is a reality. Estimates run as high as 10 million cases of food poisoning each year in the United States. Most cases, or course, are mild stomach upsets that go unreported and untreated. Some may be cases of often fatal botulism that go unreported because the symptoms resemble those of stroke.

About one-third of all food poisoning cases can be traced to food prepared at home, another third to that prepared in restaurants, and about 5 percent to the food-processing industry. The source cannot be determined in the remaining cases. Commercial food preparation, under increasingly tight supervision and regulation of the FDA, has become safer over the years (Schmidt). But since 1 in every 3 cases of food poisoning originates in the home, a major share of the responsibility for safe food falls on the individual.

OVERWEIGHT AND UNDERWEIGHT

"I look at you, Mr. Shaw," said Alfred Hitchcock to the celebrated playwright, "and I know there is a famine in the land."

"I look at you, Mr. Hitchcock," replied George Bernard Shaw to the famous film producer-director, "and I know who caused it."

Fat people and skinny people look at the world through opposite ends of the telescope. Hunger—and outright starvation—are responsible for the underweight of tens of millions around the world, but in the United States, overweight is the more common problem. Ironically, this is just as true among the poor, whose dinner plates are padded with inexpensive carbohydrates, as among the affluent with their diets rich in meats, sweets, and sauces. For most of this section, we will be peering at people on Mr. Hitchcock's end of the telescope—through we will not entirely neglect those who, like Shaw, "can't seem to gain an ounce no matter what I do."

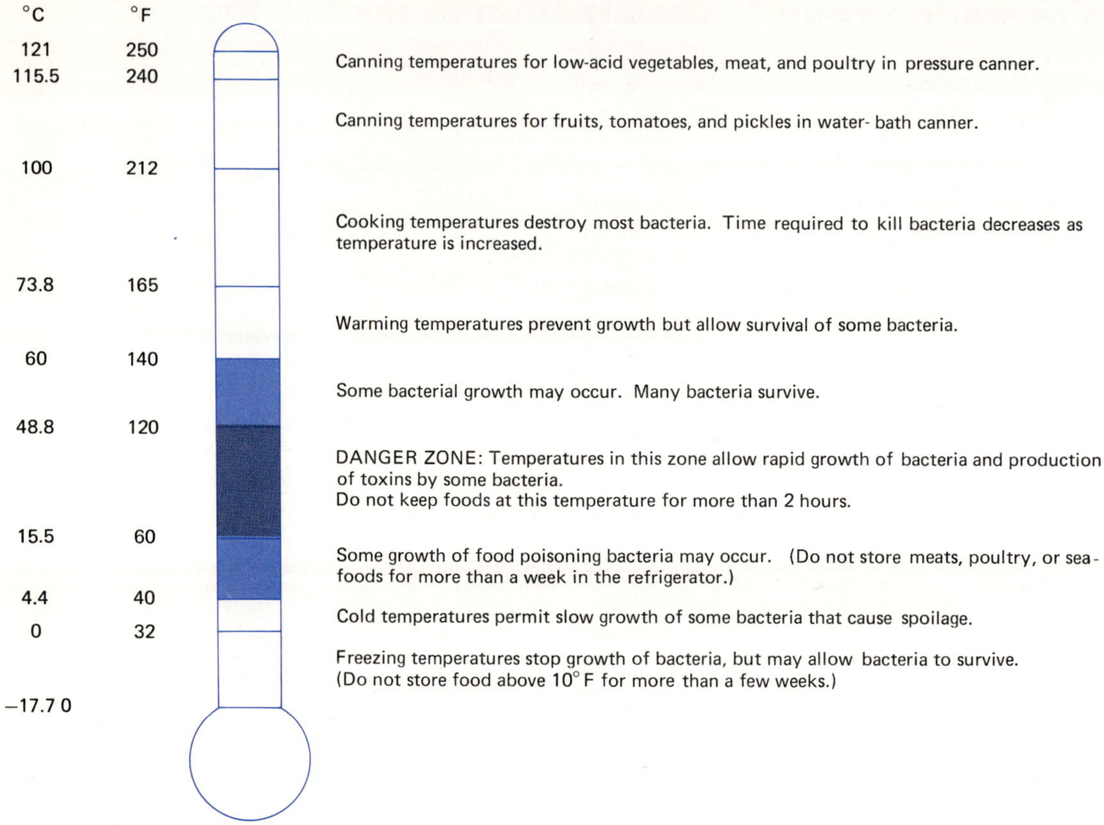

FIGURE 5.2 How temperature affects bacteria growth and safety. [*U.S. Department of Agriculture,* Keeping Food Safe to Eat, *p. 7.*]

Who Are the Overweight?

According to the Metropolitan Life ideal weight charts (Table 5.7), which are based on the weights at which people live longest, the average American is overweight—women by 15 to 30 pounds, men by 20 to 30 pounds—and is becoming more so every year. The overweight man, woman, or child is nothing like the familiar stereotype of the "jolly fat person." Overweight people may be either jolly *or* sad on the outside, but according to Dr. Richard Stuelke of Duke University's innovative "fat clinic," they often suffer from feelings of worthlessness, loss of esteem, social isolation, depression, anxiety and panic, guilt and anger, suicidal tendencies, and insecurity. The most frequent lifestyle pattern revealed by Dr. Stuelke's research is one of insufficient exercise, lack of assertiveness, and lack of structure in daily life.

Fat people are neither immoral nor weak-willed. They can, however, often be categorized as "external reactors," dominated by outside forces and their environment, rather than as "internal actors" who control their own environment. They have fallen into habit-traps that lead downhill to obesity.

What Causes Overweight?

Very simply, taking in more calories each day than the body burns results in weight gain. The following are the most common contributing factors.

Lack of activity For many years, experts proclaimed that the only useful exercise for dieters was "pushing away from the table." But recent studies show that many people are overweight not because they eat more than others, but because they are much less active and burn many fewer calories. They also show that exercise may do more than burn calories. Exercise may be necessary for the proper functioning of the appetite control center in our brains, called the "appestat" by the late nutritionist Dr. Norman Joliffe. It appears that having little or no exercise actually increases appetite (Mayer, *a*).

Glandular malfunction This is an often-used excuse for overweight, but is rarely the true cause. Some few people, however, are fat because of "glandular" problems—most often inadequate production of thyroid hormone. Carefully supervised thyroid supplements, diet, and exercise can correct this type of obesity.

Childhood overfeeding Parents proud of their bouncing baby with dimpled elbows may be sorry to learn their adorable infant is en route to becoming an obese adult. Recent studies suggest that overfeeding in infancy may lead to the development of extra fat (adipose) cells that persist for life. There is further evidence that additional fat cells can build up during puberty—ages 9 to 13 (N. M. Kaplan).

Heredity Animal breeders have long recognized the genetic component in fatness; when they want plump offspring, they select fat parents. In humans, two normal-weight parents have only a 7 percent chance of having overweight children; if one parent is fat, 40 percent of the children are likely to be obese; and if both parents are fat, 80 percent of their children will probably be overweight (Mayer, *b*). The theory that this might be due to family eating habits rather than hereditary factors has not been proved. But good eating and exercise habits can prevent even an inherited tendency to fatness from showing up.

Psychological conditioning Some people eat when upset (usually fat people); others can't eat a thing when upset (usually thin people). Eaters are usually those who have been conditioned to think of food as comfort and consolation. ("You scraped your knee? Here, a cookie will make it better!") Diets attempted during a period of depression, anxiety, or boredom rarely succeed for such people. Many parents, like animal trainers, also use food as a reward. ("An A on your report card? You deserve a big piece of chocolate cake!") Children grow up to reward themselves.

Hazards of Overweight

The overweight person can expect a shorter lifespan and an increased risk of illness, including heart disease, diabetes, high blood pressure, and gallstones (Duncan). Fat people have a higher incidence of cancer than thin ones (Rundles). Being overweight also carries added risks during pregnancy, childbirth, and surgery—as well as from exposure to fad diets and the great physical and psychological strain of repeatedly removing pounds and putting them back on.

Perhaps the greatest hazard faced by the overweight is the misery of loneliness, rejection, lack of self-esteem—an unhappiness that can probably only be understood by those who experience it. Fortunately, the hazards of obesity can be reversed by permanent weight loss.

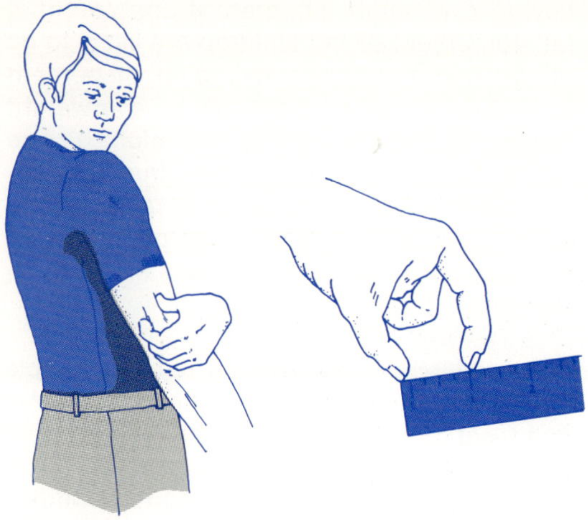

FIGURE 5.3 The pinch test for obesity. An easy way to measure for excess fat or obesity is this pinch test. The physician may perform the test with a "caliper"—an instrument that measures the pinched area precisely. Individuals can, however, do the test themselves with a ruler:

1 Pinch up a fold of skin and fat from the back of the upper arm; do not include the triceps muscle beneath the fat (see picture).

2 Remove your fingers, keeping the same distance between them. Measure this distance with a ruler. If this distance is more than an inch you—or the person you are measuring—are obese or fat, even if you are not overweight according to Table 5.7.

Approaches to Weight Reduction

Is weight loss necessary? The first step is to determine whether one is truly overweight or obese. Overweight is commonly described as heaviness above average body weight for size of 10 percent or more. Obesity refers to deposits of fat from 10 to 20 percent or more above normal range for age, sex, and height. In other words, a person can be overweight—because of heavy muscle and bone—without being fat. The obese person is fat (Solomon; GMD).

Height-weight charts (Table 5.7), the pinch test (Figure 5.3), and an honest self-appraisal while standing stripped in front of a mirror are ways of determining at home whether or not weight loss is necessary.

How is weight lost? In spite of what many books and magazine articles proclaim, calories do count. Unless glandular or other physical problems are present, losing weight means cutting down on the number of calories taken in, and/or increasing the number burned. A sensible approach is to cut about 500 calories a day—250 through diet, 250 through exercise. That represents 3500 calories a week—or 1 pound in weight. A slight increase in the ratio of protein to carbohydrate and fat in the diet may help, too. The body uses 5 to 7 calories to process 100 grams of fat or carbohydrate, but 30 calories to process the same amount of protein.

Can you do it alone? People who are no more than 10 percent above the recommended weight for sex, age, size, and build according to Table 5.7, and who are in good health, can probably go about a weight-reduction program on their own. Others should see their family physicians or visit the school health service for a physical checkup and individualized diet. Doctors who specialize in weight reduction often do an excellent job, but a few appear to run "diet mills" with little concern for the individual health needs of their patients. Be sure you select a doctor carefully.

A dieter in need of further support—as many are—can join a diet club or group. Some are nonprofit and attached to hospitals or clinics. Others are branches of broad commercial networks—such as Weight Watchers International—and charge a fee. Group philosophies vary, and the dieter should choose one that feels comfortable.

The role of exercise Dieters who exercise 30 minutes a day show a greater fat loss than matched dieters who do not exercise. They also gain in improved heart condition and

TABLE 5.7 Desirable body weights*

MEN				
HEIGHT (WITH SHOES ON)		WEIGHT IN POUNDS, AS ORDINARILY DRESSED, INCLUDING SHOES AND SUIT		
FEET	INCHES	SMALL FRAME	MEDIUM FRAME	LARGE FRAME
5	2	112–120	118–129	126–141
5	3	115–123	121–133	129–144
5	4	118–126	124–136	132–148
5	5	121–129	127–139	135–152
5	6	124–133	130–143	138–156
5	7	128–137	134–147	142–161
5	8	132–141	138–152	147–166
5	9	136–145	142–156	151–170
5	10	140–150	146–160	155–174
5	11	144–154	150–165	159–179
6	0	148–158	154–170	164–184
6	1	152–162	158–175	168–189
6	2	156–167	162–180	173–194
6	3	160–171	167–185	178–199
6	4	164–175	172–190	182–204

WOMEN				
HEIGHT (WITH SHOES ON; 2-INCH HEELS)		WEIGHT IN POUNDS, AS ORDINARILY DRESSED, INCLUDING SHOES AND DRESS		
FEET	INCHES	SMALL FRAME	MEDIUM FRAME	LARGE FRAME
4	10	92–98	96–107	104–119
4	11	94–101	98–110	106–122
5	0	96–104	101–113	109–125
5	1	99–107	104–116	112–128
5	2	102–110	107–119	115–131
5	3	105–113	110–122	118–134
5	4	108–116	113–126	121–138
5	5	111–119	116–130	125–142
5	6	114–123	120–135	129–146
5	7	118–127	124–139	133–150
5	8	122–131	128–143	137–154
5	9	126–135	132–147	141–158
5	10	130–140	136–151	145–163
5	11	134–144	140–155	149–168
6	0	138–148	144–159	153–173

*These are desirable weights for men and women over 25, graded according to body frame. These tables, prepared by the Metropolitan Life Insurance Company, are based on weights associated with the lowest mortality. The charts allow about 8 pounds for men's clothing and 4 pounds for women's. To arrive at the normal weight of women 18 to 25, subtract 1 pound for each year under 25. These charts may be useful in determining overweight or underweight, but they are less reliable than water weighing or the pinch test.

The young adult who is moderately active requires about 15 calories per pound of *desired* body weight each day. The very active individual requires more calories, the sedentary fewer. Calorie needs decrease with age.

Source: Burton, p. 245.

TABLE 5.8 How quickly can you burn calories from common foods?

		BURNING RATES, IN MINUTES								
FOOD	CALORIES (APPROX.)	RECLINING IN BED	BATHING, SHAVING, ETC.	WALKING 2.5 MPH	TENNIS	RUNNING 7.5 MPH	BICYCLING 13 MPH	SWIMMING 45 YD/MIN	SKIING, HARD-PACKED SNOW	GARDENING
1 apple	75	60	23	15	11	5	7	6	8	15
1 banana	130	104	40	26	19	9	12	11	13	26
1 grapefruit	70	56	22	14	10	5	6	6	7	14
1 egg, scrambled	120	96	38	24	17	8	11	10	11	24
1 slice bread	65	52	20	13	9	4	6			
1 strip bacon,	60	48	19	12	9	4	5	5	6	12
½ cup tuna	225	180	70	45	32	15	19	18	23	45
1 chicken leg and thigh, fried	325	260	101	65	46	22	30	29	33	65
4 oz hamburger	195	156	61	39	28	13	18	17	20	39
½ cup string beans	25	20	8	5	4	2	2	2	3	5
1 ear fresh corn	180	144	56	36	26	12	17	16	18	30
¼ head lettuce	15	12	5	3	2	1	1	1	2	3
1 baked potato	100	80	31	20	14	7	9	9	10	20
8 pieces french fries	150	120	40	30	21	10	14	13	15	30
6 potato chips	95	76	30	19	14	7	9	8	10	19
8 oz whole milk	166	133	52	33	24	11	16	15	17	33
8 oz skim milk	80	64	25	16	12	5	7	7	8	16
8 oz cola	105	84	33	21	15	7	10	9	11	21
8 oz beer	115	92	36	23	16	8	11	10	12	23
1 oz milk chocolate	140	112	44	28	20	9	13	12	14	28

general fitness (Kenrick et al.). Thus good advice to the healthy overweight is: Don't ride when you can walk. Don't use an elevator when there are stairs. Don't use a power tool when you can use person power. To calculate your own calorie burning, see Table 5.8.

Appetite versus hunger Hunger and appetite are not one and the same. Hunger speaks through stomach pains, headache, faintness, weakness, and a sensation of emptiness in the stomach. Prolonged hunger leads to death by starvation. Appetite is a craving for food often stimulated by psychological or physical factors, but not necessarily related to hunger.

The appestat—the body's appetite signal system—appears not to work properly in the obese. In one study, fat people who had first been given a heavy meal and/or had been made anxious were able to eat as much (or more) food during a testing situation later on as when they had not eaten or not been made anxious. Normal people, however, who were given a heavy meal or made anxious before the test meal could eat very little. Apparently, the appetites of the normals were controlled by the fact that their stomachs had signaled, "I'm full," or "I'm too upset to eat." The obese seemed to receive no such signal. Their appetites seemed totally unrelated to the state of their stomachs or their minds. People of normal weight were controlled by internal signals, the obese by externals such as the smell and sight of food (Schacter).

Changing eating habits Modification of eating behavior is now believed by some authorities to be the best way to lose weight and *keep it off* (Stunkard, *b*). Reward—the chance to see a new show, a new dress, a tennis racket, anything appealing except food—can increase motivation. But the reward should be for the behavioral change, not the weight loss.

Drastic Measures for Weight Reduction

When weight seems impossible to lose, people are often willing to try anything. But drastic measures often lead to drastic results, and they do not change eating habits. Wise patients, in consultation with their physicians, will carefully weigh risks against benefits before deciding to use any of the following extreme measures.

Lopsided diets Some obese people find it easier to stick to very limited diets—grapefruit or egg diets, Atkins or Mayo. If weight is lost, it is because total calorie intake in relation to calories burned has been reduced, often because of the monotony of the diet. But eating habits are not altered in most cases, and any lost weight is quickly regained when the diet is discontinued. Mayer has

Locking the jaw is a radical weight loss measure, with safety and long-term effectiveness still under study.

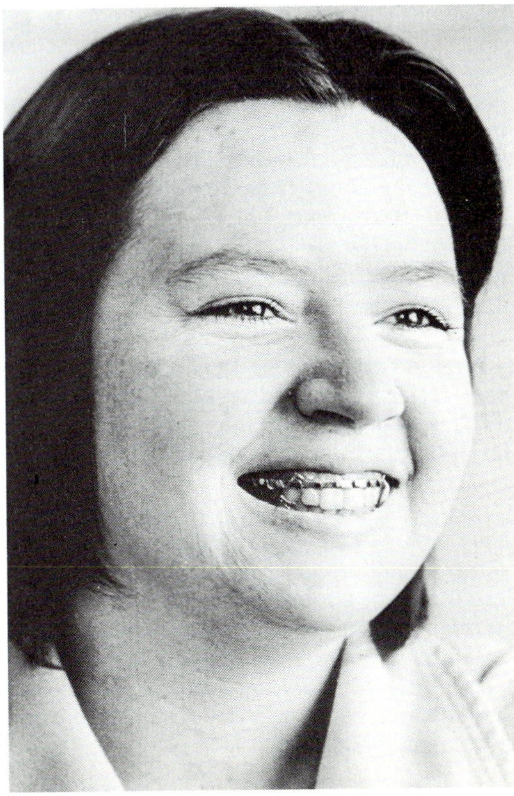

United Press International

aptly dubbed this the "rhythm method of girth control"—loss, gain, loss, gain, ad infinitum. Since lopsided diets are almost always deficient in several nutrients, they can upset the metabolism and other body systems and can be harmful to health as well as ineffective in weight control. The predigested liquid protein diet, popular in 1977, for example, was reportedly linked to several deaths.

Fasting A few physicians have successfully employed this most extreme diet, allowing only water, vitamins, and other supplements for extended periods in reducing the *extremely* overweight. But such diets can be fatal and must be carried out only under close medical supervision in a hospital setting. Any diet of 500 calories or less can seriously upset body balances (N. M. Kaplan).

Surgery Two kinds of surgery have been used to reduce weight. In one, a portion of the intestine is removed, allowing less space for absorption of food and calories. This "short circuiting" of the digestive system, called the *jejunoileal bypass*, has come under fire for overuse and abuse by many medical people. Results are not always good and serious complications are common (Winkelman et al.). Many authorities believe "diet by scalpel" should be limited to cases in which overweight itself is immediately life-threatening and all other weight-loss measures have failed.

Another surgical method slices away excess fat and skin and resutures the skin. In this method there is a major risk: that a new fat buildup can cause the incision to open.

Locking the jaw More than 5000 Americans have already lost weight by having their jaws wired together, forcing them to live on a liquid diet of soups, juices, milks. Digestive problems often occur because of lack of bulk, and jaws become inflamed and painful. Conversation is as limited as calories. Safety and permanence of the weight loss are still to be evaluated.

Hypnosis Less hazardous than the above methods, hypnosis is also less likely to work because only about 1 in every 3 or 4 adults is susceptible to hypnotic suggestion. Even in those who are, the will to eat often triumphs. Therapist Nathan Fleischer suggested to one overweight woman that she would no longer enjoy desserts because they would all taste like burnt rubber. But when she returned some time later, she had lost no weight. "What happened?" he asked. "I've learned," she replied, "to enjoy the taste of burnt rubber."

Drugs Drugs are not the easy street to weight loss they once promised to be. Stimulant amphetamines lose their effectiveness as appetite suppressants after a few weeks. They are, like other methods employed by "diet doctors," such as the use of unneeded thyroid pills and diuretics, subject to serious abuse. According to obesity expert Dr. Albert J. Stunkard:

> In no medical condition are patients subjected to more shady practice or downright fraud than in the treatment of obesity. . . . The desperation of many obese persons has led them wittingly or unwittingly to take serious risks. Some have died as a result. (*a*, p. 33)

Among other weight-reduction frauds are injections of HCG (human chorionic gonadotropin), a hormone from the urine of pregnant women; reducing machines, belts, and suits that promise to take off weight without physical activity; and reducing pills or candies that promise weight loss without diet. Acupuncture and ear staples have been promoted, too, but are of dubious value. As long as there is money to be made in weight loss, new "miracle" diets and methods, like streetcars of old, will be along every minute. It is wise to consider carefully before climbing aboard.

The Underweight

Overweight people often enviously wonder why those who are underweight (10 to 20

A Weight-Loss Plan

The following suggestions were culled from many sources, and most weight watchers will find one or more of them useful:

1 Recognize obesity as a lifelong, incurable, but controllable disease—much like alcoholism. You can't crash diet, return to old eating ways, and remain slim.
2 Adopt a long-range plan. With fat, it's "Easy go, easy come back." So don't rush it.

- Plan to lose about 5 to 15 pounds at a time in a one- to three-month period.
- Plan for a net loss of 1 pound per week, by cutting back 500 calories a day.
- Be prepared for setbacks; don't let them throw you into a fit of despair.
- Don't give in to fads or gimmicks that promise instant weight loss; their effects usually last an instant.

3 Keep a diary of what you eat, when, under what circumstances, where, and with whom. Do you notice that you always overeat just before an exam? Or after an argument? Also note your exercise patterns. How can you change the environmental situations that encourage eating and discourage exercise? If the problem is pizza at 11:00, go for a walk at 10:45; if studying leads to snacking, study in the library.
4 Increase your level of physical activity. Walking 2 miles a day in about an hour can cause a 25-pound weight loss in a year, with *no* change in food intake. (See Table 5.8 for caloric values of other exercises.)
5 Modify your eating habits.

- Don't serve family style; serve individual portions.
- Don't go back for seconds.
- Slow down eating: Wait a minute or two before attacking food; put your fork or spoon down between bites; take occasional 2-minute breaks during the meal; try to extend the meal so it will last at least 20 minutes. (No matter how much you have eaten, you won't begin to get a "full" signal for 20 minutes.)
- Eat five or six small meals rather than three larger ones. Larger meals tend to stretch the stomach.
- Make up for occasional indulgences by being very strict the day before or after.
- Plan what you are going to eat in advance, whether you will be eating at a party, at home, or in the school dining hall. Then stick to your plan. Don't wait until you are faced with the tempting foods to make your selections.
- Don't linger at the table when you are through eating.
- When you feel like snacking, set the alarm clock to ring in 10 minutes. If you still feel like eating when it rings, try to take something low in calories. Even better, try to find something else to do: Call a friend, run up and down the hall, wash you hair, go down to the gym, write a letter, etc.
- Cover or wrap all foods in the refrigerator. Don't leave any dishes of nuts or candies around. The sight of food is the downfall of many dieters.

TABLE 5.9 A chart of food values (Including calories, cholesterol, protein, vitamins)

	MEASURE OR WEIGHT	CALORIES	PROTEIN, grams	FAT, grams	FATTY ACIDS, SATURATED, grams	FATTY ACIDS, POLYUNSATURATED (LINOLEIC), grams
MEATS						
Chicken, broiled, no skin	3 oz	115	20	3	1	1
Cod fillet, poached	3 oz	89	20	‡	‡	‡
Tuna, in oil, drained	3 oz	170	24	7	2	1
Shrimp, canned	3 oz	100	21	1	*	*
Ground beef, lean	3 oz	185	23	10	5	Trace
Lamb, roast, lean	3 oz	156	24	6	4	Trace
Veal, roast, med. fat	3 oz	230	23	14	7	Trace
Pork, roast, lean	3 oz	219	25	13	4	1
Ham, boiled	3 oz	203	17	15	6	2
Bacon, crisp	2 slices	90	5	8	3	1
Beef liver, fried	3 oz	195	23	9	*	*
Bologna	2 slices	80	3	7	†	‡
Frankfurter, (8 per pound)	1	170	7	15	†	‡
Egg	1 large	80	6	6	2	Trace
Red kidney beans, cooked	1 cup	230	15	1	*	*
Split green peas, cooked	1 cup	290	20	1	*	*
Peanut butter	1 tbsp	95	4	8	2	2
Peanuts	¼ cup	210	9	18	4	5
Walnuts	¼ cup	198	6	19	1	9
Coconut	¼ cup	112	1	11	10	Trace
DAIRY FOODS						
Skim milk, nonfat	1 cup	90	9	Trace		*
Whole milk	1 cup	160	9	9	5	Trace
Buttermilk	1 cup	90	9	Trace	*	*
Chocolate drink	1 cup	190	8	6	3	Trace
Evaporated milk, undiluted	1 tbsp	22	1	1	1	Trace
Light cream	1 tbsp	30	1	3	2	Trace
Heavy cream	1 tbsp	55	Trace	6	3	Trace
Powdered imit. cream	1 tbsp	30	Trace	3	2	0
Pressurized imit. cream	¼ cup	48	Trace	4	4	0
Pressurized wh. cream	¼ cup	39	Trace	4	2	Trace
Dairy sour cream	1 tbsp	25	Trace	2	1	Trace
Yogurt, part skim milk	1 cup	125	8	4	2	Trace
Ice milk	½ cup	100	3	4	2	Trace
Ice cream, regular	½ cup	128	3	7	4	Trace
Baked custard	½ cup	152	7	8	4	1
Cottage cheese, dry	½ cup	85	17	1	Trace	Trace
Cottage cheese, creamed	½ cup	130	17	5	3	Trace
Process. Amer. cheese	1 oz	105	7	9	5	Trace
Cheddar cheese	1 oz	115	7	9	5	Trace
Cream cheese	1 oz	107	2	11	6	Trace
FATS AND OILS						
Butter	1 tbsp	100	Trace	12	6	Trace
Margarine, regular	1 tbsp	100	Trace	12	2	3
Margarine, liq. oil 1st ing.	1 tbsp	100	Trace	11	2	4
Hydro. veg. shortening	1 tbsp	110	0	13	3	3
Lard	1 tbsp	115	0	13	5	1
Corn oil	1 tbsp	125	0	14	1	7
Cottonseed oil	1 tbsp.	125	0	14	4	7
Peanut oil	1 tbsp	125	0	14	3	4
Mayonnaise	1 tbsp	100	Trace	11	2	6
French dressing	1 tbsp	65	Trace	6	1	3

*Value unknown, but probably a measurable amount.
†Value unknown, but probably a considerable amount.
‡Value unknown, but probably very little.
Source: Family Circle, 1971.

CHOLES-TEROL, mg	CARBO-HYDRATES, grams	CALCIUM, mg	IRON, mg	VITAMIN A, I.U.	VITAMIN B/ THIAMIN, mg	VITAMIN B/ RIBOFLAVIN, mg	VITAMIN B/ NIACIN, mg	VITAMIN C/ ASCORBIC ACID, mg
				MEATS				
50	0	8	1.4	80	0.05	0.16	7.4	*
*	0	11	0.45	0	0.07	0.08	2.5	2
60	0	7	1.6	70	0.04	0.10	10.1	*
106	1	98	2.6	50	0.01	0.03	1.5	*
60	0	10	3.0	20	0.08	0.20	5.1	*
60	0	11	1.7	*	0.14	0.25	5.3	*
77	0	10	2.9	*	0.11	0.26	6.6	*
60	0	11	3.2	0	0.91	0.26	5.5	*
60	0	9	2.4	0	0.38	0.14	2.3	*
†	1	2	0.5	0	0.08	0.05	0.8	*
257	5	9	7.5	45,420	0.23	3.56	14.1	23
†	Trace	2	0.5	*	0.04	0.06	0.7	*
†	1	3	0.8	*	0.08	0.11	1.4	*
275	Trace	27	1.1	590	0.05	0.15	Trace	0
0	42	74	4.6	10	0.13	0.10	1.5	*
0	52	28	4.2	100	0.37	0.22	2.2	*
0	3	9	0.3	*	0.02	0.02	2.4	0
0	7	27	0.8	*	0.11	0.05	6.1	0
0	5	Trace	1.9	95	0.07	0.04	0.2	*
0	3	4	0.5	0	0.02	0.01	0.2	1
				DAIRY FOODS				
7	12	296	0.1	10	0.09	0.44	0.2	2
27	12	288	0.1	350	0.07	0.41	0.2	2
7	12	296	0.1	10	0.10	0.44	0.2	2
†	27	270	0.5	210	0.10	0.40	0.3	3
†	1	40	Trace	50	Trace	0.05	Trace	Trace
†	1	15	Trace	130	Trace	0.02	Trace	Trace
†	1	11	Trace	230	Trace	0.02	Trace	Trace
‡	3	3	Trace	Trace	*	*	*	*
‡	2	1	*	85	*	0	*	*
†	2	17	*	142	*	0.01	*	*
†	1	12	Trace	100	Trace	0.02	Trace	Trace
†	13	294	0.1	170	0.10	0.44	0.2	2
†	15	102	0.05	140	0.04	0.15	0.05	Trace
30	14	97	0.05	295	0.03	0.14	0.05	Trace
150	15	150	0.6	465	0.06	0.25	0.2	Trace
‡	3	90	0.4	10	0.03	0.28	0.1	0
19	4	115	0.35	210	0.04	0.32	0.1	0
24	1	198	0.3	350	0.01	0.12	Trace	0
28	1	213	0.3	370	0.01	0.13	Trace	0
34	1	17	0.06	437	0.01	0.06	0.03	0
				FATS AND OILS				
36	Trace	3	0	470	*	*	*	0
0	Trace	3	0	470	*	*	*	0
0	Trace	3	0	470	*	*	*	0
0	0	0	0	*	0	0	0	0
12	0	0	0	0	0	0	0	0
0	0	0	0	*	0	0	0	0
0	0	0	0	*	0	0	0	0
0	0	0	0	*	0	0	0	0
‡	Trace	3	0.1	40	Trace	0.01	Trace	*
0	3	2	0.1	*	*	*	*	*

TABLE 5.9 (*Continued*)

	MEASURE OR WEIGHT	CALORIES	PROTEIN, grams	FAT, grams	FATTY ACIDS, SATURATED, grams	FATTY ACIDS, POLYUNSATURATED (LINOLEIC), grams
FRUITS AND VEGETABLES						
Orange juice	½ cup	60	1	Trace	*	*
Grapefruit	½ med	45	1	Trace	*	*
Strawberries	1 cup	55	1	1	*	*
Apple	1 med	70	Trace	Trace	*	*
Banana	1 med	100	1	Trace	*	*
Avocado	½ med	132	2	13	1.4	1
Applesauce, no sugar	½ cup	50	Trace	Trace	*	*
Peaches, canned	½ cup	100	Trace	Trace	*	*
Pineapple, crushed	½ cup	97	Trace	Trace	*	*
Raisins	¼ cup	120	1	Trace	*	*
Cabbage, shredded raw	½ cup	8	Trace	Trace	*	*
Carrot, raw	1 med	20	1	Trace	*	*
Tomato, raw	1 large	40	2	Trace	*	*
Green beans, cooked	½ cup	15	1	Trace	*	*
Spinach, cooked	½ cup	20	3	Trace	*	*
Summer squash, cooked	½ cup	15	1	Trace	*	*
White potato, baked	1 med	90	3	Trace	*	*
Sweet potato, baked	1 med	155	2	1	*	*
Peas, canned	½ cup	83	5	Trace	*	*
Corn, canned	½ cup	85	3	1	*	*
BREADS AND CEREALS						
White bread, enriched	1 slice	70	2	1	*	*
Whole wheat bread	1 slice	65	3	1	*	*
Oatmeal, cooked	½ cup	65	3	1	*	1
Shredded wheat	1	90	2	1	*	*
Corn flakes	1 cup	100	2	Trace	*	*
Sugared corn flakes	1 cup	155	2	Trace	*	*
Puffed rice	1 cup	60	1	Trace	*	*
Rice, enriched, cooked	½ cup	112	2	Trace	*	*
Macaroni, enr., cooked	1 cup	155	5	1	*	*
Egg noodles, enriched	½ cup	100	4	1	Trace	Trace
All-purpose flour	1 tbsp	28	1	Trace	*	*
Pancake, 4-in	1	60	2	2	Trace	Trace
Saltines	4	50	1	1	*	*
Graham crackers	4	110	2	3	*	*
Brownie	1 med.	95	1	6	1	1
Doughnut	1 med.	105	3	5	*	‡
Angelfood cake	1/12	135	3	Trace	*	*
Yellow cake, choc. icing	1/12	366	4	13	4	2
Apple pie	⅛	306	3	13	4	3
Lemon meringue pie	⅛	269	4	10	4	2
SUGARS, SWEETS, AND BEVERAGES						
Granulated sugar	1 tbsp	40	0	0	*	*
Brown sugar	1 tbsp	51	0	0	*	*
Jelly	1 tbsp	50	Trace	Trace	*	*
Syrup, corn, blend	1 tbsp	60	0	0	*	*
Molasses, light	1 tbsp	50	*	*	*	*
Choc. fudge topping	2 tbsp	125	2	5	3	Trace
Milk choc. candy	1 oz	145	2	9	5	Trace
Cola beverage	12 oz	145	0	0	*	*
Beer	12 oz	150	1	0	*	*
Scotch, 80 proof	1½ oz	100	*	*	*	*

CHOLES-TEROL, mg	CARBO-HYDRATES, grams	CALCIUM, mg	IRON, mg	VITAMIN A, I.U.	VITAMIN B/ THIAMIN, mg	VITAMIN B/ RIBOFLAVIN, mg	VITAMIN B/ NIACIN, mg	VITAMIN C/ ASCORBIC ACID, mg
				FRUITS AND VEGETABLES				
0	15	13	0.1	275	0.11	0.01	0.5	60
0	12	19	0.5	10	0.05	0.02	0.2	44
0	13	31	1.5	90	0.04	0.10	1.0	88
0	18	8	0.4	50	0.04	0.02	0.1	3
0	26	10	0.8	230	0.06	0.07	0.8	12
0	4	9	1.4	460	0.09	0.09	1.4	6
0	13	5	0.6	50	0.03	0.01	1.0	1
0	26	5	0.4	550	0.01	0.03	0.7	3
0	25	15	0.4	60	0.10	0.03	0.3	9
0	32	26	1.5	8	0.04	0.03	0.2	1
0	2	17	0.1	45	0.02	0.02	0.1	17
0	5	18	0.4	5500	0.03	0.03	0.3	4
0	9	24	0.9	1640	0.11	0.07	1.3	42
0	4	32	0.4	340	0.04	0.06	0.3	8
0	3	83	2.0	7290	0.07	0.12	0.5	25
0	4	26	0.4	410	0.05	0.08	0.8	10
0	21	9	0.7	Trace	0.10	0.04	1.7	20
0	36	44	1.0	8910	0.10	0.07	0.7	24
0	16	25	2.1	560	0.11	0.07	1.1	11
0	20	5	0.5	345	0.03	0.06	1.1	6
				BREADS AND CEREALS				
‡	13	21	0.6	Trace	0.06	0.05	0.6	Trace
‡	14	24	0.8	Trace	0.09	0.03	0.8	Trace
0	12	11	0.7	0	0.09	0.03	0.1	0
0	20	11	0.9	0	0.06	0.03	1.1	0
0	21	4	0.4	0	0.11	0.02	0.5	0
0	36	5	0.4	0	0.16	0.02	0.8	0
0	13	3	0.3	0	0.07	0.01	0.7	0
0	25	10	0.9	0	0.12	0.01	1.1	0
0	32	8	1.3	0	0.20	0.11	1.5	0
†	18	8	0.5	55	0.03	0.01	0.3	0
0	6	1	0.2	0	0.03	0.02	0.2	0
26	9	27	0.4	30	0.05	0.06	0.4	Trace
0	8	2	0.1	0	Trace	Trace	0.1	0
0	21	11	0.4	0	0.01	0.06	0.4	0
36	10	8	0.4	40	0.04	0.02	0.1	Trace
15	22	147	0.7	0	0.12	0.07	1.0	Trace
0	32	50	0.2	0	Trace	0.06	0.1	0
69	60	68	0.6	160	0.02	0.08	0.2	Trace
‡	45	9	0.4	35	0.03	0.03	0.4	1
103	40	15	0.5	175	0.04	0.09	0.2	4
				SUGARS, SWEETS, AND BEVERAGES				
0	11	0	Trace	0	0	0	0	0
0	13	12	0.5	0	Trace	Trace	Trace	0
0	13	4	0.3	Trace	Trace	0.01	Trace	1
0	15	9	0.8	0	0	0	0	0
0	13	33	0.9	*	0.01	0.01	Trace	*
‡	20	48	0.5	60	0.02	0.08	0.2	Trace
‡	16	65	0.3	80	0.02	0.10	0.1	Trace
0	37	*	*	0	0	0	0	0
0	14	18	Trace	*	0.01	0.11	2.2	*
0	Trace	*	*	*	*	*	*	*

pounds or more below ideal weight) complain at all. But underweight persons, too, may suffer from lack of self-esteem and feelings of despondency. Underweight men usually crave the image of strength and assurance they ascribe to acquaintances of normal weight; thin women desire more curves, not more muscle. However, thin people are usually quite healthy and can expect to outlive their heavier friends. It would seem easy to put weight on—add a few cream pies and milkshakes to the diet, and presto!—but it is not at all easy for these people. Gaining weight can be more difficult and complex than losing (Mayer, *e*).

Gaining weight The first step is to see a physician to determine whether there is a physical reason—say, a glandular problem or an unrecognized acute or chronic illness—for the failure to gain weight. If there is no physical cause, the physician is likely to suggest a special diet of high-calorie, high-nutrition foods: meats and fish, fried or with gravy and sauces; cheeses; peanut butter; grilled sandwiches, on whole grain breads; milk, ice cream, and shakes; dried fruits, bananas, avocados, fresh fruits, and juices; omelettes; nuts; dressings, rice, pastas, stuffings, potatoes. Snacks should be chosen from this list, but should not be taken so near mealtime as to interfere with appetite. A bedtime snack is especially important—but it should be high in protein, low in sugar.

Exercising for about 15 minutes a day will both improve appetite and assure that new weight is well-distributed muscle, not flab. Swearing off smoking is another good weight booster. Should weight-gain efforts fail—they sometimes do—thin people can console themselves with high-fashion styles that the overweight cannot wear, and by remembering they may be the only ones on their block to live to be 100.

Temporary weight gain—using water and salt to achieve a particular weight for, say, an athletic event—is highly dangerous and can lead to serious illness, or even death in persons with unrecognized high blood pressure or kidney disease.

Anorexia nervosa A few of American's millions of constantly dieting young women carry it to extremes. The diagnosis in these cases is anorexia nervosa (*anorexia* = lack of appetite, thus, a nervous lack of appetite). Actually, some of these women suppress normal appetites, eating almost nothing out of sheer neurotic determination to lose weight. One woman subsisted on one egg and one raw vegetable a day for months. Some choose to eat, then force-vomit. In spite of starvation food-intake levels, they may appear to be highly energetic and often are compulsive exercisers.

The condition may occur in young women who were once plump and were subject to teasing. Even when they achieve an ideal weight, they view themselves as fat and compulsively continue dieting—often thinning down to 50 or 60 emaciated pounds. Some psychiatrists suggest that these young females are attempting to halt developing womanhood, and indeed, their severe weight loss is usually accompanied by a cessation of menstruation. Though there has been some evidence that an abnormality in fat metabolism may be involved (Pops and Schwabe), present treatment consists of hospitalization, forced feeding, and psychiatric treatment. The treatment is usually successful, but untreated, the condition can be fatal.

LOOKING BACK

REVIEWING CONCEPTS IN CHAPTER 5

- Good nutrition is among the easiest and most successful forms of preventive medicine.
- Malnutrition can mean eating too little, too much, or the wrong kind of food. It is common in the United States.
- Food choice is affected by many factors—societal, personal, and environmental.
- Nutritive value of human food is no longer tied to taste as in the past. Taste has thus become a poor way to choose foods.
- Our bodies need calories and the proteins, carbohydrates, and fats that provide them, as well as vitamins and minerals, water, and dietary fiber.
- RDAs of various nutrients are not designed to be rigidly followed by individuals planning a daily diet.
- Variety is one key to a healthful diet. Avoiding "empty" calories is another.
- Fad diets that do not contain all needed nutrients can be hazardous.
- Good diet is not necessarily costly.
- "Natural" in foods does not automatically mean safe; nor does "chemical" or "additive" always mean unsafe. Decisions to permit or outlaw certain food additives are based on risk versus benefit.
- Contaminated food is believed by some to be a greater hazard than food additives, and can almost always be prevented by careful handling, storage, and preparation of foods.
- Overweight is a major health problem in the United States.
- The *only* way to lose weight is to burn more calories than you take in. Reducing calorie intake and increasing exercise both contribute.
- Overweight has both physical and emotional components; it is often the result of learned attitudes and eating habits.
- Overweight people respond to sight, smell, and thought of food; people of normal weight eat when they are really hungry.
- Loss of weight and keeping it off permanently require modification of eating behavior.
- Drastic dieting can lead to drastic results, and should be undertaken only under a physician's supervision.
- Underweight people may be unhappy with their appearance but, assuming they have no underlying disease, they are healthier than overweights.
- Gaining weight is best accomplished by the addition of high-calorie, high-nutrition foods to the diet.
- Anorexia nervosa, characterized by extreme dieting, requires immediate professional care.

6

TAKING CARE OF YOURSELF— PREVENTING COMMON HEALTH PROBLEMS

WHAT'S AHEAD IN CHAPTER 6 How does intelligent care of mouth and teeth, eyes, ears, skin, back, and feet help improve the quality of life? What are the major threats to oral health? What combination of personal and professional effort is necessary to combat them? How large a role does prevention play? What should be the major goal of the dentist you select to care for your mouth? Can any disease of the mouth be fatal? How could such a disease be prevented or most easily cured? How can you use knowledge of the various factors that can damage your eyes and ears to protect vision and hearing? What is the role of the regular checkup in protecting these vital senses? What factors are likely to affect skin health? How can skin be protected? Is acne, which strikes nearly everyone and eventually clears up by itself, worth treating? What can the condition of your hair tell you about your health? Is backache the inevitable lot of creatures audacious enough to get up off all fours and stagger around on two legs? Or are there precautions we can take to prevent the aching back? How does the purchase of footwear affect one's health?

Aching back. Sore feet. Throbbing tooth. Painful ear. Tired eyes. Itching skin. Who isn't familiar with the common disorders of the sensing organs (eyes, ears, mouth, and skin), that interfere with vision, hearing, taste, and touch; and of the feet and back, that interfere with lifting and locomotion? They are responsible for distress, disability, and discomfort in millions every day.

Fortunately, however, most of these ailments are preventable through individual action. Others are often controllable or treatable. For easy access to information on how these fascinating and functional parts of the body work, what problems they are subject to, and how these problems can be prevented, controlled, or treated, this chapter is arranged in a series of convenient-to-refer-to tables, diagrams, and sidebars.

THE ORAL CAVITY

The oral cavity is the main entryway to the body. With tongue and teeth, it is involved in tasting, chewing, and digesting, and in breathing, talking, and loving. It is deserving of our attention.

Major Disorders of the Oral Cavity

The major threats to dental health and causes of tooth loss are dental caries (decay or cavities), affecting 98 percent of the population, and periodontal disease (gum disease, pyorrhea), affecting 90 percent of adults.

Dental caries Decay that forms cavities in the teeth, often leading to pain and, if untreated, to tooth loss. *Cause*: Three factors are believed necessary for decay to develop: (1) bacteria (primarily *Streptococcus mutans,* found in all mouths); (2) susceptible teeth (some are more so than others); (3) fermentable carbohydrates (usually sucrose, ordinary refined table sugar) in the diet. (See Figure 6.2.) They are believed to form caries in the smooth surfaces of the teeth this way: The sucrose is metabolized by the bacteria into a sticky complex sugar called *polyglucon* that allows the bacteria to attach themselves to the teeth in groups or colonies called *plaque*. Once the plaque beachhead is established, it becomes a secure environment for more bacteria to thrive in. Each time sugars are eaten, these bacteria act on them within seconds, producing an acid bath. Then the process shown in Figure 6.3 begins, usually unnoticed by the victim. In the pitted chewing surfaces of the teeth, the bacteria often attack directly, entering the tooth through faults and fissures. The major infectious agent is uncertain, but sugar figures prominently in forming enamel-destroying acids. *Detection*: Dental examinations and x-rays can show up early decay. Pain is often a late symptom. *Treatment*: Restoration, when possible, to make diseased teeth serviceable via: (1) making *fillings*, a process in which the decay is drilled or excavated and then replaced with silver amalgam or tooth-colored plastic resin or silicate; (2) making *inlays* of gold or *crowns* of gold, porcelain, or plastic, used to restore more severely damaged teeth; (3) doing *root canal therapy* (often performed by an endodontist), in which the inside of the decayed tooth, including pulp and nerve tissue, is removed down to the root and the tooth is then filled. When restoration is not possible, the tooth is extracted, or removed. *Prevention:* Good personal oral care. (See pages 135 to 139.)

Periodontal disease Gingival or gum inflammation (gingivitis) and later destruction of fibers and bone that anchor teeth in place (periodontitis) leading to tooth loss. May begin in childhood and progress slowly over many years. *Cause and development*: Not fully understood (Suomi); believed to be caused, at least in part, by bacteria. In early stages, bacteria in the plaque along the gum lines of the teeth manufacture irritants that inflame the gums. If the plaque is not removed by regular brushing and flossing, it hardens as bacteria die and calcify, forming *calculus* (tartar). With its rough surface, the calculus continues to serve as a nesting place for billions of live bacteria. If not removed at the dentist's office, it may contribute to further tissue breakdown, extending to the fibers that fasten gums to teeth and into the alveolar bone that supports the teeth. (See Figure 6.3.) *Detection*: Early symptoms, if any, of gum disease usually involve bleeding, redness, and puffiness. These may disappear as the disease progresses deeper into the gums, and the victim may believe that the

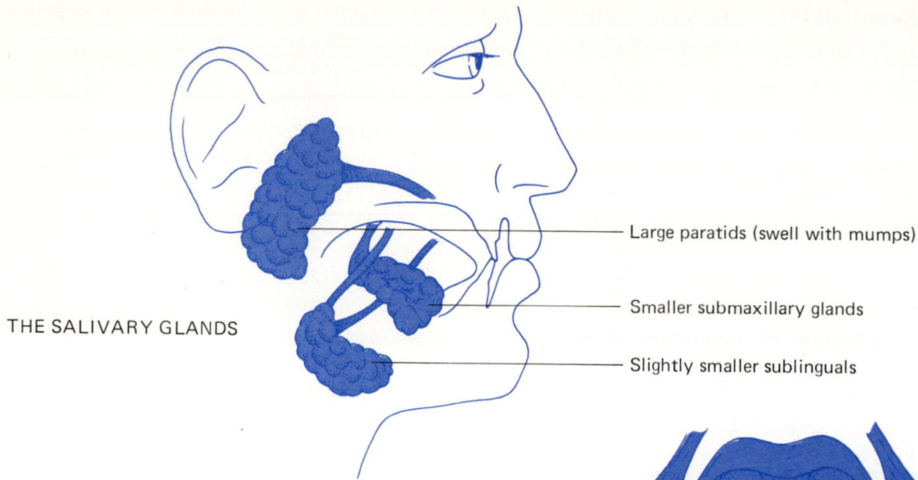

	HEALTHY	SIGNS OF ILLNESS OR ABNORMALITY
COLOR	Pink	Red, white, black, bluish, streaked, spotted (except from foods or dye)
SURFACE	Rough papillae soft, elastic	Lesions, sores that do not heal in 3 weeks, shiny, smooth
SIZE	Fits comfortably in mouth	Oversized tongue = endocrine disorder, vitamin deficiency
MOBILITY	Can stick straight out, move easily	Leans to one side, sluggish
MOISTURE	Moist	Dryness = illness or vitamin deficiency
SMELL	No odor	Food waste and bacteria in its crevices cause odor (can be prevented by gentle brushing once a day)

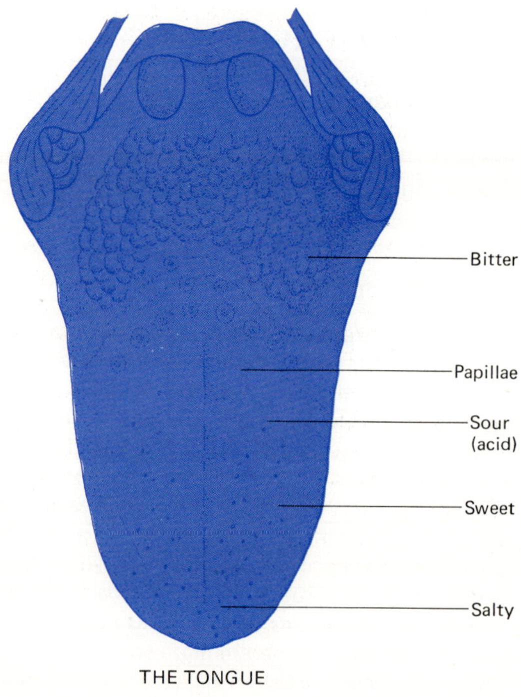

FIGURE 6.1 Major stuctures of the oral cavity:

The salivary glands. Saliva begins the digestion of starches (and possibly other nutrients), moistens food for swallowing, helps protect teeth from decay-causing bacterial acids, washes away unattached bacteria and bits of food, and may affect the ability to distinguish between different tastes. It is a combination of the secretions of hundreds of tiny salivary glands as well as of those shown. The exact content of saliva varies from person to person and from time to time. Secretions decrease during sleep and darkness, and are affected by emotions, drugs, and disease.

The tongue. Plays an important role in speech (try to talk while keeping it still); in taste (see taste buds or papillae above); in eating (chewing, mushing, pushing food to back of mouth for swallowing); and in diagnosing illness.

problem is gone. Bad breath from infected material in gum pockets, pain during chewing, shifting or loosening of teeth, or gum recession, however, may be present. The dentist can detect the current disease state by using microscopic diagnosis and the periodontal probe, a sort of dipstick gently inserted into the gingival crevice, a ditch between gums and teeth. Normally, the ditch is from 1 to 3 millimeters deep; if it is deeper, disease destruction is suspected. Previous tissue destruction can be estimated by x-ray. *Treatment*: Prompt treatment during early stages by a well-trained dentist or periodontist combined with conscientious oral germ control by the individual at home can usually halt and often reverse damage. If the condition reaches a more advanced stage, extensive treatment, including surgery, may be needed. Such treatment is often painful, expensive, and time-consuming, but it can save teeth. *Prevention*: Good personal and professional care, as discussed below.

Tooth loss *Cause*: Dental decay and periodontal disease as well as accident. *Prevention*: Good dental care. *Treatment*: Teeth, like stones in an arch, support one another. The loss of one can upset all the others, eventually leading to further loss. Dentures or some sort of prosthesis—today made of light, comfortable, synthetic materials, molded to fit the individual's mouth—to replace lost teeth are thus vital, even in small children. Should a tooth be broken or knocked loose accidentally, pack the gum with gauze to control bleeding, if any. Preserve the tooth or tooth fragment in a wet cloth or cup of water but do not clean it. Head for the dentist immediately. A broken tooth may be glued together with special dental adhesive, and a lost tooth can sometimes be reimplanted in the gum. Implantation of artificial teeth into gums and bone is being done experimentally.

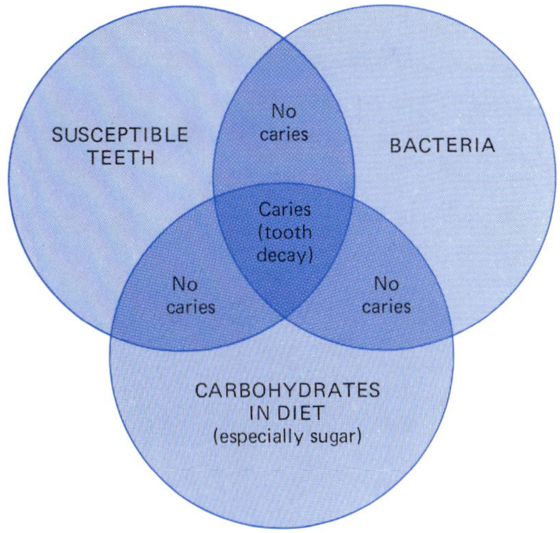

FIGURE 6.2

SELF-CARE

Gums and Teeth

Prevention is primarily the responsibility of the patient and is aimed at eliminating or weakening the effects of one or more of the three elements that contribute to decay (see Figure 6.3) and at the daily removal of the accumulating germ masses that can lead to periodontal disease.

Controlling bacteria The object of oral hygiene is to remove plaque, acid, and food debris, and to disturb the bacteria in the mouth so they cannot regroup for an attack. A good program includes brushing of teeth (Figure 6.4), preferably after each meal but at least once a day, using an effective fluoride toothpaste recommended by the American Dental Association; careful flossing (Figure 6.5) at least once daily; and thorough rinsing after brushing, possibly with a water irrigation device, to wash away debris. Rubber or wood gum stimulators or properly shaped toothpicks should be used only as directed by the dentist. Mouthwashes, chewing gum (even sugarless), apples, and water rinsing are not effective substitutes for brushing and flossing, because they are not effective either in cleaning teeth or in preventing mouth odor. In addition to daily personal care, periodic cleaning—removal of accumulated

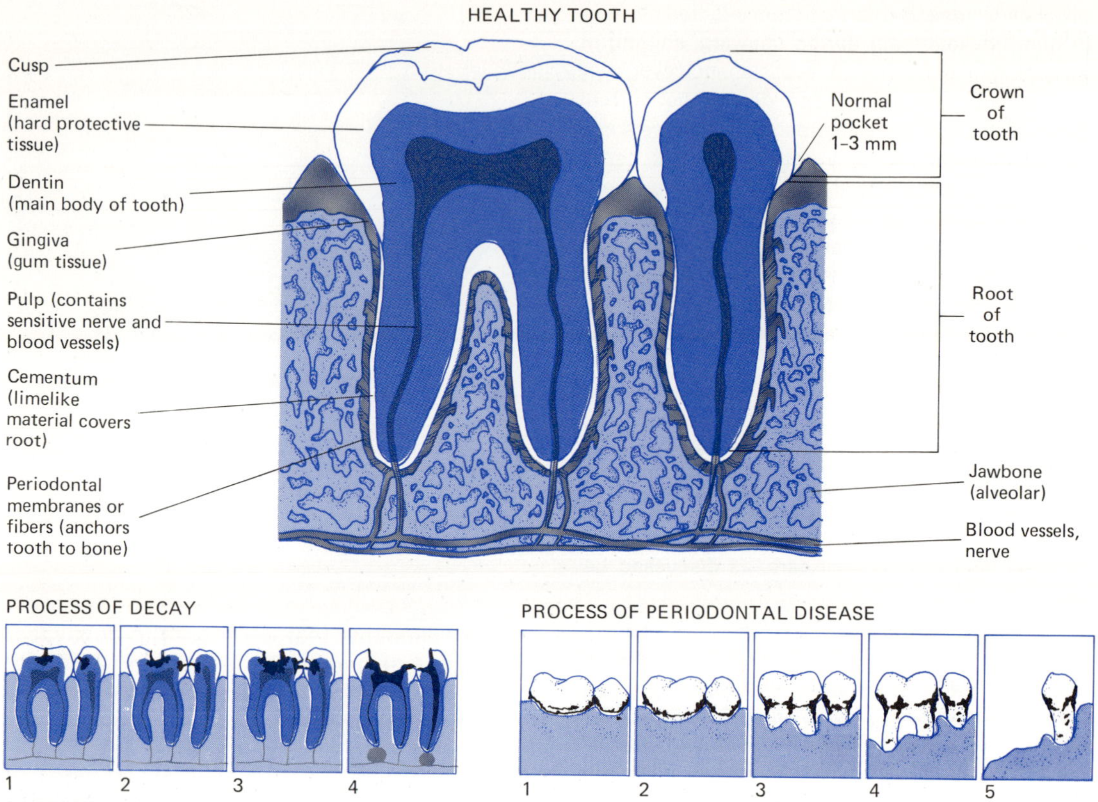

FIGURE 6.3 The human tooth in health (above) and disease (below).

In the process of decay:

1 Acid wears hole in enamel, allowing bacteria to enter dentin.
2 Decay spreads into dentin.
3 Decay attacks pulp, damaging nerve and causing pain.
4 Decay spreads down to tip of root, where abscess may form.

Treatment at any stage can stop the progression of decay. [*DHEW (i), p. 2.*]

In the process of periodontal disease:

1 Irritation causes swollen gums, which bleed easily.
2 The gums begin to withdraw from the teeth.
3 The gums withdraw further, and the disease process reaches the bone.
4 Most of the bony support for the teeth is destroyed.
5 One tooth is lost. Another is weakened.

[*After ADA, a, p. 4.*]

1 Use a brush recommended by your dentist—often a brush with a straight handle, flat brushing surface, and soft, round-ended bristles.

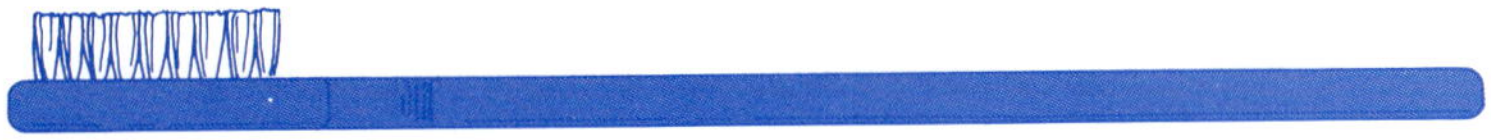

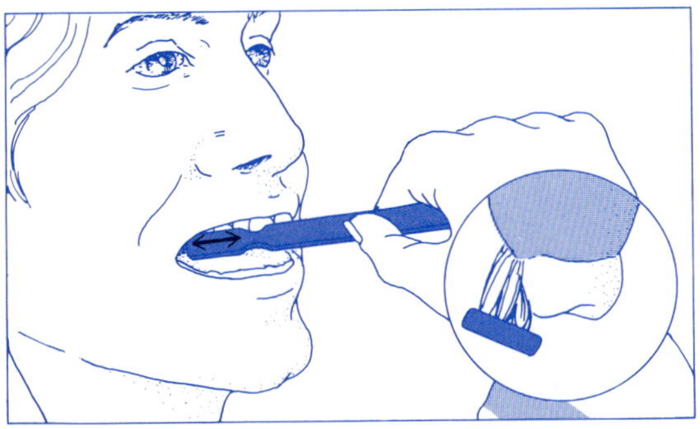

2 Place brush where teeth and gums meet with enough pressure so that you can feel the bristles, but not enough to give discomfort. Brush from side to side (see arrows on brush above). Do a few teeth at a time, using short, careful strokes.

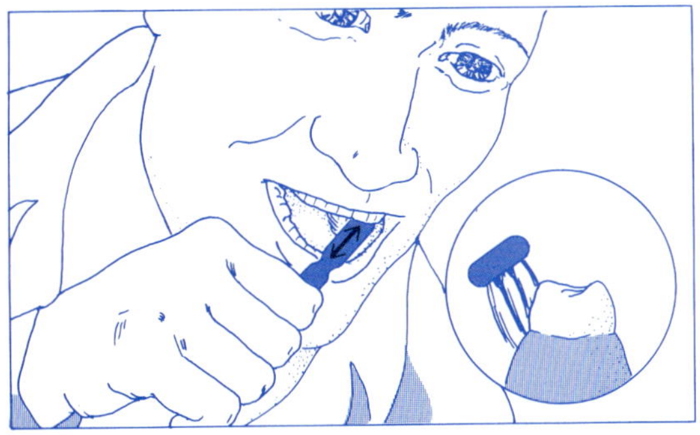

3 Use same method on inner surfaces of the teeth, brushing back and forth in short, careful strokes.

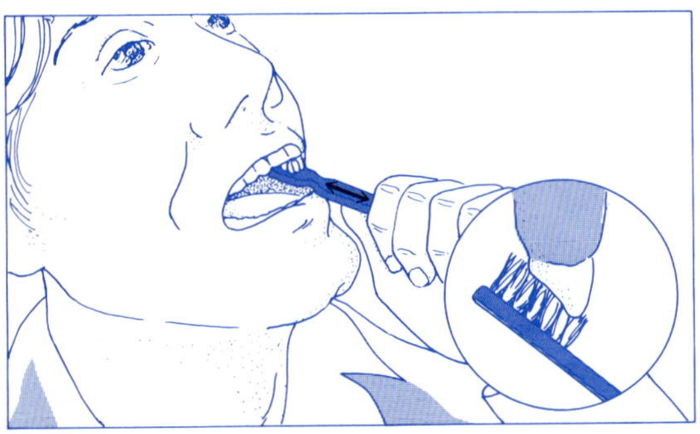

4 For inside surfaces of front teeth, upper and lower, hold brush vertically and brush up and down gently over gum and teeth, using short strokes.

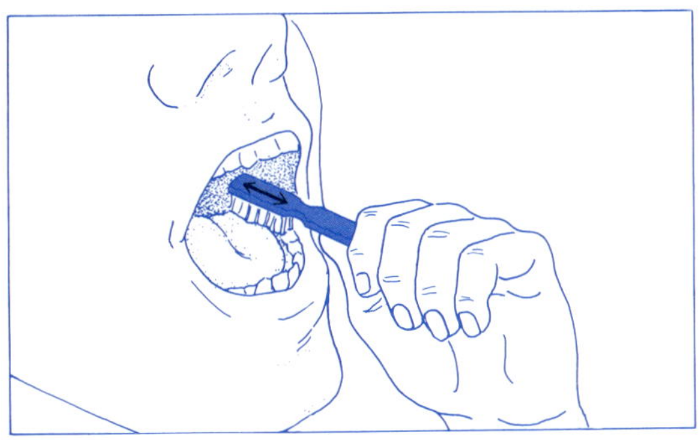

5 For chewing surfaces of teeth, hold bristles flat and brush back and forth.

6 Rinse vigorously after brushing to remove loosened debris and plaque.

FIGURE 6.4 Brushing for dental health. Shown here is the Bass brushing technique, often recommended for removing plaque. Your dentist may recommend another technique. If so, follow his or her directions. [*American Academy of Periodontology, pp. 1–7.*]

plaque and calculus—by the dentist or dental hygienist is necessary.

New weapons aimed at inactivating mouth bacteria, which are being tested but are not ready for routine use, include: a *vaccine* that would provide immunity against caries-causing bacteria and possibly periodontal disease; *enzymes*, to block the production by bacteria of substances harmful to the teeth; *antibiotic agents* that, when given orally, may reduce decay (Scherp; DHEW-*y*). Further study on the rare individuals who never get

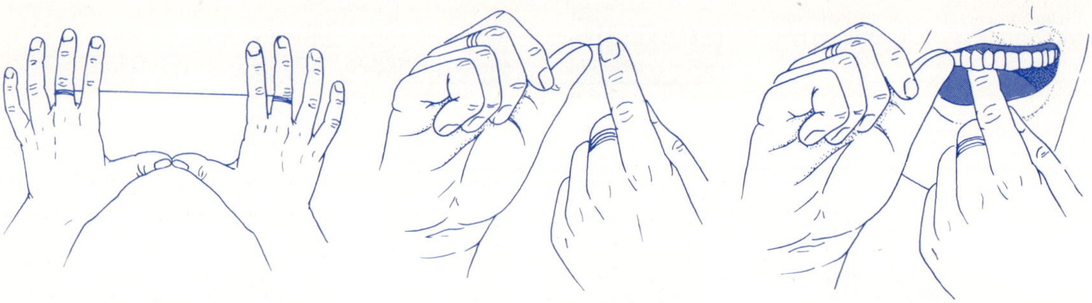

1 Break off about 18 inches of floss and wind most of it around the middle finger on one hand; wind the rest around the middle finger on the other hand.

2 Use thumb and forefinger to guide floss between upper teeth. For lower teeth, use both forefingers. Keep ½- to 1-inch distance between fingers. Do not force or snap; gently saw back and forth to slide floss into place.

3 Curve floss around tooth and gently slide it in between gum and tooth until you feel resistance. Slide floss up and down tightly against side of tooth six times. Repeat for each tooth. As floss becomes soiled or frayed, turn it from one middle finger to the other to bring up a fresh section.

FIGURE 6.5 Flossing for oral health. Continuous practice will increase flossing skill and effectiveness. Some bleeding and soreness are not unusual when you first begin a flossing program. If bleeding continues for more than a few days, consult your dentist. Rinse vigorously after flossing to be certain that all food particles and loosened plaque are removed. [*After American Academy of Periodontology, pp. 7–11.*]

tooth decay and may be caries-immune may yield additional clues to the prevention of decay.

Diet control Diet affects dental health in two ways. First it puts sugar into the three-part picture. Sugary foods—especially those that stick to the teeth (such as caramels) or that stay in the mouth a long time (such as hard candies and gum)—increase *cariogenic*, or caries-causing, activity. Such sweets, if they are eaten at all, should be eaten no more than once a day, as part of a meal. Foods taken between meals should be unsweetened, and preferably should be crisp and require thorough chewing (carrots and celery, for example). Apples and other fresh fruit are more nutritious snacks than candy, but their fructose (fruit sugar) may be involved in caries production. Dried fruit is rich in sugar and has been linked with caries formation; and acid foods, such as citrus fruits and juices, can damage tooth enamel. Teeth should be brushed and rinsed after these foods are taken.

Second, diet affects another part of the caries-formation diagram: resistance. Though resistance also depends upon such factors as heredity, composition of saliva, and possibly the body's defense system, good diet—of the mother during pregnancy when baby teeth are forming, and of the infant while permanent teeth are forming—leads to stronger teeth.

Strengthening resistance with fluorides U.S. Public Health Service studies begun in 1938 have shown that 1 part of the trace mineral fluoride per million parts of water reduces tooth decay in children by about 60 percent. In comparing children in fluoridated Newburgh, New York, with children in unfluoridated Kingston, New York, public health authorities found that 41 percent of

Newburgh 5- and 6-year-olds had no cavities while only 17 percent in Kingston were so fortunate. The mean annual cost for dental treatment was almost 3 times as much in Kingston as in Newburgh (ADA, *c*).

A 1975 fluoridation census by the Center for Disease Control found that 105 million Americans—49.4 percent of the population—live in areas where water is naturally or artificially fluoridated to optimum levels (MMWR, *a*). Millions of others around the world do, too. Though the subject has aroused great controversy—much of it political—about the safety and propriety if not the efficacy of fluoridation programs, dental authorities strongly defend fluoridation as the single most important factor presently known for strengthening resistance to decay.

Though water fluoridation programs are the most successful way to reach large numbers of people, fluorides can also be administered: (1) topically, to the surfaces of the teeth, using ADA-recommended fluoride toothpastes, or in the dentist's office; (2) with concentrated gels in a custom-fitted mouthpiece inserted daily (expensive and time-consuming); and (3) as fluoride tablets, chewed and swished before swallowing, taken regularly.

Sealants to strengthen resistance Fluorides tend to protect against smooth surface caries, but are less effective against decay in the pits and fissures of chewing surfaces. The discovery of organic polymer, a type of plastic that can be bonded to dental enamel, has given dentists their first shield against these cavities. Plastic coatings can protect teeth from acids and bacteria for as long as 5 years, the length of time depending on conditions in the patient's mouth (ADA, *d*).

HEALTH CONSUMER TIP

Selecting a Dentist

The modern dental practice is patient-centered and biologically oriented, with a program of prevention at its heart. Yet there are still dentists who spend most of their time

WHO'S WHO IN HEALTH CARE

Dentistry

Dental specialists All these specialists are required to have a minimum of 2 years of graduate training beyond dental school:

- *Endodontist* Treats the tooth pulp and tissues inside the roots of the teeth.
- *Oral surgeon* Performs extractions or other surgical procedures in and around the mouth; treats fractured jaws, takes biopsies.
- *Orthodontist* Inserts braces and moves teeth to prevent or correct bad bite, i.e., crooked or badly spaced teeth.
- *Periodontist* Treats problems of gum and supporting structures of the teeth.
- *Pedodontist* Treats children's dental problems.
- *Prosthodontist* Designs and fits replacements for lost teeth and parts of the mouth, jaw, and face.

Dental aides

- *Hygienist* Cleans teeth and teaches home hygiene.
- *Assistant* Works closely with dentist, often serving as an extra pair of hands.
- *Laboratory technician* Makes dentures, crowns, and the like.

Bill Anderson/Monkmeyer

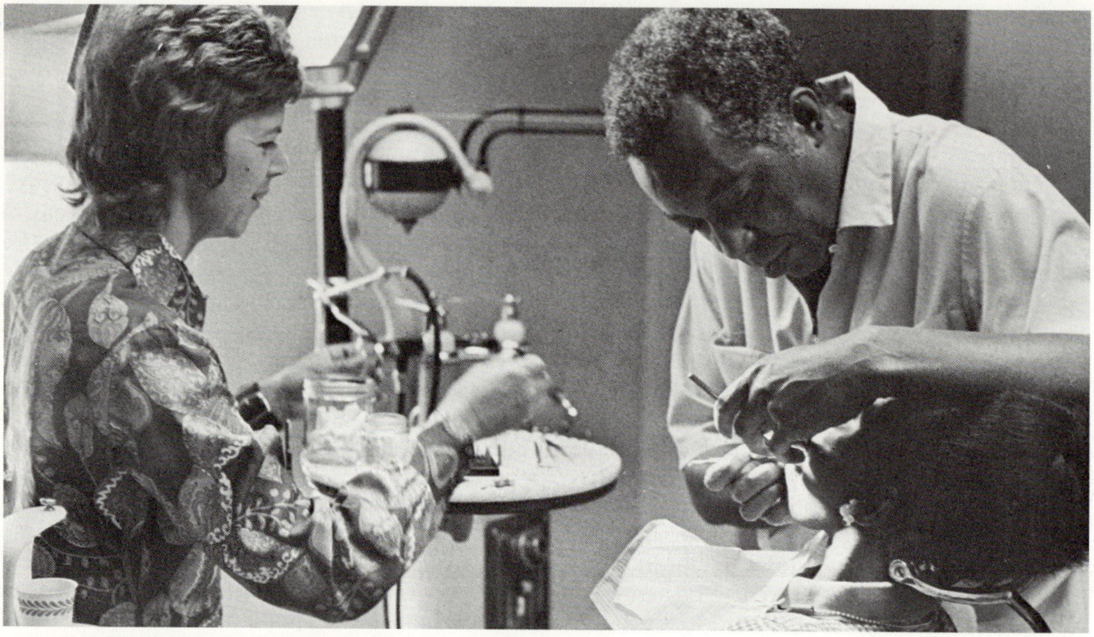

The alert health care consumer selects a dentist who gives a thorough oral examination and is prevention-oriented.

repairing and extracting teeth and pay little attention to prevention. Wary health consumers are learning to identify the minority of incompetent dentists, and in some instances, dental societies are helping.

Names of local dentists are easy to come by from friends, dental associations, or the yellow pages. But there are several things careful health care consumers look for and avoid in evaluating the potential dentist.

They look for the dentist who: (1) takes time to give advice about oral hygiene—how to brush, floss, remove plaque; (2) gives a thorough dental exam (see below), rather than just checking for cavities; (3) explains what is being done and why, offers alternative treatments when they exist, and explains benefits and possible complications of procedures; (4) checks gums as well as teeth at every visit; (5) is well-organized, and spends uninterrupted spans of time with patients.

They are wary of dentists who: (1) refuse to discuss fees in advance or put them in writing; (2) never refer patients to specialists, but do all work—whether or not qualified to do it; (3) are extraction-oriented (removal of a tooth should be viewed as the ultimate dental disaster and every possible effort made to avoid it); (4) appear primarily interested in filling holes in teeth.[1]

Evaluating the Dental Exam

The most effective dental exam includes:

1 A complete medical and dental history so that the dentist is aware of medical problems as well as dental problems.

2 A check of external structures, the jaw joint, and the entire oral cavity for signs of irritations and tumors.

[1]Adapted from *Consumer's Guide to Dentistry*, Connecticut Citizens Action Group in concert with the Connecticut State Dental Association.

3 A thorough examination of all visible tooth surfaces, air-drying them in order to get a better look.

4 A complete examination of gum tissue using the periodontal probe to measure the separation of gum from teeth and detect spontaneous bleeding.

5 Molds of teeth made when necessary for accurate diagnosis.

6 A full set of x-rays every 2 to 3 years (some dentists prefer these more or less often); briefer x-ray survey as needed for diagnosis. A special x-ray shield apron should cover the patient, and x-ray should be avoided if the patient is pregnant.

7 A thorough evaluation of bacterial accumulation on the teeth (microscopic if possible).

8 An explanation of prevention techniques to be carried out by the patient at home.

9 A clearly spelled-out patient treatment plan—explaining what the problems are, what the options for treatment are, and what the cost of treatment will be. Extensive plans should be in writing.

Other Problems in Oral Health

Oral cancer This is the only common oral condition that can be fatal. Of an estimated 15,000 persons with oral cancer diagnosed each year, 7000 die, often because the symptoms go unrecognized, and medical help is sought too late. *Cause*: Primarily, high temperature of smoke from cigarettes, cigars, pipes, aggravated by excess alcohol use. *Treatment*: Drugs, x-ray, surgery. Regular self-examination (see Figure 4.3) and dental checkups may turn up early cancers or precancerous conditions when chances of cure are best.

Orofacial defects

- *Cleft lip or palate* Malformation of the lip or palate occurs in one of every 750 babies born, and may range from mild to very severe, causing difficulties in chewing, swallowing, hearing, speaking, and sometimes breathing. *Cause*: Not definitely known. May be genetic, chromosomal, environmental (x-ray, drugs, poor diet during pregnancy). (See the discussion of congenital defects in Chapter 23.) *Treatment*: New surgical procedures and a multidisciplinary approach aimed at improving the child's and family's emotional health, improving speech and hearing, and correcting dental problems.
- *Malocclusion, or bad bite* An irregularity in tooth position, or in the way teeth fit together when jaws are closed. Occurs most often when permanent teeth erupt, but can occur at any time of life. Can interfere with chewing, detract from personal appearance, and cause strain on jaw joints and muscles leading to pain and deformity. Crowded teeth are hard to clean and especially subject to caries and periodontitis. *Cause*: Can be hereditary—as when a child inherits large teeth from one parent, a small jaw from the other. Also influenced by sucking, biting, tongue thrusting, shifting of teeth due to tooth loss, and possibly, sleeping on the face. *Treatment*: Many mild cases require no treatment. Often, early dental care can avoid later malocclusion problems. Treatment for children and adults is usually provided by a specialist, an orthodontist, who employs a variety of metal or plastic appliances (braces) in order to straighten the teeth and correct their position in the jaws. Treatment may completely eliminate malocclusion, may provide partial improvement, or may not help at all.

Other Common Disorders of the Oral Cavity

Trench mouth Necrotizing ulcerative gingivitis (NUG), most often observed in young adults, and is characterized by: foul breath, inflammation and ulceration of the gums, pain, bleeding, sensitivity to salty and acid foods, increased flow of saliva; sometimes a general feeling of sickness with fever. *Cause*: A combination of bacteria. Poor oral hygiene, poor diet, smoking, and stress may contribute. *Treatment*: Varies depending upon extent and cause of disease. May include: improved diet; better oral hygiene; reduced stress; local treatment of the inflammation with minor surgery, rinses, and calculus removal; sometimes penicillin.

Canker sores *Aphthous stomatitis* (*aphthous* = set afire + *stoma* = mouth) is characterized by burning sores, like punched-out holes with red edges inside mouth and lips, that occur anywhere from once or twice a year to almost continually. Affects twice as many women as men, with heaviest concentration in college age. *Cause*: Unknown, but hereditary element possible. Contributing factors may include stress (cankers are more common during exam periods) and allergies (particularly to acid foods). *Treatment*: Untreated lesions heal in 10 to 14 days. Severe cases may leave scarring. Tetracycline rinses and local anesthetic sprays may be useful; vitamins, special foods, and tranquilizers appear not to be.

Herpes Uncomfortable, often painful fever blister that at first oozes, then crusts over; primary infection consists of whitish blisters inside mouth that may go unnoticed or cause fever and a general feeling of illness. Following the initial attack, the individual continues to carry the virus in a latent (inactive) form and may suffer repeated secondary infections about the nose, lips, and mouth, often following colds, flu, injury, emotional stress or other periods of lowered resistance, or overexposure to sunlight. Rarely, can spread to cornea and brain, more often to genitals. *Cause*: The herpes simplex I virus. *Treatment*: Local painkillers, antibiotics to control secondary bacterial infection, and ointments to soften the crusts are all used to treat, but not to prevent or "cure." Recently, some promising new approaches have been suggested: ether or chloroform applied to the blisters; an antiviral drug, isoprinosine; and *Lactobacillus acidophilus* (used in yogurt cultures) in tablet or capsule form. They all require further study. A treatment using blue dye and ultraviolet lights has been found to be ineffective, and some believe it may possibly lead to cancer.

Herpangina Mild disease characterized by fever, loss of appetite, difficulty in swallowing, and grayish-white papules or pus-filled blisters surrounded by red rings throughout the mouth and throat. *Cause*: A virus. *Treatment*: Fluids, pain remedies, local anesthetic spray.

Bruxism Grinding or clenching of teeth during the day or while asleep, often unnoticed, which may lead to severe facial pain, headaches, stiff neck. *Cause*: Often emotional stress or tension. *Treatment*: Therapy to relieve tension, mouthpiece worn during sleep to prevent damage to teeth, and experimentally, biofeedback.

Impacted wisdom teeth Like malocclusion, impacted wisdom teeth may be the result of inheriting a small mouth from one parent, large teeth from another. If the third molars—which come in at age 17 to 21, when we are presumed to have acquired a share of wisdom—have no room to erupt, pain or other problems may occur. Surgery may be necessary to remove the impacted teeth from the gums.

HOW WE SEE

Actually, it is not our eyes that "see" at all, but rather our brains upon receiving messages from our eyes. As shown in Figure 6.6, the light rays from an image pass through the transparent covering of the eye, the *cornea* (1) or "front window," which helps to focus them. The rays then pass through the *aqueous material* (2), the watery liquid behind the cornea, and through the *pupil* (3), the adjustable opening in the colored *iris* (4). The light next passes through the transparent and flexible *lens* (5) which bends the rays and focuses them, with help from the eye *muscles* (6) which adjust the lens shape.

When the object seen is close, the lens thickens and bends or reflects the light rays quickly. When the object is distant the muscles tug on the edge of the lens, thin it out, and bend the waves more gradually. This function is known as *accommodation*. The focused rays then pass through the colorless, jellylike *vitreous material* (7) which fills the center of the eye and is received by the light-sensitive *retina* (8), the "screen" at the back of the eye, as a sharp upside-down image. When fine work such as reading is involved, the *macula* (9), the pigmented yel-

WHEN TO SEEK CARE

Dental and Oral Problems

Regular exams According to an individualized schedule set up by the dentist: yearly, semiannually, or more often.

Dental emergencies Call the dentist immediately if any of the following symptoms are present:

- *Pain or swelling* In jaws, gums, teeth
- *Pain or swelling* Around neck, ears, head
- *Bleeding* From inside a tooth

Dental problems See the dentist within a week or two if any of the following symptoms are present:

- Appearance of rough surface on tooth: broken teeth; broken filling
- Sensitivity to heat and/or cold, except when in area of recent dental work; sensitivity to sweets (probably indicates decay)
- Dark spots (might be stains, might be decay) on teeth
- Visible deposits of tartar along border of gums and teeth
- Loose teeth
- Red, puffy, sore, or bleeding gums

Early warning signs of oral cancer See a *physician* immediately if any of the following are present:

- A sore on the lips, gums, or inside the mouth that does not heal within 10 days
- Any white patch or color change in the mouth
- Any lump, bump, or swelling in the mouth
- Unusual bleeding in some part of the mouth
- Loose teeth or unusual soreness in the gums
- Pain in the jaw
- Difficulty in swallowing or talking
- Any lump or swelling in the neck or face (that has developed suddenly)
- Numbness of teeth, tongue, or lips
- Any unusual soreness or "burning" in the tongue

low center of the retina, receives the image. The retina is connected to the optic nerve (10), which sends the image to the brain—the "control room"—that turns the image right side up. Then we "see" it—just 1/100 second after the rays first entered the eyes.

SELF-CARE

Prevention of Eye Problems

Because the eye is so important, yet so susceptible to injury, it is designed with built-in protections: fluids constantly bathe it, keeping it moist and clean; lashes shield it from bright

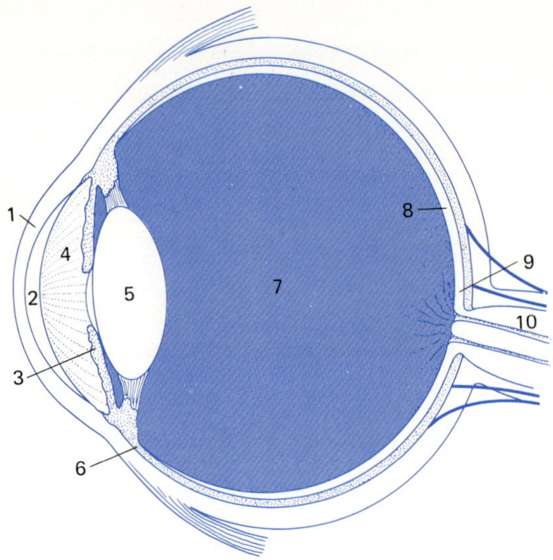

FIGURE 6.6 The human eye: side-view cross section. Parts of the eye are described in text, with references to numbers in the drawing.

light, dust, and dirt; eyebrow shields it from perspiration and other secretions from above; lids blink closed automatically when a strong light (a camera flash, for example) or foreign body (a finger or a gnat) approach suddenly. But natural protection is not enough. Individuals can further protect their eyes by following safety rules recommended by the National Eye Institute:

1 Keep dirty fingers, tissues, sleeves, etc. away from the eyes.
2 Avoid spraying, splashing, or dripping hair tints, dyes, bleaches, sprays, cleaning fluids, glues, insecticides, and chemicals in the eyes.
3 Always follow directions when using eye drops and washes.
4 Be aware of and teach children the dangers of careless use of sticks, BB guns, bows and arrows, fireworks and fishhooks, and of running or riding in a car holding sharp objects.
5 Do not expose the eyes to strong direct light from a sun or heat lamp, or to the sun itself, even during an eclipse. (Sunglasses or special filters *cannot* protect eyes from permanent sun damage.)
6 Avoid eye muscle strain by having lighting come from behind and from either side when reading, sewing, or doing other close work; by staying 5 to 10 feet away from the TV set and keeping eyes on the same level as the screen when watching TV; by resting the eyes by briefly closing them or looking off into the distance every half-hour or so when doing close work or watching TV. (*Note*: Poor lighting, close work, and TV watching do *not* damage vision.)

PROFESSIONAL CARE

The Eye Examination

A schedule of eye examinations for persons with normal vision suggested by the National Eye Institute includes examinations at birth, between $3^1/_2$ and $4^1/_2$ years of age, at puberty, and every 2 years during adulthood, particularly after 40. Persons with vision difficulties or with eye disease will, of course, need ongoing care. Anyone experiencing unusual eye symptoms should make an appointment with a family physician or eye specialist immediately.

The typical eye examination for a person with normal vision has three parts:

1 *Vision examination* Using eye charts and various lenses the ophthalmologist determines whether any vision problems exist and whether corrective lenses are needed.
2 *Medical examination* To determine eye health, and the possibility of such general illnesses as high blood pressure, diabetes, and stroke, most exams include: (*a*) check of optic nerve, blood vessels in eye, macula, and inner sides of eye with an opthalmoscope; (*b*) examination of cornea, the space between cornea and iris, and the iris itself, with a slit-lamp microscope; (*c*) examination of ex-

SELF-CARE

Eye Emergencies

Quick treatment for the following is important:

Speck of dust or other foreign particle in eye Carefully lift the upper eyelid over the lower lid; as the eye begins to water, the "tears" will wash out the speck. If not, the person should be taken to a doctor, a clinic, an emergency room, or an infirmary. *Caution*: Rubbing the eye or pressing on it might scratch the cornea and cause permanent damage.

Burn by flames, acid, or other chemical Remove contact lens, if worn. Rinse eyes immediately with cool or lukewarm water. Do not look for other chemicals to neutralize the first. Tilt the person's head so the eye can be directly under a faucet, or pour clean water into the eye from a pitcher or kettle. Continue washing the eye for 30 minutes. Then get medical help.

"Black eye" or blow to the eye Apply cold compresses (as effective as beefsteak) for 15 minutes (see Appendix). If vision is affected or eye does not begin to improve within 24 hours, seek medical attention.

ternal portion of the eye and surrounding tissues—eyelid, conjunctivae, eye muscles, and reflexes; (*d*) test of eye pressure with tonometer.

3 *Consultation* Discussion of the findings of the examination.

HEALTH CONSUMER TIP

Corrective Lenses

Well-fitted lenses to correct refractive errors can bring about remarkable changes in the lives of those who have endured the frustra-

WHO'S WHO IN HEALTH CARE

Eye Care Specialists

The ophthalmologists Medical doctors with specialized training in care of the eyes, licensed to: diagnose and treat all eye disorders and bodily disorders reflected in the eye; prescribe and fit eyeglasses or contact lenses; use drugs and perform surgery on the eye.

The optometrists Doctors of optometry (O.D.s) who have been educated, trained, and state-licensed to: examine eyes and determine the presence of, but not treat, vision problems, eye diseases, or other abnormalities; prescribe and adjust lenses; recommend visual training when indicated.

The opticians Nondoctors trained to: fill lens prescriptions written by optometrists or ophthalmologists; interpret prescriptions to determine lens specifications; prepare and deliver work order specifications to technicians who grind and mount lenses; and make necessary adjustments of the finished spectacles to fit the wearer. They may *not* examine the eyes or prescribe treatment.

WHEN TO SEEK HELP

Medical Attention for Eye Problems

Get emergency medical attention *immediately* if any of the following occur:

- Sudden loss of side vision
- Sudden blurred or fuzzy vision
- Sudden appearance of moving or floating dark spots (called floaters), a shower of bright "sparks" or "gnats," lightning streaks before the eyes, or the sensation of a curtain being drawn across the inside of the eye
- Double vision

Seek medical attention as soon as possible if you notice any one of the following:

- Gradual loss of side vision
- Gradual blurred or foggy close-up or distance vision
- Itchiness, pain, ache, or burning sensation in or around the eyes, or undue sensitivity to bright lights
- Constant frontal headaches
- Inflamed or puffy eyelids
- Styes, lumps, or growths along the edges of the lids
- Prolonged tearing or discharge from the eye or lid
- Persistent redness in the eye or lids

Make an appointment with your doctor or specialist if any one of the following occurs:

- Inability to see well at night or in dim light
- Need to change glasses more than once a year
- Inability to see printed words clearly
- Heaviness or twitching of eyelids
- Dizziness with or without nausea and headache
- Unusually dry eyes
- Lids stuck together in the morning

Medical attention should be sought for children displaying any of the following:

- Rubbing eyes frequently
- Stumbling or walking into objects often; poor eye-hand coordination
- Shutting or covering one eye regularly; tilting head sideways or forward to see better; squinting, frowning, scowling
- Appearance of difficulty when reading or doing other close work—e.g., holding books very close to the eyes, losing the place often—or avoiding close work altogether
- Blinking, irritability, fatigue when doing close work
- Eyes unduly sensitive to light
- Eyes do not appear straight, are crossed or not aligned
- Apparent inability to see distant objects clearly—e.g., blackboards
- Pupils that appear white rather than black

C. C. Kleinsorge/Editorial Photocolor Archives

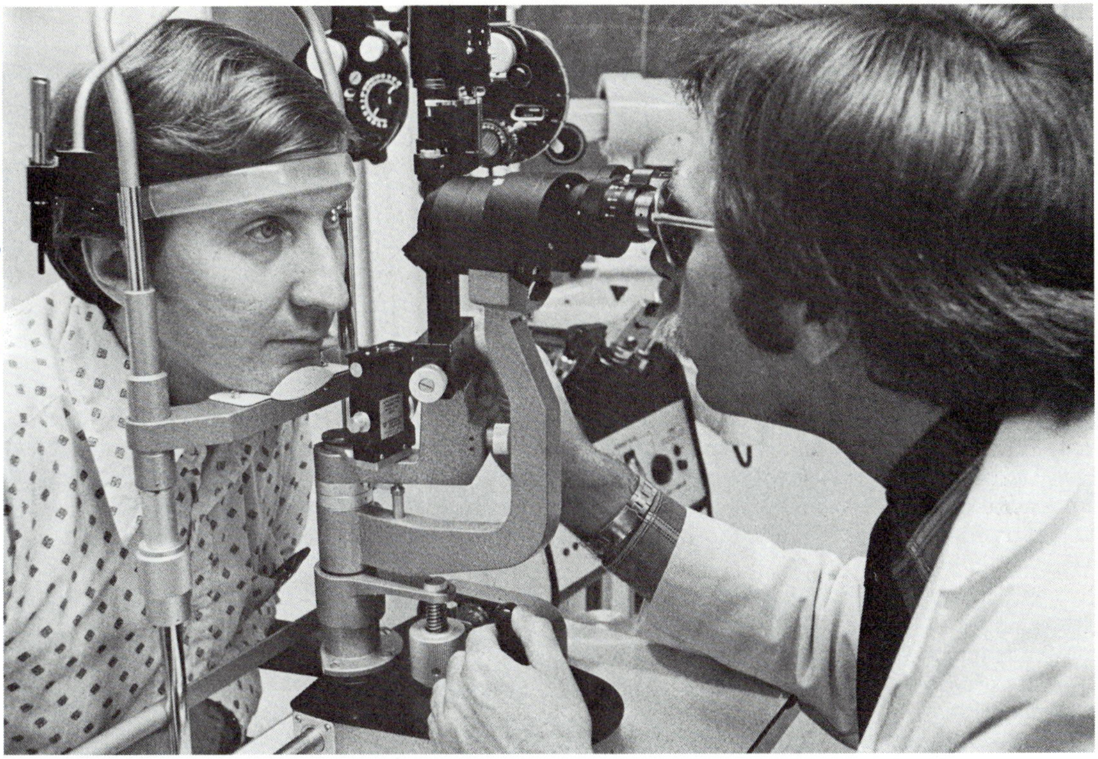

Regular eye examinations are important. They can detect eye problems in the early stages when treatment is most effective.

tion of an out-of-focus world. Corrective lenses can be framed and mounted as eyeglasses, or they can be worn directly on the eyes as contact lenses.

Eyeglasses Only an *ophthalmologist* or *optometrist* should prescribe corrective lenses, and lenses should be worn only by the person for whom they have been prescribed. The prescription is usually filled by an *optician*, who should also be sure that the frames selected are the right size, shape, and weight for the wearer, in order to ensure better vision, comfortable fit, and good appearance. They should rest comfortably on ears and bridge of nose. Federally mandated "impact-resistant" lenses are of three types: heat-treated (tempered) glass or chemically bathed glass—neither of these is shatterproof—and plastic lenses, which have greater impact resistance and lighter weight but scratch more easily. Special protective lenses should be worn by anyone exposed to eye hazards in sports, work, or play. Glasses should be stored in a lined case.

Contact lenses Contact lenses, fitted directly to the cornea of the eye and floating on a layer of tears, may be of rigid plastic or of the newer, more comfortable, softer plastics. The type that is used will depend upon the needs of the individual wearer. These lenses are worn by many for appearance's sake. They may also be recommended for vision disorders better corrected by them than by eyeglasses, or in special situations where they offer comfort, convenience, protection—such as during participation in sports.

Present lenses cannot be worn continuously (for more than 10 to 14 hours) or during sleep without irritation or infection of the eye. However, lenses that can be worn for longer periods are under investigation. Most users alternate between contacts and eyeglasses. Incorrect fitting and improper or unsanitary handling of the lenses can lead to irritation, infection, and discomfort. Contact lenses are *not* suitable for people without a high level of maturity or strong motivation for wearing the lenses; without the manual dexterity needed to handle them; with allergies or chronic respiratory problems; who are exposed regularly to irritants which might get trapped under the lenses; or whose eye structure or visual problems make fitting of lenses impossible.

Glasses to reduce glare Well-styled sunglasses may give the wearer an aura of glamour, but unless the lenses are of good quality, they may be useless in shielding the eyes from the ultraviolet and infrared rays of the sun. They may even cause eyestrain. Sunglasses should be worn only during the daylight hours and out of doors (except on medical advice). They should never be used at twilight or at night for driving or in any other dimly lit place where they might interfere with vision.

To be certain the sunglasses you select are of good quality, check these points:

1 *The lenses* The best lenses are polished or ground, but optical-quality pressed glass or plastic can be adequate. Check for bubbles, streaks, blurs, and distortions by holding glasses at arms length, focusing them on an object with strong vertical and horizontal lines—a door or window frame, for example—and moving them up and down and sideways. If the lines waver through the lenses, there is distortion.

2 *Color* Gray lenses allow the clearest color perception; green and brown tints are also good; pink, blue, yellow, purple, and other "fashion" colors are not effective.

3 *Size and design* Lenses should be large enough to shield the normal angles of vision from glare; side pieces should not be so wide that they interfere with side vision.

4 *Transmission factor* Lenses for general use should transmit no more than 30 percent light; those to be worn at the beach or on the water, where glare is great, should allow only 10 to 15 percent. Check manufacturer's tag.

Eye Disorders of Accommodation

Sometimes the distance between the cornea and the retina is abnormally short or abnormally long, so that even an elastic lens is unable to bend the light rays into proper focus. It is uncertain whether heredity, environment, or both are responsible for these conditions. All can be treated with corrective lenses.

Myopia If the distance between cornea and retina is too great, the person will be nearsighted or myopic—unable to see distant objects clearly.

Hyperopia If the distance between cornea and retina is too short, the person will be farsighted or hyperopic—unable to see near objects clearly.

Presbyopia Difficulty, beginning about age 40, focusing on very near and very far objects. *Cause*: Decreasing elasticity of lens.

Common Eye Infections

Conjunctivitis This condition (called "pinkeye") is an inflammation of the whites (conjunctivae) and lids of both eyes, characterized by swelling of lids, redness, smarting, burning, grittiness, watering, and pus in eyes. *Cause*: Usually an infectious agent, but can be an environmental irritant. *Treatment*: Depends on cause; usually ointments or drops prescribed by a physician. Warm compresses soothe. (See the Appendix.)

Styes Small boils on the eyelid that soften and

burst after a day or two, discharging infectious material, then heal. *Cause*: Infection of an eyelash hair follicle, usually by staphylococcus. *Treatment*: Antiseptics; antibiotics; 15-minute warm compresses three or four times a day; drainage by physician when necessary. *Prevention*: Correction of vision problems; vaccination of patient with own germs.

Serious Eye Disorders

Blindness and visual impairment Some 10 million Americans (1 in 20) are estimated to have an uncorrectible vision impairment. Of these, 1.5 million cannot read a newspaper even with glasses; about 500,000 are considered legally blind—they cannot read the biggest letter on the eye chart at 20 feet. Blindness is the third most frequent disabler of Americans, after heart disease and arthritis (Kupfer). *Causes*: Injury, heredity, birth defects, and most often, eye disease or other illness. *Treatment and prevention*: Early attention to underlying cause; good eye care and safety habits. Rehabilitation for the permanently blind.

Cataract Cloudiness of the lens that worsens progressively; "spots" may be seen. *Causes*: Exact process for most common type—associated with chemical changes in aging—is uncertain; can be congenital, especially following rubella in mother during pregnancy, or may result from injury, infection, chemical irritation, or other eye disease. *Treatment*: Relatively simple surgery to remove the clouded lens is 90 to 95 percent successful. Lens is replaced with contacts or glasses. New ultrasonic (high-frequency sound) technique used in selected cases, particularly in younger patients. *Prevention*: None, except avoiding eye injury and infection, and vaccinating young women against rubella before pregnancy. *Prognosis*: Without treatment, blindness; with treatment, excellent chances for regaining useful vision.

Corneal diseases Cornea becomes scarred or obscured, blocking passage of light to the retina, causing pain, impairing vision. *Causes*: Injury, infection, allergic response, or genetic defect. *Treatment*: Medication; soft contact bandage lens, or replacement of the cornea with a healthy cornea from a donor. *Prevention*: Avoidance of eye injury or infection; prompt treatment if they do occur. *Prognosis*: Blindness or severe disability and chronic pain if untreated; in some types, excellent chance of cure by surgery or medical treatment.

Glaucoma When fluid (the aqueous humor) circulating between cornea and lens fails to drain off properly (see Figure 6.6), pressure builds up and the optic nerve becomes damaged. Warnings include gradual and painless loss of side vision, frequent watering of the eyes, occasional headaches, and a need to change glasses frequently. In acute cases, there is a sudden clouding of vision, and sometimes there is severe eye pain and rainbow halos around lights. Most common in those over 35 with family history of glaucoma. *Causes*: Cause of chronic form unknown; other forms from injury to the eye, complication of other eye diseases, or inborn structural defect. *Treatment*: Surgery for acute form; lifelong medication for chronic type. *Prognosis*: Early treatment often leads to cure of acute cases and stabilization of chronic ones. Irreversible blindness in many untreated cases.

Diabetic retinopathy A disease of the blood vessels of the eye that, in advanced cases, causes bleeding. *Cause*: Diabetes (95 percent of diabetics over 25 affected). *Treatment*: Some believe good control of diabetes minimizes eye damage; lasers and other light beams are used in severe cases to seal small blood vessels and destroy abnormal new ones (photocoagulation). A promising new surgical technique—vitrectomy—is being evaluated. *Prognosis*: Good with treatment; in some untreated cases, blindness.

Childhood Eye Disorders

Amblyopia In this condition (called "lazy eye"), a child sees less well with one eye and depends upon the stronger eye. There may be no symptoms. *Cause*: Unknown. *Treatment*: *Early* detection and treatment—usually with a patch on the strong eye to force use of the weak one—corrects most cases.

Strabismus This problem can take the form of

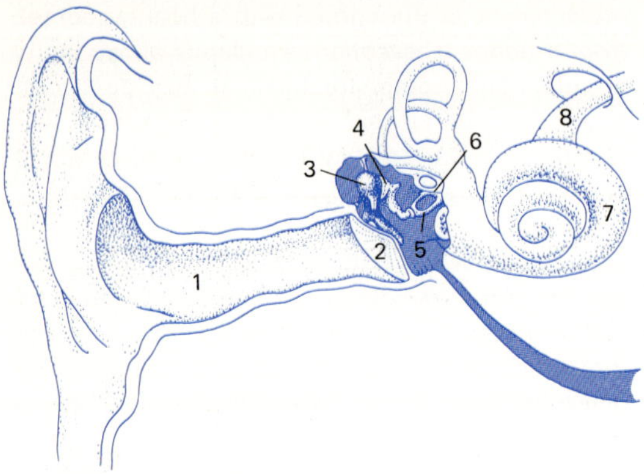

FIGURE 6.7 The human ear. The structures inside the ear are so tiny that the three bones in the middle ear can be held on the tip of the little finger. The whole middle ear is about as big as a string bean seed, about 3/16 by 3/8 inch. The cochlea is even smaller. New developments in microscopic surgery have greatly improved treatment. The text explains the hearing process, using numbers referring to this figure.

cross-eye or walleye. One or both eyes turn in, out, upward, or downward. *Cause*: Heredity, birth defect, or impairment of eye muscles. ("Playing" at cross-eyes can be habit forming.) *Treatment*: Eye exercises, glasses, surgery in severe cases. Condition is not "outgrown." *Prognosis*: If not detected and treated early, can lead to visual impairment, amblyopia.

HOW WE HEAR

As shown in Figure 6.7, sound waves pass through the auditory canal (1) and beat on the eardrum (2), causing vibrations in the chain of three small bones in the middle ear, the hammer (3), the anvil (4), and the stapes or stirrup (5). The stapes, the smallest bone in the human body, fits into the oval window (6) between the middle ear and the inner ear. When the stapes is moved by the vibrations, fluid in the inner ear carries them into the canal of the delicate, snail-shaped cochlea (7).

Inside the cochlea are thousands of sensory cells that are connected to the fibers of the cochlear nerve (8), the nerve of hearing. The movement of the fluid stimulates these cells to generate electrical impulses which are then carried up the cochlear nerve to the brain.

In effect, the sound waves are changed by the ear into electrical nerve signals which are then sent along to the brain for interpretation. A breakdown anywhere along the way—from a blockage in the auditory canal preventing the sound from entering the ear, to brain damage which prevents the brain from interpreting the sounds correctly—can interfere with hearing.

SELF-CARE AND PROFESSIONAL CARE

Prevention of Hearing Loss

Ear examination, with hearing tests for preschoolers, should be part of all regular physicals. Children with undiagnosed hearing loss are often thought retarded because they learn slowly, or disobedient because they do not come when called, or both. Early identification of hearing problems avoids misery and misunderstanding and offers the best chance for treatment, training, or cure.

Symptoms such as severe pain, fullness, ringing, other noise in the ear, loss of hearing, drainage, or discomfort after swimming should be reported to a physician immediately. Delay can lead to severe ear damage, even deafness.

A surprising amount of temporary hearing loss is caused by "wax" in the ears. This wax can easily be removed by a professional or by a lay person instructed by a physician. A very important self-care rule is the old warning: "Never put anything smaller than your elbow in your ear." If an insect should fly into the ear, don't reach in with fingers or cotton swab. Instead, try to lure the bug out with a pencil flashlight or drown it in salad or baby oil. If it doesn't fly or float out, seek medical care.

Ear and Hearing Disorders

Hearing loss Of the 13.5 million Americans classified as "deaf," 2 million are unable to understand speech at all. There are three basic types of hearing loss:

1 *Conductive*, in which sound is muffled because an obstruction (accumulated wax, a forgotten piece of cotton, a bean, or a marble) in the auditory canal or middle ear; a swelling of the eustachian tube caused by a cold or allergy; or damage or deformity of ear structure prevent adequate conduction of sound waves to the inner ear
2 *Sensorineural*, in which hearing is distorted, low pitched sounds are easiest to hear, because of damaged nerve which does not properly convert sound waves into messages for the brain (nerve deafness)
3 *Central*, in which speech may be heard, but sounds are difficult to unscramble because of a flaw in the transmission of sound between cochlear nerve and brain or interpretation of sound in the brain

Causes: Genetic or prenatal influences; viral infections (measles, German measles, scarlet fever, whooping cough, mumps, meningitis); direct blow to the ears; injury to the brain; some medications; atherosclerosis in which blood supply to ears is cut by fat clogging arteries; prolonged exposure to loud noise;[2] and many ear disorders, including those listed below. *Treatment*: Conductive hearing loss can be relieved by removal of obstruction and in some cases by correction of structural defects. Or a hearing aid can be substituted as a conductor of sound waves. There is no known treatment for nerve deafness; acupuncture is *not* effective.

[2]Dr. David Lipscomb of the University of Tennessee's Noise Study Lab, has found progressive hearing loss in young people, apparently related to exposure to loud rock music.

Documerica

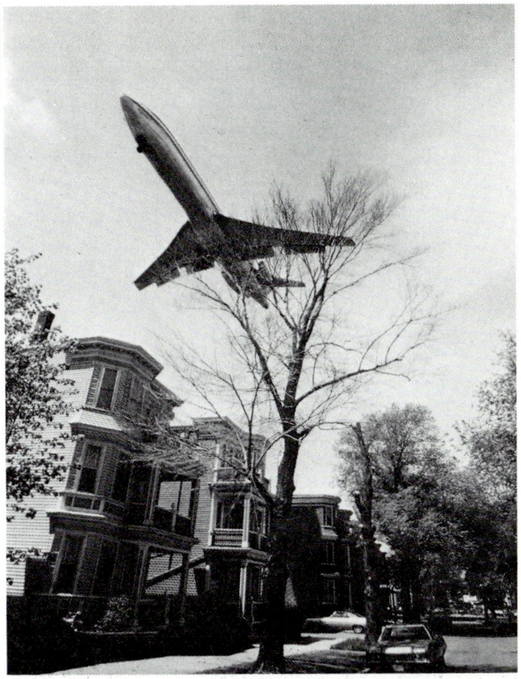

Research indicates that prolonged exposure to high noise levels can lead to hearing loss.

Otitis media (middle ear inflammation) and other ear infections Pain, swelling, and reddening of eardrum. *Cause*: Infectious agent, often secondary to colds, flu, etc. *Treatment*: Prompt medical attention; usually antibiotics to prevent complications such as deafness or possible spread of infection to brain. Aspirin and heat can relieve pain. Those with repeated infections should have follow-up hearing evaluations.

Otosclerosis New bone growth in middle ear that in about 10 percent of cases anchors the stapes (see Figure 6.7) and prevents proper transmission of sound. May cause "ringing." *Treatment*: Surgery to remove the stapes and replace it, often with a fine metal wire, is 95 percent successful.

Acoustic neuroma A benign (noncancerous) tumor, found in about 2 percent of the population, that grows behind the cochlear nerve, occasionally interfering with hearing. Rarely, it can press against the brain, causing damage, even death. Symptoms include ringing or other noise in ear, followed by hearing loss, numbness or pain in face or tongue, unsteadiness, vision problems. *Treatment*: Early diagnosis and surgical removal of the tumor may prevent serious hearing loss.

Presbycusis (*Presbys* = old man, + *akousis* = hearing.) Hearing impairment first noticed in persons over 60. *Cause*: Possible brain aging.

HEALTH CONSUMER TIP

Overcoming Hearing Loss

Early diagnosis and treatment are important. Even infants can be fitted with hearing aids—devices that amplify the intensity of sound waves—enabling them to develop linguistic skills normally. Hearing aids are not effective in every type of hearing loss, and so, whether for children or adults, federal law requires they be sold only when the patient has had a hearing evaluation examination within the past 6 months. The seller is also required to refer to a physician any prospective buyer with signs of ear disease. Though a patient over 18 can waive the examination requirement, it is unwise to use a hearing aid without first being sure that serious, but treatable, disease is not present. Information on hearing aids is available from the FDA.

If a hearing aid does not bring the spoken word into focus, other methods of communication can be used: speech (or lip) reading, sign language and "cued speech," which combines lipreading and simple gestures. The deaf can be taught speech through the use of electronic equipment. Persons who are both blind and deaf may learn to communicate through finger spelling—tracing letters in the palm of the hand—as did Helen Keller, the most reknowned and successful of such doubly handicapped individuals.

A number of electrical devices (such as a doorbell that lights up) may improve the quality of life for those with hearing loss. Friends or relatives can help, too, by speaking clearly, distinctly, and slowly, and by facing the person who depends on lipreading. They can also learn sign language.

THE SKIN

This largest organ in our bodies protects our internal parts against invasion by germs, against injury (absorbs mild shocks), and against drying out from exposure to air. Nearly totally waterproof, skin keeps internal fluids in and rain and bathwater out. In hot weather, it cools through the process of perspiration; in cold weather, blood vessels in the skin contrict, keeping body heat inside. Skin assists in respiration by absorbing oxygen and excreting carbon dioxide. By producing oily sebum, it is self-lubricating. It has a built-in protection against bacterial infection in the form of an "acid mantle," an invisible layer of perspiration combined with amino acids. It also regenerates itself, a particularly welcome trait, since the average person is estimated to suffer more than 4000 minor skin wounds in a lifetime. The skin is flexible at the joints, and is thick and coarse in the most vulnerable places, such as palms and soles. And because each person's skin forms distinctive patterns, prints from the fingers or toes can be used to establish identity.

SELF-CARE

Skin Protection

In spite of its marvelous self-protective mechanisms, the skin needs some help to stay in top condition.

Cleansing Removing dirt, sweat, bacteria and other microorganisms, oil secretions, normal skin scaling, and air pollutants from the skin is important to its health. Oily skin responds well to thorough washing with soap and water twice a day. Dry or normal skin will do better with a nondrying cleanser.

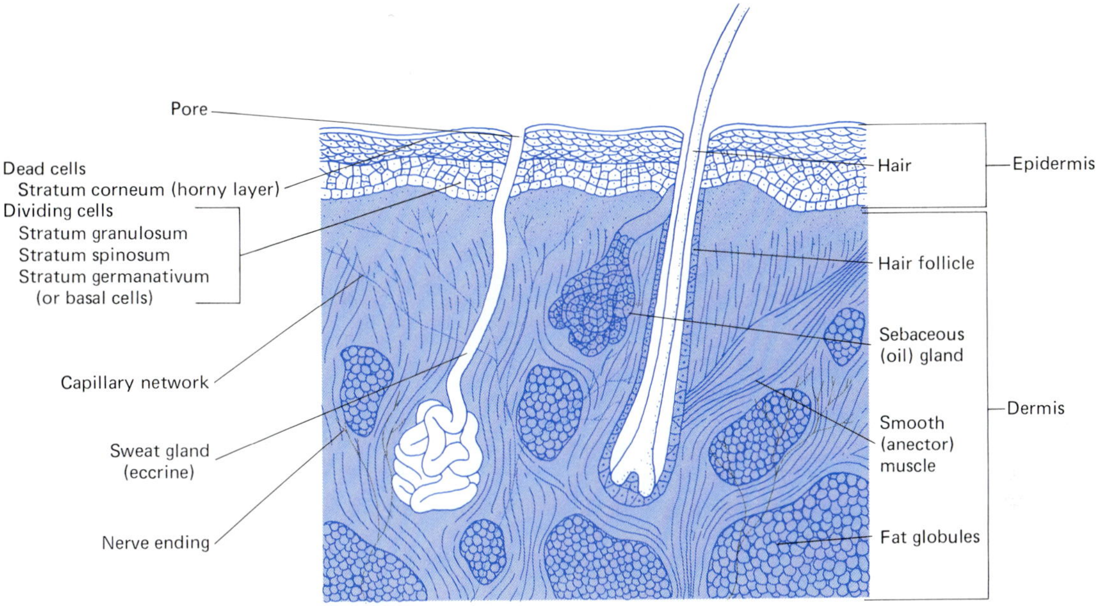

FIGURE 6.8 Cross section of a tiny area of skin. This drawing is much enlarged and very simplified. We realize how very complex the skin is when we know that in each square inch—and the average person has some 21 square feet of skin—there are approximately 650 sweat glands and 95 sebaceous glands, 65 hairs and muscles, 78 nerves with 1300 nerve endings, 13 sensory apparatuses for cold and 78 for heat, 160 pressure apparatuses for the sense of touch, 20 blood vessels, some 19,500,000 cells, as well as a variety of connective tissue and other materials. Microorganisms (such as bacteria) dwell in pores and follicles and on skin surface.

The epidermis, the outer layer of skin, is seen at the top of the drawing. It reproduces itself during a cycle of about 25 or 30 days. New cells are developed in the basal layer and then move upward during the cycle until they reach the top layer and are sloughed off as dead cells.

Preventing odor Deodorants and antiperspirants help reduce odor produced by the action of bacteria on the secretions of the sweat (apocrine) glands. But daily bathing (or showering) with soap and water does a better job because it removes some of the bacteria. Special attention should be paid to the areas with the greatest number of sebaceous glands (face, chest, back) and those where the apocrine glands are located (armpit, genital areas). In winter, however, daily bathing may be drying and may contribute (along with overheating and underhumidification) to "winter itch." Using oils or lotions in bathwater or following a shower, or using cold-cream-based soap, or bathing less often and using soap only in odor-producing areas may counteract drying.

Moisturizing Skin that is naturally dry, aging, or ravaged by sun, wind, or drying hot air needs moisturizing to keep it soft and smooth. Nongreasy moisturizers should be rubbed in well on flaky, dry skin. There is no evidence that "rejuvenating" creams containing such "miracle" ingredients as royal jelly or hormones bestow additional benefits. Some may be harmful.

Good health habits Things that tax general health also take their toll on the skin: too little rest, poor diet, emotional stress, extreme weight fluctuations.

Protection from sun damage The sun, in many ways, lives up to its reputation for being health-giving: it nourishes plant life that provides most of the world's food; indirectly it provides vitamin D; it can aid in the treatment of acne and other skin disorders; and it promotes a feeling of well-being. But our fair-weather friend is estimated to be responsible for 1 of every 3 visits to the dermatologist. Its short ultraviolet rays are the major cause of skin cancer and of wrinkled, aging skin. The sun is guilty, too, of promoting freckles, "liver spots," and actinic keratosis, the red scaly spots that, untreated, turn into cancer 20 percent of the time.

It is possible to tan without burning and damaging the skin by following these rules:[3]

1 Avoid exposure between 10 A.M. and 2 P.M. (between 11 A.M. and 3 P.M. daylight savings time), when the sun's burning rays are strongest.
2 Make your first exposure of the season brief—about 15 minutes. If you don't burn, increase the time gradually each day. If you begin exposures in April, you should be ready for full summer sun by mid-June.
3 Use a good sunscreen lotion, containing para-amino-benzoic acid (PABA), designed to filter out the short ultraviolet rays (the burning rays) while allowing the long ultraviolet rays (the tanning rays) to penetrate. Apply it frequently, especially after swimming.
4 Remember you can get a burn on a hazy day, while in the water, or while being cooled by ocean breezes, especially near sand or water.
5 Since some drugs increase sun sensitivity, check with your doctor if you are on medication.

If you do get a light burn, aspirin and cold compresses (see the Appendix) will help to relieve discomfort. If you get a severe burn, call your physician.

[3]Adapted from *Patient Care.*

HEALTH CONSUMER TIP

Cosmetics and Your Skin

The overall safety of cosmetics is considered to be quite good. Yet there have been reports of both mild and serious reactions to their use—most often to deodorants. Manufacturers are not required to prove the safety of their cosmetic products or to report any ill effects they may have. The purchaser must beware. The new labeling law that went into effect in 1975 made it easier for the consumer to evaluate a product and to be alert to ingredients to which he or she is sensitive. Do not rely upon "hypoallergenic" on the label. That only means that the perfuming agent has been removed. No cosmetic can offer 100 percent protection against allergic responses.

To home test a cosmetic for allergic reactions, place a small amount of the product on the skin and cover with a gauze patch for 24 hours. If an irritation develops, avoid use of that product and of other products containing the same ingredients. Test hair dyes, bleaches, and depilatories as suggested on the packages. Any time you think irritation, redness, itching, or tearing of the eye has developed because of a product, stop using it. Report the reaction to the manufacturer and to the Food and Drug Administration (5600 Fishers Lane, Rockville, Md. 20852). If the irritation persists, see your physician.

Cosmetic irritation can also occur owing to

carelessness: using dirty or spoiled cosmetics or applicators, using saliva to moisten makeup, applying makeup with dirty hands, or sharing cosmetics.

Skin Disorders

Acne Affects nearly everyone at some time, with blackheads, whiteheads, and pimples. Medical care required in 15 percent of cases. Most common between puberty and young adulthood, but can occur at any age. *Causes*: Not completely understood. Blemishes form when canals—through which oily sebum flows to skin surface—become blocked. Several elements are definitely related: heredity; excess of circulating male hormone (androgen) in relation to female hormone (estrogen); presence of corynebacterium acne; emotional stress; certain cosmetics and drugs. Foods (even chocolate, nuts, and greasy hamburgers) are *not* a cause of acne in most people.[4] Nor are unwashed skin, masturbation, sexual relations, lack of sexual relations. Hand-to-face contact probably plays only a minor role. *Treatment*: Cure is not known, but control is almost always possible. *Home remedies for mild acne*: Gentle washing (not scrubbing) twice a day; cleansing following heavy exercise; frequent shampooing to keep hair oils from spreading to face; nutritious diet free from foods that seem to trigger a breakout; hot water soaks for the occasional pimple to bring blood and thus more white blood cells to the area to clean up debris; avoidance of picking and squeezing, which may lead to scarring; removing noninflamed blackheads (only under directions of physician or with a commercial blackhead preparation); using nonprescription acne medications with *nonoily* bases that dry the skin (if skin becomes too dry, or peels, stop use for a few days and then resume); taking vitamin B_6 to stave off premenstrual breakouts. (Vitamin A may be useful in some types of acne but helpful doses are so large they may be dangerous.) If none of these home treatments works, professional help from the family doctor or a dermatologist—skin specialist—should be sought without delay. *Professional treatment for severe acne*: Prescription lotions, ointments, pastes applied to the skin—especially vitamin A acid (retin A) and/or benzoyl peroxide, which make the skin worse before it gets better, usually in six to eight weeks; antibiotics, particularly tetracycline,[5] which reduce the number of corynebacterium acne on the skin—used only when benefits outweigh risks of side effects; female hormones—given only to mature women who do not respond to any other treatment (the usual warnings for oral contraceptives hold); injection of certain drugs into inflamed lesions. *Prognosis*: Acne, untreated, can leave both psychological and physical scars.

Psoriasis A chronic, noncontagious skin disorder that affects an estimated 4 to 8 million Americans to some degree, most often fair-skinned persons between 15 and 35. Usually begins with a few red pinpoints followed by white scales that build on top of them. It appears that the normal process of skin cell death and production is speeded up, leading to imperfectly formed cells that scale off. The breakdown in the normal protective layers of skin leads to cracking and bacterial infection. *Cause*: None known, but several suspected. *Treatment*: Various drugs, coal tar baths, ointments covered with plastic wrap, can often bring remission. Use of psoralen pills plus light has promise as a replacement for these treatments for severe psoriasis. *Prognosis*: Untreated, severe psoriasis can be disabling; even mild cases can bring embarrassment as well as physical, psychological, economic, and social difficulties.

Skin cancers The most common and, except for melanoma, the least lethal of all cancers. There are three basic types: (1) *basal cell carcinoma*, most common and least dangerous, does not spread to other parts of the body and is not fatal, but it is disfiguring and should be treated; (2) *squamous cell carcinoma*, a slow-growing cancer on the smooth skin of the body, fast-growing and dangerous in the mucous membranes and linings of the internal organs; (3) *melanoma*, the "black cancer," the most feared of all skin cancers. A high propor-

[4]Kelp and seaweed products, extremely high in iodine, may, however, be linked to acne (Kanunester).

[5]Do not take tetracycline with food or vitamins. Take at least one hour before or two hours after meals.

tion arise in preexisting, flat black moles; they spread rapidly and are extremely resistant to cure. *Causes*: Most often, excessive exposure to sunlight or radiation. *Treatment*: Early detection through self-examination (see Figure 4.2), with careful attention to the warning signs below. Basal cell and early squamous cell carcinomas can be removed surgically. Late squamous cell carcinomas and melanomas are treated by many anticancer techniques including chemotherapy (drug therapy). (See Chapter 10.) *Prevention*: Avoidance of overexposure to sun and radiation. Prompt removal of pre-cancerous lesions.

Moles Flat or raised, smooth or hairy, from light brown to black in color and varying in shapes, these masses, spots or stains on the skin may stay the same for years, grow, or fade away. *Cause*: Believed genetic, but often do not appear until adolescence. *Treatment*: Disfiguring or annoying moles can be removed with electric current, heat, acids, or surgery. *Prognosis*: Most moles are benign (harmless), but if a mole changes shape or color, oozes, bleeds, or forms a crust, it should be examined by a physician.

Warts These horny growths appear most often on fingers, hands, on soles of feet (plantar warts, which are pushed into the skin and are painful). *Cause*: A virus transmittted from person to person or place to place on the same person, particularly through picking, scratching, biting, shaving. *Treatment*: Electrosurgery, freezing with dry ice or liquid nitrogen, use of acids or ordinary surgery. Should *not* be self-treated.

Boils Painful pus-producing inflammations of the skin (feruncles) centered around a hair follicle or oil gland, red and warm to the touch. *Cause*: Microorganism, usually staphylococcus. *Treatment*: Hot compresses (see Appendix); antibiotics or surgical drainage in more severe cases. Recurrent boils may signal underlying disease, such as diabetes.

Pigmentation problems Patches of deeper color (liver spots or chloasma) or absence of skin color (vitiligo). *Causes*: Uncertain; but liver spots are related to aging, endocrine disorders, sun exposure. *Treatment*: Difficult. Freezing or electrosurgery may remove liver spots; psoralen plus light treatment *may* bring back pigment in vitiligo.

Eczema, rashes, hives Allergic reactions showing up in skin. *Cause*: Foods, dyes, or other chemicals in clothing, cosmetics, earrings (containing nickel), poison ivy, etc. (See the discussion of allergies beginning on page 178.)

Fungal diseases Most common is *tinea* or ringworm, including "jock itch" and athlete's foot. *Cause*: Fungi. How spores are spread is not always clear, but moist, infected objects or other people are possible sources. *Treatment*: Varies with type of fungus and location. Keep area clean and dry and, when possible, exposed to light and air. Tinactin cream or other fungicide will help in most cases but must be used for long period after symptoms disappear to be certain all spores have been destroyed.

Mites and lice Head lice (transmitted by combs, brushes, hats, person to person), body lice (associated with poor personal hygiene), pubic lice (sexually transmitted), and scabies (mites transmitted by intimate body contact, bedding, towels, etc.) are all parasites that cling to and live in human skin. Can cause intense itching. *Treatment*: Prescription insecticide lotion, cream, or shampoo or nonprescription pyrethrins with poperonyl butoxide. Close contacts should also be treated, bedding and clothing washed in hot water or dry-cleaned, upholstery vacuumed.

THE HAIR

The hair is a part of the skin organ. It protects the head and scalp from sun and cold and is an excellent barometer of general health. Drab, listless hair, or hair that suddenly begins to fall out, may often be a sign of some physical or emotional illness. Microscopic and chemical studies of the hair may help in medical diagnosis.

WHEN TO SEEK HELP

Warning Signs of Skin Cancer

1 Know your skin. The average individual has forty noncancerous (benign) skin markings or tumors—moles, "freckles," "beauty marks," skin tags, warts, and the like. Become familiar with yours, their sizes, colors, locations, even those in hard-to-see spots such as soles of feet and back. (Use a mirror.)
2 Watch for changes, checking every three to six months.
3 See your family doctor, a dermatologist, or the college health service if you discover any of the following:

- Any new growth
- Change of color or shade in any existing mole or lesion
- Growth or change in size or shape of existing lesion or mole
- Development of rough or scaly "sunspots" or "red moles" on areas exposed to light
- Development of itching, burning, pain in any existing or new lesion

Do not delay. *Early treatment is important!* Many lesions can be removed before they become cancerous. And do not panic. Skin cancer has a 95 percent cure rate when discovered early.

Hair Care

Good diet, exercise, positive health habits, and shampooing as often as necessary (even daily) to keep hair clean are routes to healthy hair. Conditioners can be used to replace lost oils. Hair should be brushed just enough to keep it neat and untangled; too much brushing can be harmful. Teasing, tying with tight bands, excessive heat, bleaching, and color rinsing can also ruin hair texture temporarily.

The best shampoo to use varies from person to person and often alternating a variety of shampoos is better than sticking to just one. None of the "miracle" ingredients-of-the-month have been scientifically proven effective. FDA regulations require safety testing, but not testing for effectiveness.

Hair Problems

Hair loss—normal An estimated 50 to 150 hairs are lost each day in the normal shedding process, and the same number is replaced each day except during pregnancy or while taking oral contraceptives. (The hair is finally shed in large quantities three to six months after delivery or after the pill is discontinued.)

Hair loss—sudden, excessive *Cause*: Medication or drug use; physical or emotional trauma; insult to the body such as starvation or serious illness; use of irritating hair sprays or dyes. *Treatment*: Elimination of the cause allows hair to grow back normally.

Hair loss—hereditary "pattern" baldness Slow, progressive, permanent loss of hair is called "alopecia." In males, loss follows one of several patterns (loss at temples or at crown of head, for example); in females, there is usually a general thinning. *Cause*: Believed to be an excess of male hormones; usually hereditary. *Treatment*: Most treatments—from manure to mayonnaise, from lotions and vitamins to special brushes and electrical stimulation—are worthless. Two new procedures, however, offer hope:

1 *The hair transplant* This is an accepted and safe procedure in which plugs of skin, with about six hairs each, are punched out of the back and

sides of the head where hair is usually plentiful and "plugged"—much like zoysia grass—into the balding hair line. Performed by a dermatologist, the procedure is tedious, painful, and expensive, but the only sure way of reversing hereditary pattern baldness. It is not generally recommended for young men.

2 *Estrogen ointment and shampoo* This is still experimental. The female hormone, estrogen, taken internally, is known to restimulate hair growth—but it also stimulates growth of secondary female characteristics, such as breast tissue. Recently, however, a New York physician reported success—particularly with younger men—using an estrogen ointment and shampoo (Settel). If his results can be duplicated, baldness may become a thing of the past.

Dandruff A scaling of dead skin cells around hair follicles—anywhere on the body, but especially on the scalp. Occurs on both oily and dry scalps. It appears most often in brown-eyed brunettes, and there may be a familial and racial predilection for the condition. It appears to worsen in winter and under physical and emotional stress. *Cause*: Not known. *Treatment*: No known cure, but condition can be controlled. For mild cases, use of a commercial dandruff shampoo, which decreases cell production and resulting scaling, is often effective. Resistant conditions, and those in which itching and redness are present, may indicate more serious disease and require the attention of a dermatologist or other physician.

THE BACK

SELF-CARE

Prevention of Back Problems

Back problems can often be prevented by keeping muscles strong through exercise (see Figure 6.10). It is helpful, too, to maintain good posture (see Figure 6.11); to sleep on a firm mattress; to avoid overdoing, overbending, overlifting, and overfatigue; and to avoid positions that encourage backache (Figure 6.12). Keeping the knees bent when one is on one's feet a great deal and during sleep can relieve strain on the back. So can taking walking breaks when sitting for long stretches.

Common Back Problems

Backache Pain in the lower, middle, or upper back and neck (sometimes "referred" to legs, thighs, arms, and shoulders) is one of the most common human ailments. *Causes*: Many, known and unknown. The major cause (an estimated 80 percent) is weak abdominal muscles (Kraus). When these muscles, which support the back, are weak, or are pulled off center as in pregnancy or overweight, the spine becomes unbalanced, leaning forward slightly. This strains the stronger back muscles, causing them to become fatigued and painful. Other causes include poor posture (particularly lordosis or sway back); sitting for long periods, as when studying, typing, sewing, reading, driving; emotional tension, which can trigger muscle spasms ("a pain in the neck" or "a pain in the backside"); unaccustomed or incorrect use of the back in lifting or bending, or other stressful activities; or injury which results in a "slipped disc." Actually, the disc does not slip. (See Figure 6.9.) Rather, it is forced out of shape when two vertebrae are pinched together, usually as a result of strain too great for the muscles to handle. Less common causes of back pain are serious diseases like arthritis, ankylosing spondylitis (which occurs most often in young adult males, causing bony "freezing" of the spine and other joints), osteoporosis (a loss of bone tissue, common in elderly women, that results in brittleness). *Treatment:* Depends on cause. Liniments and patent medicines are of little or no value except as temporary pain relief. Prescribed muscle relaxants, tranquilizers, or other medications help when tension or muscle spasm is the cause. Exercise programs will help almost all types of backache. Hospitalization with traction (weights attached to head and feet so the body can be gently but steadily stretched, taking pressure off the nerves and bones and loosening up tight, cramped back muscles) is required in severe cases.

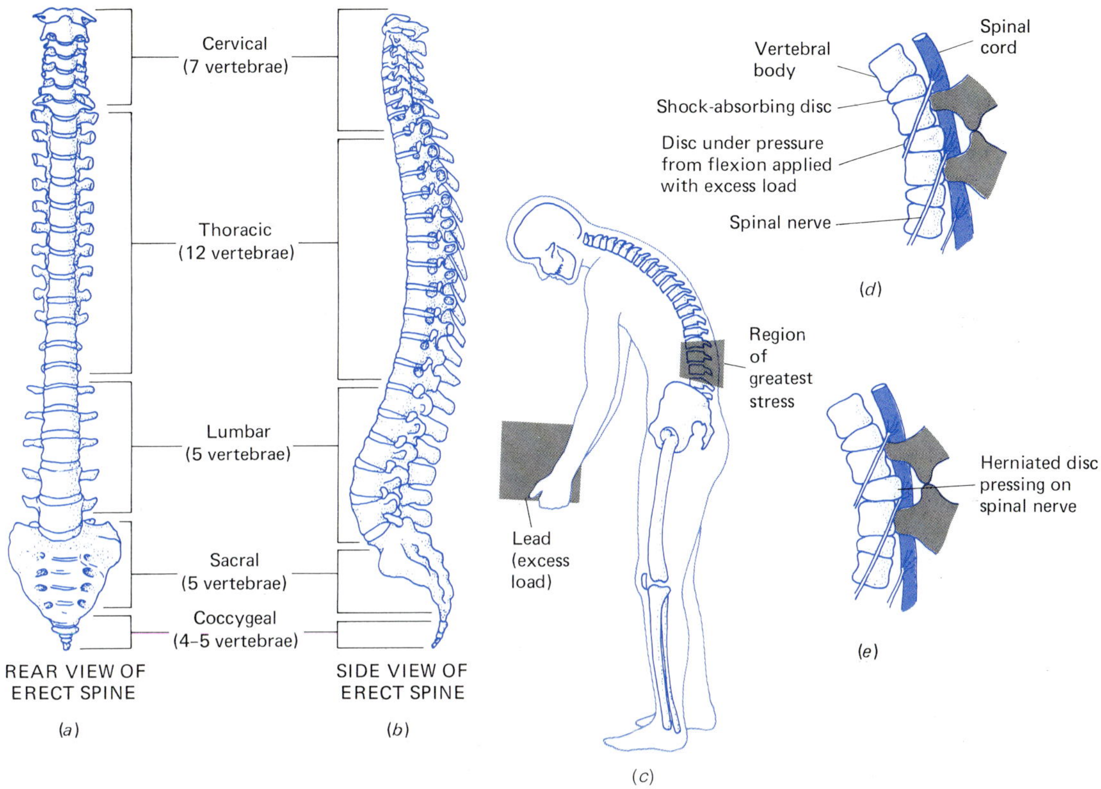

FIGURE 6.9 The human spine. (*a*) Rear view of erect spine. (*b*) Side view of erect spine. (*c*) Side view of spine bending incorrectly to lift a load—which could result in a ruptured disc (*e*). (*d*) To allow spine to bend and twist—and to cushion shocks—each vertebra is separated from the next by a shock-absorbing disc which has an oval center of springy cartilage and an outer covering of tough, heavy tissue. [*After Elson, p. 438.*]

Surgery, not always successful, may be suggested as a last resort.

THE FEET

The 52 bones of the feet support us in all our endeavors. When the feet are unhealthy, the result can be pain, fatigue, irritability, and the disruption of the pursuit of everything from buses to happiness.

SELF-CARE

Avoiding Foot Problems

Most foot problems, including athlete's foot, can be avoided by proper foot care. (The first six suggestions below are especially important in warding off athlete's foot.)

1 Give feet as much sunlight and fresh air as possible. Wear open or perforated shoes in warm weather, so that air can flow around

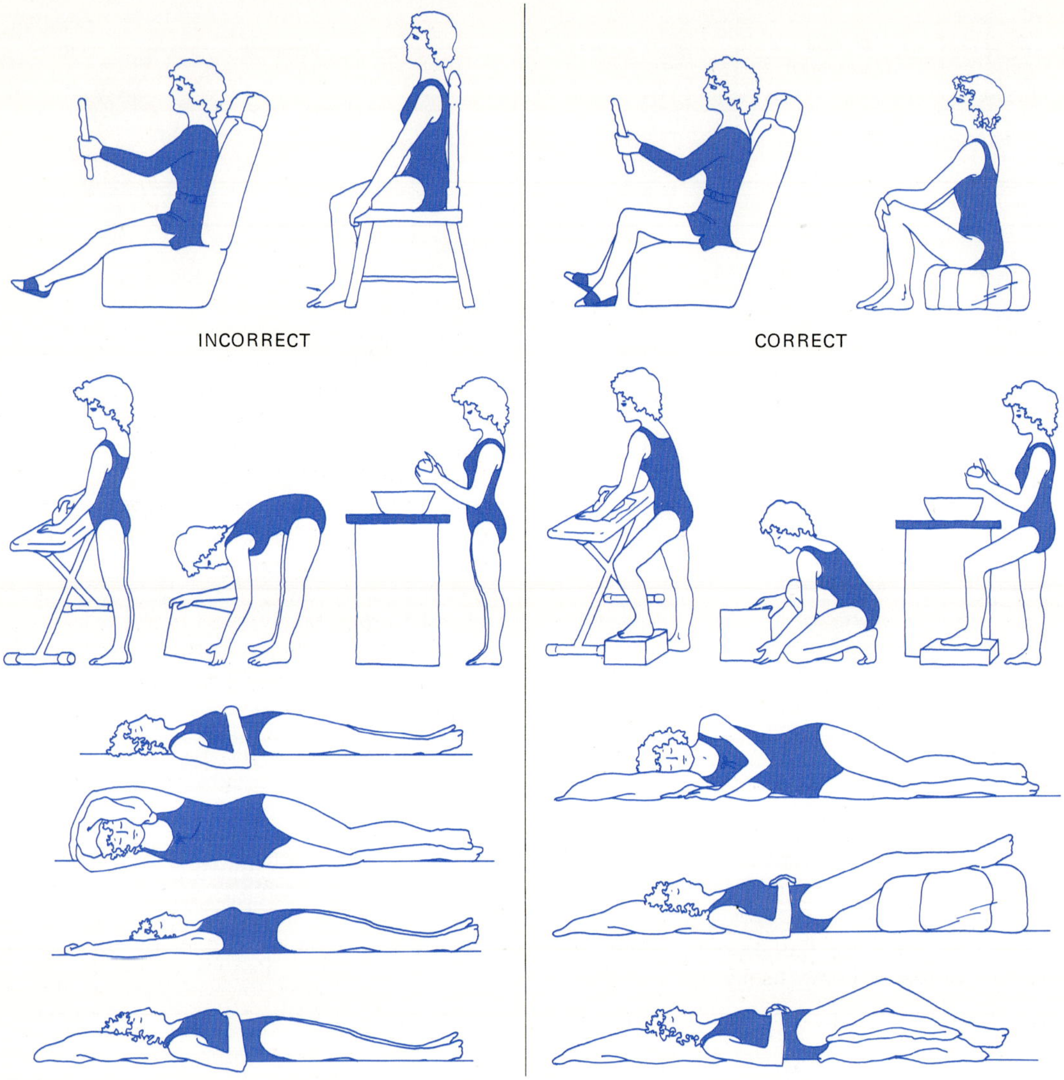

FIGURE 6.10 Incorrect and correct posture. [*Adapted from photos in Ishmael and Shorbe, pp. 10–16.*]

FIGURE 6.12 (*Opposite page*) Testing back health: Kraus-Weber tests for evaluating key muscle groups in the body. If you have back trouble or other health problems, be sure to check with a physician before testing yourself. [*Adapted from Kraus, pp. 90–94.*]

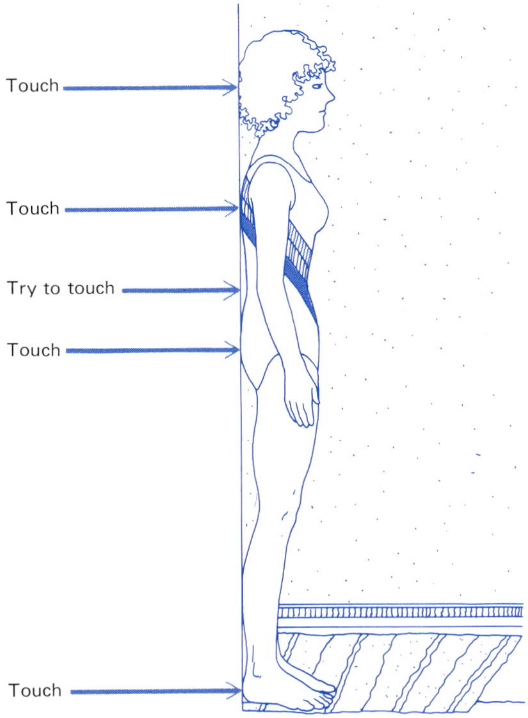

FIGURE 6.11 Good posture exercise. Stand with your back to the wall as shown here. Touch the wall with your head, shoulder blades, buttocks, and heels. Imagine a balloon attached to the top of your head gently pulling it up. At the same time, pull in your stomach muscles and tighten your buttocks muscles to bring them forward and down. Try to touch the small of your back to the wall. (If sand were poured into the back of your gym shorts, it would slide directly down into the heels of your sneakers.) Once in position, walk away from the wall, keeping yourself erect. Maintaining good posture feels awkward and difficult at first, but practiced regularly, it becomes easy and comfortable. [*Adapted from Kirk.*]

SELF-CARE

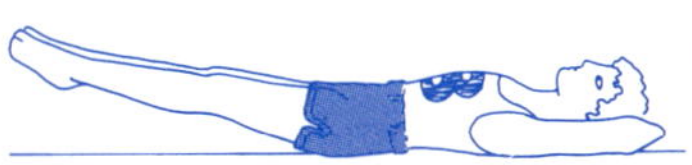

1 *Hip flexors*: Lie flat on your back on the floor with your hands clasped behind your neck and with your legs straight and touching. Now keep your knees straight and lift your feet so that your heels are 10 inches above the floor, as shown in the drawing. Hold for 10 seconds.

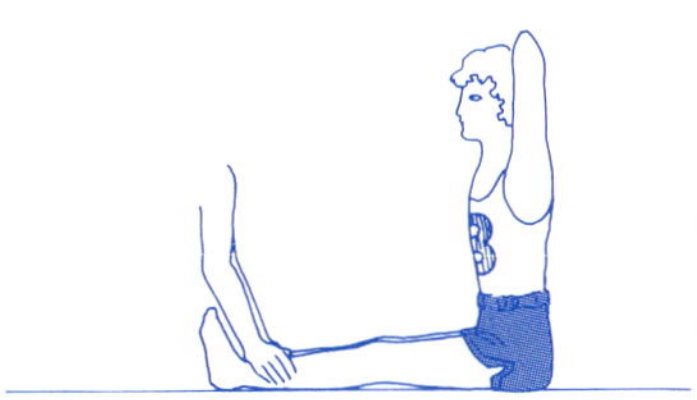

2 *Hip flexors and stomach muscles*: Lie flat on the floor with your hands clasped behind your neck. Have someone hold down your legs by grasping the ankles or hook your ankles under a heavy chair. Roll up into a sitting position.

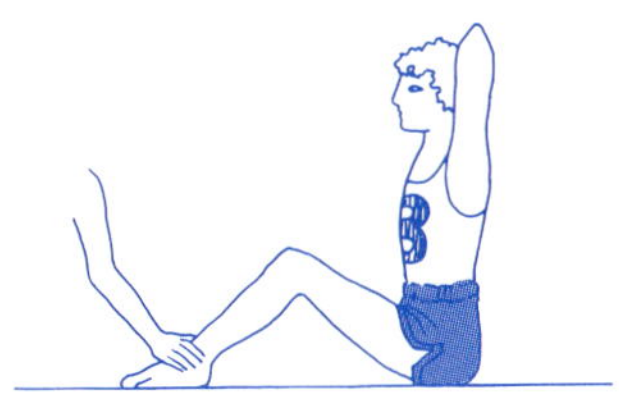

3 *Stomach muscles*: Same position as 2 but bend knees, keep heels close to buttocks. Now roll up into a sitting position again.

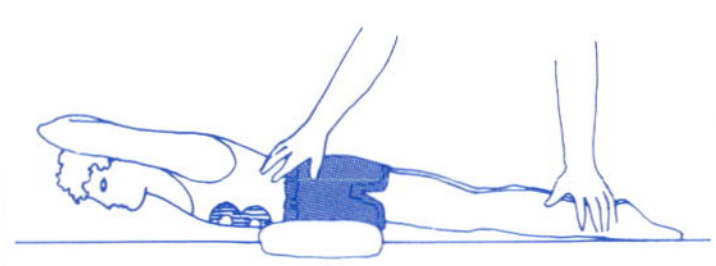

4 *Back muscles*: Turn over on your stomach. Put a pillow under your abdomen and clasp your hands behind your neck. Have a helper hold the lower half of your body steady by placing one hand in the small of the back and the other on your ankles. Now lift your trunk and hold it steady for 10 seconds.

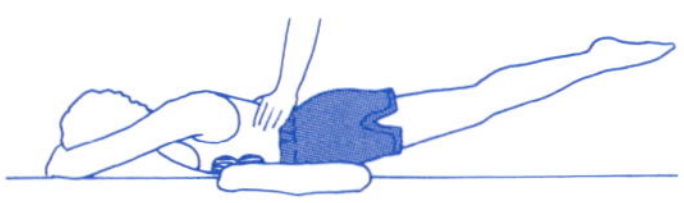

5 *Low back muscles*: Same position as in test 4, but fold your arms under your head. Have a helper hold your back steady with both hands. Now lift your legs up, be sure to keep your knees straight, and hold the position for 10 seconds.

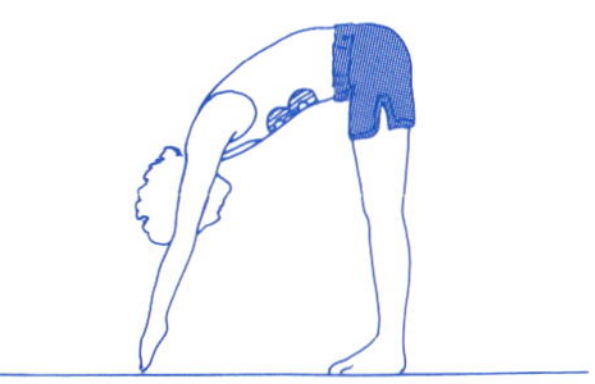

6 *Flexibility of muscles and hamstrings*: Stand up straight and make sure your feet are together. Now relax, lean over, and touch the floor with your fingertips without bending your knees.

SELF-CARE

EXERCISE 1

Lie on your back on a rug or pad on the floor, with a pillow under your knees, a pillow under each arm, and another pillow or a rolled-up towel under the back of your neck. Get comfortable.

Loosen up by wobbling your neck, shoulders, arms, thighs, legs, and feet. Raise your arms slowly, then let them drop. Do the same with your hands, legs, and feet. Let your head drop to the left, then to the right. Take a deep breath—do not strain—exhale slowly.

Now try to feel heavy—let your head, shoulders, arms, and legs rest on the floor. Do not keep them up even slightly by tensing your muscles.

Breathe again, close your eyes, let your jaw sag, try to exhale as slowly as possible, humming or hissing.

Tighten your arm muscles, then let go. Do the same with your thigh muscles and neck, then let go. The important part is the letting go—not the tightening. The tightening is important only to make you feel the difference between tenseness and relaxation.

Breathe again, slowly lift your shoulders to your ears, and then let them go.

EXERCISE 2

Sit on a chair, and do the shoulder-shrugging exercise again.

EXERCISE 3

Sit on a chair. Turn your head all the way to the left, then return it to normal front and center, and relax. Turn all the way to the right as far as you can, return, and relax. If you have a stiff neck, do this exercise again while lying down.

EXERCISE 4

Lie flat on your back with no pillows, this time with your knees flexed. Slowly draw your right knee up as close as possible to your chest. Slowly straighten your leg, let it fall to the floor limp and relaxed. Pull it up again to the flexed starting position. Now do the same thing with the other leg. Repeat the exercise several times, alternating legs.

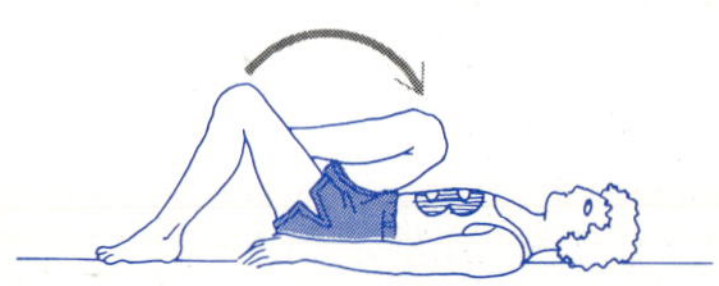

EXERCISE 5

Lie on your left side, and place a pillow under your head so it rests comfortably and your neck can relax. Keep both knees flexed and hips slightly flexed. Slide your right knee as close to your head as is comfortably possible, then slowly extend the leg until it is completely straight. Let the leg drop to the floor relaxed. Do the exercise two or three times on one side, then turn over to the other side and do the same with the other leg.

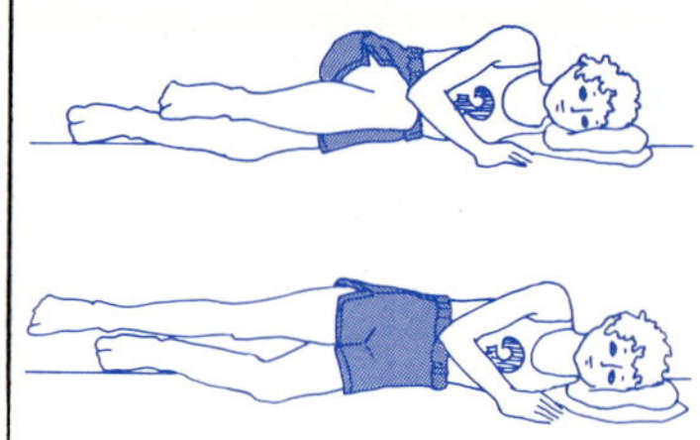

EXERCISE 6

Lie on your stomach. Fold your hands under your head and let your head rest on your hands comfortably. Then tighten your buttocks muscles. Hold for 2 seconds, then relax.

FIGURE 6.13 Exercises for the back. Wear comfortable clothing. Do each exercise two or three times, and rest after each exercise. [*Adapted from Kraus, pp. 95–99.*]

feet; choose leather, which is porous and allows air circulation, rather than plastic, which is airtight.

2 Wear white or light-colored socks of wool-cotton-nylon or orlon-cotton-nylon blends that allow air circulation and have a wick effect, drawing moisture up from moist foot to dry ankle, where it can evaporate.

3 Alternate shoes each day, if possible. If feet perspire during the day, try to switch to dry shoes.

4 Wash feet daily with mild soap and water; use a foot powder after washing, a lubricating cream for dry or flaking skin.

5 Don't wear other people's shoes or slippers.

6 Avoid walking barefoot in gyms and shower rooms; at pool areas, be sure to wade through the basins of chlorine solution before and after swimming to decrease chance of contamination.

7 Trim toenails longer than the tip of the toe; trim straight across with smoothly rounded edges.

8 Avoid so-called corn cures, harsh medications, and chemical compounds, without a doctor's prescription. Do not cut your own corns, calluses, or ingrown toenails. Instead,

seek treatment from a physician or a podiatrist (a nonmedical doctor who specializes in foot problems).

9 Be sure foot examination is included in regular checkups. Foot problems may indicate serious general diseases such as diabetes or circulatory disorders.

HEALTH CONSUMER TIP

Selecting Shoes for Good Foot Health

Millions of people walk around in shoes that are tight and uncomfortable; that cut, burn, rub, and cause a variety of foot ailments and posture problems; that cause aches and pains in legs and back; and that can even cause personality changes. Some suffer for the sake of fashion, others because they cannot afford new shoes. Foot specialists do not always agree on what is healthful and harmful in shoes.

Some foot experts believe that rigid, supportive shoes are best; others believe that soft shoes that are more like bare feet are superior. Most, however, agree that soft shoes, open sandals, and bare feet are unsafe where feet might be harmed by rocks, glass, or concrete curbs, or where they might be exposed to soil contaminated by disease-causing organisms like shistosomiasis. Many recommend soft footware or bare feet on yielding surfaces such as sand or grass, and supportive shoes on concrete or other firm ground. Very high heels are *never* recommended, since they are responsible for many leg injuries. Special shoes with wide heels, flexible soles, and shock-absorbing qualities are strongly suggested for jogging.

Whatever the type of footwear, it is important that it fit comfortably. It is best to try on shoes at the end of the day or week, when feet are most enlarged from the pressure of blood and other fluids. Left and right feet may not be identical in size, and so it is advisable to try both shoes and to select the size that fits the larger foot, padding the other if need be. Buying in a store with a sensible exchange policy gives recourse in case the fit seems wrong when you get home.

Foot Problems and Disorders

Most people have foot problems of one sort or another at some time in their lives; many suffer continuously. Still others experience backaches or leg cramps, unaware that foot problems may be the cause. Treatment should be sought from physician or a podiatrist.

Corns Horny, cone-shaped thickenings of the skin, usually on the toes. *Cause*: Pressure, friction, or bone deformity. *Treatment*: Swine dung was the preferred treatment 2000 years ago, but today flannel pads, placed around the corn to relieve discomfort, do the job with greater delicacy. The doctor can remove corns by cutting them, but unless the conditions that cause them are corrected, they will return.

Calluses Protective thickening of the horny layer of the skin (see Figure 6.8). *Cause*: Repeated or constant pressure or friction. *Treatment*: Remove pressure or friction. Soak and rub with pumice stone to remove callus. Cutting, if needed, should be done by a doctor.

Bunions Misaligned joints in the foot (particularly the big toe) which become swollen and tender. *Cause*: Weakness of muscle structure; heredity. Ill-fitting shoes may contribute. *Treatment*: Wear shoes that fit.

Ingrown toenail This condition occurs when the normally free end of a toenail grows inward and becomes embedded in the skin. *Cause*: May be improper trimming, but heredity, injury, and fungus infection (such as athlete's foot) can play a part. *Treatment*: May include packing cotton beneath the nail to keep it from growing into the skin, or in more severe cases, surgery to remove all or part of the toenail. *Prevention*: Cutting toenails properly and wearing properly fitted shoes.

Plantar warts (See page 156.)

Athlete's foot Cracking, scaling, and itching of skin. *Cause*: Fungus (ringworm of the foot) encouraged by conditions of warmth, moisture, darkness, and irritation. *Treatment*: Difficult, and must continue long after symptoms disappear to be sure all fungal spores have been killed. *Prevention*: Good foot care, as described earlier.

Flat feet A flattening of the arch of the foot, once considered serious enough to exempt men from military service, but no longer categorized as a major disability. *Cause*: May be inherited or acquired. *Treatment*: Some physicians recommend metal arch supports, but others feel that if the feet do not hurt, there is nothing to treat, and the condition is not abnormal. In fact, an Olympic runner with flat feet won a gold medal in 1972.

LOOKING BACK

REVIEWING CONCEPTS IN CHAPTER 6

- Proper care of our bodies can prevent many disorders.
- Twenty million Americans have lost all their teeth and yet today such loss is almost totally preventable. A major reason for tooth loss in young people is caries (tooth decay). In those over 35, periodontitis (pyorrhea) is a major cause.
- Dental caries are caused by a combination of bacteria in the mouth, sugar in the diet, and susceptible teeth. Periodontitis results from poor oral hygiene and buildup of plaque caused by interaction of sugar and bacteria.
- Responsibility for preventing these disorders falls primarily on the individual and includes keeping the mouth clean through flossing and brushing, eating a varied diet low in sugar, and strengthening tooth resistance with fluorides.
- The good dentist is prevention-oriented, and views tooth extraction as a tragedy that can often be avoided. When lost, teeth must be replaced to keep the rest of the mouth healthy.
- Eyes, because of their sensitivity and importance, have built-in defense mechanisms. However, we can also take other measures to help avoid eye damage.
- Vision and hearing difficulties as well as skin and foot disorders are most successfully treated when detected early. Periodic eye and ear examinations, foot checkups, and self-examination of the skin can turn up problems before symptoms are obvious.
- Hearing or vision deficiencies can be inherited; can be caused before birth; can result from disease or injury; or can simply be a consequence of aging. Hearing problems may develop from excessive exposure to noise.
- The skin is a valuable organ with many remarkable features allowing it to protect the body it encases. But it requires good care: cleansing and protection from drying elements of sun, wind, water, and smoke. Too much sun can lead to skin cancer.
- Acne, the most common skin problem, affects almost everyone at some time, but is most common in adolescence and young adulthood. Severe cases should be treated by a physician.

- Acne is believed to be influenced by heredity, hormones, skin bacteria, emotional stress, drugs, and cosmetics, but not by masturbation, nor by too much or too little sex. Food allergy probably plays only a minor part.
- Hair can often be a mirror of health. It is shed normally all the time, but sudden hair loss—except following pregnancy or stopping the Pill—can indicate illness.
- Gradual hair loss (pattern baldness) can occur in both men and women, though the patterns differ. It is hereditary and affected by hormones. No simple cures are available, though hair can be replaced by transplants.
- The best "cure" for an aching back is prevention, including: proper posture; adequate exercise to keep muscles toned; using sitting, lifting, bending, and sleeping positions that avoid back injury.
- Foot problems often cause difficulties that extend far beyond the feet. Prevention of foot problems—by good foot care, proper shoe fit, early professional care—is easier than cure.

III

DISEASE: THE OTHER END OF THE SPECTRUM

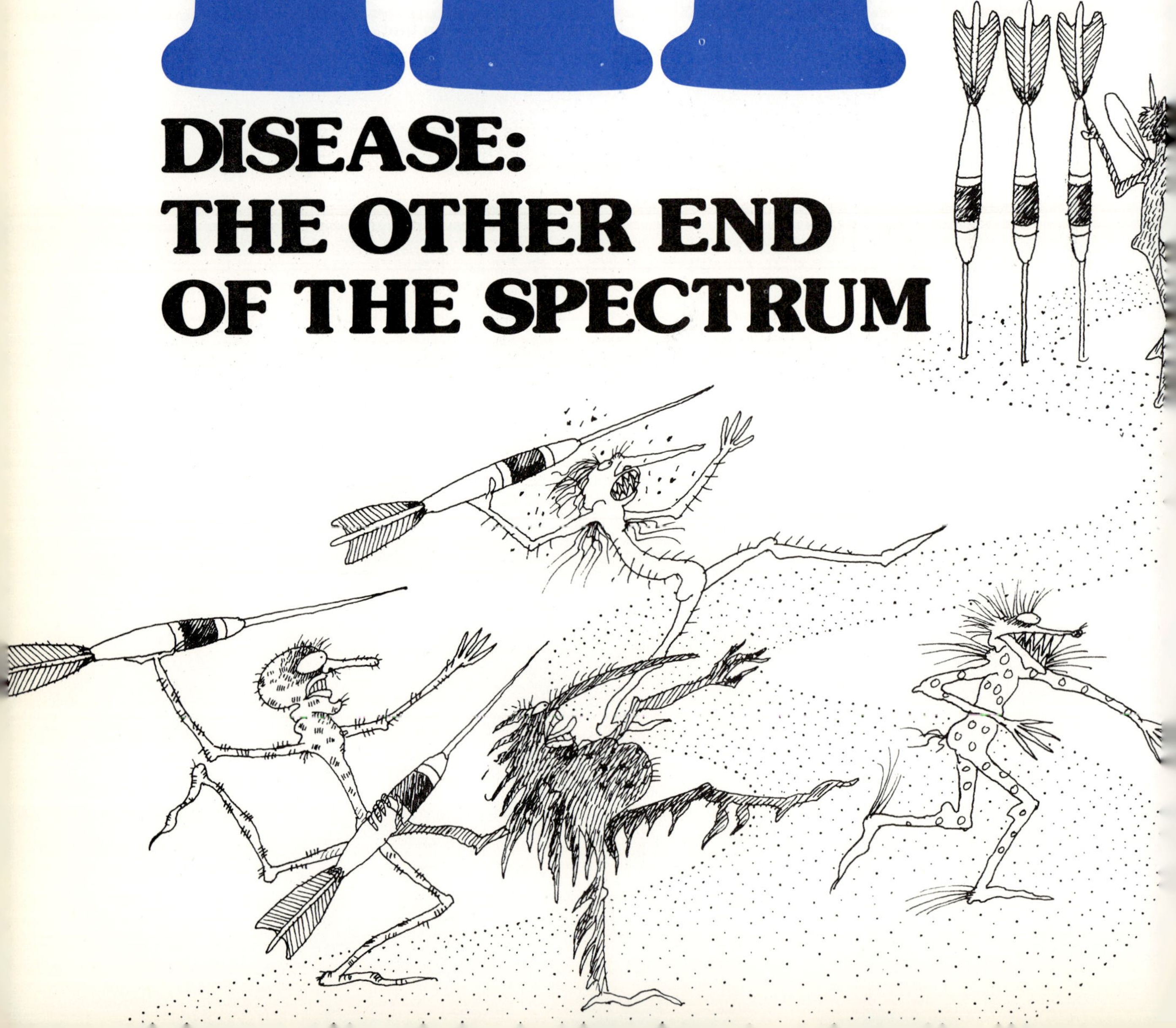

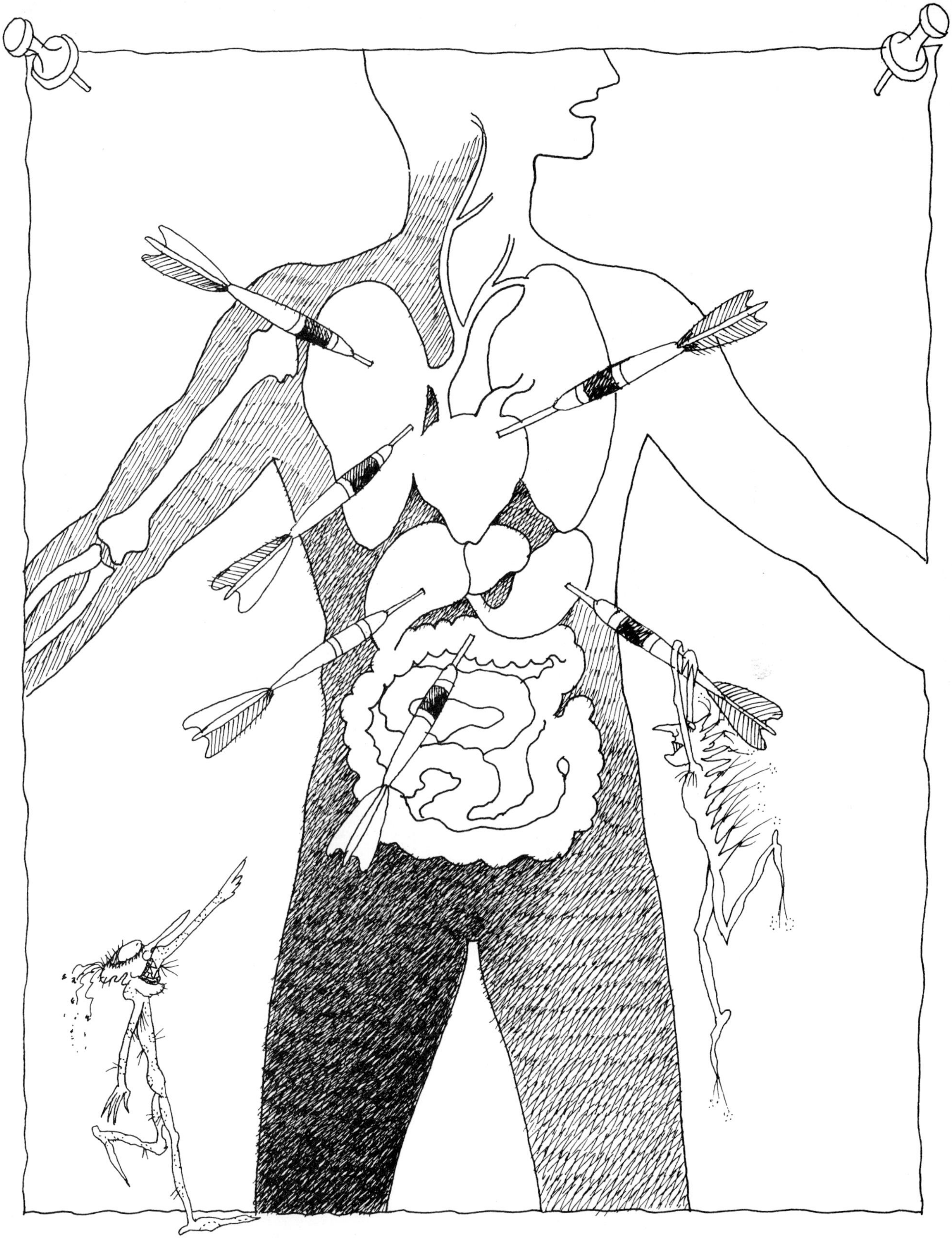

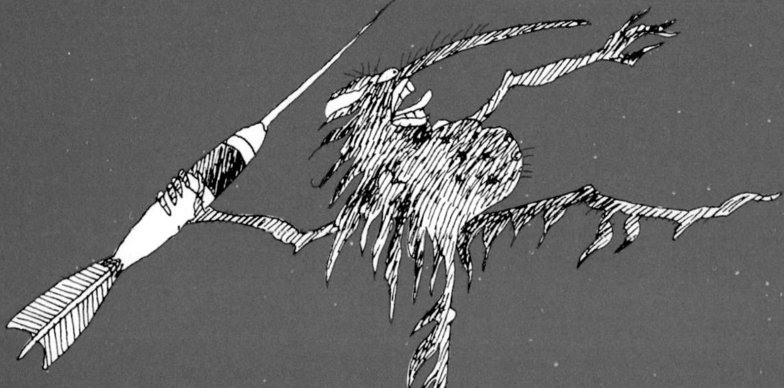

7

THRUST AND PARRY: DISEASE ATTACKS, AND THE BODY RESPONDS

WHAT'S AHEAD IN CHAPTER 7 What has happened to the patterns of human disease over the centuries? What are some of the factors that determine these patterns? What causes disease? Is there usually just a single cause for a particular ailment? Can disease-causing factors be manipulated to prevent disease? How? In what ways does the body respond to a threat to its health? What is immunological response? Why is it important? What problems result when the immunological response is underactive? How does it act *against* its own body? What happens when the body *over* reacts, is *hyper* sensitive to an invading substance? How can this hypersensitivity be controlled or eliminated? What promise does knowledge of how to depress or stimulate the immune system hold for the future?

It is difficult to know exactly when we have crossed the line from "health" to "illness." Perhaps that is because there really is no line—just a continum that runs from optimum good health on one end to death on the other, with all of us somewhere in between. Technically we are in a state of ill health (disease), when we are unable to do things we are accustomed to doing (a functional disability), or when one of our parts—a limb or an organ—is damaged (a structural disability). The disability may result from the body's failure to cope with, adapt to, or adequately counteract injury, infection, stress, or other stimuli in our environment.

CHANGING PATTERNS OF DISEASE

Archeological finds indicate that few diseases are new, that everything from cancer to cirrhosis of the liver, from sinusitis to tooth decay, plagued our ancestors. The remains of the pharoah of the Exodus (whose heart, you may remember, was "hardened" by God) showed signs of hardening of the coronary (heart) arteries.

Though diseases have not changed, the patterns of incidence have. Smallpox was so common once that the physician Lavicenna in the ninth and tenth centuries believed it to be the inherent lot of mankind, something each individual contracted in its mother's womb (Long). Yet in 1975, the World Health Organization announced that smallpox had been virtually wiped out.[1] There has also been a decline in mortality from other infectious diseases, which began early in this century. At the same time, deaths from chronic and degenerative diseases such as heart disease,[2] cancer, and diabetes seesawed upward. By 1955, more than 80 percent of all deaths were from such diseases (Wilner et al.).

Some reasons for changing patterns of disease are unknown, but others are easy to pinpoint: (1) improved living standards, including better sanitation; (2) more plentiful food supplies, leading to *over* nutrition as well as better nutrition; (3) increased lifespan, resulting in an increase in diseases of the elderly; (4) ease of travel, which causes disease to spread more rapidly; (5) new pollutants in air, water, and food; (6) occupational hazards, resulting from modern technology; (7) changing lifestyles, with less exercise, more drug use, more stress; (8) medical advances including vaccines to prevent disease, drugs to control or cure it, and better diagnostic tools (all of which present hazards as well as benefits); (9) extension of lives of those with genetic diseases, allowing them in turn to bear offspring with the same diseases; (10) effects of drugs, industry, and lifestyle on the ecological balance.

[1]In 1977, some spotty outbreaks were reported.
[2]Recently, a slight downtrend in heart disease has been noted. See Chap. 10.

FACTORS AFFECTING DISEASE

- A guest at a party arrives with a bad cold. Within three days, 4 of the other 11 guests come down with colds of varying intensity; one guest feels a cold "coming on," but never actually becomes ill.
- Twenty-nine vinyl chloride workers become victims of a rare liver cancer, and there is a general rise in tumors of all kinds in the worker population. But the vast majority of the industry's 350,000 workers are unaffected.

Clearly, exposure to a germ or a chemical alone does not always lead to illness. Ordinarily disease has a multifactorial etiology or cause; a combination of factors contribute. These factors vary widely, but in general they often include:

- *A susceptible host* An individual becomes susceptible to disease in many ways.
- *An agent that causes the illness directly* An infectious organism (bacteria, viruses), a parasite (tapeworm), an irritant (tobacco smoke), an instrument (knives, autos).
- *Environmental factors* Physical, psychological, sociological, natural, and human factors that either make the individual more susceptible to disease or directly cause illness.
- *A mode of transmission* A way for the agent and the host to come together, such as a cough spewing viral particles on all around.

Stress and Disease

Anger, fear, excitement, a threat to survival, or other stress results in an immediate rise in blood pressure and heart rate and a surge of adrenaline (epinephrine) and noradrenaline (norepinephrine) released into the bloodstream by the adrenal glands. This has an extraordinary effect on the body. Sugar stored in the liver is released and converted to glucose for energy. Blood clotting time is reduced so that, in case of injury, blood will clot more rapidly. Surface blood vessels are shut down (you turn "pale") and so are blood vessels to the digestive system. Blood is concentrated instead in the muscles and the internal organs, giving us strength we did not know we had and ordinarily do not have. We can run faster, lift more, jump further, hit harder. This reaction is part of what Hans Selye has described as the general adaptation syndrome (GAS) with which humans respond to stress.

In the early history of humankind, these physiological responses to stress were satisfactorily dissipated in one of two ways: the person either overcame the threat with physical force (fight) or ran for his or her life to avoid it (flight). Today, we rarely have the opportunity to use this extra energy physically. When we are faced with the pressure of an exam, a crucial board meeting, or a sick baby, the body is revved up for fight or flight in vain. Such situations cause wear and tear on the body and lead to gradual deterioration and disease (Selye, *a*).

By using competent coping techniques and, occasionally, defense mechanisms (see Chapter 2), however, we can often reduce stress and, with it, wear and tear. Many physicians suggest additional approaches to reducing stress such as strenuous exercise (to utilize excess adrenalin), relaxation techniques, forms of meditation, and yoga.

Failure to reduce stress often leads to diseases we call psychosomatic or psychogenic. *Psychosomatic* (*psycho* = mind + soma = body) illnesses, such as peptic ulcers, are those in which there are both mental and physical components. Psychogenic (*psycho* + *genic* = causing) illnesses have only a psychological cause. They may include some headaches, backaches, cases of upset stomach, paralysis, deafness, blindness, and inability to speak. The most common and easily recognized effects of mind on body are those on the excretory system—causing frequent urination, diarrhea, profuse perspiration.

The absence of certain factors—exercise, sanitation, good nutrition—can also contribute to disease. The more contributory or risk factors there are present, the more likely it is disease will occur.

These are the major factors known to influence whether or not people become ill:

- *Genetic makeup* Many diseases (for example, hemophilia, cystic fibrosis), susceptibility to many others (probably allergy, diabetes, heart disease, and some forms of cancer), as well as weakened defenses against still others (infectious diseases) are inherited.
- *Ethnic or racial heritage* Some disorders are more prevalent in certain groups, for example, sickle cell anemia and high blood pressure among blacks and thalassemia among Mediterranean peoples.
- *Stress* *Mental* (college health services are busiest just prior to and during exams); *social* (some people always "break out" before an important event); *emotional* (many serious illnesses follow the death of a loved one); *physical* (lack of sleep, poor eating habits, and injury increase susceptibility to disease); *sociological* (epidemics are more prevalent during or following wars, earthquakes, or other calamities or

when overcrowding or other sociological problems are common).

- *Personal lifestyles* *The way people eat* (too much, too little, or the wrong kind of food); *what they do* (smoking, drinking too much alcohol, abusing other drugs, not exercising enough, not fastening seatbelts or wearing motorcycle helmets); *where they go* (travel exposes people to unfamiliar infectious organisms against which they may not have developed protection).
- *Values* Does the immediate fulfillment a cigarette affords outweigh the risks of early disability and death from lung disease? Are brushing and flossing of teeth and giving up sweets worth the effort to avoid dental disease? Is greater protection from heart disease worth the sacrifice of bacon and eggs, and rich French ice cream?
- *Personality type* Those who are more likely to become ill are risk takers who probably share a lot in common with the accident-prone people described in Chapter 11.
- *Money* The health of the poor (who suffer from inadequate food, clothing, sanitation, and housing, from exposure to rats, peeling lead paints, and sometimes from inferior health care and less health education) and of the middle class (who are often too rich for government aid and too poor to pay for special treatment, and who must thus forego some kinds of care) is affected by economics.
- *Health care* *Iatrogenic* disease (*Iatro* = doctor + *genic* = produced) may result from poor surgical or postoperative care in a hospital, or from misguided drug prescribing. Illness may also result from lack of preventive care.
- *The environment before birth* Infection, drugs, diet, chemicals, and radiation can all affect an unborn child's future health (see Chapter 23).
- *The natural environment* Climate, season, altitude, soil type, water, humidity, natural radiation, toxic or beneficial materials in soil or water; absence or presence of essential nutrients in food, soil, or water; native disease-carrying animals, insects, and parasites can *all* affect health. Variations in these factors account in part for the fact that disease patterns differ in different parts of the world.
- *The artificial or human-created environment* Industrialization has increased the prevalence of some diseases, decreased others (see Figure 7.1). The major human-made hazards include: *heavy pollutants in the air* from automobiles, factories, power plants, home furnaces, etc.; *pollutants in the water sources* from human and industrial wastes, from accidental oil spills, corroded pipes, water softening equipment, etc.; *pesticides* sprayed on backyard gardens, campus trees, vegetables, and fruits, many of which accumulate in the body and the ultimate effects of which are unknown; *household products* such as aerosol sprays, vinylchloride food containers, some 3000 items containing free-flying asbestos, often misused chemicals and pesticides that undermine the safety of our homes; *occupational hazards* causing an estimated 100,000 disease deaths and 390,000 cases of disease annually (see Table 7.1); *perils faced by families and offspring* exposed to dangerous substances carried home on clothing and skin by workers; *noise* from traffic, from lawnmowers, snowmobiles, jet planes, machinery, and rock music. (For a discussion of how society deals with environmental problems, see Chapter 26.)

Recognition of the many factors that affect our health may at first be discouraging, but in the long run it should encourage us. Knowing the facts, we can, as informed decision makers, take steps to prevent illness and promote good health. There are a variety of ways, shown throughout this book, in which as individuals and as members of the community we can reduce risk.

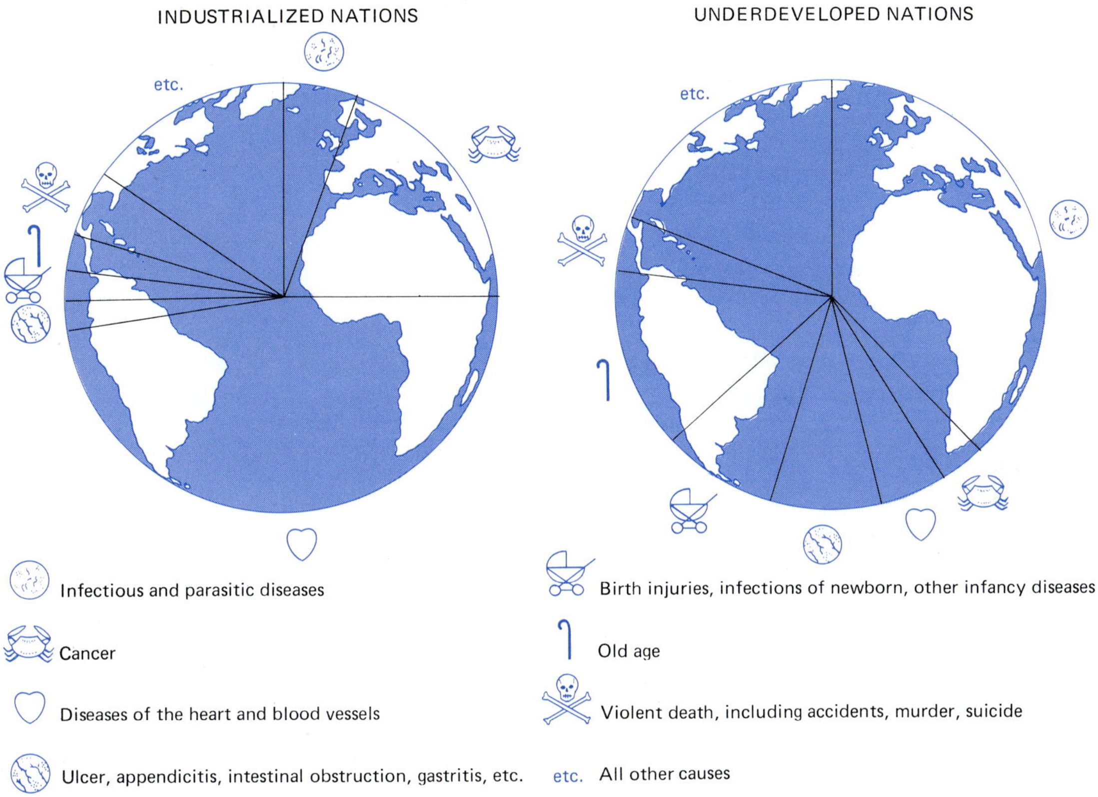

FIGURE 7.1 Major causes of death in industrialized and underdeveloped nations. [*Diagram adapted from Wilner et al., p. 306; data for 1967 from World Health Organization.*]

THE BODY'S DEFENSE AGAINST DISEASE

The most important defense we have against illness and injury is the human brain. It is our thinking brain that allows us to make decisions to alter our lifestyles, change our environments, prevent spread of disease, and so on. But even when we fail to take affirmative action to protect ourselves, a well-organized built-in system of defense often helps us avoid the many health perils that surround us.

First Lines of Defense

The five senses—smell, taste, hearing, vision, touch—constitute an early warning system for the body, signaling danger from fire, spoiled food, poisonous gases, etc. Other mechanisms block a variety of invaders: The skin protects the internal organs from germs, water, pollutants, and the like. The eyelids flick shut when a foreign object comes close. The fine hairs in the nose sift out germs and pollutants, tiny insects, dust and dirt, soot and grit, as they attempt to enter the respira-

TABLE 7.1 Dangers in the working world—some examples*

OCCUPATION	HAZARDOUS AGENT	RESULTING DISORDERS
Coal mining, other work with coal by-products	Coal dust Coal soots, tars	"Black lung" (pneumoconiosis): irreversible, progressive lung disease Various cancers (lung, skin, scrotum, larynx, urinary bladder)
Farming	Mold organisms in wet hay; insecticides (see below)	"Farmer's lung," bronchitis, pneumonia, emphysema
Asbestos mining; milling; textiles; insulation; shipbuilding	Asbestos fibers	Lung cancer in smokers; mesotheliomas and other cancers; other lung disorders
Plastics work	Vinyl chloride	Angiosarcoma (liver cancer); possibly other cancers
Insecticide production, use	Kepone, arsenic, many others (many banned)	Many, including skin, lung, liver cancer (arsenic); memory loss, liver damage, tremors, blurring vision, possible sterility (kepone)
X-ray operation	Radiation	Birth defects in offspring; cancer
Anesthesia administration; surgery	Anesthesia fumes	Birth defects in offspring; miscarriage, cancer in women; liver and kidney diseases; muscular weakness in dentists using nitrous oxide (laughing gas)
Laboratory work	Various chemicals	Cancers and other disorders
Wood, leather, chromium work; bleachers; glass, pottery, linoleum work; battery manufacture	Wood; leather; chromium	Cancers of nasal cavity and sinuses; of bladder (leather); of lung and larynx (chromium)
Dye and textile work, use; paint manufacture, use; explosives; shoe production; distilling	Several chemicals; benzene	Urinary bladder cancer, others Bone marrow cancer
Mining and smelting; work with nickel and iron oxide	Nickel; iron oxide	Lung cancer; cancer of nasal cavity (nickel); of larynx (iron oxide)
Work with petroleum and petrochemicals and by-products	Petroleum; petroleum by-products	Cancers of nasal cavity, larynx, skin, lung, scrotum
Chemical manufacture, use	Bis-chloromethyl ether; chloromethyl ether; mustard gas; isopropyl oil	Lung cancer Larynx, trachea, bronchi cancers, cancers of nasal cavity

*Job-related disorders can show up within minutes of exposure (e.g., radiation or acid burns) or may take 20 or 30 years to develop (e.g., many types of cancer). Most can be prevented if adequate safety measures are observed by both employers and employees. Serious consequences can often be avoided by regular medical screening of workers in hazardous jobs and early treatment of problems. New techniques may allow removal of toxic chemicals from the body.

tory system. Beyond the hairs, deeper in the nasal cavity, a thick spongy mucous membrane lining traps impurities that have evaded the hairs, just as flypaper catches flies. It also destroys some germs with the enzyme lysozyme.

As impurities accumulate in the mucus, a tiny army of cilia (microscopic hairs) sweeps them back toward the throat where they are swallowed and then destroyed by stomach acids. This process goes on continually, except when cilia are paralyzed by cold weather—in which case the mucus runs out the nose rather than being swallowed—or by tobacco smoke. Smoking eventually destroys cilia completely, allowing toxic agents to pass down to and accumulate in the bronchial tubes and lungs. "Smoker's cough" is an attempt by the body to rid the respiratory system of these agents.

When dangerous substances manage to slip past these initial defenses, the body often responds by expelling them automatically via a cough or sneeze, vomiting or diarrhea, which are less often symptoms of disease than of the body trying to protect itself.

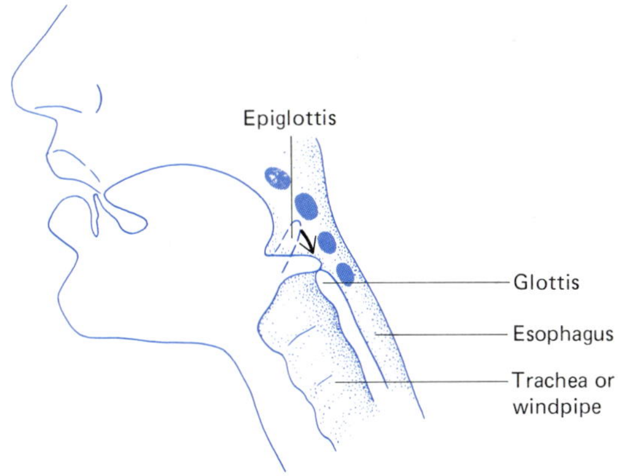

FIGURE 7.2 Keeping the airways clear. During swallowing, the epiglottis flips down to form a tight seal with the glottis, effectively preventing food or drink from entering the windpipe or trachea, allowing it instead to enter the esophagus and move toward the stomach. If you tried breathing at the moment you swallowed, you would find it impossible, for your windpipe would be closed. Occasionally, however, when a person is eating and talking or laughing at the same time, some food or liquid will slip by the glottis before it closes and "go down the wrong way." The body then responds with coughing (which sometimes has a force of 200 mph) or choking in an attempt to rid the respiratory tract of the foreign matter. (See Heimlich maneuver, Figure 11.6.)

Immunological Response

Once invaders have entered the body, the main line of defense is the vast communications system by which the body recognizes foreign substances and triggers a complex response to seek and destroy them. Important in this process is the body's ability to distinguish "self" (one's own cells) from "other" (invading cells). The immune system walks a tightrope between tolerating the harmless and destroying the harmful. If there is too little immune activity, dangerous germs and toxins cause disease, even death; too much activity, and an individual's own body tissues may be attacked. The substances that trigger the immune system—most often those like bacteria, animal cells, plant pollen that contain protein, or viruses that have protein coats—are called *antigens*.

There are presently believed to be two types of immunity, cellular and humoral, plus a variety of helping mechanisms. Both cellular and humoral immunity are dependent upon white blood cells, or *leukocytes* (*leuk* = white + *cyte* = cell), which increase tremendously in the blood when infection is present. The specific leukocytes involved are T-cell and B-cell lymphocytes which are believed to originate in the bone marrow.

Cellular immunity (cell-mediated response)

The major activity here appears to come from the T cells, which are probably processed in the thymus gland. They then move on to circulate in the blood, lymph system, and spleen, where they protect the body by surrounding and destroying invaders including various microorganisms and possibly cancer cells. They also attack cells of transplanted organs and are thought to be involved in skin allergies such as poison ivy and in mobilizing other phagocytic (*phago* = eating) cells such as macrophages to the site of an invasion by foreign cells. Some T cells (helper T cells) may assist in the production of antibodies, while others (suppressor T cells) block antibody production.

Humoral immunity (antibody-mediated response) Here the activating cells are B cells. Their major role appears to be the manufacture of antibodies to incapacitate invading antigens. Specific antibodies are designed with customized receptors to match specific antigens. Nobel laureate Gerald Edelman has described the system as a "clothing store that stocks every conceivable fit for any creature that comes in."

The antibodies are part of a group of blood proteins known as immunoglobulins. The five recognized classes include immunoglobulins G (IgG), M (IgM), D (IgD), E (IgE), and A (IgA), each appearing to have different functions.

Other aspects of immune response Also involved in immune response are: (1) *phagocytic cells* that attack and devour invaders and clean up dead cells, worn-out red blood cells, and other debris at the site of wounds, infections, or other inflammation; (2) *complement*, a complex system of interacting serum proteins that trigger in sequence to produce such effects as inflammation, the reddening seen around an infected area attacked by foreign microorganisms; (3) *interferon*, a protein produced by body cells in response to attack by viruses; (4) *the lymphoid organs*, which include the thymus, the lymph nodes, the tonsils, and the spleen. (Because of the recently discovered role of the tonsils in the immune response, it is no longer recommended that they be removed routinely.)

Immunological Memory

A nation at war keeps records of the way the enemy attacks and its style of battle to use in the next encounter. So it is with the immune system; it remembers its enemies.

When an antigen is administered or enters the body naturally, there is a latent or inactive period and then a rise in antibody production. Once the antigen is destroyed, the level of antibody begins to gradually drop. But should the same antigen return, the immunological response is much swifter than the first time around; the rise in antibodies occurs more quickly and production is higher. Cellular immunity, too, appears improved, though the precise amount of improvement is difficult to measure.

Immunological memory is the basis for vaccination and immunization for such deadly diseases as polio, smallpox, and diphtheria (see Chapter 8).

THE MANY PATHS OF IMMUNOLOGICAL RESEARCH

Immunological research promises to uncover many long-sought health secrets. Research centers on the following problems:

Disorders of the Immune System

Millions of Americans suffer from diseases caused by the immune system's acting too little, too late, too much, or in the wrong way.

Immune-deficiency diseases Hundreds of children are born in the United States each year with severe combined immunodeficiency disease (SCID), sometimes inherited, or with partial deficiencies in their immune responses. Some of these children lack all or some of the antibodies, and others have a small, abnormal, or missing thymus. Most face daily danger of death from infections against which they have no defense.

United Press International

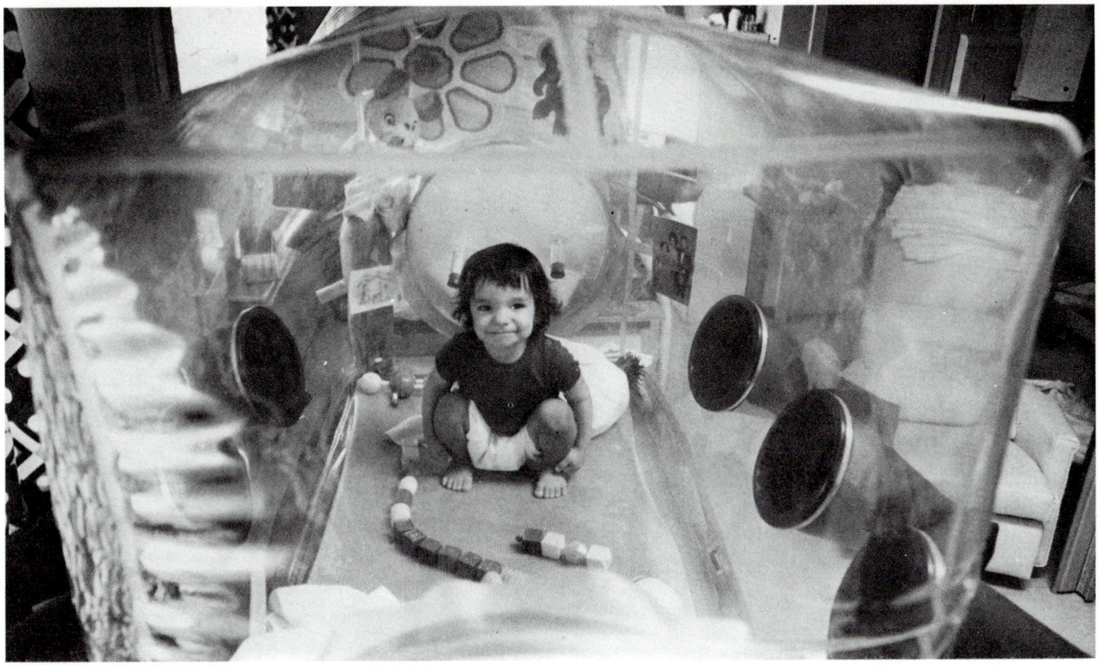

Special germ-free environments protect those with SCID or with suppressed immune systems from infection, against which they have no defense.

Autoimmune diseases In autoimmune diseases, the mechanism for telling "self" from "other" breaks down. Antibodies or sensitized cells, instead of tolerating and respecting the body's own cells, begin to attack them. Nobel laureate Sir Frank MacFarlane Burnet likens this apparently uncontrolled production of antibodies to the runaway cell production of cancer.

Conditions now believed to be autoimmune diseases include: *rheumatoid arthritis*, the painful crippler of young adults (usually aged 20 to 50, most often women), characterized by swelling, pain, and inflammation of the joints; *systemic lupus erythematosus* (SLE), a lifelong, incurable, but controllable disease that primarily strikes young women (about 80 percent of victims are female) and can be disfiguring and even fatal; *periodontitis*, a disease causing breakdown of bone and gum tissue supporting the teeth; *multiple sclerosis*, an incurable malady crippling hundreds of thousands around the world; *myasthenia gravis*, a debilitating disorder of the skeletal muscles; and some forms of *goiter* (*Hashimoto's disease*) and *anemia* (pernicious).

Stimulating the Immune System

The immune system is critical to survival. Thus learning how to stimulate it—when it is lazy or absent, or when the invading organisms are particularly difficult to overcome—is extremely important. There are several, still mostly experimental ways of doing this.

Interferon Part of the healthy immune system, this substance, produced by human white blood cells in the laboratory, may some day checkmate influenza and the common cold (Merigan et al.). Since the interferon produced by 30 to 50 pints of blood is needed to treat one patient, a more practical approach to fighting virus infection may be to stimulate the body's own production of interferon (H. Levy, et al.).

BCG Bacillus Calmette-Guerin, used as a TB vaccine since early in this century, is being widely studied for its ability to stimulate the immune system, particularly against cancerous tumors.

Bone marrow transplants Since lymphocytes originate in the bone marrow, an injection of marrow from a normal person can give a patient with deficient immunity healthy new cells for strengthening the immune system. Host and donor must be compatible (that is, their tissues must match) to reduce the risk of donated immune cells rejecting the host (graft-versus-host disease). A sibling is the best donor.

Thymus injections Injecting thymus tissue, the hormone thymosin, or T cells has shown promise in stimulating sluggish cell-mediated immunity and providing such cell-mediated response in persons born without a thymus or with an abnormal one. Thymosin has also been found to raise the immune defense in cancer and severe burn cases.

Synthetic vitamin A Retinoid, a synthetic form of vitamin A, appears to enhance the work of BCG, to reduce the suppression of the immune system by steroids, and to help the system in overcoming precancerous cells (B. Cohen).

Transfer factor Temporary immunity can be transferred from one person to another in this way. Mrs. A has had a particular disease, recovered from it, and now has immunity to it. Mr. B has the same disease, but is not fighting it off successfully. Transfer factor from Mrs. A's blood, injected into Mr. B, gives B the ability to combat the disease. As a final cancer treatment, transfer factor also appears to provide the scavenger cells to clean up leftover cancer cells.

Suppressing the Immune System

Sometimes the immune system needs to be suppressed, as when it reacts abnormally against its own body in autoimmune diseases or when it rejects an organ transplant (kidney, heart, skin). Suppression is possible with drugs and radiation prior to transplantation and experimentally by extraction of excess immune cells from the blood in autoimmune diseases. The problem, of course, is that when the immune system is suppressed, there is no defense against infection. Thus such treatment is carried out in special germ-free environments.

ALLERGY: MOST COMMON OF IMMUNE SYSTEM DISORDERS

Ellen breaks out in big red itchy hives every times she even nibbles a raw strawberry. John's eyes itch and his nose runs from August through October every year. Shelly wheezes and chokes for air whenever she enters a home that has a cat.

Like an estimated 31 million Americans and the Egyptian king Menes, who died of a hornet sting in 2641 B.C.E., these people have allergies, or *hypersensitivities*. Allergies are overly sensitive reactions by the body's immune system to a particular antigen, in this case called an *allergen*. Instead of being protective, these responses may be annoying (hay fever), disabling (asthma), even fatal (shock reaction to a drug). Allergy follows a familial pattern: 70 percent of adult asthmatics and 80 percent of hay fever sufferers have a family history of allergy. If both parents are allergic, there is almost a 100 percent certainty that the children will be. Some childhood allergies are "outgrown," and sometimes they return in another form in adulthood.

Types of Hypersensitivity

Immediate Most cases of allergy are related to the actions of the B cells and the IgE antibodies they produce, though T cells appear to play a helper role. As with other immune responses the antibody-producing cells are sensitized at one exposure, then respond immunologically on following exposures. For example, Ellen did not break out the first time she bit into a juicy red berry. Sensitization—antibody-producing cells encountering and "taking note of" a foreign substance—occurred first. It could have taken place the first time Ellen ate a strawberry, or the fiftieth time. When the allergen returned, more sensitizing antibodies were produced. The antibodies combined with the allergens and then these complexes attached to the surface of the mast cells (most frequently found beneath skin and mucous membrane) and stimulated them to release a number of biologically active compounds or chemical mediators, such as *histamines*. Histamines dilate blood vessels, contract smooth muscle, stimulate increased secretion of mucus and cause the capillaries to leak fluid into surrounding tissue, leading to tissue damage. The end result: symptoms of allergy.

Delayed hypersensitivity Some allergic responses involve sensitized T cells that directly damage tissues, or produce mediators that cause damage. Delayed hypersensitivity plays a part in rejection of skin grafts and transplanted organs, and in allergic reactions to bacteria, viruses, fungi, and such plants as poison ivy, poison oak, and poison sumac.

TABLE 7.2 Allergies

COMMON CAUSES OF ALLERGIC REACTION—ALLERGENS	MOST COMMON ALLERGIC REACTIONS*
Pollens: of grasses, trees, flowers, weeds	*Hay fever* (seasonal rhinitis): sneezing, nasal discharge, congestion, sinusitis; asthma and secondary infection in serious cases
Mold spores	*Year-round rhinitis:* same as above, but not seasonal
House dust: fabric fibers, feathers, bacteria, molds and fungi, insect bites, animal dander, algae, mites, aging fabrics, furniture stuffing	*Sinusitis:* pain in sinuses
Heat or cold	*Asthma*: breathlessness, coughing, wheezing
Sunlight	*Skin eruptions:* hives (itchy, whitish bumps); eczema (scaling, itching, crusting; moist, weeping, easily infected sores) mostly in infants; perfume allergy (dirty brown streaks)
Foods: eggs (especially raw whites), milk, nuts, chocolate, citrus fruits, cheese, alcohol, wheat, tomatoes, strawberries, etc.	*Edema:* swelling of body tissue
Drugs: aspirin, penicillin, laxatives, many others	*GI symptoms* (digestive): pain, nausea, vomiting, etc.
Chemicals: synthetics, food additives, pesticides, nitrates, dyes, perfumes, plastics	*Headache*
Metals: nickel in earrings	*Mouth and lip inflammation*
Air pollutants: tobacco smoke, gases: sulfur dioxide, CO, hydrocarbons, chlorine	*Anaphylactic shock:* can be fatal
Animal dander: hair and skin bits	*Nervous system symptoms:*† paralysis, numbness, confusion; fatigue; hyperactivity; depression; personality changes; psychotic behavior, aggression
Insect bites: especially cockroaches	
Insect stings: bees, wasps	

*Allergic response can occur immediately or hours after exposure to an antigen. Almost any tissue in the body can be affected, but the reactions listed are the most commonly experienced.
†Whether or not such symptoms can be allergic reactions is still under investigation.

United Press International

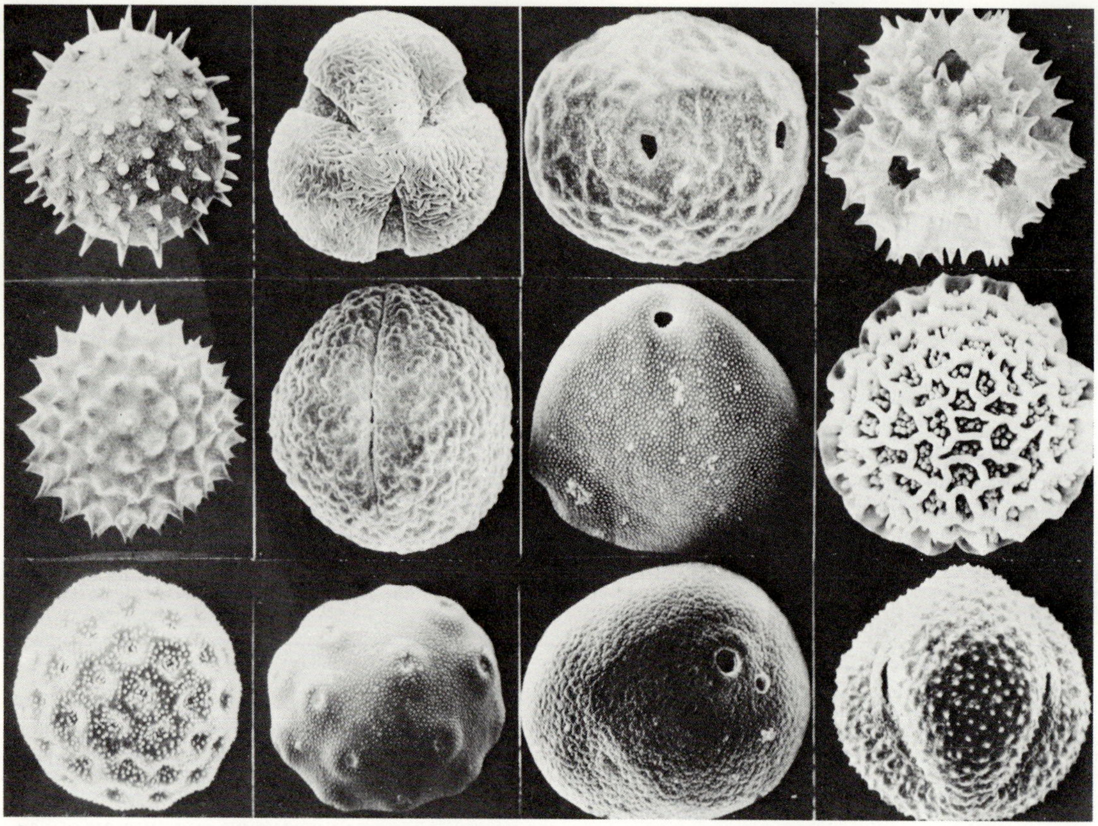

Hay fever has nothing to do with hay and does not produce fever. It is most commonly caused by pollens such as these (*left to right*): (*top*) elder, white oak, saltbush, giant ragweed; (*middle*) dandelion, American elm, Johnson grass, sagebrush; (*bottom*) pecan, hibiscus, bougainvillea, and black walnut.

The Most Common Allergic Diseases

Hay fever and asthma affect some 22 million Americans and combine to cause an average 116 million restricted-activity days and 4.5 million bed-disability days each year. About 2000 deaths are attributed to asthma annually.

Hay fever This condition, which has nothing to do with hay and does not produce fever, is most commonly caused by pollen of the ragweed plant east of the Rocky Mountains and by pollens of trees, grasses, and other weeds to the west. Weather and other factors may aggravate symptoms of pollen allergy. "Hay fever" that seems to linger all year is often caused by nonseasonal allergens—household dusts, animal dander, or feathers—and is called allergic rhinitis (*rhin* = nose).

Asthma This most serious of the chronic allergic diseases, involving severe respiratory difficulties, can begin at age 2 or 82, but most often appears in the first or second decades of life. It handicaps its victims and can impair productivity and happiness. Frightening struggles for breath may require hospitalization or emergency treatment and are sometimes life-threatening. Untreated asthma can lead to loss of lung function, leaving the patient short of breath upon light exertion or even at rest. It can also lead to physical retardation in children and to life as an invalid. Asthma can be either *extrinsic*, with allergies generally involved, or intrinsic, where no external factors can be identified. Emotional stress, air pollution, and nonallergenic irritants such as dust or fumes can trigger an episode.

Allergy and emotions Some investigators now believe that allergies, particularly to food, can affect the central nervous system, but the theory has yet to be fully proved. Symptoms attributed to such allergies include confusion, depression, anxiety, extreme fatigue, aggressiveness, poor coordination, impaired performance, amnesia, weakness, and in some cases, symptoms mistaken for mental illness (Frazier).

Diagnosing Allergy

Diagnosing allergy requires the expertise of a physician, sometimes one who specializes in allergy. The most common method of diagnosis is to apply the suspected allergen to a skin scratch or prick or through subcutaneous (under-the-skin) injection or to the skin surface under a patch. If allergy exists, a large raised red wheal will appear within 10 to 30 minutes on the test site. In a patch test, a rash will appear within 24 hours of exposure to the antigen.

Skin tests are not infallible and their use in diagnosing food allergies is still under investigation. Usually the physician will use an elimination diet to discover the food causing allergic symptoms. In some cases, just a few of the most common food allergens—chocolates, nuts, and milk, for example—will be eliminated from the diet to see if symptoms disappear. In other cases, everything may be eliminated except a few basic foods. Additional foods will be added one at a time in an attempt to pinpoint the culprit.

Individuals who believe they may have allergies can help their physicians by keeping a diary of allergic symptoms in relation to weather, food, emotional state, travel, pets, and activities.

Treating Allergy

There are presently three basic approaches to treating the allergic patient. Two of these approaches, controlling the environment and use of drugs, treat only the symptoms. The third, desensitization, attempts to eliminate the allergy.

Controlling the environment Altering the environment by removing the offending substances almost always brings relief from allergy. This would mean, for example, keeping pets out of the house if there is allergy to animal dander; using hypoallergenic cosmetics if cosmetics cause a rash; checking labels on drugs, foods, and the like to be sure the allergenic substances are not in the formula; and keeping the home—especially the bedroom—allergy-free by avoiding carpeting, upholstery, clutter, and other dust collectors. In some cases of seasonal allergy, moving to a new climate may help, but often it does not. Such a major step should be made only on the advice of a physician, following thorough allergy testing.

Drug therapy or chemotherapy Antihistamine drugs, counteracting the effects of the histamines, are the most widely used of all allergy drugs. Most effective for nasal allergies, they are often useful in skin and other responses as well, but drowsiness—a major side effect—may interfere with driving, study, or other activities. Most asthmatics benefit from regular use of drugs called bronchodilators, that shrink the mucous membranes and bronchial mucosa. Nasal drops or sprays are useful, but overuse may lead to a worsening

Camera M.D. Studios

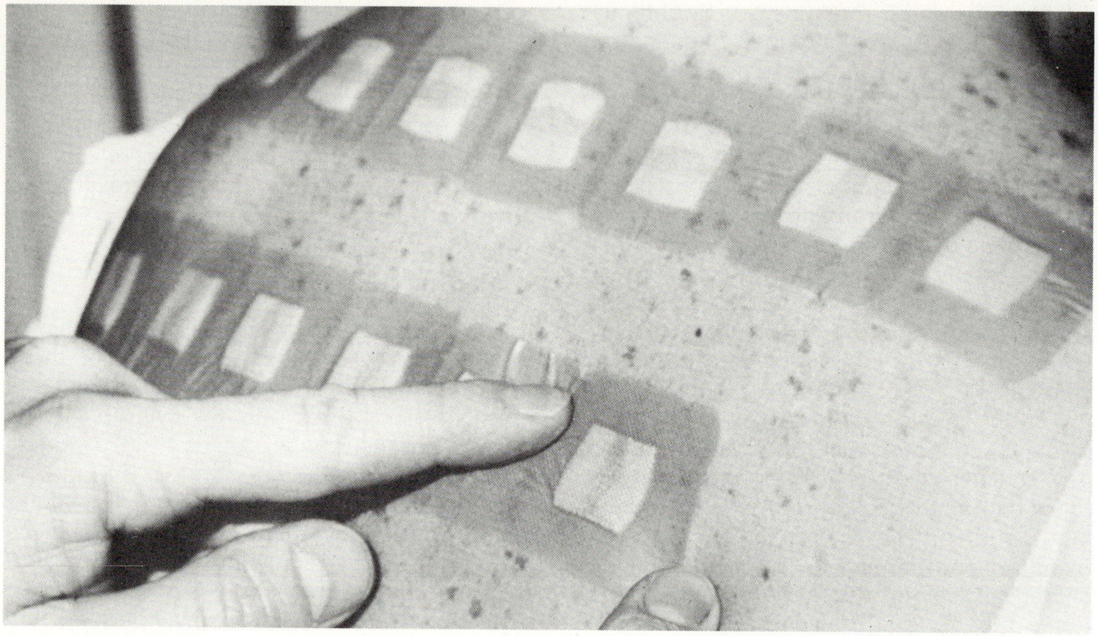

One way of determining the cause of an allergic reaction is to apply the suspected allergen to the skin, cover with a patch, and wait for a reaction. If a rash forms, the patient is probably allergic to the substance.

of symptoms after a few days due to a "rebound phenomenon." Corticosteroids, used since 1949 for asthmatic attacks, have many adverse effects and are usually recommended only for life-threatening attacks and for short-term use. Research is under way to find a chemical that can block release of histamines in allergic response.

Hyposensitization When environmental control and antihistamines fail to bring relief, the physician may consider "desensitizing" the patient. The purpose of such hyposensitization is to obstruct the activity of the IgE antibodies with blocking antibodies. This is accomplished by a series of injections of the allergen in increasing amounts, starting with tiny doses too small to cause a reaction. In anywhere from two months to a year, the patient may be free of the allergy. Sometimes, however, the process fails. Even a successful hyposensitization may wear off with time and need to be repeated.

Prevention

As always, prevention is preferable to cure. Doctors generally recommend that, when possible, infants be breast-fed—especially those with a family history of allergies or with high IgE in blood serum. Babies should be introduced to other foods very gradually, one a week, no earlier than 3 months of age.[3] A relatively allergy-free environment may help prevent allergies from developing in high-risk persons.

[3]The Academy of Pediatrics has declared there is no reason for solid foods during the first year. Many allergists disagree, believing small portions of a variety of foods should be given after 3 months to non-breast-fed infants to prevent development of allergies. The most common causes of allergy—e.g., chocolate, nuts, eggs—should not be introduced until later.

LOOKING BACK

REVIEWING CONCEPTS IN CHAPTER 7

- Though few diseases can claim to be brand-new, patterns of disease—for reasons known and unknown—change periodically.
- Disease is multifactorial. Ordinarily a variety of influences—ranging from genetic susceptibility and psychological stress to physical environment and lifestyle—contribute to ill health.
- The body responds to attack or threat to health with a variety of defenses.
- The first lines of defense include the early warning system provided by the five senses, and a wide range of physical and chemical responses that block entry of foreign agents into the body, or expel or destroy those that do get in.
- Immunological response is the major defense against certain kinds of disease. The tactics of the immune system include cellular response—in which invaders are destroyed directly—and humoral response—in which specific antibodies are produced to incapacitate specific attackers.
- Because the immune system "remembers" many types of earlier invaders, science has been able to develop immunization against them.
- The immune system can malfunction in various ways. It can be underactive, providing inadequate protection, as in immune deficiency diseases. It can also react against an individual's own tissue, as may be the case in rheumatoid arthritis.
- Many techniques have been and are being developed both to stimulate and to depress the immune system.
- The most common disorders of the immune system are the allergic responses, or "hypersensitivities." These can be handled by avoiding the allergen causing the response; by chemicals that control the response; or by hyposensitization to reduce or eliminate hypersensitivity.

8

INFECTIOUS DISEASES: WHEN MICROORGANISMS ARE THE CULPRITS

WHAT'S AHEAD IN CHAPTER 8 What factors are ordinarily necessary for the process of infection to take place in humans? Can we manipulate these factors to prevent disease? How do microorganisms affect human ecology and health? What are the major disease-causing organisms? How can we totally eliminate infectious disease among humans? What are the ways in which infectious disease can be controlled? How effective are they? What is the most widespread group of infectious diseases, other than the common cold, to afflict Americans? Who is most susceptible to these diseases? How are these infections transmitted? How can they be prevented?

■ *Example 1* It is a warm night in midsummer. A bird, with a dangerous virus circulating in its blood, dozes quietly. A mosquito lights between down and feathers, bites, sucks blood until satisfied, then flies off to shelter in a dark culvert. Here she stays for one week, digesting the blood and developing her eggs, while the newly acquired virus multiplies in her body. After laying her eggs, she searches for another meal. This time, she finds a camper sleeping beneath the stars. As she punctures the man's flesh to sip his blood, she injects virus-laden saliva into her victim. Just another mosquito bite, scratched and forgotten. But five days later, the man suddenly feels ill and headachy, has trouble thinking and moving. Diagnosis: Encephalitis, inflammation of the brain. (U.S. DHEW, *d*)

■ *Example 2* It is exam period at a small

college. An instructor with strep throat leaves his sick bed for an appointment with a student. The student, tired and dejected after averaging three hours of sleep a night all week and eating nothing but candy bars, coffee, pizza, and cokes, is further upset when told she has failed the course. Five days later, her throat becomes red and raw, swallowing is difficult, and her temperature is 102°. Diagnosis: Strep throat.

■ *Example 3* On a Navajo reservation, a 9-year-old Indian boy cuts his finger. The young brave pays little attention to the wound. Next day, he helps his father skin and clean some game for food. A day or so later, the child runs a high fever. A boil appears on his finger at the site of the cut and he becomes very ill, his lymph nodes swollen knots. Physicians at the Indian Health Service Hospital immediately recognize the disease: bubonic plague, scourge of mankind since ancient times, often called the Black Death. (U.S. DHEW, *d)*

CONDITIONS THAT LEAD TO INFECTIOUS DISEASES

There are ordinarily six factors—all active in the examples above—necessary for the process of infectious disease to take place in humans:

1 *A causative agent,* a living organism capable of invading the body and causing disease. Such agents are called *pathogens* (*path* = disease + *genic* = producing).

2 *A reservoir* in which that pathogen can live and often multiply until it is passed on to a new host. The reservoir may be: (*a*) human, someone ill with a disease caused by the pathogen, or a carrier not affected by the disease who unwittingly spreads it; or (*b*) animal, a domestic animal, rodent, insect, or bird. *Zoonoses,* animal diseases transmitted to humans, are not usually transmitted from human to human.

3 *A means of escape* from the reservoir: (*a*) through the respiratory tract, as secretions from nose, throat, bronchial tree and lungs that are coughed, sneezed, or breathed out; (*b*) through the digestive tract via feces, vomitus, or saliva in bites or on contaminated eating utensils; (*c*) through the urinary tract; (*d*) through open sores, cuts, or other body lesions. The period in which the organism can escape from the body to infect another person is the *infectious period,* and isolation and other controls are important during this period to prevent spread. Organisms with no means of escape from the human reservoir, such as the parasite that causes trichinosis, present less of a public health threat, since they are not communicable from one person to another.

4 *A means of transmission* from reservoir to new host. Transmission can be direct (from one body to another as in venereal contact, kissing, touching) or it can be indirect (via animate, live, *vectors* such as animals and insects; or via inanimate, nonliving, *fomites* such as furniture, clothing, linens, eating utensils, toilet seats, and tissues; or by water, food, air, and soil). Pathogens transmitted indirectly—capable of existing outside a reservoir host—are a greater threat to public health than those that travel only from host to host.

5 *A means of entry* into the new host, most often through the respiratory tract (breathed in), the digestive tract (swallowed), broken skin, or the mucous membranes lining the mouth, nose, anus, vagina, etc.

6 *A host susceptible* to the pathogen. Infection may not occur if immunity exists from previous exposure, or if strong body defenses ward off the organism before disease symptoms appear. Resistance depends upon general mental and physical health as well as a variety of environmental factors. (See Chapter 7.) The period before symptoms appear—during which the organism multiplies within the host—is called the *incubation period.* (Adapted from Wilner et al.)

THE MAJOR DISEASE-CAUSING ORGANISMS

Microorganisms (Microbiota)

This group comprises all living organisms too small to be seen without a microscope. The majority are so important to life that animals raised in a germ-free environment, in which there are no microorganisms, have increased susceptibility to infection and stress, more exacting nutritional requirements, and incompletely developed body cells and organs. Some microorganisms, however, cause disease, that is, they are pathogenic.

Microbiota in humans are usually divided into two classes: *endogenous* (found normally in the digestive tract, nose and throat, skin, and other body areas) and *exogenous* (invaders from outside). Endogenous microbes, the normal flora of the body, live in harmony with the body as long as the balance between them and their host is maintained. When the equilibrium is upset by stress, malnutrition, toxicity, or disease, these microbes can cause illness. Whether or not exogenous microbes cause illness depends upon the success of the body's defense system.

Bacteria The villainous public image of the bacterium is not deserved. These tiny one-celled organisms are vital to the ecology of the entire earth. They are the industrious recyclers that help the decay process along, transforming dead organic material into chemicals useful to plant and animal life. Being neither entirely animal nor entirely plant, they are categorized in a third group as *Protista*.

Like other living things, bacteria require nourishment; but unlike us, they thrive on such humble fare as snail shells, transmission grease, old rubber tires, and in some cases, nothing more than sunlight, water, and carbon dioxide. They also require a favorable environment: acceptable temperature, lighting, moisture, oxygen, and acidity levels. Some require an oxygen-free atmosphere and are called *anaerobic* (*an* = without + *aero* = air).

When conditions are unfavorable, as in a freezer or in boiling water, some particularly hardy bacteria form spores (hard shells) around themselves and thus survive until conditions are once more favorable. Then the process of sporulation is reversed and the normal life cycle begins again. Such bacteria have been known to revive and begin reproducing after as long as 60 years.

Pathogenic bacteria produce their ill effects in various ways, in such diseases as pneumonia, strep throat, and meningitis. Sometimes disease symptoms are caused by potent poisons, or toxins, secreted by the bacteria; sometimes by overwhelming growth of bacteria; sometimes by a strong reaction of the body's defense system.

Viruses or virions Viruses are much smaller and less independent than bacteria. Unlike bacteria, they are not complete cells. Nor are they, by strict definition, living things; they neither respond to stimuli nor carry on metabolic functions. Yet, like living things, they reproduce themselves. This reproductive process takes place only within animal, plant, or bacterial host cells, making viruses *intracellular parasites*. Because virus particles are small enough to pass through a fine filter, they may be referred to as *filtrable viruses*.

When the virus finds a cell that is a good match for it, having a complementary chemical design, the two may become attached. This opens the way for the virus or part of the virus to enter the cell, beginning the infectious process for a cold, flu, measles, fever blister, wart, or other viral disease. At this point, the infected cell's normal functions come to a halt and the hijacked cell machinery is turned over to the production of new virus particles under the direction of the viral nucleic acid. (Nucleic acid gives the orders for cell reproduction; see Chapter 23.) As a virus population explosion occurs, particles may begin to leak out of the host cell or the

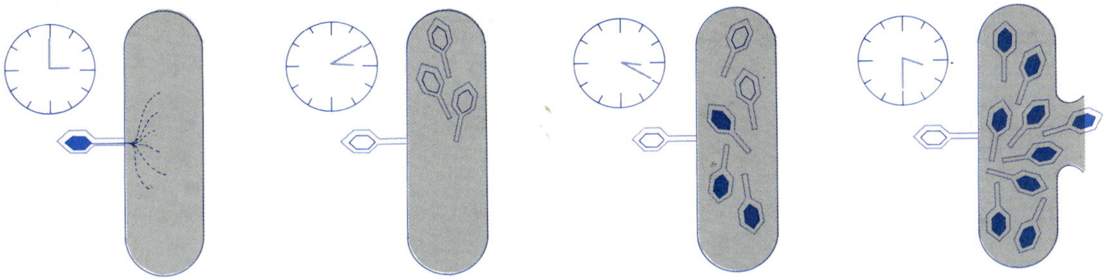

FIGURE 8.1 Reproduction of bacterial virus (coliphage T2) consists of four stages: (*a*) infection, in which the virus attaches to the host bacterium by the "tail," and the nucleic acid core is emptied into the bacterial cell; (*b*) the "dark" period during which virus nucleic acid begins to multiply and induces formation of new protein "coats"; (*c*) the "rise" period when nucleic acid appears within the protein coats; and (*d*) the burst, when some 200 new virus particles are released. The bacterium begins to disintegrate and then disappears. [*From Stent, pp. 38–39.*]

cell may swell and burst, releasing particles. In either case, the host cell is likely to have been fatally damaged and the new virus particles go on to other cells to continue the infectious process.

Some viruses, however, appear to remain "quiet" for months or years after penetrating the host. Suddenly, when conditions are favorable—perhaps when resistance is low—they become active. These "slow" viruses may be responsible for such disorders as the cold sore, in which symptoms flare up intermittently years after an initial infection, or for the puzzling and crippling multiple sclerosis.

Other infectious microorganisms Other infectious microorganisms include: (1) *mycoplasmas*, a leading cause of pneumonia in young adults, vulnerable to antibiotics; (2) *rickettsiae*, a type of bacteria that can, like viruses, reproduce only within other cells, that is susceptible to antibiotics, and that causes such diseases as Rocky Mountain spotted fever, typhus, and Q fever; (3) *fungi*, members of the Protista group, such as yeasts and molds, that can be multicellular as well as single-celled, that are larger and more independent than the other microorganisms we have discussed, and that cause such disorders as athlete's foot, jock itch, other types of ringworm, and moniliasis; and (4) *protozoa*, single-celled organisms that have complex nutritional and physical needs, and that cause such diseases as malaria, toxoplasmosis, trichomoniasis, and giardiasis.

Multicellular Parasites

These many-celled organisms, larger and more complex than microbes—many have digestive, excretory, and nervous systems—range from 1 centimeter to 10 meters in length and may survive for up to 25 years. Among them are: (1) *internal multicellular parasites*, that, like other parasites, draw nourishment from the host in which they live and cause such diseases as roundworm, hookworm, and pinworm diseases as well as trichinosis and schistosomiasis; (2) *external or ectoparasites*, such as scabies, ticks, mites, and lice, that draw sustenance from the host but live outside the body.

Unfortunately, in the words of an experienced scholar in this field, DDT went further toward the eradication of malariologists than of mosquitoes. (Dubos, p. 380)

CONTROL OF INFECTIOUS DISEASE

Wiping out all pathogens appears to be a goal which nature opposes at every front. One type of pathogen is reduced by drug therapy and others previously controlled by the first multiply rapidly and cause new illnesses. Sprays cut down on disease-carrying insect populations, until the insects wise up and avoid sprayed areas; and the insecticides themselves cause a variety of health problems. Bacteria attacked repeatedly by antibiotics change form and become resistant to the drugs. Vaccines give immunity to a pathogen, but do not destroy it; the pathogen lies in wait for an unsuspecting, unvaccinated population.

It is clear that we cannot totally eradicate disease-causing organisms. We can, however, gain a large measure of control over them through immunization, environmental control, and drug therapy.

In 1796, the Scottish physician Edward Jenner smeared pus from the sores of a milkmaid infected with cowpox on two small cuts in the arm of a healthy 8-year-old. It was the beginning of modern immunization.

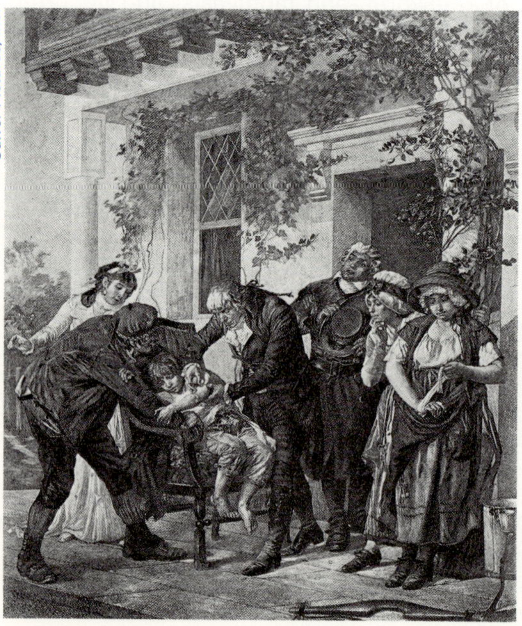

Culver Pictures, Inc.

Immunization

Historical perspective The ancients recognized that once people survived certain diseases, they would not contract them again. In Athens, recovered plague victims were used to nurse new patients. Some societies practiced a crude form of immunization: they ground up smallpox scabs and stuffed them in the nostrils, hoping to acquire a mild form of the pox as protection against future infection.

Later, in eighteenth-century Turkey, old women crudely vaccinated children by scratching the child's vein with a needle dipped in a nutshell of pus collected from pox victims with mild cases. Though some children contracted severe infections and died, most were only mildly ill for a few days and then recovered, immune from the pox. The wife of the British ambassador took the idea back to Britain where it was tested first on seven condemned prisoners—who survived and won their freedom—and then, with equal success, on six orphans. The procedure then became commonplace in Britain.

Modern immunization developed when Scottish physician Edward Jenner decided to put to scientific test the old belief that a person who contracted *cow*pox from cows would never get smallpox. In 1796, Jenner smeared pus from the sores of a milkmaid infected with cowpox on two small cuts in the arm of a healthy 8-year-old. The child developed a slight fever a week later, and then a couple of small scabs on his arm. Subsequent attempts at inoculating him with smallpox pus were unsuccessful. He was apparently immune.

Immunization today Today children and adults can be protected from a wide range of serious diseases with vaccines more scientifically prepared than Jenner's, but employing the same principle. In Chapter 7, we saw how a healthy immune system "remembers" many disease-causing antigens, and how it is ready to wipe them out with an antibody army next time they appear. Vaccination or immunization introduces the antigen intentionally with the purpose of developing long-memoried immunity. The dose is carefully gauged to be mild enough not to cause illness, yet strong enough to stimulate antibody production. This "active immunity" can be conferred with:

- *Vaccines* made from weakened (attenuated) or killed microorganisms. (The Salk polio vaccine uses killed viruses, the Sabin vaccine weakened ones.)
- *Toxoids*, toxins produced by certain microorganisms, deactivated by heat or chemical treatment so they are no longer toxic but still able to stimulate antibody production. (Tetanus and diptheria toxoids are used for immunization.)

FIGURE 8.2 Active and passive immunity. Polio vaccine and diphtheria/pertussis/tetanus combinations given to infants are examples of active immunization artificially induced. Administration of gamma globulin to pregnant women exposed to rubella is an example of passive immunization.

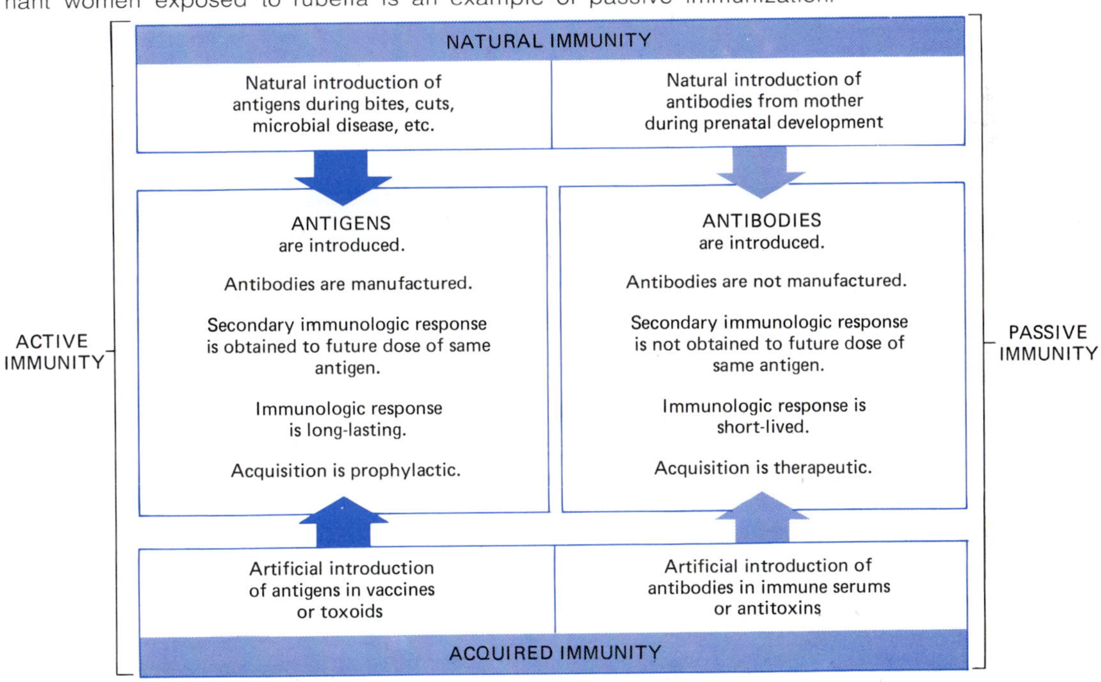

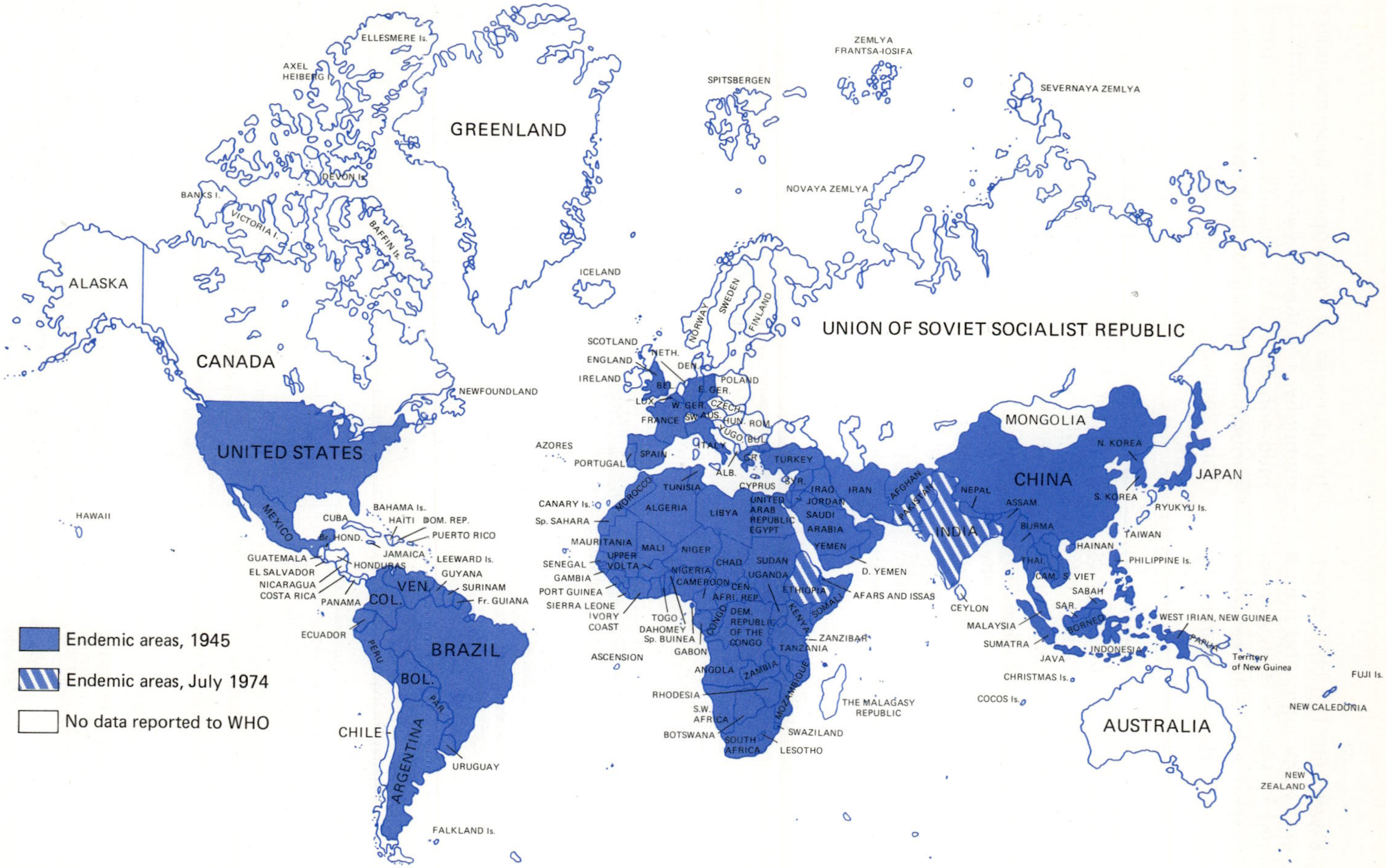

FIGURE 8.3 The effects of smallpox vaccination worldwide. Comparing endemic areas of smallpox in 1945 and 1974, this map shows how effective mass vaccination can be. A worldwide smallpox vaccination campaign virtually eliminated the disease by 1975. [*From WHO.*]

HEALTH CONSUMER TIP

TABLE 8.1 Immunization guidelines

AGE	DISEASE*
2 months	DPT (diphtheria and tetanus toxoids combined with pertussis—whooping cough—vaccine); TOPV (trivalent oral polio virus vaccine)
4 months	DPT; TOPV
6 months	DPT; TOPV
12–15 months	Measles (may be combined with rubella—german measles—or may be a measles-mumps-rubella combination); mumps (may be given later, but before puberty); rubella (may be given later, but before puberty)
18 months	DPT; TOPV
4–5 years	DPT; TOPV
Every 10 years	DT (diphtheria-tetanus booster)

*Tetanus immune globulin or antitoxin is given following a wound if immunization history is incomplete or last booster was more than 5 years earlier.

- *Vaccines* made from antigens similar to harmful ones that can stimulate an immune response against disease caused by both, as cowpox vaccination protects against both cowpox and smallpox.

A short-term "passive immunity" can be conferred with preparations containing antibodies taken from already immune persons. Gamma globulin, for example, may be given to prevent hepatitis A in exposed persons.

Immunization and public health More than 100 years ago, biologist Thomas Huxley said of his next-door neighbor: "If he is to be allowed to let his children go unvaccinated, he might as well be allowed to leave strychnine (poison) lozenges about in the way of mine." Huxley had a point. Parents who neglect to have their children vaccinated on schedule—out of ignorance, apathy, or the mistaken belief that childhood diseases have been wiped out—do a disservice not only to their own children, but to the community at large.[1] Unless 85 percent of susceptible persons are protected by immunization, there is risk of epidemic. Thus the effort to achieve total immunization coverage is a major public health thrust.

[1]Certain religious groups object to vaccination and are allowed to refuse it—except during epidemics.

Guidelines for travelers Immunization requirements for travelers change almost monthly. To obtain the latest information, check the World Health Organization booklet: "Vaccination Certificates: Requirements for International Travel." It may be available at a local library or at your travel agent, or you can buy it for $7.50 from the WHO, United Nations, Secretariat Building, New York, NY 10017. In general, however, no immunizations of any kind are required for travelers from the United States to Europe (including practically all the Soviet bloc nations), Japan, Hong Kong, and Australia and New Zealand. Travelers to South America, Africa, or Asia usually must have cholera and yellow fever shots.

Drugs to Fight Infection

A dramatic decline in the number of deaths and cases of serious disability from certain infectious diseases (pneumonia, TB, syphilis) is clearly linked to the discovery of sulfa drugs in 1937 and the subsequent development of other antimicrobial drugs. (See Figure 8.4.) To be effective, such drugs must be

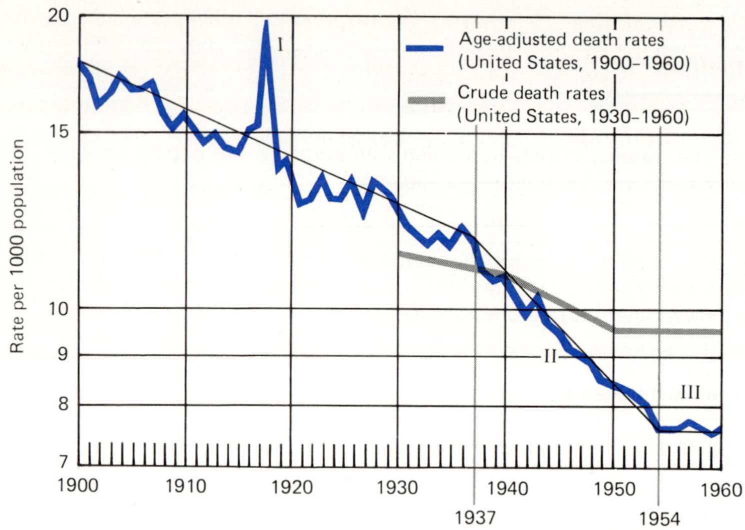

FIGURE 8.4 Influence of antimicrobial drugs on death rate. From 1900 through 1937, the death rate in the United States went through a pattern of ups and downs, but in 1937 (II) there was a sudden and steady drop that continued until 1954 (III), when it leveled out. What caused this drop? In 1936, the first antimicrobial—sulfonamide—was introduced. The peak around 1918 (I) resulted from the flu pandemic. [*Adapted from Kilbourne and Smillie, p. 14.*]

"selectively toxic"—much more damaging to the target microorganism than to the body of its host.

Antibiotics The fact that the penicillium fungus could kill bacteria was discovered quite by accident in 1928, before sulfa drugs came into use. It was not until 10 years later that the antibacterial substance was isolated as pencillin, and not until 1944 that the drug came into general use. The earliest antibiotics were produced naturally, like penicillin, by microorganisms. Today, many are produced synthetically. Some are broad-spectrum, effective against a wide variety of bacterial infections, and particularly useful when the identity of the agent causing the illness is uncertain. Others aim specifically at one type of microorganism. Neither type is effective against viral infections such as influenza or the common cold. They can, however, be useful when viral infections are complicated by secondary bacterial illness—when a cold, for example, leads to an ear infection or bronchitis caused by bacteria.

Wonder drugs versus bacteria—an ongoing battle As death rates plummeted dramatically for several bacterial illnesses, the new antibiotics were gratefully hailed as "wonder drugs." Then, suddenly, bacteria fought back. Some strains became resistant to the drugs' effects: The quantity of penicillin needed to knock out gonorrhea rose to 24 times the original dose. As some bacteria were laid low by drugs, other competing bacteria, because of inherent resistance factors, became more serious threats to health. Normally useful microorganisms dwelling in the body were often destroyed by antibiotics, leading to secondary infection by antibiotic-resistant pathogens, usually kept in check by them. And, there were many serious side effects to several of the antibiotics and allergic reactions to penicillin. Thus, a warning flag went up: Physicians should carefully weigh risk versus benefit and refrain from indiscriminate antibiotic use.

As you can see from the *Medical Tribune* debate, there is less than total agreement. Yet most authorities recommend that certain rules should be followed when prescribing antibiotic drugs: Prescribe only for illnesses caused by organisms susceptible to them; use the correct specific antibiotic when possible rather than a broad-spectrum drug; culture the organism to establish its identity; consider the patient's history.

Antiviral drugs Until 1977, no antiviral drugs were available and viral diseases were treated symptomatically—aspirin for fever, cough medicine for cough, etc. But that year three antiviral drugs were licensed for use. In addition, studies with interferon and interferon inducers were underway (see page 177).

Opinions on Antibiotic Use

In November 1975, the following letter was published in the Medical Tribune, a newspaper for physicians:

> One of the most constantly raised points in the current discussion about overprescribing of drugs is the alleged prescribing at a spinal reflex level of antibiotics for "the common cold." It is repeatedly said that in surveys of doctors in practice, a very high percentage of patients who come to the doctor's office for "the common cold" receive an antibiotic.
>
> On the face of it, this seems reprehensible. On reflection, however, it occurs to me that most patients do not visit a doctor's office, and pay good money, for advice about uncomplicated coryza. I suspect, instead, that most patients with upper respiratory complaints go to see doctors suffering from a combination of cough, stuffed nose, post-natal drip, swollen glands in the neck, earache, etc.—in other words, from secondary bacterial complications of the common cold. If this is the case, then the prescribing of an antibiotic is not wrong. . . .
>
> Louis Lasagna, Professor of Pharmacology,
> University of Rochester School of Medicine

In response to the letter came a large number of comments from practicing physicians supporting Dr. Lasagna's position. But there were several from both private physicans and eminent scientists like Albert Sabin (developer of polio vaccine) that sharply disagreed. They insisted that a culture should almost always be taken before an antibiotic is prescribed to be certain that the infecting organism is one that can be routed by the drug. They pointed out that in study after study, only a small number of patients with the kinds of symptoms Dr. Lasagna describes actually turn out to have a bacterial infection; that the unnecessary use of antibiotics can lead to the growth of resistant strains and that individuals who have taken unnecessary antibiotics will be less likely to respond to the drugs in the future when perhaps it might be a matter of life and death; that the cost of a lab culture is no more than the cost of a bottle of antibiotic capsules. They suggest the truth of the old maxim about colds: "Treated they last two weeks; untreated, a fortnight."

Environmental Control

Community decision making is a crucial factor in environmental control of disease. The community decides which public health measures will be developed and how they will be enforced. Major approaches include:

- *Sanitation* *Treatment and disposal of human wastes* to prevent diseases, such as typhoid fever and hepatitis A, which are passed through the fecal-oral route (pathogens shed by an infected person in body wastes enter a new host through food or water contaminated by those wastes); *sanitary handling of food* to prevent food-borne diseases (see Chapter 5); *sanitary disposal of food wastes* that can be breeding grounds for disease-carrying insects and animals; *purification of water supplies* through use of chlorine or other chemicals, and filtration to eliminate water-borne diseases; *safe handling of milk*, including sanitary milking procedures, mandatory disease-free status for cows, proper refrigeration, and pasteurization.
- *Control of insect vectors* *Elimination of insect breeding places* by draining and filling in marshes and swamps or other still bodies of water where mosquitos breed; *careful disposal* of organic wastes (food, for example) and manure (a favorite breeding ground of flies); *use of screens on windows; stocking of breeding waters with fish* that eat the insect larvae or eggs; *insecticide spraying* (which can, however, damage plant, animal, and human life); *prevention of successful mating of insects* through biological means harmless to other forms of life (preferred by environmentalists).
- *Control of animal reservoirs* *Vaccination of pets* capable of carrying rabies; *good veterinary care* for pets; *handwashing after handling of pets or other animals; avoidance of pets* (such as chicks, birds, turtles) *that commonly carry disease; control of wild animal populations; careful disposal of animal wastes.*

Finally, there is the *detection and control of human carriers* which may sometimes be the most difficult of all measures to enforce. Mary Mallon ("Typhoid Mary") was believed responsible for more than 200 cases of typhoid and at least 3 deaths in and around New York City at the turn of this century. Mary developed typhoid in 1901 and recovered. A month later, the laundress in the house in which she worked as a cook was stricken. In 1902, Mary moved to a new position, where 2 weeks later a servant and 7 household members came down with typhoid. In 1904, she infected 4 servants of a Long Island family. In 1906, when she infected 6 members of another family, she finally came under suspicion as a carrier. While sanitary engineer George A. Soper traced her movements, she continued to spread typhoid. When taken into custody in 1907, cultures of her stool showed she was excreting enormous numbers of typhoid bacilli.

Mary was required to sign a pledge to give up her career as a cook, be scrupulous in personal hygiene, and report to the Health Department every 3 months. She kept her bargain for 3 years, and then vanished. In 1915, an outbreak of 25 cases of typhoid occurred in the Sloane Hospital for Women, and the cook disappeared, leaving no forwarding address. Traced by the Health Department, Mary Mallon was found living under an assumed name. This time, she was detained in an institution until her death in 1938. Further study showed she may have been the source of an additional 1300 cases of typhoid in Ithaca, New York, in 1903. Today, lifetime confinement of carriers is unnecessary, thanks to antibiotics or other drugs and treatments that can clear their infections.

Epidemic Control

The Center for Disease Control The Center for Disease Control (CDC) in Atlanta, Georgia, an agency of the Public Health Service, is the coordinating center for collection and dissemination of data on disease prevalence and

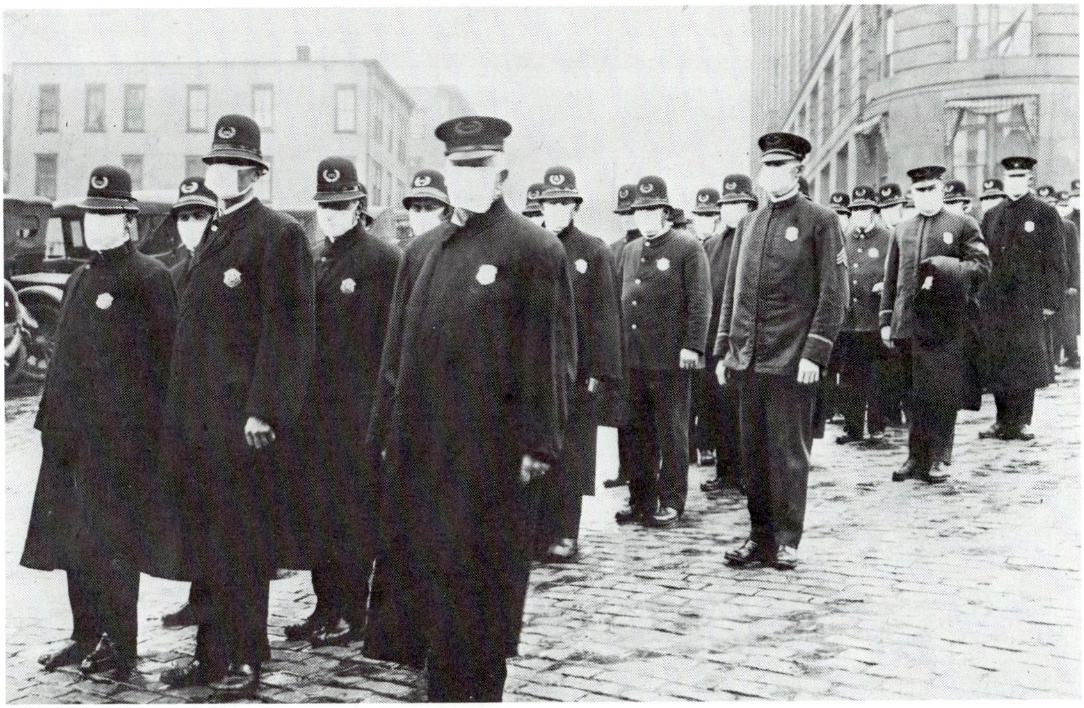

Control of infectious disease. During the influenza pandemic of 1918, schools were closed down, courts convened out-of-doors, and gauze masks were standard attire for public servants.

incidence. In concert with local and state health departments, it picks up ominous patterns that may predict epidemics, administers national and international immunization programs, enforces quarantine regulations when needed, provides investigators and laboratory facilities to track down disease sources, directs national programs for the prevention and control of communicable and other preventable diseases, and cooperates in international programs.

In 1976–1977, the CDC was involved in the development of the controversial swine flu program which aimed at immunization of millions of Americans against a potentially dangerous flu virus. But the billion-dollar program ended in confusion and recrimination when the vaccine was linked to cases of Guillain-Barré syndrome and when the threatened epidemic did not materialize.

Disease detectives When an outbreak (two or more cases of a communicable disease in an area, less widespread than an epidemic) of potentially serious infection occurs, public health officials must trace the cause and attempt to prevent further spread. Physicians, other health personnel, and coroners cooperate: (1) to isolate and identify the causative agent; (2) to find the original or index case and track all contacts this person had just prior to and during illness; (3) to discover the mode of transmission; (4) to decide whether this is just an isolated incident or one with serious epidemic potential; (5) to take steps to contain any possible epidemic.

TABLE 8.2 Selected communicable diseases

DISEASE AND CAUSATIVE AGENT	MODE OF TRANSMISSION	INCUBATION PERIOD*	SYMPTOMS†	CONTAGIOUS PERIOD	COMPLICATIONS	IMMUNIZATION AVAILABLE
Chicken pox (varicellazoster virus)	Person to person or by articles soiled by discharges of infected person	2–3 weeks (13–17 days)	Fever, headache, followed by pink spots that become pimples; blisters, then scabs form	From 5 days before to 6 days after rash appears	Rarely pneumonia and encephalitis	None
Diphtheria (Corynebacterium diphtheriae)	Contact with patient or carrier or with articles soiled by discharges of infected person; or through contaminated raw milk	2–5 days or longer	Fever, headache, sore throat, enlarged lymph nodes, grayish membrane in throat; can also affect nose or other mucous membranes	Variable; usually 2–4 weeks	Damage to central nervous system, heart muscle; 5–10% fatality rate	Yes
German measles, rubella (rubella virus)	Direct contact with infected person or freshly soiled articles; droplet or airborne transmission; congenital rubella transmitted from mother to fetus in early pregnancy	14–21 days (18 days)	Slight mottled or pimply rash; low-grade fever, headache; swollen glands in back of neck; possibly conjunctivitis	From 1 week before to 4 days after rash appears	Very rarely encephalitis; congenital syphilis in children in utero during mother's infection	Yes (women who are not immune and are exposed during first 3 months of pregnancy are given gamma globulin for passive immunity)

Hepatitis, infectious (hepatitis virus)	Person to person, fecal-oral route; contaminated food, milk, water, or needles or syringes	10–50 days (30–35 days)	Fever, weakness, loss of appetite; nausea, abdominal discomfort (upper right); then jaundice or yellowing of skin, eyes, etc.	From last half of incubation period to few days after jaundice appears	Slow recovery, disability lasting several months; fatality less than 1%	Passive only, with gamma globulin (temporary)
Measles (measles virus)	Usually droplet or person-to-person contact with infected patient	8–13 days (10 days) until initial fever	Fever, hard cough, cold symptoms, conjunctivitis; dusky red, blotchy rash appears in 3 or 4 days; white (Koplik) spots in mouth	From beginning of illness to 4 days after rash appears	Pneumonia, encephalitis; severe in adults, infants, and malnourished children	Yes (gamma globulin confers passive temporary immunity in unvaccinated exposed persons)
Meningitis (meningococcus bacteria)	By direct contact with discharges from nose or throat of carrier or patient	2–10 days (3–4 days)	Fever, severe headache, nausea, vomiting; then stiff neck; later delirium, coma; sometimes rash	Ends when meningococci are no longer in discharges; usually 24 hours after treatment begins	Possible involvement of many parts of the body; with prompt treatment, death rate as low as 5%	None (antibiotics may be given to exposed persons)

*The figure in parentheses is the most common incubation period.
†In most of these diseases it is possible to have a mild case with no symptoms.
Source: Developed from Berenson.

TABLE 8.2 ***(Continued)***

DISEASE AND CAUSATIVE AGENT	MODE OF TRANSMISSION	INCUBATION PERIOD*	SYMPTOMS†	CONTAGIOUS PERIOD	COMPLICATIONS	IMMUNIZATION AVAILABLE
Mumps, infectious parotitis (virus)	By direct contact with droplets or saliva of infected person; or indirectly through freshly soiled articles	12–26 days (18 days)	Fever, swelling, and tenderness of one or more salivary glands—most often the parotid	From 6 days before to 9–12 days after gland swells; most contagious 48 hours before swelling	Involvement of reproductive organs after puberty (can lead to sterility); other organs and systems may also be affected	Yes (should be given to all children, especially boys, be fore puberty)
Poliomyelitis (virus)	By direct contact with throat secretions or feces of infected persons; rarely, milk	3–21 days (7–12 days)	Fever, headache, intestinal disturbance, weakness, stiff neck, backache; in some types, paralysis	7–14 days before and after onset	Involvement of central nervous system; permanent paralysis; 2–10% fatality rate	Yes
Rocky Mountain spotted fever (rickettsiae)	Usually bite of infected tick	3–10 days	Sudden fever, headache, chills; mottled red rash about third day	Tick remains infective permanently	Fatality about 20% without treatment; uncommon with prompt treatment	Yes (3 doses, must be repeated annually)
Scarlet fever (streptococcus)	Usually respiratory transmission by direct or intimate contact	1–3 days	Fever, sore throat; then bright red spots and rash; skin may later peel	Mainly during illness; untreated persons may become carriers	Ear infection; rheumatic fever; kidney problems; few deaths in U.S.	None

Tetanus; lockjaw (tetanus bacillus)	Usually through puncture wound contaminated with soil, dust, human or animal wastes; also through trivial wounds	4–21 days (10 days)	Painful muscular contractions; rigidity		Fatality rate varies, 35–70%	Yes (boosters every 10 years, especially following puncture wound); antitoxin for unvaccinated
Typhoid (typhoid bacillus)	Direct or indirect contact with feces or urine of infected person usually through food or water; flies may be vectors	1–3 weeks (2 weeks)	Continued fever, weakness, lack of appetite, slow pulse, rose spots, involvement of spleen and lymph tissue	Variable; 2–5% become carriers	Fatality rate 10% without therapy; 2–3% with	Yes
Whooping cough (pertussis bacillus)	Directly by droplet spread; indirectly through articles freshly soiled by discharge from infected person	5–21 days (usually within 10)	Irritating cough becomes paroxysmal; lasts 1–2 months; each series of violent coughs is followed by high-pitched whoop	From 7 days before development to 3 weeks after	Fatality low in U.S., mostly occurs in infants; as high as 15% in some countries	Yes

*The figure in parentheses is the most common incubation period.
†In most of these diseases it is possible to have a mild case with no symptoms.

Mononucleosis—The College Disease

Infectious mononucleosis can strike at any age but is most common among young adults. It is probably caused by the Epstein-Barr (EB) virus and may be transmitted in the saliva during kissing, whence the nickname "kissing disease." Symptoms, which generally appear about 2 weeks to 2 months after exposure, at first include low-grade fever, headache, and fatigue. After a few days, severe sore throat and swollen neck glands appear. Blood tests showing elevated white blood cell count and characteristic changes in the structure of blood cells can confirm the diagnosis. The acute phase of the illness may last from a week to 10 days, but the patient often doesn't feel well for up to 2 or 3 months. Because mononucleosis is caused by a virus, antibiotics are of no use in treatment. Symptoms can be relieved by aspirin, bed rest, lozenges, and saltwater gargles, but this treatment does not appear to alter the course of the disease.

These procedures were followed when, in the summer of 1969, an entire New England college football team had to cancel its season because every member, including coaches and managers, mysteriously tested positive for hepatitis. Disease detectives discovered that children living adjacent to the field had had hepatitis during the summer and had contaminated pools of water near irrigation spigots while playing on the field. When water pressure dropped as hydrants in the area were opened, the disease-carrying water was sucked through the irrigation spigots and then back into the water system, down to the lower level of the playing field water faucet used by the players.

In this instance, there was clearly no threat of epidemic. The water contamination was so brief that the freshman football squad, arriving for pracice one week later, was unaffected. But the information gained was useful in restructuring the water system to avoid future contamination, and as a warning to others with similar water layouts. The incident was routine for public health officials but important in the battle against disease.

SEXUALLY TRANSMITTED DISEASES

Other than the common cold, the most prevalent communicable diseases in the United States are the venereal diseases. Ironically named in honor of the Greek goddess of love, Venus, these diseases are transmitted by close heterosexual or homosexual contact—most often by contact of moist mucous membranes during intercourse, but during oral and anal sex and deep kissing as well. They can also be passed on to a newborn moving through its mother's infected vaginal canal at birth. Because most of the organisms (bacteria, viruses, fungi) that cause these diseases cannot survive very long outside the warm, moist tissues of the body, the diseases are very rarely transmitted by toilet seats, towels, or bedsheets.

Just a few years ago, only two maladies would have been listed in Table 8.3: syphilis and gonorrhea. But scientists have since identified many new disease-causing organisms in the reproductive tracts of humans. These have been grouped, along with syphilis and gonorrhea, in a new category called sexually transmitted diseases, or STD.

Who Contracts Sexually Transmitted Diseases?

Anyone who has intimate contact with an infected person can contract a sexually transmitted disease—from commoners to kings like Richard II of England and Charles V of France. It is possible that Napoleon and Columbus, too, were victims. These diseases have been diagnosed in physicians and homemakers, in professors and students, in bank presidents and dishwashers, in people of all ages and occupations. STDs are, however, most common in the most sexually active age group, 15 to 30.

In 1977, epidemic levels were reached for several STDs with up to 1 million cases of nonspecific urethritis, 1 million cases of trichonomiasis, 200,000 cases of genital herpes, 80,000 cases of syphilis, and 2 million cases of gonorrhea estimated (Blount). Many reasons have been suggested to explain the epidemic: increased sexual activity by both heterosexuals and homosexuals; a longer period between first intercourse and marriage for many, allowing time for more partners; a decrease in the use of the VD-inhibiting condom; and an increase in the use of oral contraceptives that encourage the growth of infectious organisms in the vaginal canal. Venereal infections in mouth, throat, and rectum, formerly rare, have increased dramatically as a result of increasing oral and anal sex acts by both heterosexuals and homosexuals. A major federal effort at control of sexually transmitted diseases, however, does appear to have slowed the rapid increase of these diseases in the late 1970s. (See Figure 8.5.)

Diagnosis

Though several blood tests (see Table 4.3) can diagnose syphilis, and microscopic examination of culture of genital secretions can diagnose gonorrhea and other veneral diseases, many cases go undiscovered. Many who suspect a problem—because of pain, itching, burning, discharge, sores in the genital area, difficulty in urination or intercourse, or because they know they have been exposed to an infected or possibly infected person—will go to a physician or clinic immediately. Others, fearfully or foolishly, just "wait and see." If symptoms disappear, they forget about the problem. They are unaware that syphilis has several stages, and that it

FIGURE 8.5 Reported gonorrhea and syphilis in the United States, 1960 to 1976. Cases of early syphilis, and to a lesser extent gonorrhea, continued to decline in 1977. [*U.S. Department of Health, Education, and Welfare/Public Health Service,* Morbidity and Mortality Weekly Report, *Jan. 14, 1977.*]

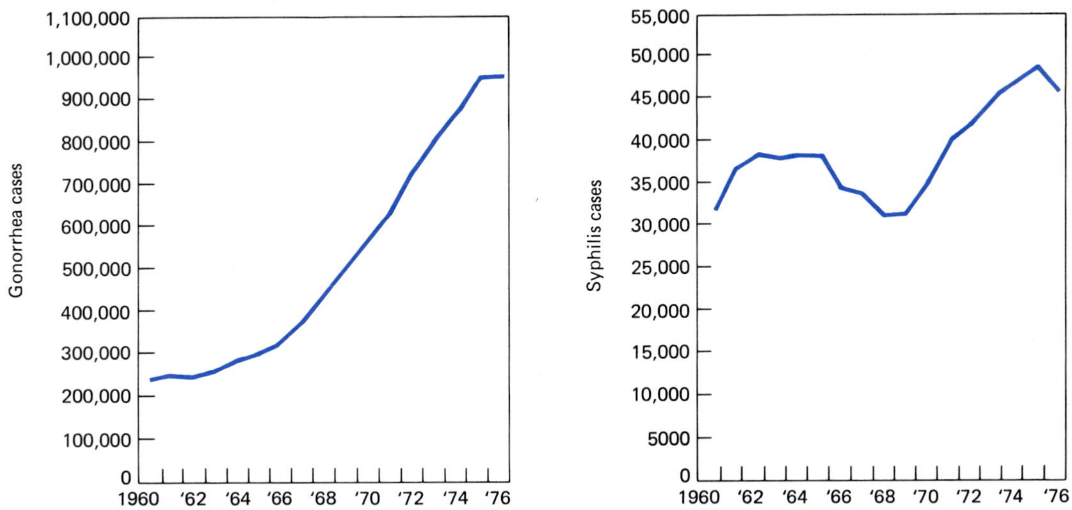

TABLE 8.3 The most common sexually transmitted diseases*

DISEASE AND CAUSATIVE ORGANISM	INCUBATION PERIOD	SYMPTOMS	COMPLICATIONS	TREATMENT	COMMENTS
Gonorrhea† (gonococcus, *Neisseria gonorrhoeae)*	2–8 days or longer	*Males* Infection of urethra; pain, inflammation of urinary canal, yellowish discharge; 7–20% have *no* symptoms. *Females* *Stage 1:* 60–80% have *no* symptoms; mild inflammation of urethra or cervix, lower abdominal pain, painful or frequent urination, vaginal discharge, joint pains and abnormal menstruation all possible. *Stage 2:* Invasion of pelvic region.	Pelvic inflammatory disease which can lead to sterility; arthritis; inflammation of heart lining; spread to prostate; epididymitis in males.	Penicillin; tetracycline in allergic patients	Untreated patients may become carriers; no immunity develops; reinfection possible
Syphilis† *(Treonema pallidum,* a spirochete)	10 days to 10 weeks (usually 3 weeks)	*Stage 1:* Primary lesions (pimples) usually on genitals, but can be anywhere. *Stage 2:* Secondary skin and mucous membrane eruptions. *Stage 3:* Latency or inactive period; may continue for life or may advance to stage 4. *Stage 4:* Lesions of skin, bone, nervous or cardiovascular systems, digestive tract.	In final stage: brain disease, heart disease, death	Penicillin or substitute in sensitive persons; *followup needed*	Untreated patients may be contagious indefinitely; no immunity develops; reinfection possible
Herpes† (herpes simplex II virus)	Up to 2 weeks	Blister-type eruptions on penis, female genital area, cervix; usually painful	Linked to cancer of cervix in women, of penis in men; damage to genitals	None proven, but disease seems self-limiting	More common in uncircumcized males
Chancroid *(Haemophilus ducreyi* bacillus)	3–5 days, plus or minus	Genital infection; ulcerations; painful inflammatory swelling; swelling of lymph nodes; may be *no* symptoms in women	Can do extensive damage to genital area	Sulfa drugs and other antibiotics; disease is self-limiting	Infection usually lasts several weeks and is communicable during that time

Lymphogranuloma venerum (bedsonia, chlamydia; also known as TRIC agents)	5–21 days (secondary stage 10–30 days to several months)	*Primary stage:* Small painless lesion. *Secondary stage:* Inflammation and swelling of lymph nodes in groin and of genitals; may also be fever, chills, headache, aches and pains, loss of appetite	Serious complications involving rectum can be disabling	Tetracycline and other antibiotics	Communicability can vary from weeks to years as long as disease is active. Can be transmitted on contaminated clothing, linens, etc.
Nonspecific urethritis (chlamydia and others)	3–4 days	Milder than gonorrhea; discharge may only be noticed on awakening in morning		Antibiotics; lots of water to flush out system; salt restriction	
Trichomoniasis (*Trichomonas vaginalis,* a protozoan)	4–20 days (7 days average)	Heavy, foul-smelling discharge in females; may be frothy and green; there may be redness around vagina; itching		Metronidazole (Flagyl); both partners should be treated	Both sexual and nonsexual transmission
Candidiasis (*Candida albicans; Monilia albicans,* a fungus)	Varies	Itching primarily; may also be inflamed vagina, white patches, rashes, thick cheesy discharge	Uncommon; but can spread to brain, heart, lungs, GI tract	Local topical ointments or suppositories	Certain medications and illnesses increase susceptibility; sexual and nonsexual transmission
Genital warts (virus)	3 months, plus or minus	Painless warts—dirty gray or red; bleed easily if bruised		(1)Clear up any discharge; (2) destroy warts chemically or surgically	Grow best in warm, moist genital area; cotton underwear helps prevent growth

*Can sometimes be transmitted in other ways. Any symptoms described above should be reported to a clinic or a physician even if there is no possibility of sexually transmitted infection.

†May be passed on to fetus by infected mother; see Table 23.4.

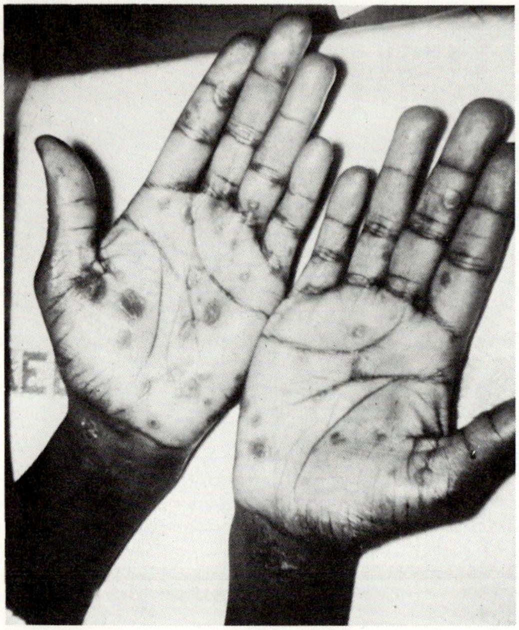
Center for Disease Control

When syphilis is untreated, the inactive third stage may be followed by a virulent fourth stage in which lesions of skin, bone, and the cardiovascular, nervous, and digestive systems occur. These can lead to damage to the heart, central nervous system, and brain, and finally to death.

can remain quiet for years and then suddenly reappear, more virulent than ever. They are also unaware that genital herpes, too, can return, and that, even if all symptoms disappear, the infection can be harmful to an expected newborn. (See Table 8.3.)

Sometimes there are no symptoms at all to warn the victim. It is believed that at any given time there are approximately 800,000 women without symptoms (asymptomatic) in the United States who are infected with gonorrhea, but do not realize it. An unknown number of men, perhaps 12 percent of those infected, are similarly unaware of their disease. The only way they will learn of it is by undergoing testing by a physician or at a public health facility or free clinic. (The individual's privacy is protected by these organizations.)

Hazards of Venereal Diseases

Does absence of symptoms mean absence of danger? Not at all. Some untreated victims of gonorrhea, for example, develop serious, even irreversible complications such as pelvic inflammatory disease (PID), arthritis, and gonorrheal infections of the skin, throat, and rectum before any symptoms are noted. Complications of gonorrhea are a major cause of sterility.

Untreated syphilis can lead to heart damage and central nervous system and brain deterioration. Before the advent of penicillin, more than 10,000 Americans (14,064 in 1940) died of advanced syphilis each year, and thousands more were admitted to mental institutions because of syphilitic brain disease.

An unwelcome newcomer to the STD scene is the herpes simplex II virus, a cousin to the more familiar herpes simplex I that causes annoying cold sores and fever blisters. Some physicians are finding it more frequently than other STDs. Although the symptoms (sores and pain) seem to be self-limiting, frequently disappearing within a few weeks, they often recur. Recurring infection in young persons with active sexual lives has been linked with cervical cancer and may also be linked with prostate cancer. Newborns carried by mothers infected with herpes, gonorrhea, or syphilis are at high risk of serious malformation, illness or death. (See Table 23.4.)

Treatment

The development of antimicrobial drugs and their use against venereal disease has dramatically reduced rates of serious illness and death. But the microorganisms are again gaining on us as they become increasingly resistant to drug therapy. Gonorrhea, for example, which once responded to 200,000 units of penicillin now requires 4.8 million units to do the job. The introduction into the United States of a new, totally penicillin-resistant strain of gonorrhea further complicates the picture. To combat these setbacks, scientists are working on new and potent drugs they hope will be effective against gonorrhea and other STDs.

Daniel S. Brody/Editorial Photocolor Archives

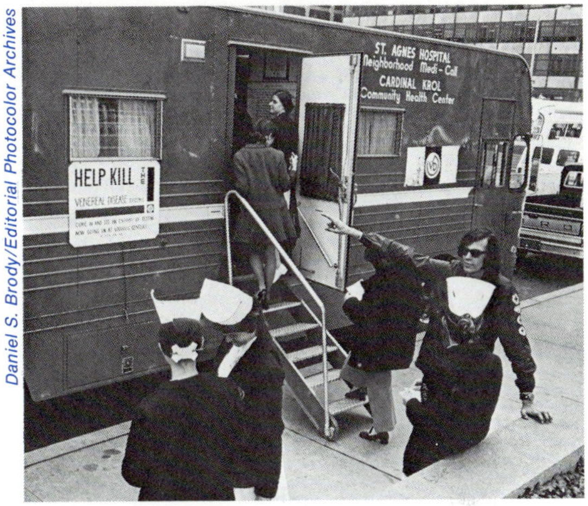

Control of STDs. Regular testing of sexually active individuals, to identify and treat potential carriers of gonorrhea and syphilis, could greatly reduce the spread of these diseases.

Preventing the Spread of STDs

It has been suggested that one way to eliminate the STDs would be to ban all sex outside of marriage. It has been reported that the Republic of China does this successfully. In a society where individual freedoms are valued, however, other steps seem more practical:

- *Use of condoms* During World War I, the U.S. Army reduced gonorrhea from 625 cases per 100 to 35 per 1000 by providing condoms and encouraging their use. The failure rate of properly used condoms in disease prevention is a low 1.3 percent, and some authorities believe that both males and females who are likely to have unexpected sexual activities should carry them routinely.
- *Choosing partners with care* Unlike some infectious diseases, STDs do not stimulate immunity to reinfection. Partners believed to be sexually active with many people should be avoided like the plague they may carry.
- *Improved reporting* Many people do not report symptoms to their doctors out of embarrassment or ignorance. And many physicians fail to report cases to disease control authorities so contacts can be traced and treated. This allows further spread of disease. It is recommended that individuals know the names and addresses of sex partners so they can be traced if necessary.
- *Routine diagnosis and treatment* If individuals who are sexually active were routinely checked for gonorrhea and syphilis when undergoing medical examinations, there would be a great increase in the number of asymptomatic cases picked up and treated and a corresponding drop in the number of persons spreading VD.
- *Development of vaccines* None are yet available though some work is being done.
- *Good hygiene* Washing thoroughly with soap and water immediately after intercourse or other sexual experience can remove some of the microorganisms that may be present. Urinating as soon as possible can wash them out of the urinary tract before they advance further. These measures, however, lower risks only slightly and are more effective for males than for females.

LOOKING BACK

REVIEWING CONCEPTS IN CHAPTER 8

- Six factors are ordinarily necessary for the process of infection to take place among humans: (1) a causative agent or pathogen; (2) a reservoir or source; (3) a means of escape; (4) a means of transmission; (5) a means of entry; (6) a susceptible host.
- Though microorganisms such as bacteria—found both inside and outside the human body—may sometimes cause disease, they are vital to human ecology.
- The major disease-causing microorganisms are: bacteria, viruses, mycoplasmas, rickettsiae, fungi, and protozoa.
- Multicellular organisms, larger and more complex than microbes, also cause disease. Examples are hookworms, pinworms, roundworms, and tapeworms.
- Though infectious disease can never be totally eradicated, it can be controlled in several ways: (1) Immunization, used against certain bacterial and viral diseases, to enhance the body's immune response to a particular invading organism—making the individual "immune." (2) Drug therapy to combat many types of infection. (Overuse or careless use of these drugs can, however, be hazardous.) (3) Environmental control: improved sanitation, cleaner food and water, control of animals and insects that carry disease, and control of human carriers.
- The most widespread infectious diseases in the United States (other than the common cold) are venereal or sexually transmitted diseases. They can strike anyone who has intimate physical contact—e.g., intercourse, deep kissing, anal or oral sex—with an infected person.
- Selectivity in sexual partners, getting immediate medical attention for any possible symptoms of VD, reporting of all sexual contacts by persons who are infected, and use of condoms are all ways of preventing spread of VD.

9
DISORDERS THAT AFFECT OUR MAGNIFICENT MACHINE

WHAT'S AHEAD IN CHAPTER 9 How can knowing about the way the body functions help you to keep it working better? Why is the respiratory tract so susceptible to assault by microorganisms, smoke, soot, and other pollutants? Is there a known cure for the common cold? Why is prompt attention to colds and other minor respiratory illnesses important? How are growth, body temperature, amount of physical energy available, sex drive, and reproduction regulated? What are the symptoms of *hyper*glycemia? *Hypo*glycemia? Why is it important to report such symptoms to a physician? What role do brain and spinal cord play in the operation of the human body? What are some of the disorders that disable the nervous system? How does rehabilitative therapy help individuals suffering from nervous system disorders? What is the part of the digestive system in keeping the body in good health? Which symptoms of digestive disease indicate serious illness and a visit to the doctor?

In 1711, Joseph Addison, British essayist and critic, described the body as ". . . a system of Tubes and Glands, or to use a more Rustick phrase, a Bundle of Pipes and Strainers, fitted to one another after so wonderful a manner as to make a proper Engine for the Soul to work with." Though his understanding of the body was a bit thin scientifically, Addison possessed the scientist's awe for the magnificent machine that is the human body. Most of the rest of us take this machine for granted, as long as it is functioning smoothly. When it is not (marvelous as it is, it does break down), we want to know more.

To make a large amount of information easily available, this chapter, like Chapter 6, has been designed as a series of diagrams, charts, and sidebars. These explain the functions of four major body systems—respiratory, digestive, nervous, and endocrine—the disorders that most affect these systems, self-care tips for illnesses that are easily self-treatable, and modes of disease prevention when these are known. With the body, as with the automobile, if you know a little about the way the machinery functions, take care of routine maintenance on schedule, and see that small problems are remedied before they become big ones, you can expect that the machine will operate better, with fewer breakdowns, and for a longer time.

THE RESPIRATORY SYSTEM

The lung, a pinkish, spongy, elastic organ at birth, has, by adulthood, been darkened to gray by its constant exposure to outside air, much like a room with an always-open window. The dirt, pollutants, and germs that enter with every breath can cause both acute (sudden, brief) and chronic (long-term) illness, and eventually irreversible damage to the lungs. (See Chapter 7 to find out how the respiratory system defends itself.)

The function of the lungs is respiration: the breathing in of oxygen and out of carbon dioxide (CO_2) and other wastes about 16 times every minute for adults. This function is essential to life. Even short periods without fresh oxygen lead to death of the brain, the heart, and of cells throughout the body.

Breathing is both voluntary (like walking) and involuntary (like the beating of the heart). Thus we can hold our breath briefly while swimming under water or when exposed to noxious fumes. But if we hold our breath long enough to become unconscious (small children sometimes do), we automatically begin breathing again. The same involuntary control takes command when we hyperventilate (take in too much air) in an anxiety attack. By breathing too hard, we blow off an excess of carbon dioxide, causing temporary neurological changes and symptoms, such as dizziness, muscle spasm, and twitching. When unconsciousness ends this hyperventilation, respiration slows down, we produce enough CO_2, and the body returns to normal. Hyperventilation can be ended quickly by getting the patient to breathe into a paper bag—where the needed CO_2 is reinhaled and normal equilibrium rapidly achieved.

Strong emotions or physical activity can increase breathing rate involuntarily by increasing carbon dioxide production, which leads to rapid "panting" to dispose of the CO_2 wastes and take in more oxygen. Nonstimulating surroundings can slow breathing down, making us sleepy. If we fight to stay

FIGURE 9.1 (*Opposite page*) How we breathe. Air inhaled through nose (1) or mouth (2) is drawn into *pharynx* (3) and *trachea* (4). It then moves on into right and left primary *bronchi* (5), and then into smaller bronchi (6) and into tiny *bronchioli* (7). Seconds after it enters the nose, the air is in the microscopic little sacs, *alveoli* (8), at the ends of the bronchioli. Oxygen from the inhaled air passes through the walls of the alveoli and into the capillaries (9), tiny blood vessels, surrounding them. The oxygen is then transported to the heart, from which it is pumped to the rest of the body. While oxygen is moving out of the alveoli, carbon dioxide wastes collected throughout the body by the blood pass into them and are eliminated from the body when the

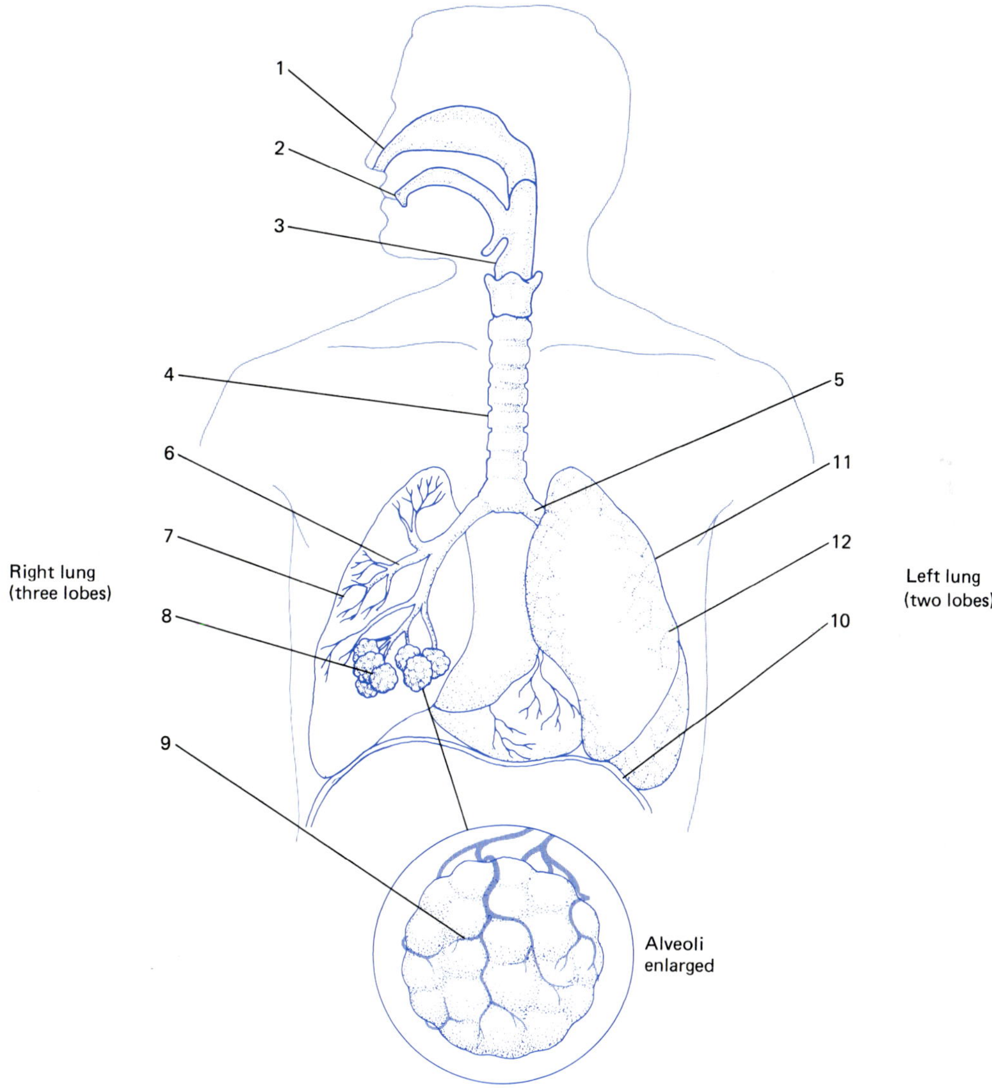

air in the lungs is exhaled. When trachea, bronchi, and alveoli become damaged (see Figure 17.3), as from smoking, the breathing process becomes labored and eventually may become impossible.

The diaphragm (10) is the muscle that controls the expansion and contraction of the chest (thoracic) cavity, allowing us to exhale and inhale. Each lung is covered with a thin membrane, or pleura (11). The surface of the chest wall is lined with a similar membrane (12). These fluid-lubricated membranes make breathing comfortable by sliding and gliding over each other as lungs expand and contract.

awake, the automatic response is a yawn, an attempt to draw in more oxygen and break the shallow breathing pattern.

Disorders of the Respiratory System

Disorders of the respiratory system are the most frequent afflictions of human beings. They include the common cold, influenza, and pneumonia, caused by microorganisms; asthma and hayfever, caused by allergens; emphysema and chronic bronchitis, brought on by exposure to irritants and pollutants, particularly inhaled cigarette smoke. Asthma and hay fever are discussed under allergies in Chapter 7, and emphysema and bronchitis in Chapter 17, "Tobacco." This section deals with major infectious respiratory diseases.

The common cold Sneezing, coughing, runny nose, headache, aches and pains, and sometimes fever are symptoms of this "mild" illness that costs billions in medical expenses and lost income from absenteeism every year. *Cause*: Not wet feet or going without a hat, but rather one of at least a hundred already identified cold viruses. *Transmission*: From someone with the infection (most contagious during the first 24 hours), either by direct contact (kissing), direct contact with nasal discharges (handshakes, soiled tissues, etc.), or less often, through droplets coughed or sneezed into the air. Most easily transmitted in winter when people cluster indoors in hot, dry air. Some believe that fatigue, poor general health, stress, irritants such as cigarette smoke, and possibly even chilling may make people more susceptible to colds. Symptoms usually appear 1 to 3 days following exposure. *Treatment*: Americans spend $750 million yearly on some 50,000 cold and cough preparations. Yet a 1976 FDA study declared that there is *no* treatment generally accepted as able to prevent, cure, or even shorten a cold. Symptoms, however, can be treated with: (1) aspirin for headache, fever, achiness (although some studies indicate it may increase contagiousness); (2) antihistamines, *only* if allergic reaction accompanies the cold (they are ineffective on colds themselves); (3) a humidifier to add moisture to the air (some prefer a cool-mist type); (4) saltwater gargle or cough lozenges to soothe throat; (5) nasal decongestants—spray, drops, inhalants used for a limited time only as directed, or tablets, capsules, or liquids; (6) fluids—juice, tea, or soup—at the rate of about one cupful per hour to thin secretions. Bed rest is not necessary unless

HEALTH CONSUMER TIP

Cures and Noncures for the Common Cold

Vitamin C, in varying doses, has been suggested to prevent or lessen cold symptoms, and its most celebrated champion has been Nobel prize–winning chemist Linus Pauling. Though studies funded by the National Institutes of Health have found that ascorbic acid (vitamin C) can prevent the multiplication of some cold-causing germs in the lab, studies on humans to this point have been inconclusive—partly because it is so difficult to control for all factors in such studies. There is some evidence that people who are well-nourished are most likely to benefit from vitamin C.

Among popular treatments that definitely do *not* work in curing a cold are: mouthwash, aspirin, laxatives, "sweating it out," cold baths, and exposure to cold air. Antibiotics have no effect on a cold virus, but they play an important role should secondary infection by bacteria occur. Over-the-counter (nonprescription) cold remedies are of questionable value. The 1976 FDA study of the ingredients in such products found only one-third could be classified as "generally safe and effective," relieving cold symptoms.

there is fever, but taking it easy may help to fight complications. Staying away from others early in the infection may keep it from spreading. *Prevention*: Because of the large number of cold viruses and the short-term immunity they confer, cold vaccines are not practical. Since adults suffer fewer colds than children, it may be that some modest protection is built up over time.

Influenza or "flu" More serious and more highly contagious than a cold and often longer lasting, generally 9 to 15 days. Early symptoms include weak and aching muscles and sore throat, followed by chills, fever, headache, backache, muscle pain, loss of appetite, and finally coldlike symptoms. A nagging cough and tired feeling may hang on for weeks. *Cause*: Three main types of viruses: A, B, and C, with several strains within each type, changing slightly from year to year. Type A is most virulent and seems to occur in epidemic cycles about every 10 years; the milder type B can also cause epidemics; type C usually does not. *Treatment*: Bed rest until 2 days after temperature returns to normal, plus symptomatic treatment as for a cold. The new drug amantadine may be prescribed to relieve symptoms and shorten illness. Complications, such as earache, sinus pain, or persistent cough, require medical attention. *Prevention*: Flu vaccine may be recommended for the high-risk population—the elderly, pregnant women, the chronically ill. Because of the variation in strains, vaccination must be repeated yearly.

Sinusitis A pressure buildup in the sinuses resulting from a blockage or swelling of the drainage canals (Figure 9.2), causing excruciating pain around eyes and in neck, ears, top of head, jaws, and forehead; as well as inflammation, swelling, pain, and tenderness around eyes and in cheeks; loss of smell; stuffy nose, and postnasal drip. Location of pain depends upon the sinuses affected; pain is worse on bending over. *Causes*: Infection, allergy, alcohol, chlorine in pools, tobacco smoke, or polyps or tumors blocking canals. Forceful nose blowing, swimming, diving, or change in pressure in airplanes can force infected material into sinuses. *Treatment:* If bacterial infection, antibiotics; if allergic response, antihistamines or de-

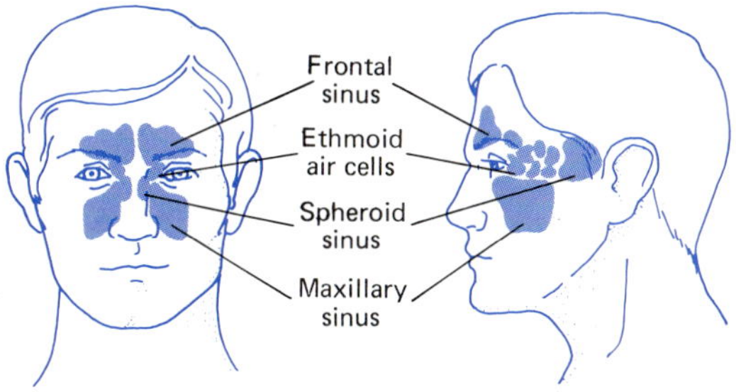

FIGURE 9.2 The sinuses. The paranasal sinuses are mucous-membrane-lined hollows or cavities that produce mucus that drains down into the nasal cavity, helping to moisten incoming air.

congestant sinus tablets. Nasal sprays and drops can be used for a day or two. Alternating cold and hot compresses and increasing fluid intake may improve drainage. (See Appendix.) Aspirin can relieve pain. Severe cases may need mechanical drainage or surgery.

Pneumonia An infection of the lungs, pneumonia (*pneumo* = lung) can start without any sign of previous illness, or can come on as a "complication" or "secondary infection" after a cold or other respiratory infection. There are three major types:

- *Bacterial pneumonia*[1] Often strikes when resistance is lowered by stress or illness. Symptoms may come on suddenly or gradually and include: shaking chills, chattering, severe chest pain, cough that brings up greenish or rusty sputum, and high fever. The skin may take on a bluish tinge from lack of oxygen; breathing may become rapid in an attempt to increase oxygen intake. *Treatment*: Antibiotics make most bacterial pneumonia cases—formerly 25 percent fatal—relatively easy to cure. But the disease still takes its toll in those with lowered resistance, and death rates of hospitalized patients whose pneumonia is caused by the staphylococcus bacterium are rising.

[1]Legionnaire's disease is a newly identified type of bacterial pneumonia.

WHEN TO SEEK HELP

Respiratory Symptoms

Anyone who has the following symptoms should see a doctor: (1) severe headache; (2) chest pains; (3) hard coughing; (4) earache; (5) rusty, bloody, or very thick sputum (collect in a jar and take to physician for examination); (6) high fever (over 101°F for a day or two, in adults); (7) wheezing (noisy rattle heard when patient breathes through mouth); (8) cough that lasts more than 10 days; (9) pulse rate more than 100 or less than 50 beats per minute (in adults). *Note*: Anyone who is over 60 years of age, who has a chronic disease, or who smokes should see a physician for *any* respiratory symptoms.

- *Viral pneumonia* About half of all pneumonia cases—more in children—are caused by viruses. Symptoms include fever, dry cough, headache, muscle pain, prostration. After 12 to 36 hours, there is increased breathlessness, cough worsens, and sputum may become bloody. Though most victims recover without special treatment, a few viruses can cause severe, even fatal, pneumonia. In "walking pneumonia" there may be no fever and only a mild cough. *Treatment*: Bed rest, aspirin for fever and pain, cough medicine for cough. Antibiotics are valueless, unless there is secondary bacterial infection.
- *Mycoplasma pneumonia* Usually mild, this form is most common in young adults. Symptoms include chills, violent cough, fever, and sometimes nausea and vomiting. Heartbeat may slow, and in severe cases there may be breathlessness and bluish skin. *Treatment*: Specific antibiotics.

Prevention: Good health habits to increase resistance to infection; proper care of minor respiratory infections; early treatment for suspicious symptoms; following physician's instructions, including finishing antibiotic medications even after symptoms are gone. New vaccines for mycoplasma and some bacterial pneumonias are under investigation.

Tuberculosis A serious infectious disease most frequently affecting the lungs. Incidence in the United States has dropped considerably in this century due to improved living conditions and new treatments that render patients noninfectious to others. Still, an estimated 16 million Americans have dormant TB germs encapsulated in their lungs—most without knowing it. Symptoms in an active case include: chronic cough, coughing up of blood, constant tired feeling, weakness, unexplained weight loss. In an inactive case there are no symptoms. *Cause*: Tuberculin bacillus. *Transmission*: Through day-to-day close contact with an active case; bacilli sprayed into air by cough are breathed into lungs of new host. If the new host is run down, infectious process begins immediately; if he or she is strong and healthy, bacilli are walled up in tiny hard capsules, or tubercles, until such time as resistance is low. Then TB germs break out and active case begins. *Detection*: Due to risk of excessive radiation, the "annual chest x-ray" is no longer recommended. A single TB (tuberculin) test in childhood, provided it is negative, should suffice unless or until there is exposure to an active case. Positive tests are followed by x-ray and other examination. An important part of the prevention process is tracing and testing all contacts of active cases. The preventive vaccine BCG, very commonly used in Europe, is not widely used in the United States. *Treatment*: Active cases are treated with isonazide, usually in combination with other drugs, for a period of 2 years. Isolation in sanitoria and disruption of normal life patterns are not usually necessary today. Inactive cases may be treated or simply kept under observation.

Other respiratory infections Infection can occur anywhere along the respiratory tract, from nose to

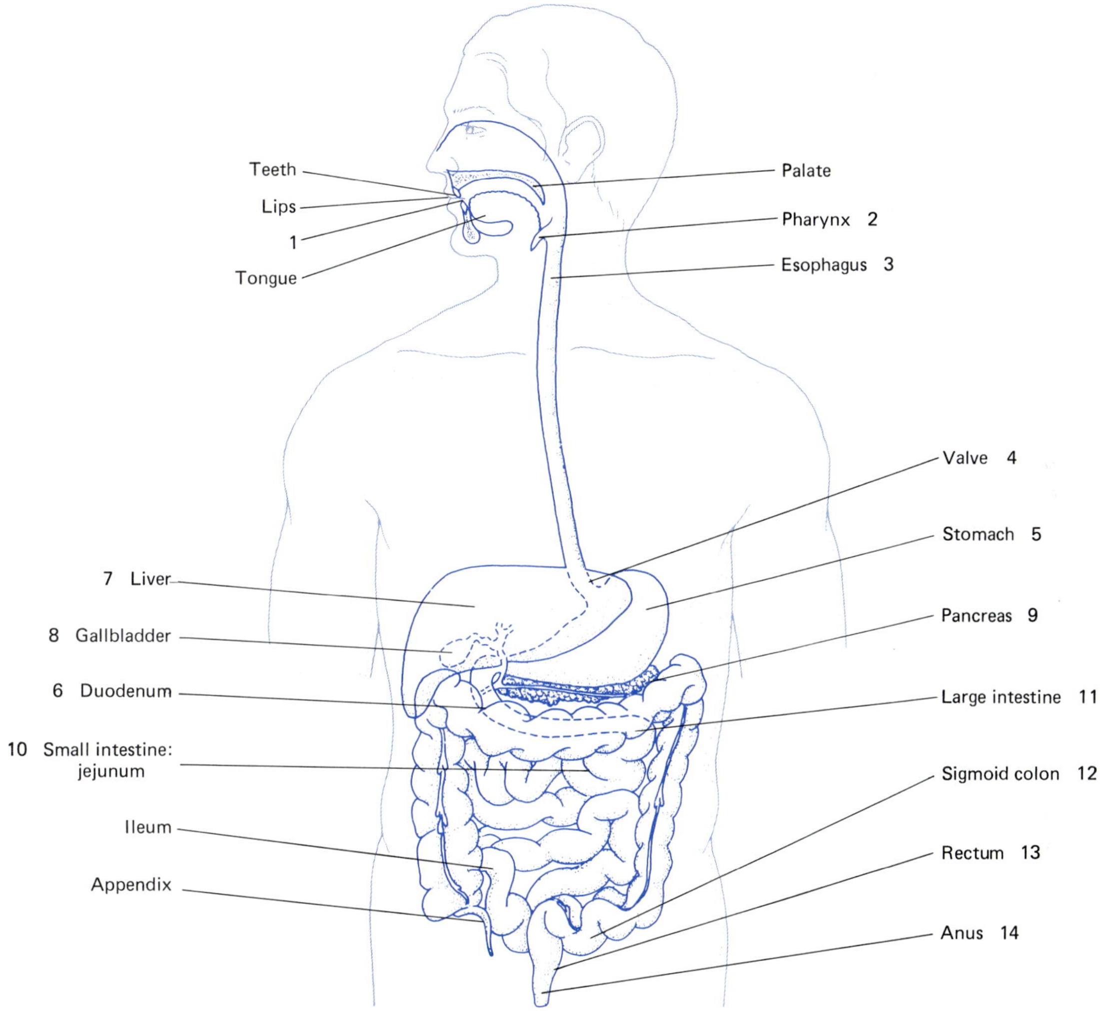

FIGURE 9.3 The digestive system.

lungs. It can attack the trachea (tracheitis), the pharynx (pharyngitis), the nasopharynx (nasopharyngitis), the larynx (laryngitis), or the bronchial tubes (bronchitis).

THE DIGESTIVE SYSTEM

As shown in Figure 9.3, digestion begins in the mouth (1). Mechanical digestion starts as teeth and jaws crush food into smaller particles; chemical digestion begins when salivary glands (see Figure 6.1) secrete an enzyme that breaks carbohydrates into simpler sugars and when the breakdown of fat, protein, and other substances begins. When it is well mixed with salts, enzymes, and mucus, the ball of food, or bolus, is passed through the pharynx (2) to the esophagus (3) by a complex reflex mechanism called swallowing.

Wavelike contractions (peristalsis) of the muscles in the esophagus move the bolus down toward the stomach. The bolus is then propelled through a valve (4) and into the stomach (5) where the next phase of digestion begins. Rhythmic contractions of the muscles of the stomach wall mechanically mix and mash the bolus. Stomach enzymes and hydrochloric acid chemically break it into smaller molecules called peptides.

From 1/2 hour to 4 hours after the bolus has entered the stomach, it is ready to move into the first section of the small intestine, the duodenum (6), where the third phase of digestion begins. Bile, produced by the liver (7) and stored in the gallbladder (8), and pancreatic (9) juices and enzymes finish the job of breaking down the chemical bonds of the food. The carbohydrates are broken down into simple sugars such as glucose, the proteins into amino acids, and fats into fatty acids and glycerol. As those materials pass, by peristaltic contractions, through the remainder of the 20-foot-long small intestine (10), the nutrients are absorbed by the walls of the intestines and pass through them into the bloodstream or lymphatics to be distributed to the cells of the body. What is left in the alimentary canal is indigestible material which passes into the large intestine (11), where water is removed and absorbed into the body. Bacteria act on the remaining material to decompose it and to produce some important vitamins, including vitamin K and a number of B vitamins, for body absorption. The totally useless remainder passes through the final length of the 5-foot-long large intestine, the S-shaped sigmoid colon (12), into a short, muscular tube, the rectum (13). Contraction of the muscles of the rectum results in defecation, the elimination of the feces through an opening called the anus (14). The bulk of the feces is derived from bacterial products rather than food, except in persons eating diets high in "fiber."

Digestive Disorders

Serious digestive diseases, such as ulcers, diverticulitis, ileitis, and irritable colon, affect about 13 million Americans. Less disabling digestive disorders—indigestion, heartburn, nausea and vomiting, constipation and diarrhea, and intestinal gas (which was described by Benjamin Franklin as "whirlwinds in the bowel," and the venting of which in public

WHEN TO SEEK HELP

Digestive Problems

Consult a physician for any of the following:

- Vomiting, nausea, or diarrhea that continues for more than 6 to 8 hours in young children, the elderly, or the chronically ill; or for more than 24 hours with treatment, 36 without, in others
- Vomiting or diarrhea, or other digestive distress accompanied by fever over 101°F
- Vomiting or nausea related to head injury within the past 48 hours
- Persistent or severe pain in the abdomen
- Any change from your normal bowel habits that continues for more than 2 weeks
- Persistent or intermittently recurrent indigestion, or other gastric distress
- Rectal bleeding or black spots (tarry blood) in stool

was banned in Rome in A.D. 40)—affect everyone at some time.

Vomiting, nausea "Throwing up" or feeling like throwing up. *Causes*: Viruses, or less often bacteria or other parasites transmitted in food or by food handlers; overindulgence in alcohol, rich foods, foods to which one is sensitive; emotional stress; pregnancy; motion of ship, car, airplane; serious illness such as gallbladder infection, appendicitis, hepatitis, and so on. *Treatment*: Depends upon cause. Home treatment includes abstaining from food and drink while vomiting continues; sucking on ice cubes for fluid replacement; bed rest (upright position increases fluid loss); clear liquids once vomiting has stopped (cola, ginger ale, sweet tea, broth, or "special drink"; see Appendix); soft diet resumed gradually (custard, gelatin, cooked cereal, baked potato, etc.). When all symptoms are gone, fatty or highly seasoned foods and alcohol should be avoided for 5 days.

Diarrhea Frequent loose or liquid bowel movements. *Cause*: Same as for vomiting, plus a variety of lower digestive tract disorders. *Treatment*: Depends on cause and duration. A kaolin-pectin preparation can help when the cause is emotional and after 6 to 8 hours (to allow the natural purging effects of diarrhea to work) in other cases. Fluids (see "Vomiting, nausea" above) should be taken in quantity; plain boiled rice may help.

Constipation Excessively hard, difficult-to-pass stools (bowel contents). Normal frequency of bowel movements varies from 3 times per day to once in 3 days.[2] *Cause*: Illness of many kinds; medication; hormone imbalance; psychological stress; lack of dietary fiber; poor muscle tone. *Treatment*: Relief of underlying cause; addition of bran or other high-fiber foods, prunes, raisins, or figs to diet; regular exercise. Laxatives, suppositories, or enemas should be used only for short-term problems in adults, *never* regularly or in children.

[2]There is a documented case of a man who did not have a bowel movement for an entire year.

Gas pain or flatus Pockets of gas somewhere along the digestive tract can cause pain, distention, and discomfort. *Cause*: Excess air swallowed (aerophagia) when food is gulped or when under nervous tension. Other causes are less well understood but may be related to bacterial metabolism of sugars that are eaten. *Treatment*: Relief of underlying cause. Antigas medication, prescribed or off the druggist's shelf, may provide temporary relief; a low-carbohydrate diet may be helpful.

Heartburn A burning sensation in upper abdomen or chest an hour or so after eating. *Cause*: Often related to obesity, smoking, coffee, spicy food, iced drinks, hard-to-digest foods, or stress, which can stimulate production of excess acid, irritating stomach lining. *Treatment*: Weight reduction; abstention from smoking; neutralizing acid with food, milk, or antacids. Antacids should be used with caution; many have side effects. *Prevention*: Elimination of cause.

THE NERVOUS SYSTEM

The nervous system, the body's communications network, oversees and coordinates the activities of the complex organization that is the human body. Its job description is threefold: (1) it collects data from the environment; (2) it interprets, analyzes, and files this information in its memory banks for future use; and sorts and refiles as new information comes in; and (3) it swiftly directs the body to respond appropriately to the world around it (to pull a hand away from a hot pot for example, or blink an eye when a finger comes toward it). If this description seems to apply to a computer's functioning, that is not surprising. The computer is designed to mimic the function of the human nervous system.

Information gathering is accomplished by a remarkable array of complex receptors in the eye, ear, nose, and mouth for sensing light, sound, smell, and taste, supplemented by

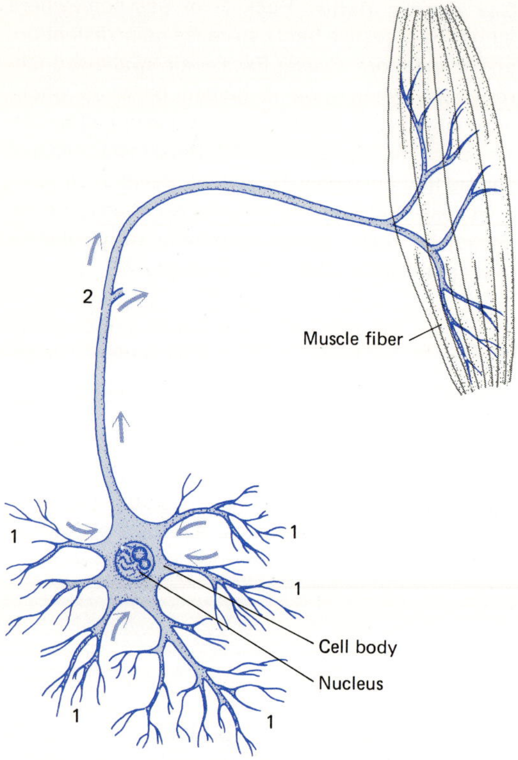

FIGURE 9.4 A motor neuron, a nerve cell that controls movement-producing impulses. Dendrites (1) conduct nerve impulses to their own cell bodies. Axons (2) conduct nerve impulses away from their own cell bodies. [*Adapted from Elson, pp. 86–87.*]

highly specialized sensory receptors located throughout the body whose job it is to detect changes in temperature, pressure, touch, and pain, and to relay this information to the command posts of the system—the brain and spinal cord. The working unit of this system is the nerve cell or neuron (see Figure 9.4). Extending from the neuron cell body are fibers along which messages, as nerve impulses, travel to and from the central nervous system at speeds as high as 225 miles per hour (100 meters per second). The neuron is so specialized for this one function that it has lost the ability to reproduce itself. Thus, the complete set of neurons provided at birth must serve a lifetime.

The brain, protected within the bones of the cranium, or skull, can be likened to a large mushroom with the cerebrum perched on top like a cap (see Figure 9.5). The brain is divided into three areas: the *cerebrum* (1), or new brain made up of right and left hemispheres, which controls speaking, walking, performance of other conscious acts, perception of sensations (touch, smell, sight, hearing), and storage of thoughts and memories; the *cerebellum* (2), which controls coordination and allows awareness of the position of one part of the body in relation to others; the *brain stem* (3), or old brain, a more primitive area concerned with those body functions that cannot easily be controlled by will: respiration, heart rate, blood pressure, emotions such as rage and the physiological response to them, and sensory information from the viscera, such as hunger and thirst.

The spinal cord (4), protectively encased in the bony vertebral column, begins as the continuation of the brain stem and extends down to about waist level. Impulses such as pain travel along the spinal cord to and from the brain from neurons and receptors throughout the body. The spinal cord also directs reflexes, such as pulling the hand away from a fire even before one is consciously aware of the sensation of heat.

Disorders of the Nervous System

Should the brain stop functioning for more than 4 minutes because of illness, injury, or lack of nourishment, permanent damage almost always follows (see Chapter 13). The individual personality may be forever altered. Damage to brain or spinal cord can lead to such difficulties as convulsions, deafness, vision deficiencies, dizziness, nausea, diarrhea, muscular weakness, and loss of ability to talk, walk, or reason, depending upon the location of the injury. Damage can be caused

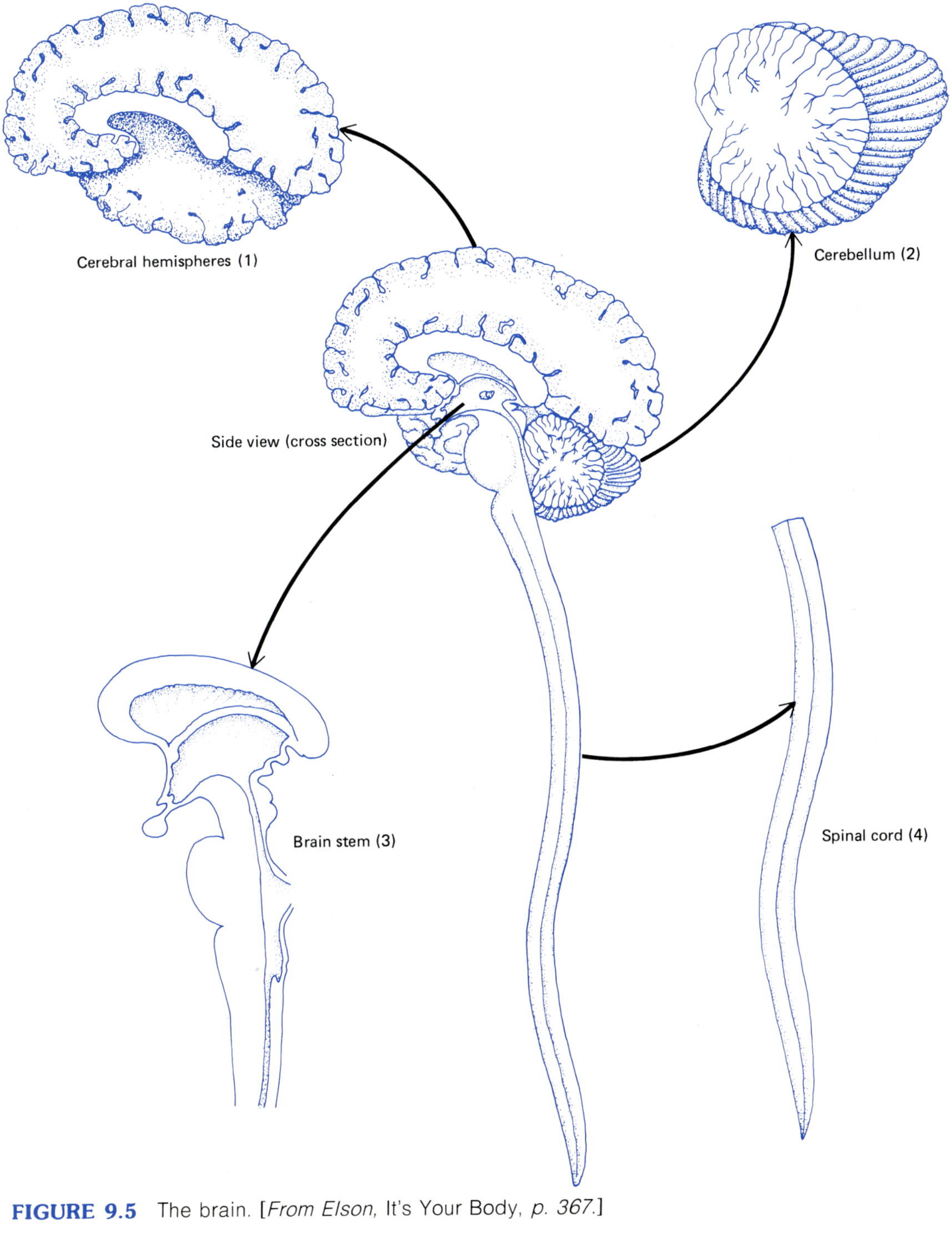

FIGURE 9.5 The brain. [*From Elson,* It's Your Body, *p. 367.*]

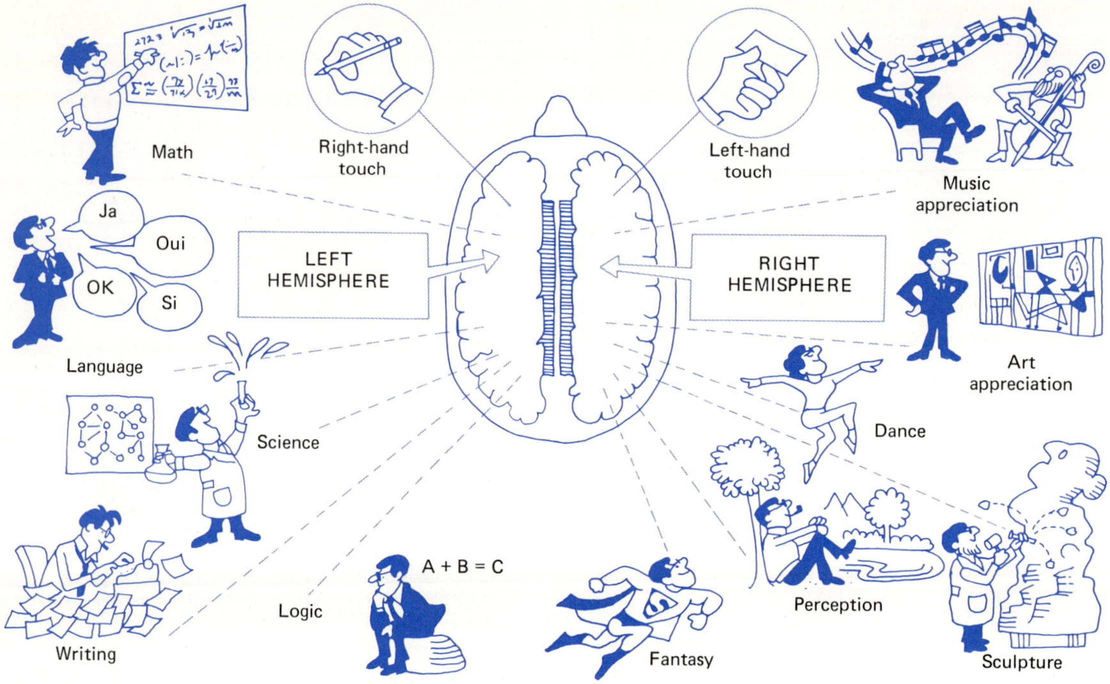

FIGURE 9.6 How the brain divides its work (top view showing both hemispheres). [*Adapted from* Newsweek, *Aug. 6, 1973.*]

by any of the entire spectrum of disease factors, from heredity (Huntington's chorea) to microorganisms (encephalitis) to injury (a blow to the head) to environment (exposure to lead paint). Stroke, a blood vessel disorder that cuts off the blood supply to the brain, can also cause brain damage.

Though much remains to be learned about the functioning of the brain and the nervous system, present knowledge allows physicians to treat many of these disorders using drugs, brain pacing (an electrical timing device inserted in the brain), and highly skilled rehabilitative therapists to retrain healthy parts of the brain to take over for damaged sections. Still, poor coordination, speech difficulties, and other problems often set victims of such disorders apart. The discrimination that results from this "differentiation" is, in many cases, more disabling than the disorder itself. (see "Rehabilitation" in Chapter 12). Yet these individuals are frequently capable, productive human beings.

Many of the diseases affecting the nervous system are discussed elsewhere: stroke in Chapter 10, cerebral palsy, Huntington's chorea, and mental retardation in Chapter 23, and nerve deafness in Chapter 6. Others include the following.

Epilepsy *Epilepsy* comes from the Greek for "seizure," because it was believed the victim was "seized" by evil spirits. It occurs in several forms and can range from mild to disabling. *Causes*: Brain cells discharge energy abnormally due to injury, infection, tumor, or possibly heredity or unknown causes. *Treatment*: Wide variety of drugs can control seizures completely in 60 percent of victims and partially in another 20 percent, allowing such persons normal, or nearly normal, lives. The remainder cannot be helped by drugs. Surgery may work for some of these. Having others behave normally toward the victim is an important part of therapy.

Muscular dystrophies A group of chronic neuromuscular diseases characterized by progressive weakening of muscles, occurring in various forms in adults and children. *Cause*: Mostly genetic defect inherited through various patterns. *Treatment*: None presently, but physical therapy, braces, and exercise can slow crippling, and psychological counseling may ease stress. *Prognosis*: Children rarely survive to adulthood: the disease progresses more slowly in adults, who may live 10 to 20 years after diagnosis.

Multiple sclerosis Periodic attacks of progressively worsening loss of coordination, disturbances of speech and vision, numbness, muscle weakness and spasms, pain and paralysis. MS is most common in young white adults, usually between ages 20 and 40. *Cause*: Unknown, but a slow-acting virus and/or an autoimmune reaction or cellular immunity deficiency may be involved in the loss of the protective myelin or nerve endings that leads to short circuits in the nervous system and causes the symptoms. *Treatment*: Presently, there is no way to prevent or reverse underlying nerve damage, but physicians can treat the whole patient and minimize disabilities. *Prognosis*: Symptoms usually progress from mild to debilitating over many years, leading eventually to death. Typical lifespan is about 75 percent that of unafflicted persons.

Shingles Shingles is also called herpes zoster (*herpes* = creeping + *zoster* = girdle). It is an acute inflammation of nerve cells causing pain and, after several days, a rash of small blisters on reddened skin following the path of the affected nerve. Persons in run-down condition are most susceptible. *Cause*: Probably the *Varicella zoster* virus, which also causes chicken pox. *Treatment*: Usually none is needed, but pain relievers, powders, or liquids applied to the rash ease the symptoms, and antibiotics can prevent complications. Any involvement of eyes or ears requires expert medical help. Gamma globulin is under study as a treatment.

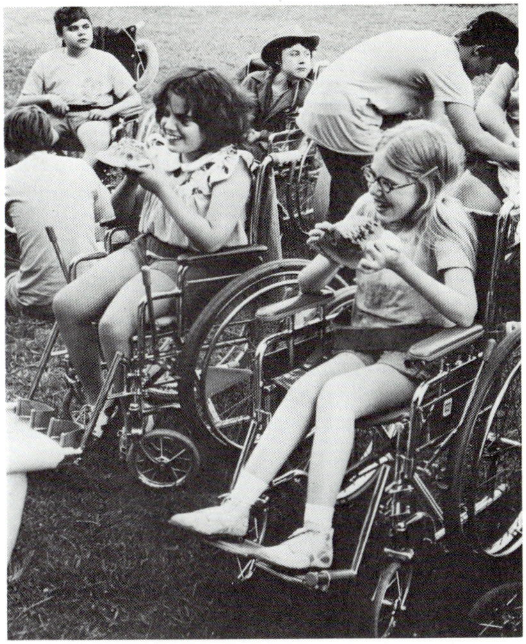

Muscular Dystrophy Association

The muscular dystrophies, characterized by progressive weakening of the muscles, present a challenge to medical researchers still seeking an effective means of treatment.

Myasthenia gravis Myasthenia gravis (*my* = muscle + *asthenia* = weakness + *gravis* = heavy or serious) is a weakness of voluntary muscles which worsens after activity, lessens with rest. It most often attacks women from 15 to 35 and men after 40. *Cause*: Unknown, but there appears to be a defect in the transmission of nerve impulses to the muscle. *Treatment*: Drugs can help patients recover 80 to 90 percent of strength. In some cases, removal of the thymus is indicated. *Prognosis*: All symptoms disappear spontaneously in 10 to 15 percent of patients, and in 38 percent of those with thymuses removed. The remainder live nearly normal lives, although activity is sometimes limited. Death may come from a "crisis," in which the patient is unable to breathe or clear airways because of muscle weakness.

Encephalitis and meningitis Encephalitis (inflammation of brain) and meningitis (inflammation of membranes of the brain or spinal cord) are two groups of diseases that cause many types of brain-damage symptoms and sometimes death. *Cause*: A wide variety of infectious organisms, toxins, and chemical substances; may follow as complications of milder diseases such as measles. *Treatment*: Varies with cause and extent of damage. *Prognosis*: Death in severe cases, permanent coma or vegetative state in others, no or few aftereffects in many others. Rehabilitative techniques are very valuable.

ENDOCRINE GLANDS—THE BODY'S REGULATORY SYSTEM

The endocrine system keeps the human body and its many functions within certain norms, regulating blood pressure, growth, metabolism, appetite, water and mineral balance, weight gain and distribution, sex drive, reproduction, bone demineralization and remineralization, and how much energy we have for daily tasks.

The endocrine glands, also called *ductless glands* because they secrete their products (chemical substances called *hormones*, from the Greek word for "to arouse") into the bloodstream directly rather than through

FIGURE 9.7 Endocrine glands and secretions. [*Adapted from* Gould Medical Dictionary.]

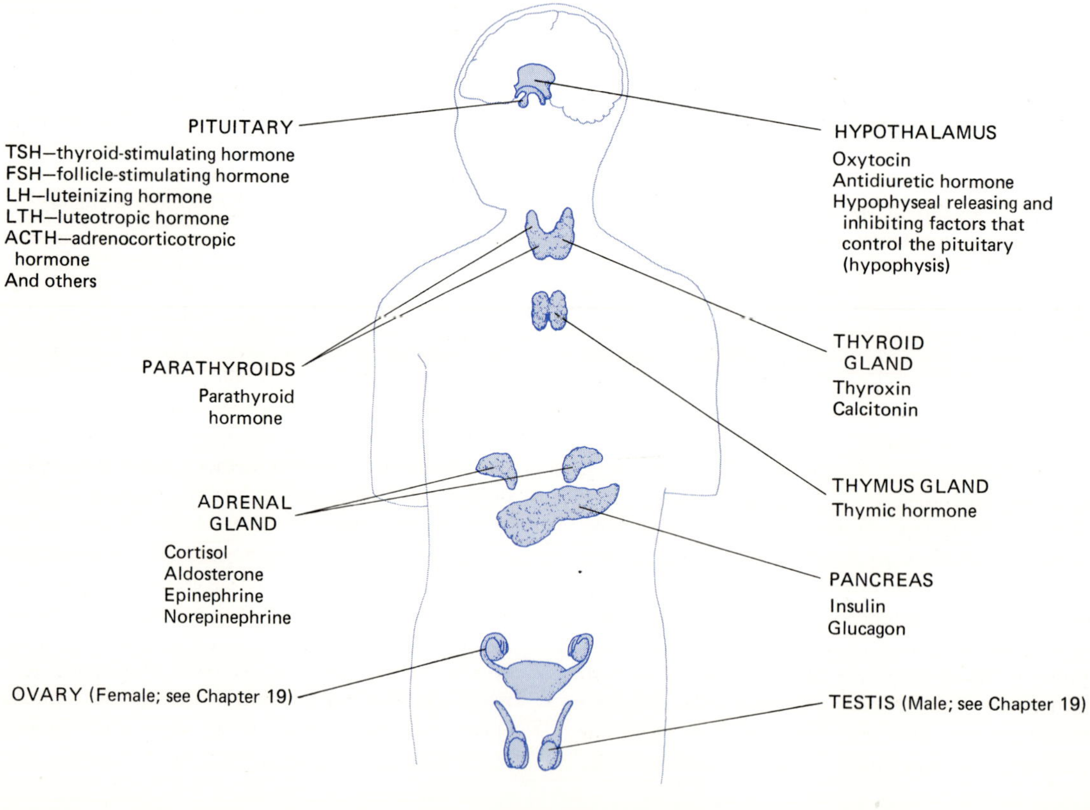

TABLE 9.1 Disorders of the endocrine system

GLAND; HORMONES	RESULT OF DEFICIENCY; TREATMENT	RESULT OF EXCESS; TREATMENT
Pituitary or hypophysis; at least 10 different hormones	Extreme thinness; sexual abnormalities; intolerance of normal variations in temperature; growth failure resulting in dwarfism. *Treatment:* Pituitary extract.	Giantism in childhood; acromegaly (continued growth of hands, feet, jaw) in adults. *Treatment:* Radiation of pituitary gland; estrogens for girls, testosterone for boys; surgery.
Thyroid; thyroxin, calcitonin	Cretinism in infants (lack of normal growth and development, physical and mental); in adults, mild to severe lack of energy, depression, constipation, dry skin, low body temperature, tissue swelling, easy weight gain. A deficiency of calcitonin results in abnormal levels of calcium and phosphorus in the blood. *Treatment:* Natural or synthetic thyroid hormone.	(Can be brought on by stress.) Fatigue, jitteryness, alertness, staring or bulging eyes, hand tremors, weight loss along with increased appetite, rapid pulse, sweating, and intolerance of hot weather. Also, goiter, or swelling of thyroid, because of inadequate iodine intake. *Treatment:* Medication to slow production of thyroxin, or surgery to remove part of malfunctioning gland. Iodine in salt or pills.
Adrenals; 50 or more hormones or hormonelike substances	*Acute* (can be caused by infection, hemorrhage, or obstruction of blood flow to gland): High fever, mental confusion, collapse, even death. *Chronic* (Addison's disease): Weakness, hair loss, increased skin coloring. *Treatment:* Replacement hormones and salt.	(Can be caused by adrenal or pituitary tumor.) Cushing's syndrome (weakness, loss of muscle tissue, purple skin streaks, "moon" face). Excess of sex-regulating hormones (increased sexuality in females, early puberty). *Treatment:* Surgery and hormone replacement therapy, if needed.
Parathyroids; parathyroid hormone	Calcium in blood drops, phosphorus increases; can lead to tetany (prolonged painful muscle spasms). *Treatment:* Regulation by increasing calcium and reducing phosphorus in diet; administration of parathyroid extracts.	Excessive calcium and phosphorus are withdrawn from bones, leaving them soft and fragile. *Treatment:* Surgical removal of gland may be necessary, especially if tumor is present.
Islets of Langerhans; insulin	Diabetes. See pages 222–223.	Hypoglycemia. See page 223.

ducts. Through an intricate "feedback" system, the hormones balance body functions much as a thermostat keeps the room temperature at a preset level. Too much of one hormone triggers another to turn it off; too little triggers a hormone to stimulate production. The hypothalamus, located in the brain, directs the entire regulatory operation. Because the hypothalamus is easily affected by emotions, the same is true for glandular balance. For example, a woman who is worried that she is pregnant may have her menstrual cycle thrown off, and her period may be late.

The mystery of how hormones accomplish their designated tasks has recently been unfolding. Scientists now believe that hormones activate enzymes within cells that in turn lead to the development of cyclic AMP (adneosine 3',5'-monophosphate). Cyclic AMP then takes over the messenger role, activating genes and controlling cellular enzyme activity.

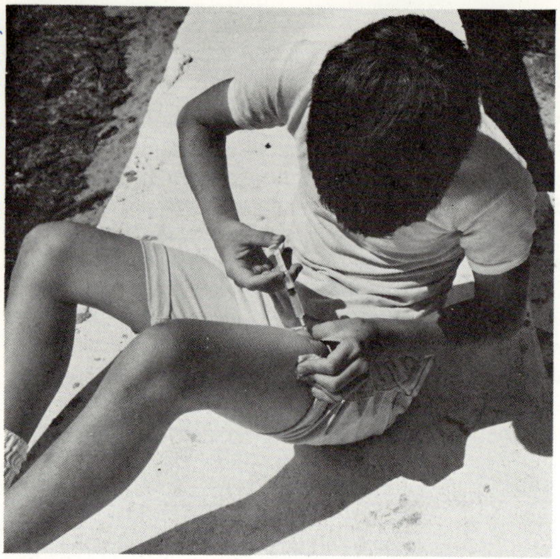

Michal Heron/Monkmeyer

Victims of a disorder of the body's regulatory system, diabetics must monitor their diet and exercise, and in many cases take daily doses of insulin to control levels of sugar in the blood.

HEALTH CONSUMER TIP

What You Should Know about Diabetes

This most common and puzzling of endocrine disorders involves, at least in part, the hormone insulin, produced by the beta cells of the islets of Langerhans, located on the pancreas. Some recent research indicates that overproduction of glucagon by pancreas alpha cells may also be involved (Gerich et al.). If this is so, diabetes should be redefined as a *bi*hormonal disorder.

In diabetes, supplies of insulin, used to metabolize sugar, are inadequate or cannot be utilized by the body, causing sugar to pile up in the blood. Some of the excess is excreted in the urine, sweetening it—thus, the name diabetes mellitus (*mellitus* = sweet).

The disease affects some 10 million Americans—women more often than men, nonwhites somewhat more often than whites, the poor 3 times more often than the middle class or wealthy. Though most diabetics live a relatively normal life, diabetes rose in 1976 to be the third leading cause of death in the United States. There are two forms of diabetes. Some physicians believe that they are two separate diseases.

Childhood-onset diabetes Also known as juvenile diabetes, this more severe form of the disease is most common in children and teenagers but is seen in adults as well. It is usually characterized by little or no production of insulin. Its symptoms include: weakness, rapid weight loss, abnormal thirst and hunger, frequent urination. Tests show sugar in the urine and high blood-sugar levels. Coma may occur in severe, untreated cases. Serious complications, such as heart and circulatory problems, kidney damage, and vision difficulties, cut the lives of victims to an average of 27 years following onset. Control includes diet and insulin injections.

Maturity-onset diabetes Victims are most commonly over age 40 with a family history of the disease. They may have a relatively large insulin output but lack the ability to utilize it effectively. Symptoms include overweight, tiredness, frequent urination, periods of abnormal thirst and hunger, and giving birth to babies 9 pounds and over. The condition can often be controlled without insulin simply by following a diet in which starch and sugar intake is carefully regulated. Oral diabetes drugs may be used in more difficult cases, but there has been considerable controversy over their safety.

Research goals When injectable insulin was discovered, it was hailed as the ultimate solution for the diabetic, and research in the field was all but halted. It was many years before it became apparent that although insulin could control sugar levels, it did not prevent the diseases's many complications. Today, NIH and other researchers are engaged in an all-out effort to solve the puzzle of diabetes.

SELF-CARE

Handling a Diabetic Emergency

Insulin reaction or hypoglycemia[3] (rapid onset) *Cause*: Too much insulin, not enough food, too much exercise, delayed meal. *Symptoms*: Excessive sweating, faintness, headache, hunger, pounding of heart, trembling, irritability, confusion, drowsiness, personality changes, coma. *What to do*: Give sugar or any food containing sugar (candy, juices, soft drinks); call the doctor; do not give insulin;[4] give glucagon if there is loss of consciousness.[4]

Diabetic coma (slow onset) *Cause*: Too little insulin, failure to follow diet, infection, fever, emotional stress. *Symptoms*: Increased thirst and urination; large amounts of sugar and ketones in urine on test;[4] weakness, abdominal pain, generalized aches; loss of appetite, nausea, vomiting. *What to do*: Call the doctor at once; put patient to bed, keep warm, give fluids without sugar; continue usual urine tests.[4]

[3] *Low* blood sugar.

[4] For those who are regularly involved in the care of diabetics.

What You Should Know about Hypoglycemia

While diabetes is *hyper*glycemia, or an overabundance of sugar in the blood, it is also possible to have too *little* sugar in the blood, or *hypo*glycemia. This disease has been overplayed in the popular press, encouraging many persons to self-diagnose. This is dangerous because the symptoms of hypoglycemia resemble those of several more serious ailments. Low blood sugar is sometimes caused by malfunction or tumor in an organ such as the liver, the pancreas, or the brain, and may require surgical or other medical treatment.

Symptoms of hypoglycemia include trembling, sweating, and a growing hunger within a few hours of eating (especially a high-carbohydrate meal), as well as personality changes, yawning, a drop in energy, headache, fatigue, and a drop in blood-sugar levels. Alcoholic beverages, caffeine, a high-carbohydrate diet, lack of sleep, fad weight-loss diets, emotional stress, or an organic defect can cause blood sugar to drop. Treatment involves eliminating the causes (including possible organic disorders), modifying the diet so that it will be high in protein and low in carbohydrates, and use of tranquilizers and psychotherapy to ease emotional stress.

LOOKING BACK

REVIEWING CONCEPTS IN CHAPTER 9

- Understanding how the various body systems function may help us to keep them functioning properly.
- The respiratory tract—from nose to lungs—is exposed to the open air and thus subject to attack by a host of microorganisms, as well as by soot, smoke, and other air pollutants.
- There is presently no cure for the commonest of respiratory disorders, the common cold. But symptoms can sometimes be controlled.

- Prompt attention to minor respiratory infections can avert more serious complications, such as pneumonia.
- The brain and the rest of the nervous system make up the communications network of the body. Various parts of the brain are involved in all our conscious acts, in our five senses, in coordination, and in involuntary functions such as breathing, heart rate, blood pressure, hunger, and thirst.
- The spinal cord, with its many nerve fibers, is in charge of reflexes—instant responses to stimuli such as heat and pain.
- Disorders of the brain can be severely disabling. But new types of therapy can help retrain many who are thus handicapped.
- The digestive system—from mouth to rectum—breaks food down mechanically and chemically into units small enough to be used for nourishment by the cells, then discards the remaining waste.
- Digestive system ailments range from the mild, common case of indigestion to severe, life-threatening cancers and ulcers.
- The "ductless" endocrine glands—the pituitary, thyroid, parathyroid; adrenal, and reproductive glands, and the islets of Langerhans—regulate many of the body's functions, including growth, weight change, sex drive, reproduction, and energy levels. Too little or too much of a hormone from these glands can lead to a foul-up in body functioning.

10

THE KILLER DISEASES: CORONARIES AND CANCERS

WHAT'S AHEAD IN CHAPTER 10 Why should young adults be concerned with diseases like heart disease and cancer that most often strike in middle age and beyond? In what ways can individual decision making affect the chances of becoming a victim of one of these diseases? What are the early symptoms of high blood pressure? Which factors contribute to its development and which can be controlled? What is stroke? Can risk of stroke be reduced or is it inevitable? What is the relationship between atherosclerosis and "heart attack"? What are the heart attack risk factors? What kind of life can a person who has had a heart attack expect to live? What techniques can lay people learn to help in heart attack emergencies? What is cancer? What are the factors that are known to be associated with the development of cancer? Which are suspected? What part does early detection play in the treatment of cancer? Can treatment really cure cancer? What are the most common approaches to treatment? How do psychological problems affect the lives of cancer victims and their families? Why are they often easy prey for purveyors of quackery?

Why should heart attacks, hardening of the arteries, and cancer be of concern to young adults—except as a way of understanding some of the dangers that threaten their parents and grandparents? After all, only middle-aged men and elderly people keel over with heart attacks, become senile from hardening of the arteries, and get most kinds of cancer. But once the mechanisms behind the development of these most common killers of Americans are understood, it becomes clear that anyone interested in living a long and healthy life stands to benefit from a knowledge of the subject.

Take Ralph, for example, a bright college freshman determined to succeed. He is in school on a partial scholarship, and his folks work hard to pay the rest. He works a couple of nights at a local drive-in to earn spending money and devotes nearly every other waking hour to studying. He never finds time for a game of touch football or to shoot some baskets. In the college dining hall, he loads his tray with eggs, red meats, and unlimited quantities of milk and ice cream—all luxuries when he was growing up. He skips salads, considering them food for rabbits and dieters. He started smoking when he was 14 because that made him a big man; now he smokes out of habit. When the pressure gets to him, he sometimes overdoes the alcohol.

Ralph is making some well-thought-out decisions about his future career. What he does not realize is that by his pattern of rich foods, smoking, stress, and lack of exercise he is making some important decisions about his future health as well. Scientists are now convinced that heart disease, though it seems to strike suddenly, takes a lifetime to develop; and that many kinds of cancer are related to dietary habits, smoking, and excessive alcohol consumption—though, again, the resultant diseases take years to develop. In this chapter we will look at each of these major illnesses and see why it develops.

THE HUMAN CIRCULATORY SYSTEM

To understand how heart and blood vessel diseases develop, we must first understand how the circulatory system functions. In ancient times, the heart was believed to be the seat of the soul and the mind. Later, it was thought of as the source of love. William Harvey's idea that it was a pump that sent blood on a circular route though the body was ridiculed by the seventeenth-century medical establishment. Of course, he was on the right track, though he did not realize that the heart pumps blood through *two* completely separate circulatory systems, as can be seen in Figure 10.1.

The heart, a muscular organ the size of a fist, weighing about 8 ounces in women and 10 in men, pumps blood at an average rate of 72 times a minute. Each minute's work is equivalent to lifting a 70-pound weight a foot off the ground. Though the muscles of the arms and legs would quickly tire from this kind of exertion, the heart muscle does not seem to tire. An electrical system located in the SA (sinoatrial) node is a natural pacemaker. It sets the rate of heartbeat by sending electrical impulses to the AV (atrioventricular) node, which in turn signals the ventricles. Though 72 beats per minute is average, the normal range is between 60 and 80. Generally, the smaller the person, the faster the heartbeat. Good physical conditioning slows the heartbeat. (If you would like to check your own heartbeat, turn to Figure 4.6.)

Should the heart stop pumping blood for more than a few minutes, the body would cease to receive the life-supporting nutrients and oxygen the blood transports. As little as 4 minutes without oxygen can destroy the ability of the brain to function normally. Recognizing the importance of the heart, nature protects it by placing it behind the breastbone and surrounding it with a tough multiple membrane, the pericardium (*peri* = around + *cardium* = heart). Fluid between the membranes cushions the heart from shocks and cuts down friction as the heart beats against the breastbone and diaphragm.

CARDIOVASCULAR DISORDERS

Cardiovascular (*cardio* = heart + *vascular* = blood vessel) diseases are responsible for

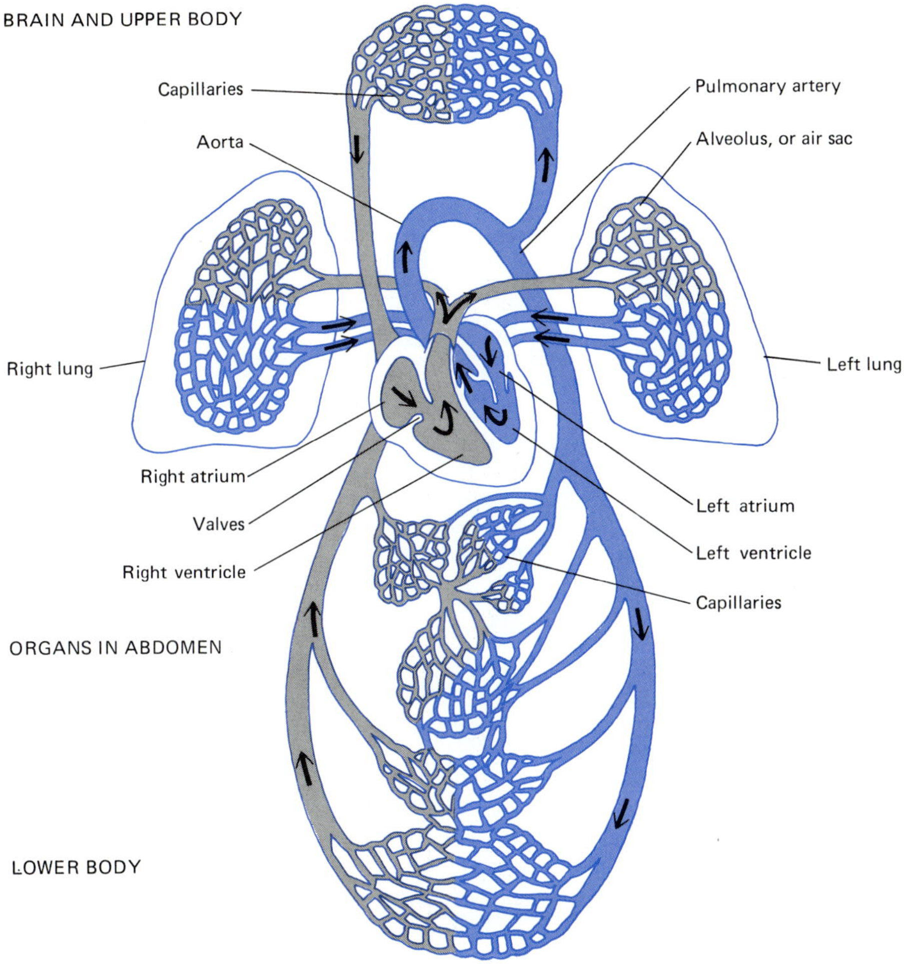

FIGURE 10.1 Human circulation. Freshly oxygenated blood arriving in the left atrium from the lungs is pumped by the left ventricle to all parts of the body. It passes from larger arteries into smaller ones and finally into microscopic capillaries where cell wastes are picked up and oxygen and other nutrients are deposited. The waste-laden blood, now bluish, moves into small veins and on into larger ones. It arrives back at the heart in the right atrium, is pushed to the right ventricle, and is then pumped to the lungs. There it discards waste products and picks up oxygen and returns to the left atrium, where the process begins anew.

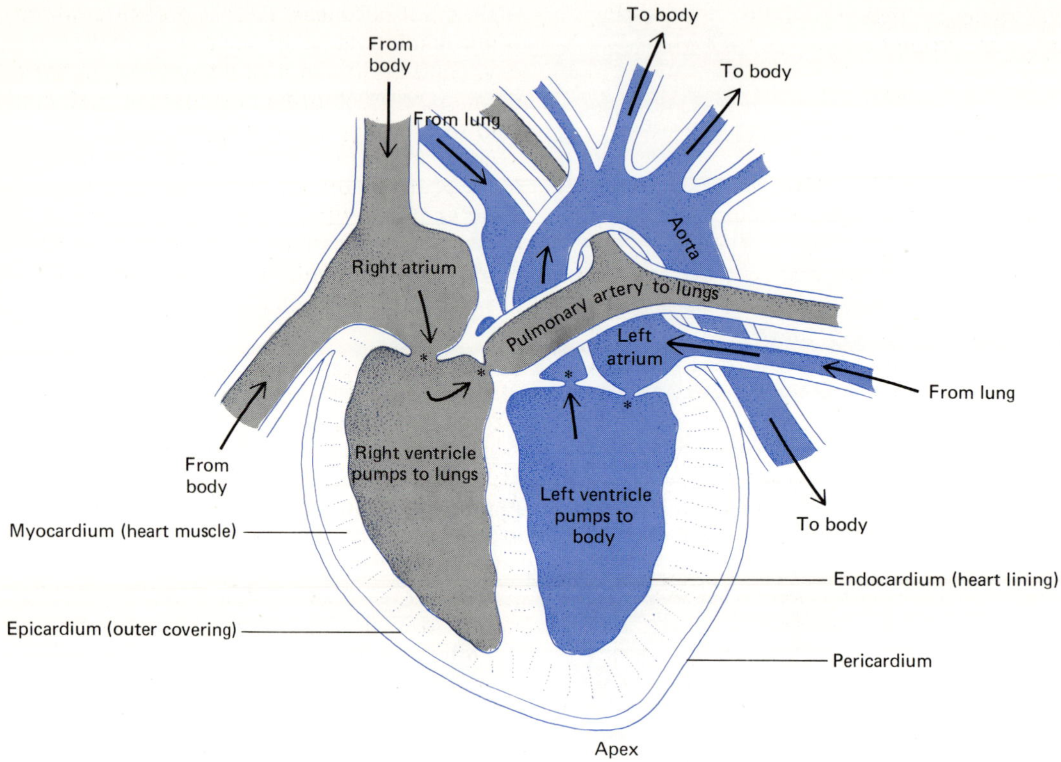

FIGURE 10.2 The human heart. Valves (*) prevent blood from leaking backwards and keep it moving in the right direction; they give the heartbeat its characteristic lubb-dubb sound. Coronary arteries return from aorta to bring blood to nourish heart muscle.

more deaths in the United States each year than all other causes combined, and for much disability as well. Deaths are most common among older people, but more than 1 in 3 occur in persons under 65. Cardiovascular diseases are responsible for 31 percent of all deaths in the 35 to 44 age category, and for 70 percent of deaths after 75. At all ages under 75, males are more likely to be affected than females.

Though still high, the rate of deaths from heart disease has been dropping since the early 1970s. The reasons are unclear. There is some speculation that changes in lifestyle aimed at reducing risk of heart attack, improvement in the treatment of high blood pressure, and better emergency and long-term care of heart attack victims may be factors. There may be other unknown reasons as well.

Although cardiovascular diseases have long been categorized as degenerative disorders of the elderly, it is now recognized that the degeneration or wearing out of the circulatory system begins early in life. It is probably during childhood and young adulthood that these diseases can best be controlled and prevented by medical leadership and by conscious decision making by the community, parents, and young adults themselves.

HIGH BLOOD PRESSURE

The pressure at which blood is pumped through the arteries is kept level by built-in regulators, such as the carotid sinus in the neck. Body hormones also play a role in regulating blood pressure, speeding it up in emergencies when the body needs added energy and nourishment, slowing it down at night during sleep.

When regulating mechanisms go awry for some reason (often unknown), the blood pressure becomes much greater than normal, putting stress and strain on the arteries. This is the condition called hypertension or high blood pressure (HBP). Unfortunately, since you cannot feel a change in your blood pressure the way you can in your heartbeat, it is possible to have high blood pressure for years without knowing it. Despite its silence, HBP is not harmless. Excess pressure on the veins leading to such organs as heart, kidneys, and brain can eventually cause serious damage to those organs. Untreated HBP can lead to both heart disease and stroke.

Some individuals have blood pressure that is lower than normal. Unless serious disease is present, low blood pressure is harmless. It may even be beneficial because it lessens the strain on the circulatory system and lowers the risk of heart attack.

Who Gets High Blood Pressure

There is a widespread impression that HBP is a disease that strikes only the tense, "uptight" person—possibly because of the name hyper*tension*. Actually, there are many people with calm temperaments among the 20 to 25 million Americans presently believed to have above normal blood pressures. ("Normal" is about 120/70, with some disagreement on what figure above that point requires medical attention.)

FIGURE 10.3 (*a*) Causes of death in the United States. (*b*) Deaths due to cardiovascular diseases. [*From* Vital Statistics of the United States, *1975*.]

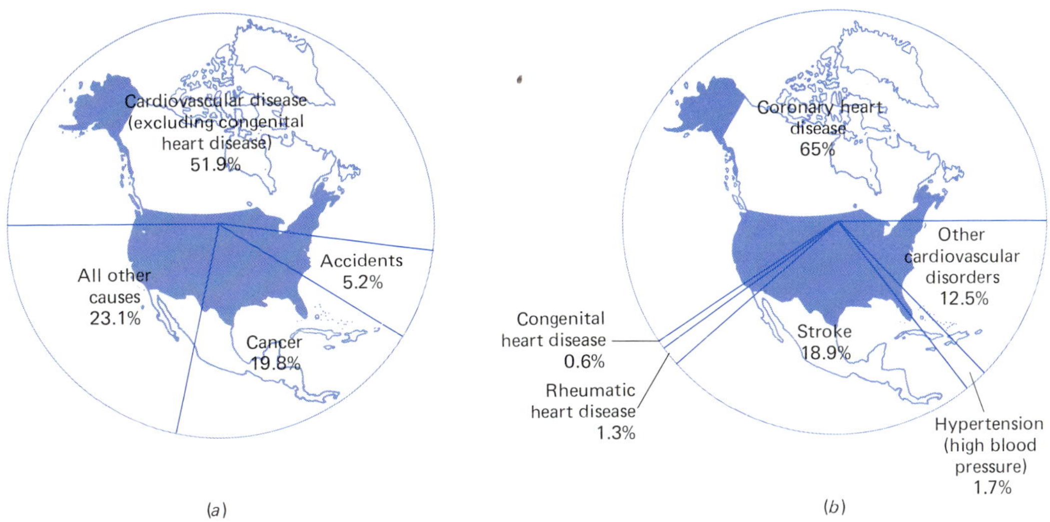

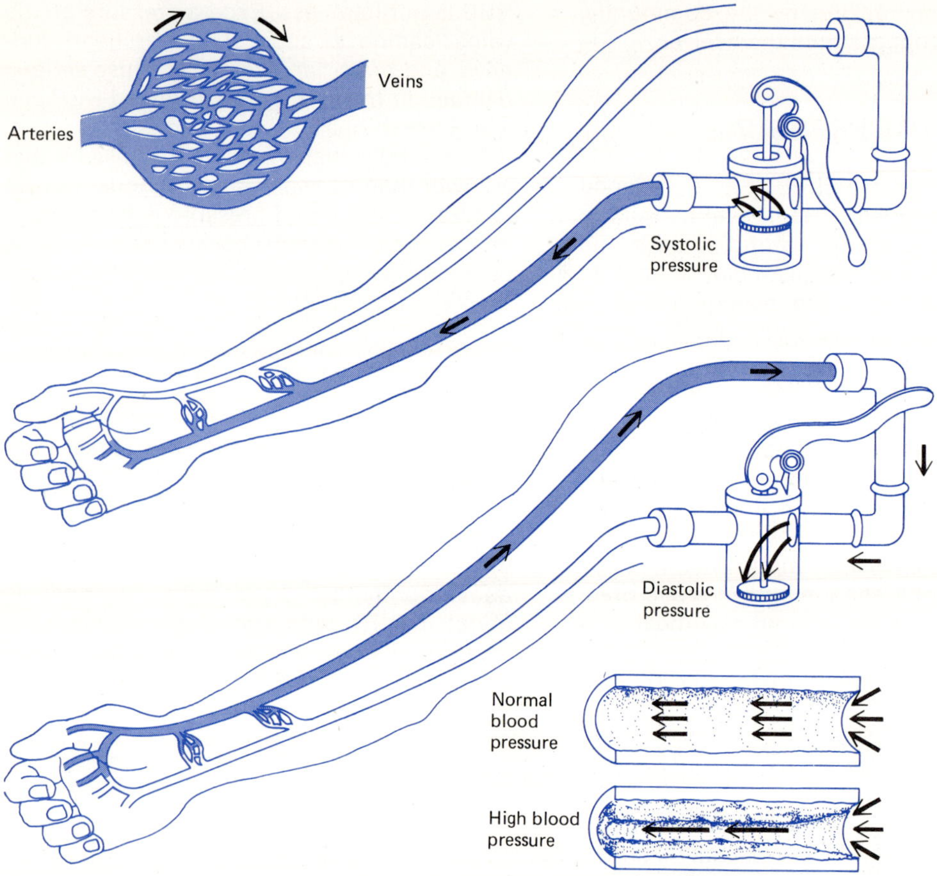

FIGURE 10.4 The mechanics of blood pressure. When the heart is pumping blood into the circulatory system, blood pressure is at its highest point and is called *systolic pressure*. When the heart is at rest and filling between pumping beats, blood pressure is at its lowest point and is called *diastolic pressure*.

High blood pressure (over 150 systolic and 95 diastolic in most people) occurs when the arteries become partially blocked, inflexible, or both, thereby increasing pressure in the arteries and making the heart work harder to pump blood through the system. [*Adapted from* Patient Care, *Nov. 15, 1973.*]

The disease strikes high-powered executives and unemployed laborers, teachers and homemakers, doctors and mechanics—even children. It strikes blacks more often than whites, though the difference may be more environmental than genetic. It affects women as often as men, but females seem to suffer the consequences less frequently, possibly because of the protection of female hormones.

Causes

In 5 to 10 percent of cases, hypertension is the result of some organic malfunction, usually of the kidneys or the adrenal glands. This is called *secondary hypertension*, and can often be cured by surgery. The remainder are idiopathic (of unknown cause), called *essential hypertension*. Though the mechanism is not understood,[1] many risk factors have been associated with this type of HBP:

- *Inherited susceptibility*
- *Overweight*
- *Stress* It is probably not the amount of stress one is subjected to but a recurrent inability to cope with increasing stress that upsets the blood pressure regulatators and eventually causes them to be reset upwards.
- *High salt intake* Epidemiological studies, confirmed by animal tests, seem to correlate the incidence of hypertension with salt intake. (Eskimos take 1 to 2 grams a day and have a 1 to 2 percent hypertension rate; Americans consume about 7 to 10 grams and have a 15 percent HBP rate; Japanese ingest a whopping 40 to 50 grams day and nearly half the population show high blood pressure readings.)[2]
- *Oral contraceptives* Some women also develop temporary HBP during pregnancy.

[1]Enzymes called kallikreins may be involved.

[2]Studies of monkeys show high sugar intake may also be involved.

Detection and Treatment

Although the National High Blood Pressure Education Program increased awareness of the disease, nearly 30 percent of Americans with high blood pressure in 1976 were unaware of it and only half of those who knew were being treated properly. Yet early detection and treatment can greatly reduce the risk of illness and death from the complications of high blood pressure. (See Figure 10.5.) Detection is by means of a simple instrument called a sphygmomanometer or blood pressure cuff (see Figure 4.7). Treatment usually consists of weight loss, exercise, salt-free or low-salt diet, and when necessary, drugs to reduce blood pressure directly or to remove excess fluid and salt from the body. Yoga, transcendental meditation (TM), behavior modification, and biofeedback may also help to lower blood pressure in some patients.

Stroke—A Major Result of Untreated HBP

Interference with blood flow to the brain—known as *cerebrovascular accident* or *stroke*—may have many causes, but is most often related to high blood pressure. The five major ways in which blood flow may be cut off are shown in Figure 10.5. A permanent cut-off of blood causes the death of cells in that area of the brain affected and loss of bodily functions controlled by it. A temporary shortage can cause a "little stroke" which may warn of a major stroke ahead. A stroke causing a great deal of brain damage can be fatal.

Risk factors Factors other than high blood pressure which may contribute to stroke are overweight, high-cholesterol or high-fat diets, diabetes, atherosclerosis, stress, infection, an inborn weakness in a cerebral artery, a variety of heart disorders, and possibly smoking.

Effects Symptoms vary depending upon the

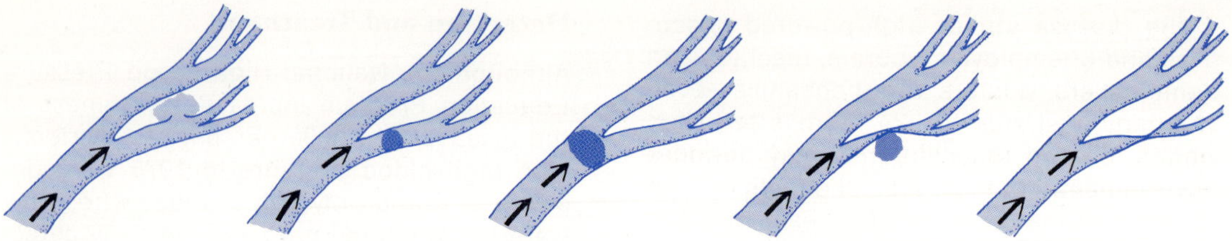

FIGURE 10.5 Types of strokes. There are five major ways in which strokes occur:

1 Hemorrhage (bleeding). The wall of an artery to the brain or in the brain may rupture, allowing the blood to escape and damage the surrounding brain tissue. The break may be caused by an inborn weakness in the artery wall or by hypertension.

2 Thrombosis (clotting). A clot of blood may form in an artery of the brain and stop the flow of blood to the area of the brain the artery serves. This is most likely to happen in arteries that have been narrowed by atherosclerosis.

3 Embolism (a floating clot). A clot formed elsewhere in the body, usually a diseased heart, may be pumped to the brain and may clog one of the brain's arteries, especially if it has been narrowed by atherosclerosis.

4 Compression (pressure). A tumor, swollen brain tissue, or something else may press upon a vessel, cutting off the flow of blood to the brain.

5 Spasm (tightening and closing down of the walls of an artery). A constriction of the artery by spasm can reduce the flow of blood to the brain. Brief spasms usually cause no permanent damage.

part of the brain affected. They may include: headache, vision difficulties, dizziness, fainting spells, numbness of hand or face, weakness, paralysis, difficulty in speaking and/or thinking, personality changes, and mental disturbances. Similar effects may occur with little strokes, but they last just a short time—perhaps minutes.

Long-term effects of stroke vary from none at all to total disability, depending upon the amount and location of damage to the brain. Recently it was discovered that when a part of the brain is damaged by stroke, it releases chemicals (catecholamines) that damage surrounding areas, greatly worsening the effects of the stroke. If a drug could be developed to prevent the release of these substances, stroke damage could be greatly reduced. Until that time, rehabilitative therapy (see Chapter 12) and large quantities of encouragement and support to counteract the depression brought on by the disabilities of stroke are the best medicine.

Prevention Intelligent decision making can often help to prevent stroke through controlling or eliminating such key risk factors as high blood pressure. Drugs to prevent blood clots can be prescribed for patients with a tendency to clotting or with arteries narrowed by arteriosclerosis. Surgery can be performed on defective blood vessels before they burst, and to remove clots or other blockages in blood vessels to the brain.

ATHEROSCLEROSIS

Atherosclerosis is the form of arteriosclerosis (hardening of the arteries) most damaging to health. Like hypertension, it inflicts its damage silently over a long period of years.

Development

In atherosclerosis, the thickening and hardening of the arteries are caused by a type of deposit called *atheromas*, or *atheromatous plaque*. Some believe these plaques begin with the yellowish fatty streaks found in the aortas (major arteries) of nearly all children by the age of 3. Over the years, plaque buildup continues, with a core composed mainly of the fatty substance cholesterol covered by a cap of fibrous scar tissue. The rough surface is ideal for blood clots or other matter to adhere to and block the artery.

Plaque development may be quite well developed by young adulthood. Autopsies of United States casualties in Vietnam showed 70 percent of young men, mean age 22, had atherosclerosis in their coronary arteries and 5 percent had at least one totally blocked artery. But symptoms of disease usually do not appear for 20 to 40 years.

Effects

The narrowing of the pathways through the arteries by atherosclerotic plaque is our nation's most serious health problem. It can lead to the following major disorders.

Coronary heart disease As the arteries to the heart become narrowed, blood flow to the heart is reduced. Normally the lessened flow, the *ischemia*, does not disturb the heart's function. But when pressure is put on the heart to pump more blood—as during exercise, fright, or other stress—the shortage of blood causes pain. This pain is called *angina pectoris*, and the condition *ischemic heart disease*.

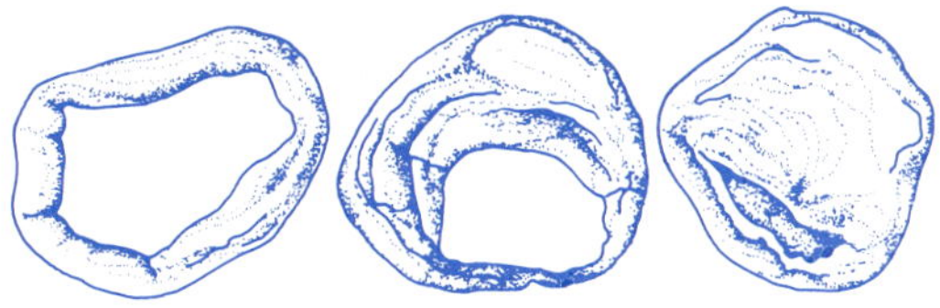

FIGURE 10.6 Formation of atherosclerotic plaque. The deterioration of a normal artery (*a*) is seen as atherosclerosis develops and begins depositing fatty substances and roughening the channel lining (*b*) until a clot forms (*c*) and plugs the artery to deprive the heart muscle of vital blood. Heart attack results. [*From American Heart Association,* Heart Facts, *1976.*]

Should a coronary artery become totally blocked—by plaque or by a blood clot lodged in the narrowed artery—the blood supply to that part of the heart supplied by the artery is cut off and the affected portion of the heart dies. This is called a *myocardial infarct*, or MI. A small infarct may be silent, with the affected area healing and scar tissue forming over the spot. It may go unnoticed until revealed by an electrocardiogram (ECG or EKG) months later that differs visibly from those taken at past checkups. But if the MI area is large, the patient will experience the symptoms of a "heart attack." If a major coronary artery is blocked and blood flow to all or most of the organ is cut off, sudden death may result.

Cerebrovascular disease Narrowing of the arteries to the brain caused by atherosclerosis is one of the common causes of stroke.

Atherosclerosis in other arteries Atherosclerosis in the aorta, in the arteries leading to the kidneys and lungs, or in those leading to the legs may also cause serious illness—including kidney damage, hypertension caused by kidney damage, leg cramps, numbness, and eventually gangrene (tissue death) possibly leading to amputation.

TABLE 10.1 Risks of developing coronary heart disease within 6 years, with selected risk factors

	CHANCES PER 100		
RISK FACTORS	MALE, AGE 35	MALE, AGE 60	FEMALE, AGE 45
None	0.3	4.8	0.4
High blood pressure (195 syst.)	1.0	13.4	1.7
High blood pressure plus high cholesterol (335)	7.5	21.0	5.8
High blood pressure plus high cholesterol plus diabetes	9.6	25.7	8.5
High blood pressure plus high cholesterol plus diabetes plus abnormal ECG reading	18.2	42.1	12.6
High blood pressure plus high cholesterol plus diabetes plus abnormal ECG plus smoking	25.9	53.3	13.2

Source: Coronary Risk Handbook, American Heart Association.

HEART ATTACK

"Heart attack," though not a scientific term, is commonly used to describe the symptoms of a myocardial infarction and of several other heart conditions. In this section, we will be discussing primarily MI and how it can be prevented and treated.

Prediction and Prevention

Atherosclerosis is a major factor in the development of MI, but what are the factors that contribute to this form of hardening of the arteries and to heart disease directly? As you can see in Table 10.1, there are several that appear to be related to increased risk of heart attack: high blood pressure, high serum cholesterol levels, and smoking—the most firmly established and most significant factors—as well as high serum triglycerides, obesity, lack of exercise (see Chapter 4), diabetes, and abnormal ECG readings. In women over 50, the combination of smoking and birth control pills is a major risk factor, multiplying the chance of death from heart attack manyfold. From Table 10.1, developed from results of the Framingham study, you can see that the more risk factors, the greater the risk of heart disease. You can also see the effects of age and sex on the risks.

More difficult to measure, but often mentioned as a risk factor, is stress. Stress and cholesterol have become the centers of both interest and controversy in the medical community and are of great concern to individual health decision makers.

The cholesterol controversy Epidemiological studies show that countries in which inhabitants have high levels of certain kinds of fats (lipids) in their blood usually have a high rate of heart attack. In most instances, this *hyperlipidemia* (*hyper* = over + *lipid* = fat +

American Heart Association Recommendations for a Prudent Diet

- Eat no more than three eggs a week—alone or in cooking.
- Limit use of shellfish and organ meats.
- Limit beef, lamb, pork, and ham (including bacon) to five medium portions per *week*; substitute fish, chicken, turkey, and veal at other meals.
- Choose lean cuts of meat, trim visible fat, and discard the fat that cooks out of the meat; skim the fat off gravies and sauces that are made from meat juices.
- Avoid deep fat frying and substitute instead cooking methods that help remove fat—baking, broiling, boiling, roasting, stewing.
- Restrict intake of fatty luncheon meats and cold cuts like sausage and salami.
- Instead of butter, lard, or other fats that are solid or completely hydrogenated, use liquid vegetable oils and margarines that are rich in polyunsaturated fats.
- Instead of whole milk and cheese made from whole milk and cream, use skimmed milk and skimmed milk cheeses.

emia = condition of the blood) is directly related to high intakes of cholesterol and saturated fats in the diet.

Still, it cannot be said that high blood cholesterol levels are always caused by high-cholesterol diets. Nor can it be said that heart attack always strikes those with high blood cholesterol levels.[3] Some questions remain incompletely answered: Does reducing blood cholesterol levels with drugs or dietary change reduce the risk of heart attack? Are some people able to consume high cholesterol diets without ill effects? Does a high sugar intake raise triglyceride levels and increase heart attack risks? Do other factors—stress or exercise—raise or lower cholesterol levels?

The puzzle of cholesterol may be considerably clarified by recent evidence that suggests it is not blood cholesterol levels but rather levels of the fat-protein complexes that *transport* cholesterol that are the significant factor in heart attack. These studies (Castelli) indicate that heart attack risk is heightened by high levels of LDLs (low-density lipoproteins) which carry cholesterol from the liver to the cells, or VLDLs (very low-density lipoproteins) which transport triglycerides. On the other hand, high levels of HDLs (high-density lipoproteins) appear to protect against heart attack by removing excess cholesterol from tissues and returning it to the liver to be excreted.

Despite the unanswered questions, the American Heart Association and most authorities believe that evidence contraindicating high dietary intakes of cholesterol and fat is impressive enough for Americans to adopt a "prudent diet," one that is low in cholesterol and saturated fats.

Stress and heart attack If you have ever had your blood pressure taken while you were upset, you know that stress can affect blood pressure. Some experts believe that a stressful life can also affect heart health. A strong medical community consensus supports the contention of cardiologists Raymond Rosenman and Meyer Friedman that "type A" personalities—characterized by a compelling sense of urgency ("Gotta get it done now!"),

[3]Hereditary hyperlipidemia appears unrelated to either diet or heart attack.

Some Typical Type A Traits You Might Recognize in Yourself or Others

1. Explosive accenting of key words in ordinary speech when not appropriate.
2. Moving, walking, eating rapidly.
3. Impatience at the rate with which things are happening.
4. Difficulty in refraining from talking about subjects of own special interest.
5. Feeling vaguely guilty when relaxing and doing nothing.
6. Loss of appreciation of things beautiful or important.
7. No time for "becoming," only for "getting."
8. Scheduling more and more in less time, no time for interruptions.
9. Frequently challenging others, especially other type A's.
10. Thinking more about quantity than quality, numbers rather than people.
11. Intense dedication to job or work or cause.

aggressiveness, and competitiveness, usually combined with a marked amount of free-floating hostility—are at greater risk of heart attack than others.

Can heart attack be prevented? It is widely believed that informed decision making aimed at reducing risk factors can reduce risk. But, cautions Dr. Basil Rifkind of NIH: "Degenerative diseases are not like infectious ones, where you apply a treatment and people stop dying. These diseases take years to develop and preventing them is very complicated." Two major studies are presently under way—one to determine whether reducing cholesterol by means of a drug (cholestryamine) reduces chance of heart attack and the other to determine the effect of reducing the three key risk factors, blood cholesterol levels, blood pressure, and smoking. These studies and several others in progress may soon tell us more about what we can do to prevent heart attacks.[4]

[4]Finland, the only country in the world with higher heart disease rates than the United States, succeeded in dramatically reducing these rates in its most coronary-prone county by reducing the three major risk factors: HBP, high serum cholesterol, and smoking.

Treatment

Only a generation ago, a heart attack meant death or a life as a "cardiac cripple"—to some "a fate worse than death." Today many heart attack patients train for and successfully run the 26½-mile Boston Marathon. Thousands have returned to their former jobs; many claim to have more energy and be more active than before their attacks.

The reason? A new approach to treatment. In the past, 6 weeks to 3 months of bedrest were commonly prescribed for heart patients, leaving them both physically weakened (nurses spoon-fed them) and psychologically depressed. Today, many hospitals, recognizing that long periods in bed weaken even healthy people, put patients with uncomplicated MIs on a phased exercise program within days of their attacks. By the time the patients leave the hospital, usually after the third week, they can walk up and down a flight of stairs and take care of their personal needs. The treatment, in sharp contrast to earlier approaches, clearly transmits the message: "Heart attack is not the end of the line."

Modern rehabilitation programs continue with:

- *More exercise* Patients progress from simple household chores to driving, sexual activity, and in many cases, brisk walking, jogging, or bicycling for miles at a clip (something most could not do before their coronaries).
- *Vocational therapy* Between 80 and 90 percent can return to jobs they formerly held with proper training and encouragement. (Employers may need encouragement, too.)
- *Education* Both patient and family need to learn to understand the condition, what caused it, and how to prevent a recurrence. Families must also be taught not to make invalids of patients by continually saying, "Don't do that!"
- *Medication* Appropriate drugs can control heart pain, reduce clumping of blood platelets that can lead to blood clot,[5] lower blood pressure, etc.
- *Lifestyle changes* The patient can learn to reduce such risk factors as smoking and overweight, to cut down stress and striving, and to create a healthy balance of relaxation and activity.
- *Surgery* A bypass may be performed to replace blocked arteries with segments of blood vessels from elsewhere in the body or other types of surgery may be done when necessary. When the heart is so damaged as to be unable to function, a heart transplant from a compatible donor may be a solution.

Cardiac Emergencies

A 64-year-old physician, en route to a convention, experienced crushing chest pain that radiated to his left shoulder. For 2 hours, he dismissed the possibility of heart attack, and he even stopped at a drug store for some antacid tablets. Not until he called his office for messages, mentioned the pain "in passing" to his nurse, and was urged to go straight to the nearest hospital did he acknowledge the possibility he had suffered an MI.

[5]Recent studies indicate aspirin may be effective in reducing risk of blood clot and thus of heart attack and stroke, particularly in men.

Why is it that even those who should readily recognize heart attack symptoms often ignore them? Many people simply find it difficult to face that "It's happening to me." Others fear it *is* a coronary, and would just as soon die as become cardiac invalids. So they delay medical care.

If you are with someone who appears to have heart attack symptoms, doctors recommend that you not delay, plead, or cajole. Just follow the procedures outlined in Figure 10.7.

If the patient's heart stops (if there is no pulse), only immediate emergency treatment—within 3 or 4 minutes—can prevent permanent damage or death. For this reason it is recommended that as many lay people as possible be trained in revival technique—cardiopulmonary resuscitation (CPR). (See Figure 10.8.)

OTHER CARDIOVASCULAR DISORDERS

A variety of other disorders can affect the heart and the blood vessels. Among the most common are:

Heart block When the natural pacing of the heart's electrical system breaks down, weakness, blackouts, very slow pulse, and even death may occur. *Cause*: Congenital (inborn) defect, infection, or injury of electrical pathways during heart surgery. *Treatment*: Surgical insertion of an externally powered replacement for the body's natural pacer—an electronic pacemaker.

Arrhythmias The heart may beat too quickly, too slowly, or too erratically, or may seem to flutter or skip a beat. *Cause*: Fatigue; emotional upset; use

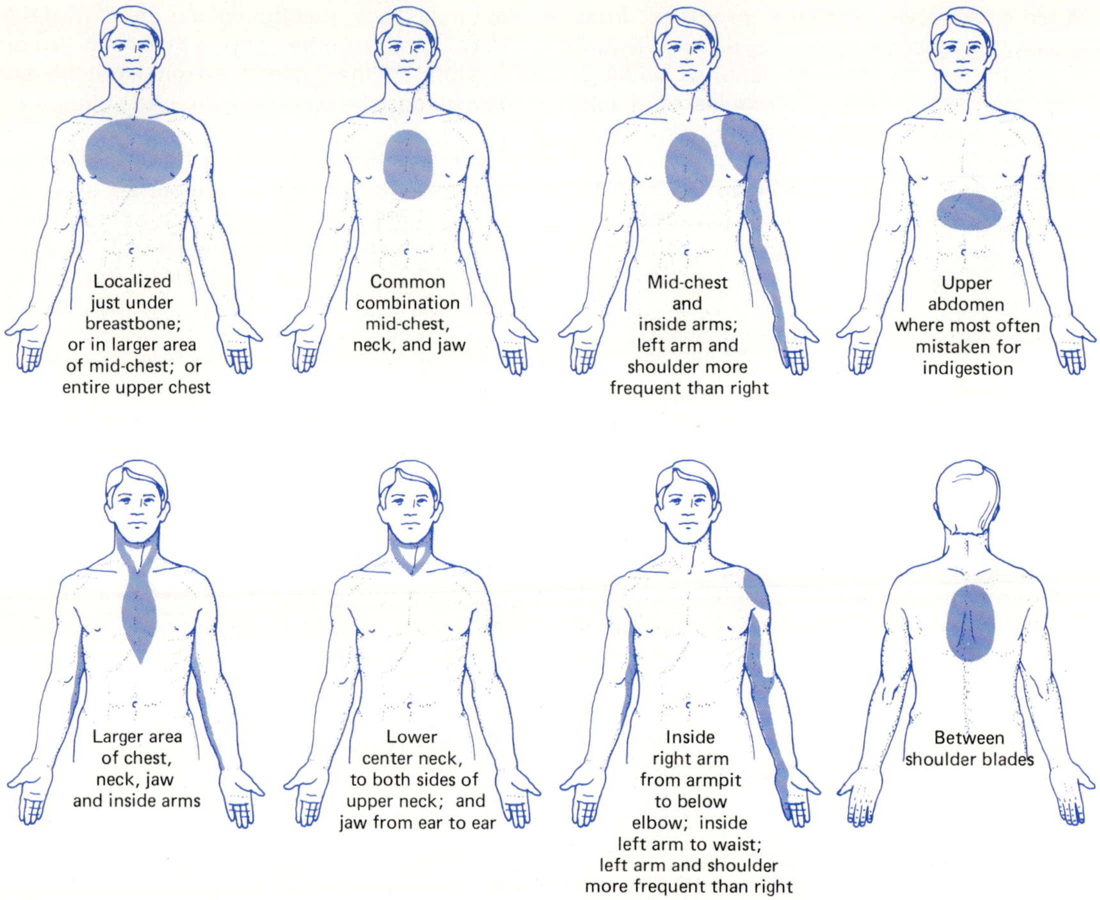

FIGURE 10.7 Early warnings of a heart attack. Pain, in one form or another, almost always accompanies a heart attack, and can range from a mild ache to pain of unbearable severity. When severe, the pain often feels constricting, like a vise on the chest. Pain also often includes the burning and bloated sensations that usually accompany indigestion. The pain may be continuous and then subside for a while; but it should not be ignored just because it subsides. Heart attack pain can occur in any one of the locations shown in the drawings, or in a combination of several locations.

Symptoms that may accompany the pain include: difficulty in breathing, palpitations, nausea, vomiting, cold sweat, paleness, weakness, anxiety. (Anxiety that one is having a heart attack may also bring on these symptoms.) None of these symptoms is conclusive proof of a heart attack. But the more of them present, the more likely it is that the individual *is* undergoing a heart attack.

of caffeine (in coffee or cola drinks), tobacco, or marijuana; or serious disease. Physician must diagnose. *Treatment*: Avoidance of triggering factors; drugs to regulate heartbeat; for very rapid heartbeat (tachycardia), relaxation techniques. A doctor may suggest a self-help technique for interrupting the vagus reflex that stimulates the tachycardia.

Fibrillation When the heart beats so rapidly that it can no longer be effective—400 to 600 beats per minute—the patient is in extreme danger. *Cause*: Myocardial infarction or other heart problems. *Treatment*: Drugs; electric countershock—defibrillation—to shock the heart's electrical system back into working order.

Congestive heart failure A congestion or accumulation of fluid in various parts of the body (lungs, abdomen, legs, etc). *Cause*: Weakness of heart muscle, resulting in inability to pump out all the blood that returns to it and maintain satisfactory circulation. *Treatment*: The drug digitalis, restricted salt intake, and use of diuretics.

Varicose veins This problem, in which the veins become swollen, is characterized by increased leg fatigue, cramps, soreness, itching, burning, and the characteristic knotting and bulging blue veins beneath skin surface. It occurs when faulty valves in leg veins cause a backup of blood. *Cause*: Inherited valve weakness, pregnancy, pressure of standing or sitting for long period daily, heavy lifting, abdominal pressure, aging. *Treatment*: Immobilization of the swollen and inefficient vein by injecting it with a sclerosing (hardening) solution, or surgery to remove or tie off the vein. Other veins gradually take over the work of those blocked or removed. In mild cases, support hose or elastic bandages, adequate periods of rest with feet elevated, and exercises such as walking, swimming, or "bicycling" while lying down with the feet in the air may be all that are necessary.

Hemorrhoids Also called "piles," this disorder, estimated to affect 1 of every 3 people at some time in their lives, is actually varicose veins of the rectum. The swellings (which often look like a

---

You can best help a heart attack victim—and possibly save a life—if you know in advance: (1) the nearest hospital equipped to handle heart attack emergencies; (2) how to do cardiopulmonary resuscitation (CPR), taught by local chapters of the American Heart Association and the American Red Cross; (3) how to call a doctor, the hospital, and/or an ambulance quickly; (4) the fastest route to the hospital. Knowing these things, you should:

1 Help victim to least painful position—usually sitting, with legs up and bent at knees. Loosen clothing around neck and midriff. Be calm, reassuring.

2 Quickly call ambulance to get victim to hospital via local rescue squad, police, fire, or other available service. Once the ambulance is on the way, notify family physician, if known.

3 If ambulance is coming, comfort victim while waiting. Otherwise, help victim to car, trying to keep victim's exertion to minimum. If possible, take another CPR-trained person with you. Victim should sit up.

4 Drive cautiously to hospital. Watch victim closely (or have other passenger do so). If victim loses consciousness, check for breathing, and feel for neck pulse under side angle of lower jaw to check for circulation. If no pulse, start CPR. Call for help. Continue CPR until trained help arrives to take over.

5 If patient retains consciousness to hospital, make sure he is carried, not walked, to emergency room.

[*Metropolitan Life Insurance Company.*]

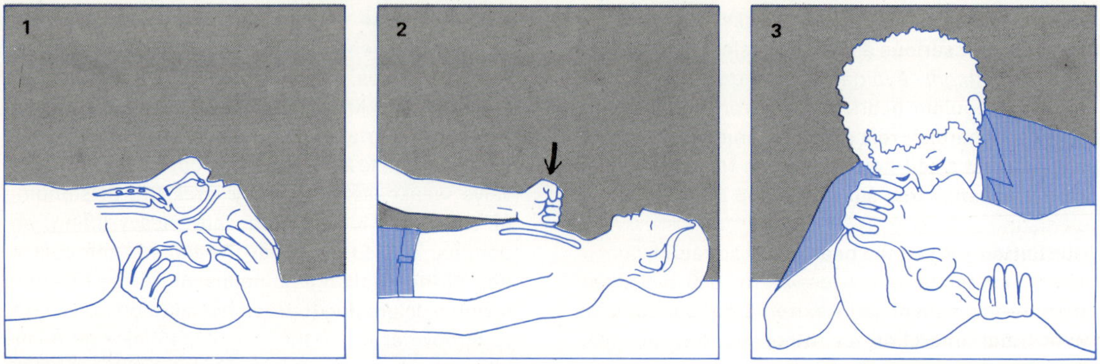

1. Open the airway by placing one hand under victim's neck and the other on his or her forehead, tilting back the head to lift the tongue from the back of the throat. Remove any obstructions—solids, liquids, vomitus. If victim is not breathing, proceed to step 2.

2. If no pulse can be felt, strike a sharp, quick single blow to the mid-chest with the fleshy portion of your fist, starting 8 to 12 inches above the chest. This must be done within 60 seconds of cessation of heartbeat.

3. To restart breathing, pinch nostrils closed, put your mouth over victim's to form tight seal, and inflate lungs with four quick, full breaths, without waiting between breaths. If no pulse is felt, proceed to step 4. Otherwise continue rescue breathing 12 times a minute until breathing resumes or help arrives.

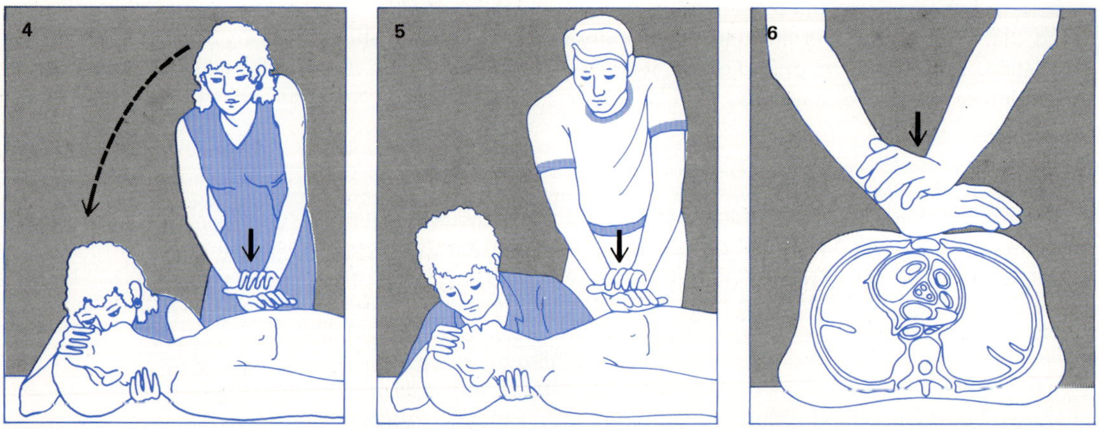

4. Begin CPR. If alone, use 15 chest compressions (80 per minute) as shown in drawing 6, followed by 2 very quick inflations of victim's lungs as shown in drawing 3.

5. If you have help, begin CPR in a 5 to 1 ratio — 5 chest compressions to 1 lung inflation, without pause.

6. Effective cardiac compression in adult requires enough pressure to depress sternum (breast bone) at least 1½ inches. Hold fingers free of chest wall.

FIGURE 10.8 Cardiopulmonary resuscitation (CPR) for heart attack victims and others who stop breathing and/or whose hearts have stopped beating (no pulse is felt). The basic aims or ABCs of CPR are: *A, airways*, clear them; *B, breathing*, get it restarted; and *C, circulation*, restart it through compressions of the chest. CPR is best administered by someone who has been trained in the technique, but in a life-or-death emergency even an untrained person should try it. [*Adapted from* Patient Care, *Dec. 1, 1974.*]

bunch of small grapes) can be internal (within the rectum) or external; they can be painful and they often bleed. *Cause*: Sitting or standing for long periods, pregnancy, childbirth, and most commonly, constipation. *Prevention*: Good diet with sufficient roughage to prevent constipation, combined with careful, regular bowel habits. *Treatment*: Sometimes relatively simple office surgery, but on occasion the more radical hemorrhoidectomy. Many doctors prefer conservative home treatment with frequent warm "sitzbaths" to reduce swelling and discomfort, careful cleansing of the anus with water or wet tissue following bowel movements, and pain-relieving ointment. *Any bleeding from the rectum—even if hemorrhoids are obviously present—requires immediate medical diagnosis.*

CANCER

Early in this century, August Bier said, "There is a tremendous literature on cancer, but what we know for sure about it can be printed on a calling card." Today, theories and suppositions could fill a library, but there are still a great many unanswered questions about cancer. What is known and understood about this disease that kills 1000 Americans each

An implanted pacemaker has enabled this heart patient to enjoy normal activities such as swimming, rescuing her from life as an invalid.

Ben Ross

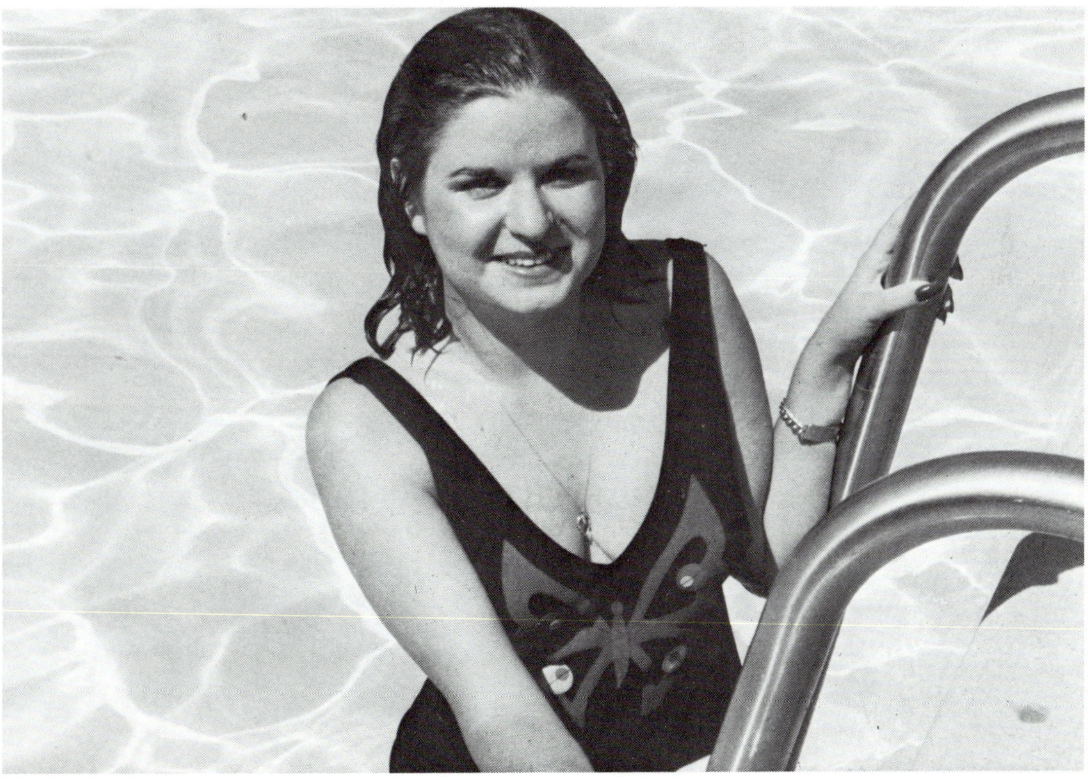

day is, however, growing daily. And with understanding come improved chances for prevention, treatment, and cure.

What Is Cancer?

Though the word "cancer" conjures up a single stereotype in most minds—of an insidious growth that cruelly and silently kills its victims—it actually describes at least 100 different diseases. Some grow rapidly, causing death in weeks. Others grow slowly and harmlessly for years. Some can be cured easily; others are rarely cured. Suspected causes differ widely.

The word "cancer" was taken from the Greek *karinos*, meaning "crab," because the cancer often reaches out in a crablike fashion to other parts of the body. In every cancer, there is a group of malignant (mischief-working) cells that grows and spreads uncontrollably, becoming life-threatening. This group of cells is called a *tumor*, or *neoplasm* (*neo* = new + *plasm* = growth). Nonmalignant, or benign (harmless), tumors have more controlled growth, do not spread throughout the body, and are not life-threatening unless they block a vital body function. Removing them cures any problems they are causing.

Differences between normal and cancerous cells Nobel prize winner James Watson has suggested that it may be 50 years before biologists can totally map the essential differ-

Varicose veins, the result of faulty valves, can cause fatigue, discomfort, and disfigurement. A variety of treatments and preventive measures are available to relieve the condition.

Randy Matusow

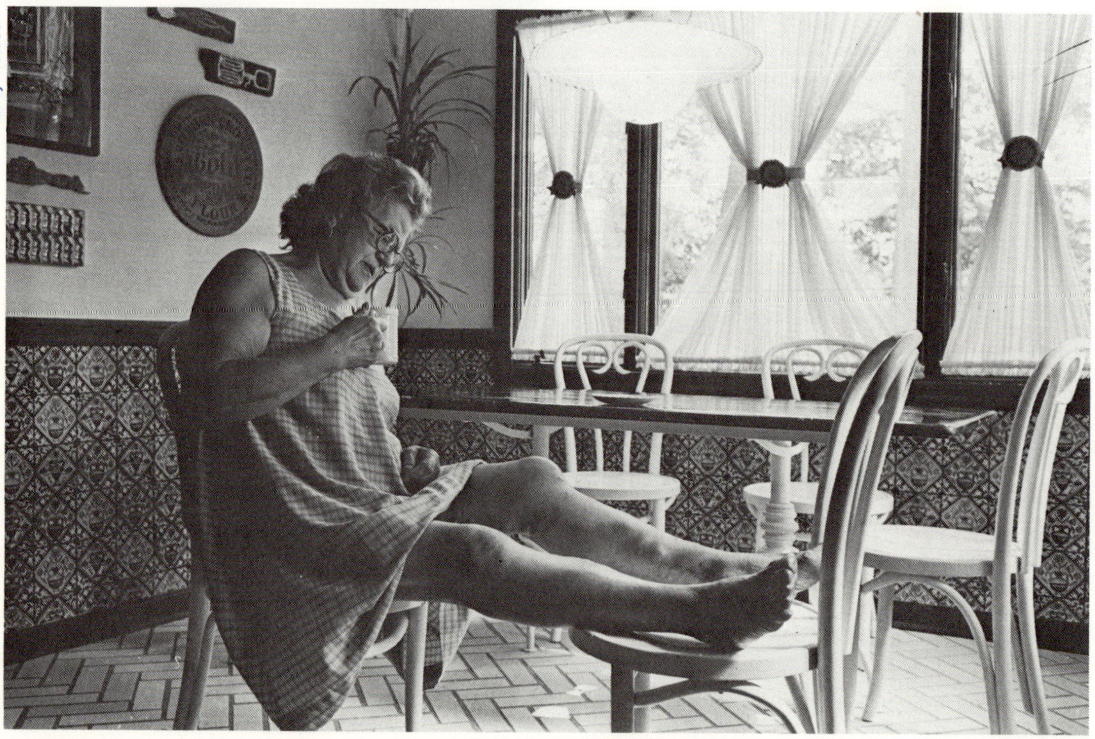

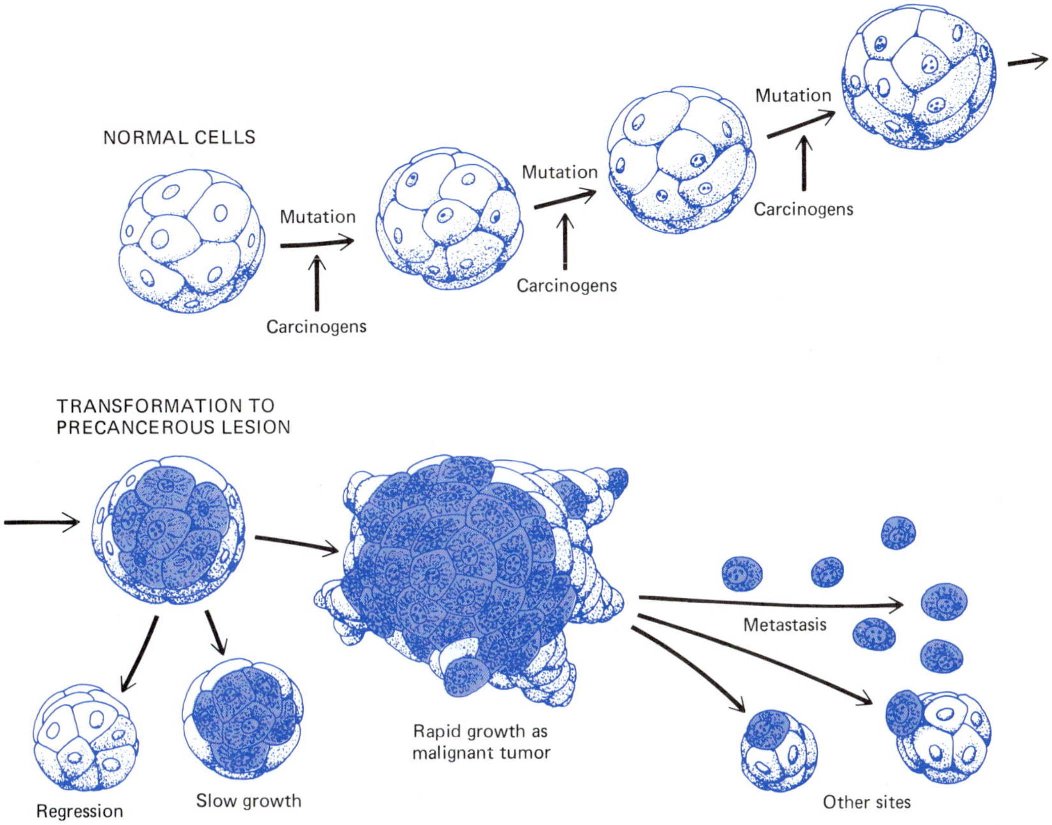

FIGURE 10.9 The change from normal cells to cancer cells: a theory. This theory of carcinogenesis states that cells are restrained from becoming cancerous by several independent genes and that tumors develop only when mutations accumulate in all those genes within a line of cells. The mutations (black dots within cell nuclei) are seldom spontaneous but are apparently caused by carcinogenic factors in the environment. Once a precancerous lesion has formed, one of three things probably happens: (1) it regresses, probably because of self-repair of the cell DNA; (2) it grows very slowly and goes unnoticed; (3) very occasionally, it progresses to an invasive, metastasizing tumor. [*Adapted from Cairns, pp. 68–69.*]

ences between normal and cancerous cells. Several basic differences have already been observed. Normal cells grow and divide in a very disciplined fashion. Each cell is programmed to follow a sequence of events for carrying out life processes—as a skin cell, a nerve cell, a blood cell, etc. When a cell becomes cancerous, it rebels against body programming; it acts on its own and grows in a disorganized fashion. Some scientists, including Nobelist Sir Frank MacFarlane Burnet, believe that cancer cells are always developing in the body, but cancer occurs only when the immune system fails to overwhelm them; this is called the *surveillance theory.* Dr. Edmund Klein, noted cancer researcher,

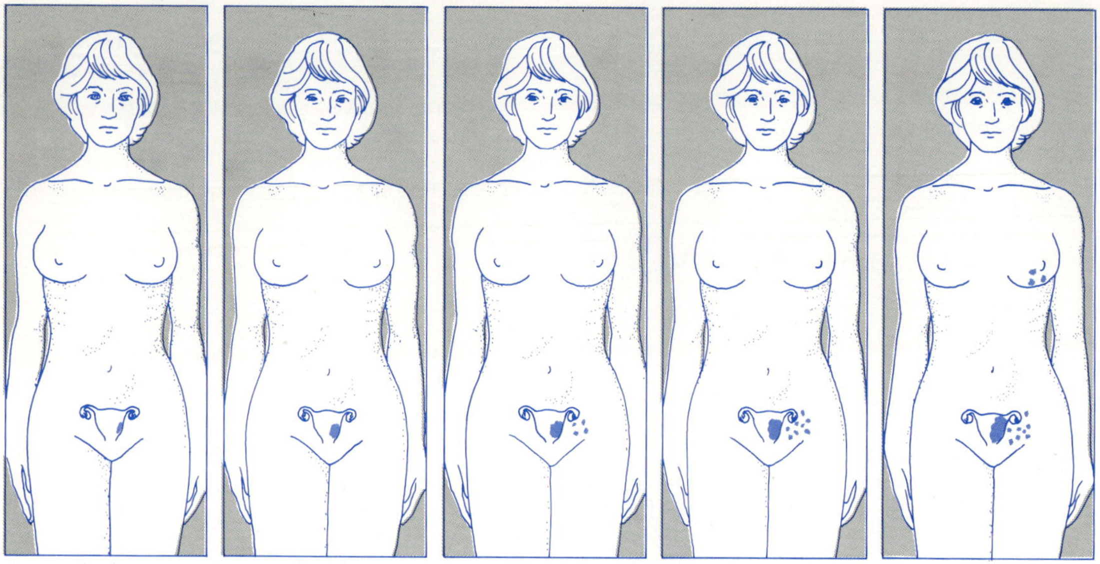

FIGURE 10.10 Stages of tumor growth: uterine cancer spreading to breast.

- *In situ* The solid tumor usually begins with a group of cells on the surface of the tissue involved. At first they remain on the surface, localized in one spot. This is the most curable stage.
- *Invasive* Eventually, in most cases, the cancer cells begin to penetrate beyond the surface and to invade underlying tissue. This happens very quickly in some types of cancer, very slowly in others.
- *Metastatic* In most cancers, if the growth is not removed or destroyed, a few cells eventually break off from the tumor and start to move or "metastasize" through blood or lymph systems to other parts of the body.
- *Regional* Often the body's defense system will trap the runaway cells for a while in one or more lymph nodes near the site of the original growth, keeping the cancer "regional."
- *Advanced* Without treatment, the cancer continues to spread, overwhelming the body's defenses completely, taking hold in other tissues. For example, a breast tumor may spread to the lungs, a lung tumor to the brain. This advanced stage of cancer is the most difficult to cure.

has reported that malignant tumors appear to have a defense against the body's specific immune response. It has also been suggested that a mild immune response might actually stimulate multiplication of cancer cells. More research is needed in these areas.

Types of tumors Malignant tumors developing in the epithelial tissues (skin, linings of mouth, stomach, intestines, bronchial tubes, or ducts in breast or prostate) are called *carcinomas*. Those that arise in connective tissue (bone, cartilage, adipose, for example) are called *sarcomas*. Carcinomas and sarcomas are "solid tumors." Cancers that occur in the lymph system (*lymphomas*) or in the system that produces white blood cells (*leukemias*) are "generalized" tumors.

Risk Factors

There may be as many cancer causes as there are kinds of cancer. Many of the factors discussed in Chapter 7 as generally involved in disease have been implicated in some way in cancer: genetic susceptibility, immune deficiency, microorganisms (viruses), environmental hazards, hormone imbalance, diet, and possibily even mental health. Many scientists now believe that no case of cancer is due to a single cause. One theory suggests that a cancer-causing agent—a chemical, the sun, a virus—damages a cell in a susceptible individual. Then, as the cell tries to repair itself, an error occurs, leading to uncontrolled growth.

Environmental factors A striking report by the World Health Organization states that 80 to 90 percent of cancers are associated in some way with environmental hazards. Little, however, is understood about how these cancer-causing (carcinogenic) hazards do their work. Some apparently require a *co*carcinogen. Asbestos, for example, seems to cause lung cancer only in those workers who smoke. The development of environmentally caused cancers may also depend on such variables as dosage and length of exposure to the environmental factor, as well as the individual's genetic background, sex, age, and physical and mental health. The major environmental hazards believed to cause cancer include:

- *Tobacco* Tobacco, smoked in cigarette, pipe, or cigar form, is the single greatest known cause of cancer deaths, related to cancers of the lung, mouth, lips, esophagus, larynx, kidneys, and bladder. (See Chapter 17.)
- *Alcohol* Excessive use of alcohol greatly increases the cancer activity of tobacco. It also appears to be related to an increase in cancers of the mouth, pharynx, pancreas, esophagus, and liver. (See Chapter 16.)
- *Other drugs* Some cancer-treatment drugs, immunosuppressive drugs, and amphetamines have been linked to the development of cancer. Since the tars of marijuana cause cancer in rats just as do the tars of tobacco, it is suspected that marijuana, too, may turn out to be carcinogenic.
- *Radiation* Long-term exposure to radiation in small doses or single exposures to very high doses (as from atomic explosion) are known to cause cancer. All living things are exposed to certain amounts of natural cosmic radiation. How much can be added safely in on-the-job exposure or for diagnosing or treating illness is not yet clear. (See page 69 for a discussion on x-ray diagnosis.)
- *Sunlight* Cancers of the skin are most common in sunny climates, and in fair-skinned persons who spend a great deal of time exposed to the ultraviolet rays of the sun.
- *Chemicals* The first example of a chemical carcinogen was noted in 1775 by a perceptive British surgeon, Dr. Percival Pott, who attributed the frequent incidence of cancer of the scrotum in chimney sweeps to intimate contact with soot as they shimmied up and down the interior of smoke stacks during work. Today, about 30 chemicals and other substances have been associated with cancer causation in humans, and many others are suspect. Many have already been banned or restricted. Carcinogenic substances include: (1) pesticides such as DDT, Aldrin, Dieldrin, chlordane, and Heptachlor; (2) industrial chemicals such as vinyl chloride, asbestos (found in 3000 products), silica (the second most abundant element on earth, used in talc, dishes, etc.), chloroform, bis (chlormethyl) ether, benzene, arsenic, beta-naphthyl-

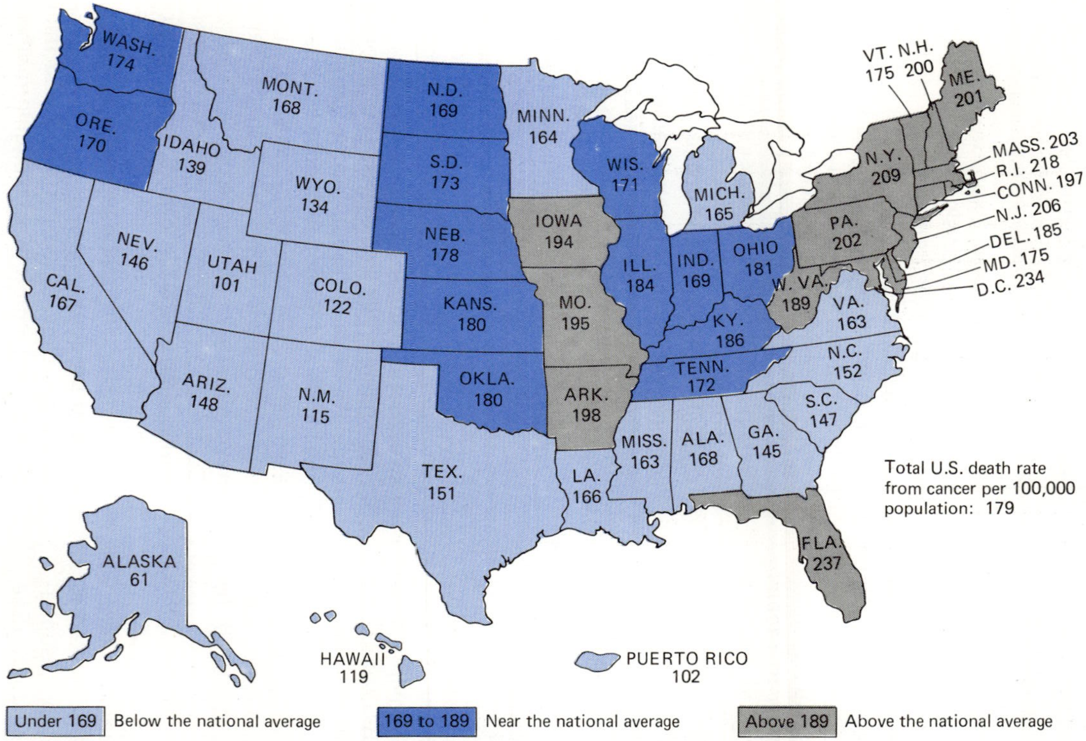

FIGURE 10.11 Estimated United States cancer death rate per 100,000 population by state, 1978. Cancer rates are highest in the Northeast, lowest in the Southwest. They are higher in urban areas than in rural regions. The death rate from skin cancer is highest in the South, with its year-round sunshine; respiratory and esophageal cancer are more prevalent in cities. Utah, with a large population of Mormons, whose lifestyle (described in Chapter 4) includes many preventive health practices, has the lowest cancer death rate in the nation. Florida, with a high proportion of older citizens more susceptible to cancer, has the highest. Cancer epidemiologists study data such as these for clues relating lifestyle and environment to causes of cancer. [*American Cancer Society*, b, *pp. 1, 12.*]

amine (used in dyeing); (3) chemicals, such as PCBs, dumped in waterways; (4) air pollutants (their effects are still being debated); (5) polycyclic aromatic hydrocarbons such as benzopyrene; (6) Tris, used to make children's sleepwear flame retardant. Recently, hair dyes (Ames) and tear gas (Dyer) have come under suspicion.

It is hoped that new short-term tests (such as the Ames test; see page 115) for determining the carcinogenic and mutagenic (birth-defect-causing) qualities of new chemicals will help manufacturers and the government to screen out substances that are potentially dangerous even before they are put into production and to screen inexpensively the many untested substances already in use. Costing only about $2000 per test, they are superior for screening purposes to standard 2- and 3-year animal studies costing from $200,000 to $3 billion each.[6]

- *Diet* Accumulating epidemiological data seems to point to a relationship between dietary habits and some types of cancer—for example, between stomach cancer and smoked fish consumption in Japan, between bowel cancer and beef consumption, between breast cancer and high-fat diets, between lack of bulk and intestinal cancers, between very hot foods and beverages and throat cancers, between barbecued foods and foods cooked on metal grills and various kinds of cancers. Excesses and deficiencies of certain nutrients also seem to be associated with cancer, as do a variety of natural and synthetic ingredients in food, discussed in Chapter 5.

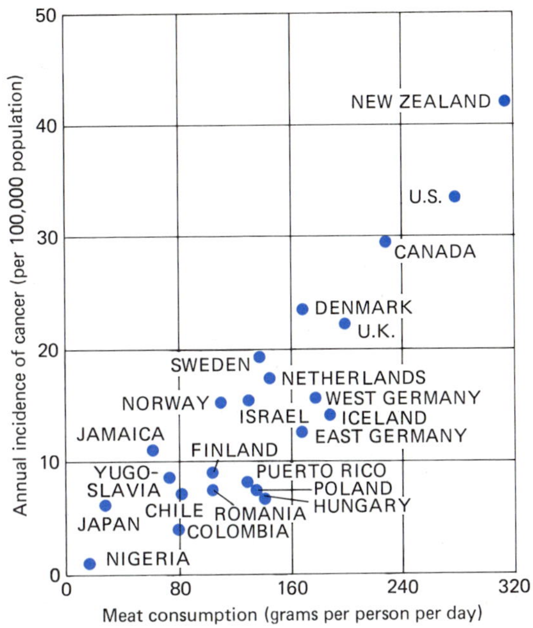

FIGURE 10.12 Cancer and epidemiology. The geography of a cancer suggests a probable cause of the disease. The incidence of cancer of the large intestine among women in 23 countries is closely related to per capita meat consumption in those countries. The data are adjusted to eliminate differences in age distribution in the populations. An alternative explanation attributes cancer of the large intestine to a low consumption of cereals. The two hypotheses are hard to distinguish from each other because high meat consumption and low cereal consumption tend to go together. This graph gives a good visual picture of how possible causes of cancer are pinpointed epidemiologically. [*Adapted from Cairns, p. 78.*]

Hormone imbalance There is strong evidence that estrogen preparations (most often given to ease the unpleasant symptoms some women experience at menopause) are associated with increased risk of uterine cancer (Weiss). The synthetic estrogen DES (diethylstilbesterol) has definitely been tied to rare cancers of the vagina and cervix in daughters of women who took the drug dur-

[6]Tests that show that a substance causes cancer in animals do not prove conclusively that the substance will also cause cancer in humans. But since tests on humans are ethically impossible, animal tests remain our best guide.

Photo Trends

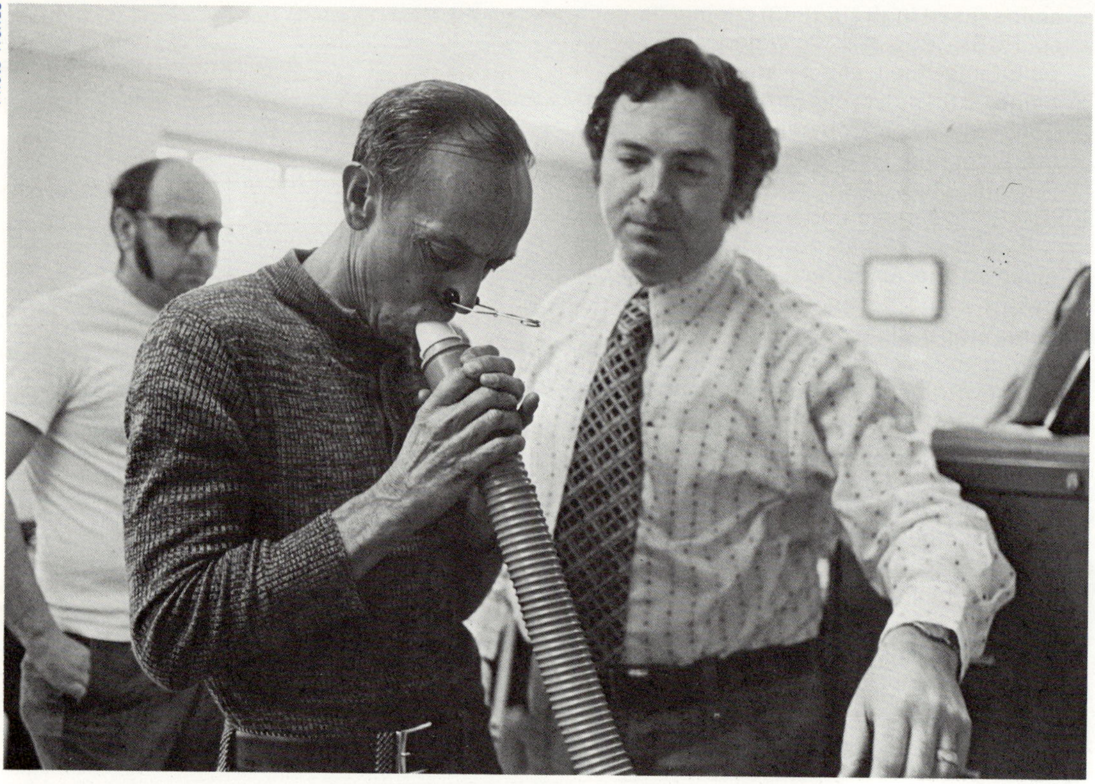

Many workers, like this plastics factory employee, must be tested for contamination by the chemicals to which they are exposed in their work.

ing early pregnancy.[7] Hormones may, on the other hand, be preventive (Lemon). Estriol, which increases greatly in women who become pregnant before age 25, seems to reduce risk of breast cancer.

Immune deficiency Transplant patients and others who have had their immune systems suppressed intentionally—as well as those who are immune-deficient because of illness or lack of a thymus—have higher than usual levels of cancer.

[7]All women born since 1940 should check with their mothers to see whether they may have been exposed to DES in utero. If exposure is a possibility, the women should see their family doctors or gynecologists.

Viruses The virus first became a suspect in 1911, when Peyton Rous of the Rockefeller Institute (who received a Nobel Prize for his work 55 years later) reported he was able to transmit chicken cancers from one chick to another by means of a cell-free, bacteria-free solution that could pass through a filter. The filtrate did contain tiny particles (called *filterable viruses*) which were subsequently named Rous Sarcoma Viruses. It has since been shown that more than a dozen other animal cancers can be stimulated by viruses.

Proof that a viral agent causes cancer in humans, however, is lacking, though there is some circumstantial evidence. As with the testing of possible carcinogenic chemicals, tests of cancer viruses on humans are impossible. A scientist cannot ethically inject a suspect virus into a human subject to see whether cancer will develop. Thus the question remains an area of major dispute among oncologists (cancer scientists).

Some believe a viral cause for human cancer is certain to be discovered; others believe the route is a dead end in cancer research. Dr. Timothy O'Connor, virologist, believes that the disagreement lies in differing views of the virus itself. Cancer virologists, he explains, do not see the virus as a noxious little bug that gives us a cold, but rather as a bit of genetic material that penetrates the cell and causes it to go haywire. The viral gene, it is now believed, may be latent in the cell for a long time before it causes trouble and may be activated by a cocarcinogen. The cancer viruses may be defective particles to start with, or they may be modified or made defective by a cocarcinogen.

If the virus is involved in human cancer, there is no evidence that it is communicable in the way that measles and flu are. Husbands who are afraid to have sexual relations when their wives are stricken with uterine cancer, wives who are afraid to kiss husbands with throat cancer are misguided. They cannot "catch" cancer. Most present scientific opinion suggests that instead that the transmission of a cancer-causing virus takes place either genetically, from parent to child, or from mother to child in the uterus.

Other factors In women, early and frequent sexual activity with many partners and infection with herpes simplex II virus appear to be linked to uterine cancer, while late or no childbearing seems related to cancer of the breast. In males, penis cancer is more prevalent among men who were not circumcised in early infancy—possibly because smegma, the cheesy secretion that accumulates under the foreskin, is carcinogenic. Smegma may also be related to the higher incidence of cervical cancer in wives of noncircumcised men.

Psychological factors—particularly significant trauma such as the loss of a loved one—appear to be related to cancer, but further study is needed to substantiate this relationship. The idea that physical trauma, such as a hard blow to the breast, will result in cancer attracts little or no support scientifically. Only 1 in 700 injured persons get cancer, which equals the rate in the general population.

Prevention

Though we often think of cancer as a relentless adversary, with present knowledge it is possible to prevent 3 or 4 of every 10 cases—almost 100,000 a year (Schneiderman).

Personal decision making Much of the effort to prevent cancer involves personal choices. Some decisions require rather serious changes in daily lifestyle; others involve periodic matters such as physical examinations. They include:

1 Avoiding unprotected exposure to direct sunlight during the middle of the day, especially if you are fair-skinned (see Chapter 6)
2 Never smoking cigarettes, pipes, cigars, possibly even marijuana—or quitting if you already smoke
3 Avoiding regular heavy doses of alcohol, including beer
4 Eating a varied and prudent diet low in fats, additives, and contaminants and high in bulk[8]
5 Limiting x-ray exposure to situations where benefit outweighs risk
6 Reducing to a minimum exposure to known or suspected carcinogens including air and water pollutants, chemicals, and so on (see pages 245 and 246); careful adherence to safety rules where risk is great
7 If an uncircumcised male, careful daily cleaning under foreskin to remove smegma
8 If female, avoiding having a large number

[8]Studies are under way to see whether or not sugar is involved in cancer causation.

WHEN TO SEEK HELP

Cancer Warning Signs

If any of the following symptoms persist for more than 2 weeks, a physician should be seen immediately.

1 *Change in bladder or bowel habits* A sudden stretch of diarrhea or constipation, not connected with an illness, may be caused by an obstruction—a tumor blocking the lower digestive tract. Other symptoms of a tumor may be gas pains and rectal bleeding. Bladder or prostate cancer may be signaled by difficulty with urination; a weak or interrupted flow of urine; lower back, thigh, or pelvic pain; burning or painful urination.

2 *A sore that does not heal* These sores are most likely to be on the skin or in the mouth. Cancers in the mouth may also be raised, irregular, warty areas, lumps or thickenings in the cheek, gums, or tongue. Usually they are painless. White patches in the mouth may be precancerous.

3 *Unusual bleeding or discharge* Any bleeding from a body cavity is a warning that something is wrong. Bleeding from the vagina is an early sign of uterine cancer, and a late sign of cervical cancer. Bleeding from the rectum is often a sign of cancer of the bowel. If the blood in the stool is tarry (black), there is the possibility of cancer higher up in the digestive tract. Examination should be made for cancer when there is bleeding, even when hemorrhoids (which also bleed) are present. Bleeding in the mouth or from the nose may signal leukemia. Bleeding under the skin—seen as black-and-blue marks with no apparent cause—can also indicate blood cancer. Blood in the sputum may warn of lung cancer.

4 *A thickening or lump in the breast or elsewhere* Lumps are often not noticed unless self-examination is practiced. Lumps and thickenings that say "See your doctor" may be found in breasts, testicles, lymph node areas (groin, armpits, neck, and jaw). They are generally painless and most often are not cancerous. But only a physician can determine which are malignant and which benign. (See Figure 4.4 on breast self-examination.)

5 *Indigestion or difficulty in swallowing* Indigestion is usually "just something you ate." But when it appears suddenly and recurs regularly, it can be a symptom of stomach cancer. That is true, too, of persistent discomfort or mild pain, fullness, or bloating; slight nausea; heartburn; loss of appetite; sometimes belching or vomiting. Difficulty in swallowing may indicate a tumor in the esophagus.

6 *Obvious changes in a wart or mole* Cancer of the skin can develop in an existing mole or wart, but it can also appear suddenly anywhere on the skin. It may be a dry, scaly patch, or a pimple which persists, or an inflamed red area with a crusting center, or a pale, waxy, pearly nodule which may eventually ulcerate. Malignant melanoma, an uncommon but serious cancer of the skin, usually occurs as a dark brown or black molelike growth which becomes larger and ulcerated and often bleeds. Some skin lesions are precancerous. (See Chapter 6.)

7 *Nagging cough or hoarseness* When a lung cancer is located in the bronchi (or air passages), it will cause an obstruction, irritation, and probably a cough. There may also be some blood in the sputum that is coughed up. Cancers deep in the lung, however, may show no early symptoms. All coughs that "hang on" should be checked by a physician. So should hoarseness with or without difficulty in swallowing, soreness in neck, or a lump-in-the-throat feeling—all of which may signal cancer of the larynx or voice box.

Many other generalized symptoms of illness can indicate cancer, as well as other serious diseases. These include fatigue, loss of appetite, and persistent fever or pain. Unfortunately, many cancers are silent, no symptoms appear until it is too late for effective treatment of the disease. Thus, the search for early detection methods—such as new blood tests that are under investigation—is critical.

It is also critical that persons who detect a possible cancer symptom seek immediate help. Unfortunately, most do not get help early; yet for those who do, there is a much better chance of cure if the diagnosis is cancer—and relief from worry if it is not.

of sexual partners, especially when young; bearing a child before age 25; having an annual pap smear for detection of precancerous cells and having follow-up treatment if they are found

9 Doing self-examinations for precancerous skin or mouth lesions and having them treated immediately

10 Having annual or biannual proctoscope examination of the rectum and lower intestine after age 40, so that precancerous polyps can be detected and removed

Community decisions Some decisions are not directly ours to make: how many chemicals are poured into our rivers and other waterways; how much chemical pollution circulates in the air we breathe; how well protected we are on the job. But as community members we can make our voices heard, can join environmental and "people's" lobbies, and can pressure employers, legislators, industry, and the President to improve conditions. (See Chapter 26.)

Future techniques Scientists are doggedly exploring a variety of ways to prevent cancer, including use of: (1) synthetic vitamin A and antioxidants such as vitamin E, BHT, and BHA to block action of carcinogens; (2) vaccines and other substances to stimulate the immune system to destroy cancers before they become menacing; (3) antidotes to counteract the effects of carcinogenic chemicals after exposure; (4) blocking agents to prevent reverse transcriptase (the enzyme that allows RNA viruses to give directions to DNA to grow uncontrollably) from doing its job.

Screening and Detection

Early detection cannot prevent cancer, but it can prevent a fatal outcome. The American Cancer Society's highly publicized "seven common warning signs" (see sidebar) are familiar to most of us. But we often do not understand what they mean, and why they are important. Nor do we always recognize that the appearance of one of these signs suggests only the *possibility*, not the inevitability, of cancer. Nor do we know that pain is not generally an early sign of cancer.

Screening tests As you saw in Chapter 4, there is no little medical controversy about the value of screening programs aimed at picking up disease before symptoms become obvious. A study by Blue Cross of mass screening for cancer is under way, with the goal of determining whether or not it can save both money and lives. Some screening procedures are already known to save lives: breast self-examination augmented by annual examination by a physician, the Pap smear for cervical cancer in women, and genital self-examination for men. (See Chapter 4.)

Screening for most cancers is not yet available, but a blood test for cancer is under study and holds promise of an easy and inexpensive screening procedure. (See Table 10.2 for present screening methods).

Making a definite diagnosis Screening tests and physical examinations suggest the possibility of cancer, but only a biopsy yields a definite diagnosis. The physician removes a bit of suspicious tissue from the tumor

TABLE 10.2 The most common cancers

SITE	ESTIMATED NEW CASES, 1977[a]	ESTIMATED DEATHS, 1977[a]	WARNING SIGNALS—SEE YOUR DOCTOR	DIAGNOSIS AND SCREENING	COMMENT
Breast[b]	91,000	34,000	Lump or thickening in breast	Monthly self-exam (Fig. 4.3) Annual checkup Mammography[c] GST[d]	The leading cause of cancer deaths in women.
Colon and rectum[b]	102,000	52,000	Change in bowel habits; bleeding	Annual checkup including proctoscopy, stool exam, esp. for those over 40	Highly curable when detected early, through routine checkups; high-bulk, low-fat diet may be preventive.
Lung	102,000	92,000	Persistent cough, or lingering respiratory ailment	Sputum test[e]	The leading cause of cancer deaths among men and rising mortality among women; 80% would be prevented if no one smoked cigarettes.
Oral (including pharynx)	24,000	8000	Sore that does not heal; difficulty in swallowing	Self-exam Annual checkup (dentist, physician)	Avoidance of smoking may prevent.
Skin (melanoma)	10,000[f]	5000	Sore that does not heal; change in wart or mole	Self-exam Annual checkup Readily detected by observation and diagnosed by simple biopsy	Avoidance of overexposure to sun may prevent.

[a]All figures rounded to nearest 1000.
[b]Five-year survival rates increased between 1950 and 1973.
[c]Recommended only for women over 50 or those 40–49 with family cancer history or under 40 with personal cancer history.
[d]New graphic heat telethermometry technique, using heat detection, may prove to be a good, safe screening method for breast cancer.
[e]See Table 4.4 for screening and diagnostic test descriptions.
[f]Estimated new cases of nonmelanoma skin cancers about 300,000.
[g]If carcinoma in situ is included, cases total over 87,000.
Source: Adapted in part from *Cancer Facts and Figures,* American Cancer Society, 1978, p. 13.

SITE	ESTIMATED NEW CASES, 1977[a]	ESTIMATED DEATHS, 1977[a]	WARNING SIGNALS—SEE YOUR DOCTOR	DIAGNOSIS AND SCREENING	COMMENT
Uterus[b]	48,000[g]	11,000	Unusual bleeding or discharge	Annual check-up including pelvic exam with Pap test[e]	Uterine cancer mortality has declined 65% during last 40 years with wider application of Pap test.
Kidney and bladder[b]	45,000	17,000	Urinary difficulty or bleeding (see doctor at once)	Annual check-up with urinalysis	Protective measures for workers in high-risk industries helping to eliminate.
Larynx[b]	9000	3000	Hoarseness, difficulty in swallowing	Annual check-up including laryngoscopy	Readily curable if caught early.
Prostate[b]	57,000	21,000	Urinary difficulty	Annual check-up including palpation through rectum,[e] urinalysis	Occurs mainly in men over 60.
Stomach	23,000	15,000	Indigestion	Annual check-up, x-rays when needed	A 40% decline in mortality in 25 years, for reasons yet unknown.
Leukemia, chronic form[b]	22,000	15,000	Leukemia is a cancer of blood-forming tissues and is characterized by the abnormal production of immature white blood cells. Acute leukemia strikes some children but more adults, and is treated by drugs which have extended life from a few months to as much as 10 years. Chronic leukemia usually strikes after age 25 and progresses less rapidly.		
Lymphomas[b]	33,000	21,000	These cancers arise in the lymph system and include Hodgkin's disease and lymphosarcoma. Some patients with lymphatic cancers can lead normal lives for many years. The 5-year survival rate for Hodgkin's disease has increased from 25 to 54% in 20 years.		

A story circulated (at a medical meeting) about a man who had decided gradually to give up everything that scientists have linked with cancer.

The first week, he cut out smoked fish and charcoal steaks.
The second week, he cut out smoking.
The third week, he cut out having relations with women.
The fourth week, he cut out drinking.
The fifth week, he cut out paper dolls.

Boston Herald, Sept. 4, 1965

by scraping, cutting, or extracting it with a needle. The specimen is microscopically examined—usually by a pathologist specializing in identifying disease in human tissues—for the characteristic irregularity of size and shape and the disorganized appearance of cancer tissue. (See Figure 10.9.)

Treatment

During the early twentieth century, even cancer scientists feared the disease was incurable. Today there are more than 1.5 million Americans who have gone through the crisis of cancer and survived for the length of time free of disease needed before the patient can be considered cured—most often 5 years. As of 1975, 2 of every 6 of the nation's 650,000 annual cancer victims are cured. If all cancer patients received the best care available, with early diagnosis and the latest in treatment, the figure would be 3 in 6. Cures for the other 3 patients are not yet available, but the odds in their favor improve with each new advance in cancer therapy and understanding.

There may well prove to be as many treatments and combinations of treatments as there are types of cancer. It seems clear that no single "wonder drug" will prove effective against all forms of cancer. But one common denominator exists: The earlier the disease is diagnosed and treated, the better the chances of patient survival. Major treatment methods today include cutting out the tumor (surgery), destroying it with radiation, attacking it with chemicals or the body's own immune system, altering the body's hormone defense, and most effective, treatment with combinations of these methods.

Surgery Alice was 44 and had two children in college when she found a lump in her right breast. The breast was removed along with lymph nodes and surrounding muscle. Alice lived nearly 40 years more, long enough to see her grandchildren in college. Surgery, used even in ancient times, is the most common treatment for cancers that have not metastasized (spread) and can be entirely removed without crippling the function of vital organs.

Cancer surgery is employed in four general ways: (1) *specific*, in hope of removing all the cancerous tissue; (2) *supportive*, to prolong life by removing some of the cancer, to remove or relieve pain or discomfort, to treat complications; (3) *preventive*, to remove precancerous lesions such as polyps or nodes in the colon, rectum, skin, mouth, cervix, etc; (4) *in combined therapy*, to get the cancer down to a manageable size, so that drugs, radiation, and immunotherapy (which is under investigation) can be used in an effort to eliminate it entirely.

Like all cancer therapy, surgery has its risks: (1) from the surgery itself, (2) from spillage of cancer cells into the blood and lymph systems, (3) from infection following surgery. In addition, there are the hazards of life with one lung or one kidney, with half a stomach or no thyroid, as well as the trauma of life with no tongue, without reproductive organs, with one breast, or with no scrotum.

HEALTH CONSUMER TIP

Breast Cancer: Which Way Is Best?

Treatment for breast cancer has aroused great controversy in the 1970s for several reasons: (1) This disease is the No.1 killer of women between ages 40 and 44, and the major cause of cancer deaths in women of all ages, striking 90,000 American women annually; (2) it involves a part of a woman's body considered by many (rightly or wrongly) to be a symbol of femininity, womanhood, motherhood; (3) the most common treatment—radical surgery—is disfiguring and to some degree disabling; (4) several prominent women, including the wives of a President and Vice President of the United States, have made public their breast surgeries.

Ever since Dr. William Halsted first devised the radical mastectomy—removal of the affected breast, the muscle tissue of the chest beneath it, and the lymph nodes in the adjacent armpit—in 1882, surgeons have been performing this type of surgery on breast cancer patients almost routinely. Survival statistics for breast patients, however, have not improved much since Halsted's time, leading many physicians to try other approaches:

Radiation Radiation, usually following radical or other surgery, but occasionally used without surgery, often destroys malignant tumors. But this treatment is controversial since radiation may lead to the development of a new cancer later on.

Chemotherapy The use of drugs for breast cancer patients is relatively new. But recent studies indicate that a combination of three powerful drugs following surgery may offer a major improvement in survival rates, at least for premenopausal patients. The final results are not yet in, however.

Other types of surgery Many physicians, often responding to the demands of their patients, have begun using less radical forms of surgery when possible. These include: the *modified radical*, in which the breast and lymph nodes are removed but the chest muscles are not; the *simple or total mastectomy*, in which the breast is removed; the *partial mastectomy*, in which overlying skin, a wide section of the breast around the tumor, and sometimes some muscle beneath it are removed; and the *lumpectomy*, in which only the tumor and surrounding tissue are removed, leaving the breast only slightly smaller.

These procedures are less disfiguring and disabling than the radical mastectomy, and several studies have shown that survival rates are as good. But many surgeons continue to use radical surgery, awaiting stronger evidence for long-term survival. Some physicians individualize treatment in accordance with the size and spread of the tumor, the woman's age, and her physical condition. Often they will do the biopsy (sometimes in the office), analyze it, and then, if the lesion proves cancerous, allow the woman to participate in the decision about treatment. These physicians hope that the possibility of less severe disfigurement and in many cases of reconstruction through plastic surgery will lead more women to seek earlier evaluation of suspicious lumps.

Radiation Donald T, a long-time pipe smoker, noticed a painless sore on his tongue that did not seem to heal. A biopsy showed it to be malignant. Had his physician chosen to remove the cancer surgically, Donald would have been permanently handicapped. Instead

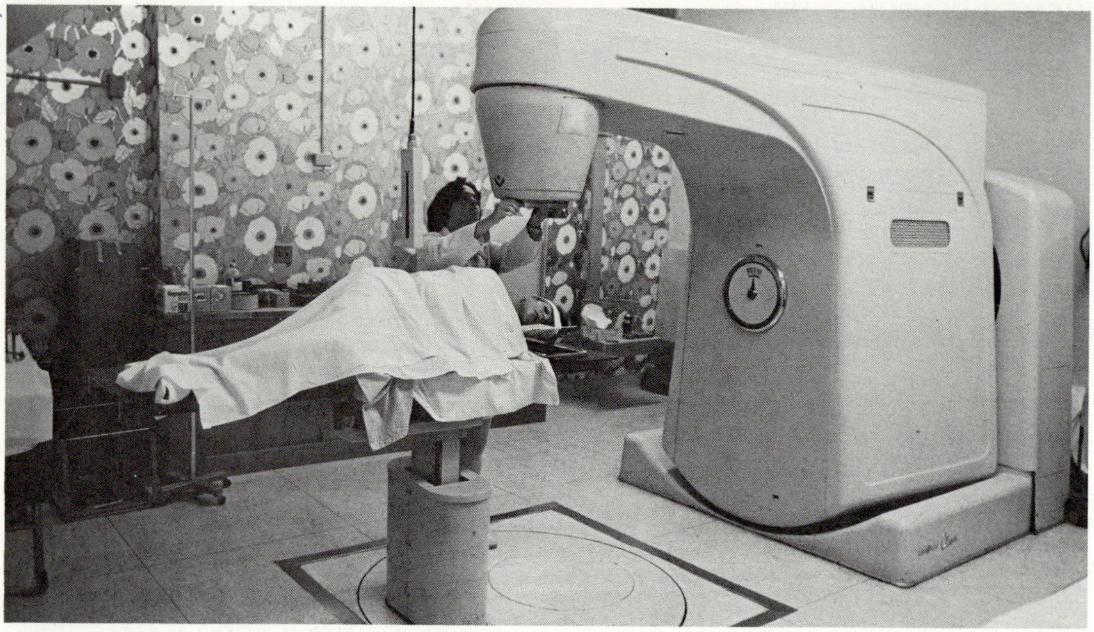

American Cancer Society

Radiation therapy, like other forms of cancer treatment, involves both risks and benefits.

he inserted a radium needle in Donald's tongue. The radiation destroyed the cancer, but left the tongue intact.

Between 50 and 60 percent of all cancer patients now receive radiation at some time during treatment from x-ray, radioactive isotopes of uranium, radium, cobalt 60, beta rays and neutrons, and several other experimental sources. Radiation can be external (aimed at the cancer from an outside source); or it can be inserted, implanted, or injected directly into the cancer or swallowed in a radioactive cocktail. Use of internal radiation is usually less hazardous to surrounding tissues and makes it possible for radiation to reach less accessible parts of the body, such as the uterus or the thyroid.

The goal of radiation therapy may be to cure, to prolong life, to ease discomfort, to delay the spread of cancer, or after surgery, to destroy stray cancer cells. It is superior to surgery in cases like Donald's where it is important to retain appearance and function. Valuable too, in treating systemic cancers that invade the entire body, it produces long-term remission in 1 of 3 chronic leukemia patients (Johnson).

But some cancers resist radiation. And since radiation damages healthy tissues, too, it must be applied in carefully focused and measured doses with the aim of doing more good than harm. Those who receive radiation treatment usually must be monitored for life to guard against possible new cancers that might develop as a result of treatment.

Drug therapy, or chemotherapy Jane was 17 and in her first year at a community college when she started feeling tired and "run down" all the time. She seemed to catch one cold after another, she bruised easily, and her gums bled. Her family doctor diagnosed leukemia. Jane was treated with a combination of four anticancer drugs plus blood transfusions at a major cancer center near her home. A few weeks after beginning treatment, she went into remission, showing no signs of leukemia.

Anticancer drugs were not available before the mid-1940s, but today more than 40 are in use, and about 15 percent of cancers treated with them are considered cured. The lives of thousands of other cancer patients are prolonged and their pain relieved. Drug therapy seems most successful against new cancers that are still growing rapidly, and against metastases.

The anticancer drugs are extremely toxic, but because cancer is a life-threatening disease, potential benefit outweighs risk. The use of antidote drugs—such as citrovorum rescue factor, which counteracts the toxicity of the drug methotrexate by "rescuing" normal cells from its action—has increased the safety, effectiveness, and lifesaving of chemotherapy. The use of ordinary antibiotics and other drugs to cure infection is another part of cancer therapy, because both the disease and the drugs used to treat it lower resistance, and a large percentage of patients die not from their cancers but from subsequent infections.

Combination therapy The 19-year-old college sophomore had just made his college football team when his leg began to bother him inexplicably. The university medical center discovered a malignant tumor of the right thighbone, the femur. Until the mid-1970s, the diagnosis of *osteosarcoma* would have meant immediate amputation of the entire leg, and only a 17 percent chance of survival. But work was being done at the medical center with a metal (vitalium) "bone" to replace such diseased femurs. One teenage girl had already regained use of her leg following this surgery. In addition, doctors were beginning to boost 1-year disease-free survival rates to over 80 percent with the use of ultrahigh doses of the drug methotrexate, followed by a "chaser" of citrovorum factor. Thus, with cautious optimism, the young athlete was treated with the same one-two punch.

More and more cancer specialists are finding that such combination treatments offer the greatest hope for cancer victims, even for some hard-to-treat lung cancer patients. One scientist likened it to orchestrating a string quartet: Each treatment has its part to play and together they do better than each singly.

Immunotherapy Stimulation of the immune system is being used in many ways, mostly investigationally at the moment, to treat cancer. Because the immune system is most effective against small or early tumors, drugs, surgery, or radiation to reduce the size of the tumor usually precede immunotherapy, which, simply stated, aims at stimulating the cancer patient's immune system to wipe out tumor cells.

Other therapies Cancer is also being treated with heat (used by Hippocrates), cold, cryosurgery, organ and bone marrow transplantation, and manipulation of hormone balances. These treatments are all investigational, but some show promise.

Spontaneous regression Very rarely—fewer than 200 cases are reported in modern medical literature—there is a partial or complete disappearance of a tumor without treatment. Just why and how these regressions take place may hold the clue to cures for some cancers. Many believe the body's immune response may be responsible, but other explanations have also been put forth: hormonal factors; the effects of infection, fever, or medications; the elimination of a carcinogen; even malnutrition in the patient, which may "starve out" the tumor.

Availability of Treatment

Cancer care in the 1970s offers considerable hope of cure or, at least, prolongation of life. Too often, however, this advanced care is not available in local communities, where most cancer patients are treated. Thus, a major federal thrust is to get the latest information

WHERE TO GET HELP

Cancer Information

Contact:

- Local Cancer Care or American Cancer Society Office

Or call:

- California: from area codes 213, 714, and 805: (1-800) 252-9066; rest of state: (213) 226-2374
- Colorado: (1-800) 332-1850
- Connecticut: (1-800) 922-0824
- Delaware and New Jersey: (800) 523-3586
- District of Columbia (including Maryland and northern Virginia suburbs): (202) 232-2833
- Florida: from area code 305: (547) 6920; rest of state: (1-800) 432-5953
- Illinois: from area code 312: 346-9813; rest of state: (800) 972-0586
- Maine: (1-800) 225-7034
- Maryland: (800) 492-1444
- Massachusetts: (1-800) 952-7420
- Minnesota: (1-800) 582-5262
- Montana and Wyoming: (1-800) 525-0231
- New York: from area code 212: 794-7982; from area code 716: 845-4400; rest of state: (1-800) 462-7255
- North Carolina: from area code 919: 286-2266; rest of state (800) 672-0943
- Pennsylvania: (800) 822-3963
- Texas: from area code 713: 792-3245; rest of state: (1-800) 392-2040
- Washington: from area code 206: 284-7263; rest of state: (1-800) 562-2875
- Wisconsin: (800) 362-8038
- Rest of nation: (800) 638-6694

Or write:

- National Cancer Institute, Besthesda, Md 20014
- Roswell Park Memorial Institute, Buffalo, NY 14263, for list of available telephone messages on (800) 462-1884

on cancer treatment and rehabilitation into the hands of community physicians and hospital staffs. This is being done through many avenues, including regional Comprehensive Cancer Centers for research and treatment that will also serve as resources for local physicians and hospitals, and treat many outpatients under the supervision of the family's physician. They will work in conjunction with clinical cancer centers concentrating on such special areas as radiation therapy, and with community cancer centers which, it is hoped, will bring the latest fruits of cancer research to Main Street physicians and their patients.

This complex network will not mean that all cancer patients will be assured treatment at a major cancer center, nor is such treatment always necessary. Local physicians will, however, be able to consult with skilled oncologists, and sophisticated facilities will be available in cases requiring them. Meanwhile, many authorities urge cancer patients to get a second independent opinion (the names of several qualified specialists can be obtained from a nearby university medical center or the American Cancer Society) before beginning treatment, and to encourage their physicians to take advantage of the assistance offered by existing cancer centers and the National Cancer Institute.

Coping with Cancer

Since earliest antiquity, cancer has aroused deep fear in humans. How well we cope with that fear can affect the outcome of the disease. The ability to cope depends on many factors, including the kind of cancer and the chances of cure, age, family situation and support, responsibilities, and personal coping style. Patients who fare best generally have strong inner resources and self-image and confidence in their medical team. Hope is another essential ingredient. It is most often found in self-confident persons who feel they exert some influence on the world around them and are not just puppets of fate. (Scientifically, of course, there is always hope, even if it is slim.)

Most cancer patients respond courageously, even to the most pessimistic diagnosis. After going through rage, envy, resentment, and "Why me?" stages, they begin to adjust, to seek information, to make plans. Often their most serious problems center on employment and finances, and on strained family relations. The pressure on families is often overwhelming, particularly when the patient is a child. These difficulties are discussed further under "Chronic and Catastrophic Illness" in Chapter 12, and in Chapter 13, "Death and Dying."

Cancerphobia Many person's fear cancer irrationally. The editor of the *New England Journal of Medicine*, Dr. F. J. Ingelfinger, has described cancerphobia as a "disease as serious to our society as cancer is to the individual—and morally more devastating." There are, he adds, two ways of dying in the eyes of the American public: "the ordinary and reasonably good way and the bad cancer way."

At first, I couldn't even say the word cancer without feeling very frightened and getting teary. I'd always thought of myself as a healthy person, and shifting from that self-image to being a cancer patient was difficult. . . . But my husband and I talked it over, and we decided it would be best to be open as we could with our eight-year-old son and our friends and relatives. . . .

Many people can't look you in the eye when you say you have cancer. They don't seem to believe what they're constantly hearing from the American Cancer Society—that it can be treated successfully if it's detected early enough. Once they hear the word "cancer," they're ready to dig a hole and bury you.

A young woman with cancer, *Rockland Journal–News*

I gave up. . . . I went to bed to await the inevitable. I even considered suicide as an easy way out. . . . Old friends were uneasy around me, afraid they would say the wrong thing. . . . One young visitor . . . exclaimed, "I've just been dying to meet you," and then she immediately apologized for saying the wrong thing.

At home things became pretty bad. My wife was sleeping in another room, and I discovered later she didn't want me to hear her crying. I spoke little about my problems because I didn't want to worry my family. There was little communication. They were trying to protect me, and I was trying to protect them. It didn't work.

Orville E. Kelly, founder of Make Today Count, a self-help group for cancer patients, p. 9

Cancerphobia can be incapacitating, preventing those who find lumps in their breasts, an enlarged mole, or blood in the urine from seeking help. But the absence of fear of cancer, too, can keep persons from acting. The healthiest response is the feeling of anxiety that takes one to the doctor.

Cancer quackery Irrational fear of cancer impels many victims and their families to turn to unproved medical and nonmedical approaches to treatment: quackery. (The danger of such recourse is discussed fully in Chapter 25.) Quack treatments for cancer run the entire gamut from special diets or foods or vitamin therapy to "psychic surgery" and faith healing. A drug called *krebiozen* was briefly touted as a cure for cancer without any scientific evidence of its effectiveness. The most controversial such treatment today is the use of the drug *laetrile*, also known as amygdalin or vitamin B_{17}, an extract of apricot pits that generates the poison cyanide. A small number of patients claim to have been helped by this extract, which has led to several states legalizing the drug over medical opposition. But repeated animal studies since the mid-1950s by the FDA and reputable independent medical scientists have been unable to show an anticancer benefit for laetrile. There is even some evidence it might be harmful, particularly in oral doses. Because of public pressure and the fact that thousands are using the drug, further FDA investigation is under way.

LOOKING BACK

REVIEWING CONCEPTS IN CHAPTER 10

- Cancer and heart disease develop over many years; preventive steps should begin in childhood and continue for a lifetime.
- The circulatory system consists of the heart, a four-chambered muscle that pumps the blood, and two separate sets of blood vessels—one nourishing the body, the other carrying waste products to the lungs and exchanging them for oxygen.
- High blood pressure affects 20 to 25 million Americans—many of whom are unaware of their disorder, since it is often symptomless. The causes of most cases of HBP are unknown, but factors appear to include high salt intake, heredity, obesity, oral contraceptives, and an inability to cope with stress.
- Stroke—a cerebral vascular accident which can be disabling and even fatal—has been related to a variety of factors, including HBP. Control of these may prevent stroke.
- Atherosclerosis—a form of hardening of the arteries—develops silently over a period of many years. It is a major cause of myocardial infarction or "heart attack." Control, where possible, of factors associated with atherosclerosis—heredity, high serum lipids, obesity, lack of exercise, HBP, smoking, diabetes—may reduce the risk of heart attack.
- Heart attack need not be the end of the line; new techniques can rehabilitate many cardiac patients. Many heart problems can now be dealt with by surgery, medication, and other treatments.

- "Cancer" is a name for at least 100 different diseases, which have in common abnormal, uncontrolled cell growth.
- Causes of cancer may be as various as its types. Risk factors probably include environmental elements (tobacco, alcohol, radiation, chemicals, diet, sunlight); hormone imbalance; and viruses (proved in animals, not in humans).
- Though cancer is a relentless adversary, many varieties can be prevented through intelligent personal decision making. Early detection—through self-examination, screening, and awareness of warning signs—can greatly increase chances of survival. All too often, however, the fear of finding out for certain that one has cancer prevents early treatment.
- Today 2 of 6 cancer patients are cured; with the best current care, 3 of 6 could be cured. Major treatment strategies are surgery, chemotherapy, radiation therapy, combinations of these, and more recently, immunotherapy.
- Coping with cancer can be traumatic for a family, but, with help, patients often bear up well. Cancer patients often become victims of charlatans and cancer quacks.

11

TRAUMA: A MODERN PLAGUE

WHAT'S AHEAD IN CHAPTER 11 What factors generally contribute to accidents? Why is it important to reduce the number of accidents that take place daily? Besides reducing accidents, how else can we decrease the number of severe injuries and the deaths that result from them? What role can personal and community decision making play in these efforts? How can a home be made safer for those who live in it? What basic rules lead to increased safety in sports and games? What are the routes to increasing safety on the road, in automobiles, and on bicycles, motorcycles, mopeds, and skateboards, as well as for the pedestrian? How does the quality of emergency care affect the chances of survival following an accident? How can emergency care be improved in a community? How can you contribute to improved emergency care?

- A middle-aged woman, upset because her husband stormed out of the house after a fight, is chain-smoking. The phone in the next room rings. Dropping her cigarette butt hurriedly into the wastebasket, she goes to answer the phone. By the time she returns, the basket is aflame, the room full of smoke.

- Two friends are about to drive home from a party on a rainy night. One insists upon taking the wheel, though his companion argues he has had too much to drink. They arrive at a dark intersection at the same moment as an elderly pedestrian. The driver doesn't see the old man in the dark coat until the instant of impact.

- A couple of students mount their bikes to do some shopping in town. As they approach a heavily trafficked corner, one of them, riding a bike she had picked up for $5 at a garage sale, cries: "Oh, my God, the brakes aren't holding!" She slams into the side of a moving car.

Each of these events resulted in injury, called "trauma" by physicians. On the basis of these accidents, and of others with which you may be familiar, would you consider accidents to be: unavoidable? the result of chance or bad luck? uncontrollable? unpredictable? the aftermath of carelessness? no one's fault? the fault of the injured person? How is personal decision making involved?

The why and how of accidents is of particular importance to college students, for trauma is the leading cause of death from ages 1 to 38. It ranks fourth, trailing only cancer, heart disease, and diabetes, as a cause of death in the general population. In addition, some 60 million or more Americans are injured severely enough each year to seek medical aid or to restrict their activities one day or more. The financial cost of trauma, fatal and nonfatal, is staggering. But as you will see, a large proportion of these injuries can be prevented by both personal and community decision making.

TABLE 11.1 Accident fatalities in the United States, 1977

Public accidents:	22,000
Drowning	4,600
Falls	4,800
Firearms	700
Fires; burns, fire-associated	900
Water transport	1,100
Railroad	400
Air transport	1,200
Other transport	200
All other public	8,100
Home accidents*	24,000
Motor vehicle accidents	49,500
Accidents at work	13,000

*A breakdown of home accidents can be found in Table 11.2

Source: National Safety Council.

CAUSES OF INJURY OR TRAUMA

On the surface, there appears to be little relationship between disease and injury. Yet on closer examination, there is a strong similarity. Injury, like disease, involves a combination of factors, including the following.

A Susceptible Host

Accidents and the ordinary person We are all susceptible to accident sometimes, and most accidents occur to ordinary persons caught up in a web of circumstances leading to ultimate entrapment. Mental and physical condition—fatigue, anger, worry, tension, fear, illness, use of drugs (medications as well as alcohol or marijuana)—all make us more susceptible to accident. Lack of strength or size or physical disabilities are less likely to. Disabled persons are particularly careful when working or driving and thus have fewer accidents than able-bodied young males, who tend to be overconfident and less cautious.

Values also influence our susceptibility. Do we choose a flashy little car with lots of chrome over a more sedate but safer model? Or 7-inch platform heels for fashion's sake, though they may lead to leg injury? Do we take "one more drink" before driving home? Or choose pretty but fire-hazardous curtains to hang near the gas range?

Accident repeaters A small proportion of the population always seems to "be getting into accidents." They often exhibit certain traits in common:

- *Behavior patterns* that include lack of adequate preparation for the task assigned, tendency to use tools incorrectly, unsanitary practices, unsafe practices, failure to follow directions (Guilford).

- *Attitudes* such as impulsiveness, desire for immediate pleasures, resentment toward authority, insecurity and poor self-image, a need for attention, feelings of rejection, overconfidence leading to inattention to safety rules, and the need to vent aggressiveness in the form of reckless behavior.

Accident repeaters also exhibit a need to punish themselves or others or to escape from problems or responsibilities. It is said that when one of Freud's children suffered a cut or bruise and went to him for sympathy, Dr. Freud would ask, "Why did you do it?" If Freud was correct, many accidents are subconsciously intentional.

Also prominent in accident repeaters is a conflict between a conscious desire to be brave and grown-up and a repressed desire to remain a baby. Such an individual jumps over the widest ditch to prove courage, then slips on the edge as the deep desire to be dependent surges up. Another major factor is the need for risk taking, either to prove oneself, or as a response to the popular notion that taking risks is admirable. This notion was realistic in pioneer days, but today few persons have the opportunity to take risks either on the job or in the course of everyday living. Thus, many people, especially males who cling to the concept of machismo, seek thrills in activities like motorcycling, hunting, skydiving, snowmobiling, or fast and reckless automobile driving (Klein).

The Causative Agent

A paring knife, the windshield of your own car, the bumper of someone else's, the blade of a power mower, a flight of stairs, a brick wall, a body of water, a sheet of flames, and an almost infinite list of other objects can cause injury when brought into contact with the susceptible host.

The Mode of Transmission: Bringing Host and Agent Together

An accident, sometimes an intentional act, brings host and agent together. Your car hits the one in front of you, and you are thrown into the windshield; your foot tangles in a line on the sailboat's deck and you tumble into the bay; the knife slips as you try to cut a frozen English muffin, and sharp knife meets finger.

Consumer Product Safety Commission's "Public Enemy" List

- Bicycles and equipment
- Stairs
- Football activity, equipment
- Baseball activity, equipment
- Swings, slides, playground equipment
- Nonglass tables
- Swimming pools
- Beds
- Liquid fuels, kindling
- Nails, tacks, screws
- Basketball activity and equipment
- Chairs, sofas, sofa beds
- Bleaches and dyes, cleaning agents
- Architectural glass (including doors)
- Floors and flooring material
- Cooking ranges, ovens
- Power lawn mowers
- Skates, skateboards, scooters
- Furnaces and floor furnaces
- Bathtubs, nonglass shower enclosures

*Derived from estimated number of injuries treated in emergency rooms for product category and the severity of these injuries. *Source*: U.S. Consumer Product Safety Commission.

HEALTH CONSUMER TIP

Reporting a Product Hazard

Individual consumers play an important role in the detection and eventual elimination of hazardous products when they report such hazards as well as product-related injuries. Reports should be made to the U.S. Consumer Product Safety Commission. Call the toll-free hotline 800-638-2666 (800-492-2937 for Maryland residents only) or write to the CPSC, Washington, DC 20207. The consumer can also, individually or as part of a group, become involved in the development of standards for a particular manufactured product by submitting suggestions according to the CPSC regulations to the Commission. Petitions asking for changes in safety standards must be written in English (preferably typewritten); include the name, address, and telephone number of the petitioner; indicate the product involved; and request a specific rule change. All possible information and documentation should be provided. The heading should specify the petition is filed under Section 10 of the Consumer Product Safety Act. Five copies are preferred.

Environmental Factors

Environmental conditions may well decide whether or not an accident will actually occur. Is it rainy and slippery? Is it dark? Is it so cold that gloveless hands are numb? Are the road signs snow-covered? Is the gas range designed so you have to reach over the flame to turn it off? Is the top rung of the ladder cracked? Are safety rules ignored on the job? Is lead paint peeling from the walls and ceilings in a room in your home?

PREVENTING ACCIDENTS AND REDUCING OR MINIMIZING INJURY

Whose Responsibility?

Personal behavior and decision making play an important role in accident prevention. But many accidents are beyond individual control. Susan Baker, public health and safety authority, points out:

> A driver may keep his car in good repair, wear safety belts, and keep his eyes on the road; but the limits to his field of vision, the blowout of a new tire, the blind curve without a guardrail, the glass window beside his face, and the inadequate emergency room are all outside his control. Effective action against many elements in the injury-producing sequence may come only through public intervention. (p. 4)

The precedent for such intervention has been set for many years. For example, milk pasteurization and immunization to prevent the spread of infection are regulated by law. Public intervention has been on the rise in accident prevention, too. The Consumer Product Safety Commission, established in 1972, sets safety standards for manufactured products ranging from bicycles to baby cribs and from TV sets to radar ranges. Federal legislation sets standards for automobile safety and a variety of other products. Local communities develop building codes so that homes, schools, and public places will be safe. OSHA (Occupational Safety and Health Administration) and NIOSH (National Institute of Occupational Safety and Health) are directed to improve the health and safety of workers in all kinds of jobs. The Department of Transportation has begun to show increased interest in the safety of roads and highways. But the job of creating a safe environment has only just begun.

Ladder Safety Rules

- When you prop a ladder against a wall, always make sure the distance from the wall to the base of the ladder is at least one-quarter the height of the ladder.
- Never place a ladder on a slippery surface.
- Do *not* stand on the top rung of a ladder.
- Do *not* lean away from a ladder you are standing on.
- Totally destroy a damaged ladder, so that it can never be used again.

Even with the best efforts of individuals and community, we will not totally eliminate accidents. That is because safety is not our only priority. Human beings also seek pleasure and progress, and these require taking some risks that may lead to accident and injury. Trying to eliminate *all* risks is actually an impossible task and could be considered pathological, or sick. But we can reduce risk and still enjoy the benefits we seek.

Injury can be prevented or minimized on three levels: (1) *prevention of the accident* that causes injury; (2) *reduction of risk of injury* if the accident cannot be prevented (wearing automobile seat belts and shoulder harnesses, for example); and (3) *provision of immediate and high-quality care and treatment*, so minor injuries will not become major ones.

Accident and Injury at Home

Home—crowded urban tenement, isolated farmhouse, suburban split-level, college dorm, or off-campus apartment—is the site of some 25,000 accidental deaths and approximately 20 million injuries, 110,000 of which are disabling, annually.

It might be said that there is no place like home for accidents. But it might also be said that there is no other place where intelligent decision making can have a greater impact on health and safety. For those interested in improving the odds against accident and injury where they live, Table 11.2 should be helpful. Provisions for children and the elderly, the people most likely to suffer accident trauma, merit special attention.

Injury from Fire

If you live in a college dorm or rooming house, learn the fire regulations, and check with people in charge if they seem inadequate. If you live in an apartment or house, you can protect your life by making the improvements shown in Table 11.2.

Wherever you live, have a planned-in-advance escape route, in case the usual exists are blocked by fire. You can often

Smoke Detector Checklist

- Is your smoke detector approved by a national testing lab?
- Are batteries included? How long will they last? How much will replacement batteries cost? Are they readily available?
- Is there a warning signal to tell you when batteries need replacing?
- Is there a testing switch? Or can the smoke detector be tested by blowing smoke into it?

TABLE 11.2 Home accidents and their prevention

ACCIDENT STATISTICS (1977)	PREVENTION
	FALLS
Deaths: 7500 Most susceptible age group: over 75	Use skid-resistant mats or stripping in tubs and showers. Install sturdy grab bars in tubs and showers. Wipe up spills on floors immediately. Don't string wires and cords across rooms. Have lamps within reach of each bed. Have stairs and halls well lighted. Use night lights for kids and elderly people. Be sure small rugs have skidproof bottoms. Don't put small rugs at top or bottom of stairs. Have handrails on stairs; keep stairs clear of junk and in good repair. Use ladders, not chairs, for climbing. (See the ladder safety rules on page 266.) Clear outdoor walks and steps of snow and ice. Avoid overwaxing floors. Don't wear sloppy slippers, high platforms and heels, or thongs that can snag. Don't walk in stockings on smooth floors. Don't leave toys, skates, etc., around on the floor.
	FIRE-RELATED INJURIES (BURNS, OTHERS)
Deaths: 5200 Most susceptible age groups: under 4; over 65, esp. over 75	Be sure home wiring is properly installed and in good condition; same for all appliances and equipment Use all equipment according to directions. Buy only UL-approved electrical appliances. Buy only AGA-approved gas appliances. Replace damaged or frayed electric cords. Enforce a no-smoking rule, or use large, deep ashtrays. Don't empty ashtrays before going to bed; never empty them into wastebaskets. Don't permit smoking in bed. Check for smoldering butts after parties. Don't leave space heaters unwatched or near flammables (things that burn). Don't allow "kindling" (paper, etc.) or flammables (oily or paint-soaked rags) to collect; they feed fires. Have escape routes from bedrooms; practice using them. Have on hand a homemade knotted, heavy rope ladder, or a purchased escape ladder. Install UL-approved smoke and heat detectors. (See the smoke detector checklist on page 266.) Have UL-approved fire extinguishers on hand. (The all-purpose type is best.) Avoid wearing loose, floppy clothes near a stove or fireplace.

TABLE 11.2 *(Continued)*

ACCIDENT STATISTICS (1977)	PREVENTION
	POISONING FROM SOLIDS OR LIQUIDS
Deaths: 3000 Most susceptible age groups: 15–24, over 65 Causes: internal medicines, cleaning agents, commercial products, pet products, plants, insecticides, cosmetics, external medicines, lead-based paints, newspaper (colored)	Keep medicines locked up, out of reach of children. (See the special safety rules for homes with small children on page 271.) Don't take medicines in the dark; read labels. Keep original labels. Don't tell children medicine is "candy." Keep poisons, cleaning fluids, aerosols, etc., out of reach of children and in well-marked containers (never use soft-drink bottles or others that might confuse children or adults). Use medications only according to directions (see Chap. 14).
	POISONING FROM GASES OR VAPORS
Deaths: 1000 Most susceptible age group: over 75 Causes: carbon monoxide from stoves, heaters, cars; cleaning products; aerosols	Don't run car motor in garage with the door closed; or for more than a minute or two even with the door open. Don't use spray paints, cleaning fluids, etc., in closed areas without ventilation. Don't mix cleaning products, e.g., chlorine and ammonia, chlorine and toilet bowl cleaner. Don't inhale (or allow children to inhale) spray from aerosols of any kind. Be sure stoves and heaters are properly exhausted to keep fumes out of the house.
	LACERATIONS, CUTS
Data on deaths and age groups not available; most such accidents not fatal Causes: knives, glass doors, power saws, power mowers	Keep knives sharp (less risk of injury). Use the proper knife for each job. Store knives properly, out of reach of children. Use a cutting board; cut away from yourself. Don't use knives to open jars or separate frozen hamburger patties. Use bright decals on sliding glass doors. Glass doors should be of safety glass. Follow directions in using power tools. Don't touch blades of power tools unless disconnected. Don't remove safety guides. Don't point a power mower ejection chute at anyone. Don't let children use tools without supervision.
	SUFFOCATION FROM INGESTED OBJECTS
Deaths: 1800 Most susceptible age groups: over 75, under 4	Always cut meats, etc., into small bites (see Fig. 11.7). Keep small, swallowable objects away from young children; cut up their food.

ACCIDENT STATISTICS (1977)	PREVENTION
	MECHANICAL SUFFOCATION
Deaths: 900 Most susceptible age group: under 4 Causes: bedclothes, thin plastics, confinement in closed space such as refrigerators, cave-ins, strangulation	Never allow small children to play with plastic materials. Avoid drawstring nightclothes. Remove doors before discarding refrigerators. Keep children barred from construction sites.
	FIREARM ACCIDENTS
Deaths: 1200 Most susceptible age group: 15–24	Never leave firearms where children can get at them. No one should handle firearms without knowing all safety rules.
	DROWNING
Deaths: 800 Most susceptible age group: under 4	Never leave a young child or disabled adult in a tub alone. Never leave a young child near a swimming pool or other body of water alone. Learn water safety rules, apply them, and teach them to others.
	ALL OTHERS (2600 DEATHS IN 1977)
Electric current	Don't touch or use electrical devices of any kind (hair dryers, lights, radios, etc.) when wet or standing in water. When using tools or appliances with grounded plugs, never remove the third prong. Don't use electrical appliances that make odd noises, give little shocks, or don't work properly. Never insert a knife in a plugged-in toaster. Don't pull the plug when an appliance is turned on. Use only "outdoor" lighting outdoors.
Explosives	Explosives should be handled only by experienced, trained persons. Don't touch suspicious items; call police. Don't use firecrackers, etc.
Blows by falling objects	Don't leave anything on a windowsill that might fall and injure someone below.

determine whether they are blocked by putting your hand against your bedroom door (which should always be closed when you sleep). If it is hot, or if smoke is seeping under it, there is fire on the other side. Keep close to the floor as you move toward a window or another escape route, with a piece of cloth over your mouth and nose. (Poisonous gases that kill most fire victims rise, and the lowest concentration is near the floor).

Injury at Play

The benefit side of the recreational activities scale is crowded: healthful exercise, relaxation, challenge, and just plain fun. Professional sports adds another: financial gain. The risk side varies depending on the activity. About 3200 people die in swimming accidents each year, but only a handful from jogging. Football, with 120,000 injuries and 20 deaths

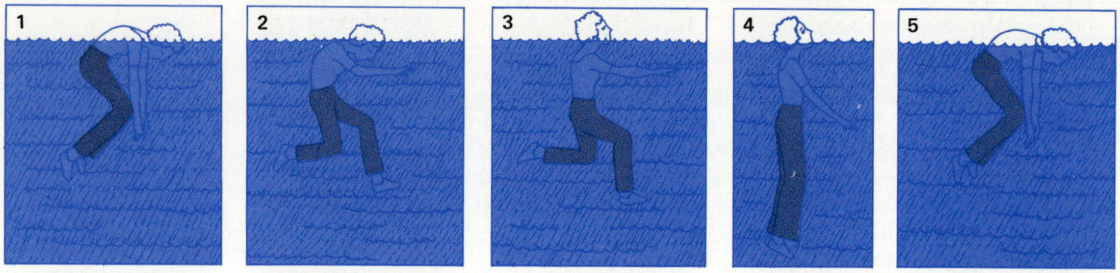

Resting position | Preparing to exhale | Exhaling | Inhaling | Return to the resting position

FIGURE 11.1 Drownproofing: a simple technique that can save your life. Half of all drowning victims *never intended to enter the water*; they fell into it from docks, bridges, boats, or the shore. If instead of panicking they had used the lifesaving technique called *drownproofing*, their chances of survival would have been greatly increased.

Drownproofing combines rhythmic breathing with floating, and it requires so little motion that it can be done for hours without fatigue. (It was originally designed for the survival of downed pilots during World War II.) Clothing need not be removed; it adds buoyancy and helps conserve body heat.

No matter what your size, shape, or swimming ability, you can learn drownproofing. Practice the five steps in the water, preferably with the supervision of an expert and *never* alone, until you know them by heart.

1 Hold your breath and relax forward into the water. Let your arms and legs dangle, and keep your face down so that only the back of your head and neck are above the surface. Relax and float in this position until you begin to feel the need to take a breath. (If you are afraid to put your face in the water, practice in a shallow place until you are used to it. You will be less disoriented if you keep your eyes open under water; this, too, comes with practice.)

2 Slowly raise your arms to shoulder height and let your legs drop down, all the while keeping your face in the water and the back of your head and neck above the surface, as in the resting position. If you feel yourself beginning to sink, gently kick your legs or press your arms downward. All movements should be slow and deliberate because vigorous activity hastens the loss of precious body heat.

3 Make sure the back of your head is still at the surface of the water; then exhale through your mouth and nose into the water while slowly raising your head. (You can also exhale through the mouth only or nose only.) Your eyes should be open so you can orient your head and body to the water level. Water in your eyes may cause discomfort, but do not try to wipe them as this will only waste energy.

4 As soon as your head is vertical, press your arms downward and your legs together gently. You will rise just enough to take a breath through your mouth, but not so high that your chin is out of the water.

5 Slowly relax forward again, arms and legs dangling, face in the water. Start the breathing cycle over when needed.

Special Safety Rules for Homes with Small Children

- Block off all stairways.
- Keep dangerous, breakable, swallowable items and plastic bags or materials out of reach.
- Use nontoxic paints on furniture, toys, etc.
- Buy safe, washable toys with no swallowable pieces.
- Never leave a young child alone at home or near water or a trafficked road.

each year, claims the greatest numerical toll in competitive sports. But exotic sports like hang gliding are proportionately more hazardous.

A decision to take up a particular recreational activity involves weighing the risks against the benefits. But it should be recognized that the risks are often less serious than they appear from the statistics, because those who most often make the casualty lists have ignored elementary safety precautions that can lower risk considerably.[1]

1 Have a medical checkup before beginning a program of strenuous or competitive activities.
2 Keep in good physical condition, warm up before strenuous activities, and cool down afterward.
3 Learn how to play the game or participate properly, and take lessons if necessary.
4 Use appropriate protective gear when needed, such as life jackets on boats, helmets for motorcycling or horseback riding.
5 Use good equipment and keep it in good condition.
6 Know your limitations; for example, don't go out on a ski slope beyond your skills or wrestle someone who outweighs you heavily.
7 Follow safety rules for the particular activity.
8 Use the "buddy system" where being alone can be a hazard, as in swimming, or in skating on a frozen pond.
9 Be a good sport, for an angry player is more likely to be injured.
10 Quit when you are tired or feeling pain.
11 Stay away from potentially hazardous activities when not in top physical or mental form.
12 Allow for your own mistakes and those of others, and be prepared for them.
13 Have first-aid equipment on hand and know how to use it for the kinds of accidents most likely to occur.

[1]Many of these same rules apply to the hobbyist or do-it-yourselfer, too.

Caution: In cold water (below 70°F) the drownproofing method is not recommended because too much heat will be lost through the head. Unconsciousness can result. For safety, whenever you are near deep water, wear a life jacket. [*From* Good Housekeeping, *May 1978.*]

Good swimmers drown, too! In fact, a large percentage of all drowning victims are teenaged males either showing off or testing their endurance (Modell). The practice of taking extremely fast, deep breaths (hyperventilating) before swimming underwater in order to increase distance has led to the drowning deaths of many strong swimmers. The practice is dangerous and should be avoided.

TABLE 11.3 Out-of-doors safety tips

SOURCE OF INJURY	PREVENTION*
Poison ivy, oak, sumac rash	Avoid contact with plants, even if you have never had a reaction before. Wash site of contact immediately for 5 to 10 minutes; change and wash clothing.
Lightning (burns, electrocution)	During electric storms, avoid standing in open field, or under trees or other tall objects; stay out of water; find shelter indoors or in car if possible.
Insects (bites that may carry disease, stings that cause allergic response)	Use insect repellents and screening. Keep arms and legs covered; use hat with netting when needed. Check for ticks after a day in the woods.† Carry antidote supplies if you are allergic to insect stings or bites.
Wild animals (bites, disease)	Avoid even if friendly; they can be dangerous and may carry disease.
Snakes (bites)	Know which are poisonous; wear boots; avoid snake-infested areas.
Fire (burns, forest fires)	When camping, smoke only at rest stops, using a hole dug in ground as ashtray; crush out and bury all cigarettes when finished. Build fires only on level ground, sheltered from high wind and away from burnables such as brush or tents. Clear a circle 10 feet in diameter; build a small fire in the center. Never leave fires unattended; always put fires out before retiring. Put fires out with water, stir, drown again.

*See Table 11.4 for emergency treatment procedures.
†Ticks spread disease. Do not touch them with bare hands. Do not try to pull them off the skin, for you may leave the head with its toxic juices still attached. Instead, force the tick to let go by covering it with alcohol, nail polish, grease, petroleum jelly, or gasoline, or by very carefully holding a lighted match near it. Then gingerly lift it off with tweezers. After removal, wash the area with soap and water.

14 Care for minor injuries before they become major ones.

Injury Out-of-doors

The outdoors is exhilarating, but it, too, has its hazards—even, as can be seen in Table 11.3, in one's own backyard. There are added hazards for the more than 40 million Americans who annually venture into the wilderness as campers, hikers, and backpackers. Most outdoor injuries can be prevented, however, by making adequate plans and preparations, having experienced leaders, wearing appropriate clothing and shoes, carrying adequate equipment and supplies (especially for emergencies), paying attention to water purity, and heeding fire safety rules. Successful campers take the limits of the weakest camper in the group into consideration. They check with forest rangers or other authorities before entering an area, and tell someone back home their expected route and estimated time of return.

When experienced campers lose their way, they do not panic. Instead they determine whether to stay put or push on. Usually, they will make camp if one of the party is injured or near exhaustion, if the terrain is rugged, if night is falling or the weather is bad, if shelter is available, or if they know someone will be looking for them. Otherwise they will push on, trying to find the trail by climbing to a high point with an overview of the area. Or they will follow a drainage ditch or other running water downstream, which usually leads to civilization.

Automobile Accidents

While 4204 of our young men were dying in Vietnam in 1970, another 17,360 Americans

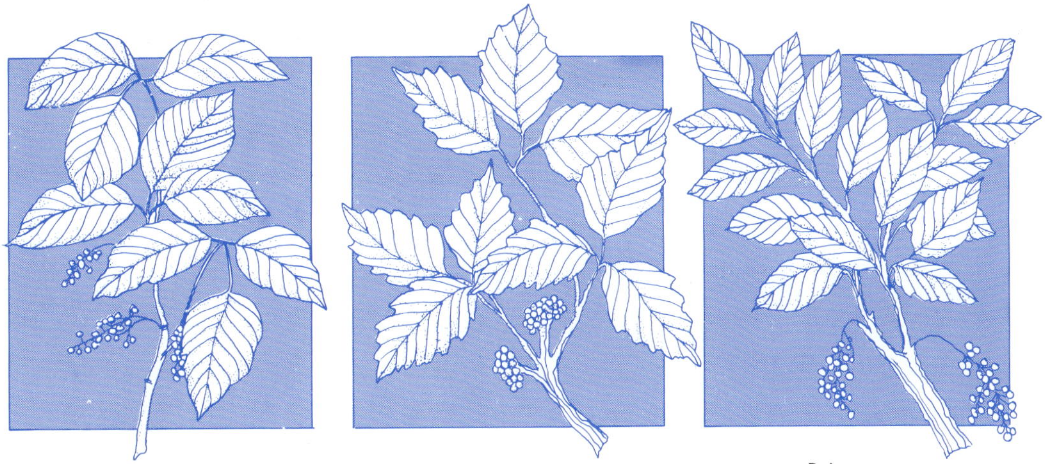

FIGURE 11.2 Poison ivy and its cousin poison oak are found almost everywhere in the United States and Canada, in backyards as well as wooded areas. Poison ivy can grow as a vine or as a shrub. Its leaves, grouped in threes and varying from smooth-edged to randomly notched, are shiny green in summer, red in fall; its berries are greenish white. The leaves of poison oak are also grouped in threes but are shaped more like oak leaves; the plant is more shrublike. Poison sumac is less common, is found mostly in wooded areas, and can be distinguished from ordinary sumac by its drooping green berries. The sticky sap of these plants can be transmitted directly or by clothing or other persons or animals who have touched it.

between 15 and 25 were dying on our streets and roads. Yet there were no marches, no sit-ins, no picketing of GM, Ford, or the Department of Transportation to protest the highway deaths. Road deaths seem to be viewed as inevitable. Yet they can often be prevented by conscious decisions of the driver, the automobile manufacturer, and the community about the factors that lead to car accidents.

The driver's condition Many accidents involve persons who are ill or who have taken drugs—legal or illegal, but especially alcohol and, increasingly, marijuana—as well as those with chronic illness, or the deterioration of reflexes and vision that comes with aging. Distractions of all kinds, from emotional upset to lighting a cigarette, turning on the radio, or kissing your passenger, can cause accidents.

Fatigue can also cause accidents. The driver who begins a long drive after a week of cramming for exams, or after heavy eating or drinking, may be en route to disaster. Stopping for 10 minutes every 2 hours, opening the window to admit cold air, listening to a lively radio show (not soft music), playing word games (even with yourself), singing, talking, and munching on pretzels or nuts can all help a driver to fight fatigue. When these measures do not work, the driver should get off the road as soon as possible. Light food, a coke or coffee, a short nap, and a short jog are refreshing. But nothing helps like a good night's sleep.

Miriam Reinhart/Photo Researchers

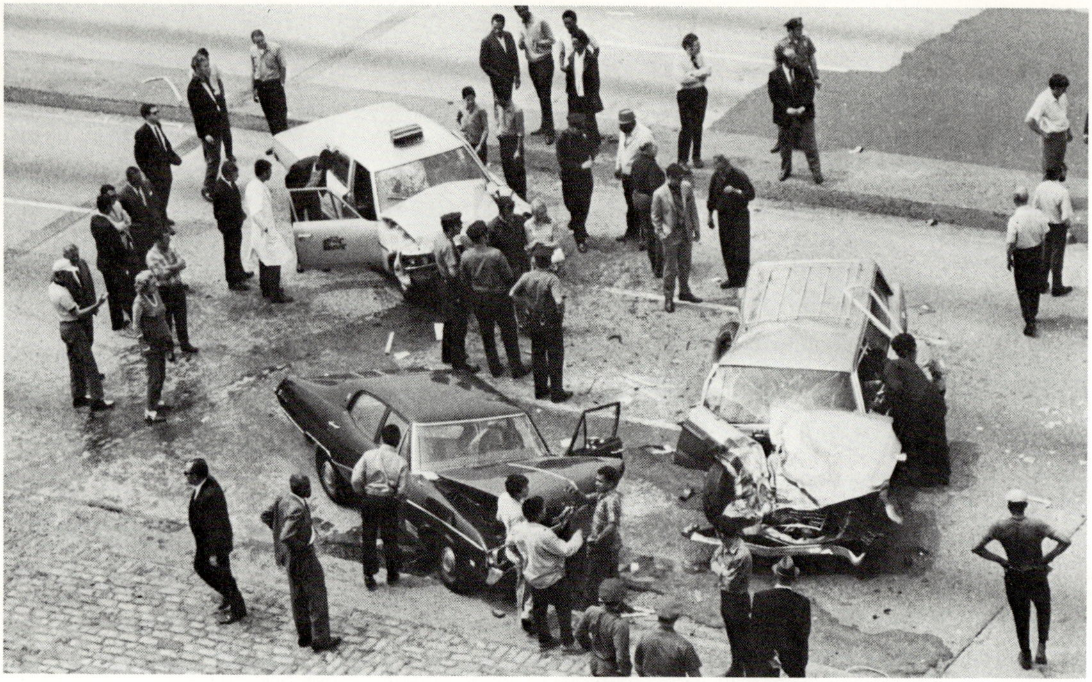

Among the factors involved in an accident are the driver's mental and physical condition, drug use, behavior patterns, and attitudes and values, and the environment.

Driver training, experience, and behavior Characteristics common to those frequently involved in motor vehicle accidents include inexperience, speeding, failure to signal, and failure to drive defensively. Becoming a good driver takes plenty of practice, but getting that practice is risky. Accident rates for new drivers are unusually high. Better driver training that offers experience in simulated emergency situations could reduce accident rates for new drivers.

Automobile condition Every driver, male or female, who is interested in safety needs to

You Don't Have to be Smashed to Smash Up

Bob Bondurant, a winner of the Riverside Grand Prix, and several other expert drivers participated in a study of the effects of even small amounts of alcohol on driving. In every test run, driving performance on the precision course deteriorated after drinking.

"I was surprised," said Bondurant. "I thought I was doing a good job." But his driving score dropped from 1.39 while sober to 2.18 after drinking—although he was not legally "drunk." A woman driver's score dropped from 1.58 to 2.10 after 2 ounces of alcohol raised her blood level to only 0.02 (0.10 is the legal intoxication level in most states).

learn what makes a car run, and how to keep it in good shape. State inspection cannot be relied on to do the job. In one Southern state, a driver died in a car state police termed a "coffin on wheels"; 10 days earlier, an inspector had pasted a "passed inspection" sticker on the car's windshield.

Even careful car owners and mechanics often overlook exhaust problems. When a tailpipe is too short (sometimes because the end has rusted off), odorless, invisible, deadly carbon monoxide is vented *under* the car and may infiltrate it through cracks. Unconsciousness, even death, can occur even before symptoms are felt. Anyone experiencing sudden dizziness, nausea, headache, or blurred vision while driving should open the windows wide, pull off the road at the first opportunity, get out, and breathe in fresh air. The exhaust system should then be thoroughly checked.

Automobile design There is no doubt that the American ingenuity that built a fail-safe space vehicle could build the perfect safety car that would take into account both preventing accidents (better brakes, better visibility, quicker response) and protecting the occupants in case accident does occur (seat belts, padded dashboards, hydraulic bumpers, effective air bags,[2] etc.). Indeed, several prototypes have been designed, including the Liberty Mutual Survival Car II. But car manufacturers, insisting that "safety doesn't sell" and declaring such cars to be prohibitively expensive, crash head-on into consumerists like Ralph Nader, who assert that a safe car can be built at an affordable cost. Because of lack of pressure from the public, there has been little effort to move forward.

Road design Dangerous curves and turns, poor visibility, slippery surface or confusing signs, even monotonous straight-and-level turnpikes increase the risk of accidents.

[2]Air bags, unlike seat belts, require no action on the part of car occupants, but their effectiveness has not been completely proved.

Driving environment Ruts and potholes, poor lighting, construction barriers without adequate warning, overcrowding, ice or snow cover, and pouring rain compound hazard.

Other Road Accidents

Safety on two wheels The number of two-wheeled vehicles on the road has increased immensely in the past decade. Motorcycles have grown in popularity because they offer low-cost transportation, low fuel consumption, easy maneuvering and parking, and excitement and thrills. Bicycles, which in several recent years outsold automobiles, are attractive, too. They do not pollute, offer excellent exercise, are the easiest way to travel short distances (5 to 8 miles) in cities, do not use fuel, and are a good way to use growing leisure time. Most recently, mopeds, or motorized bicycles, offering some of the benefits of both motorcycles and bicycles, have become popular.

Two-wheeled vehicles offer benefits, but they offer the riskiest form of popular transport as well. Reducing the high rates of injury and death from the use of these vehicles will require an alteration of rider habits, vehicle design, and riding environment.

- *The safe bike* Seventeen percent of bicycle accidents are the result of mechanical or structural failure. Figure 11.3 suggests what to look for when buying a bicycle and how to maintain it for maximum safety.
- *The safe biker* Most bike accidents are due to error of either the cyclist or the driver of another vehicle. Cyclists and moped riders can avoid such accidents by: (1) observing all traffic laws and signals; (2) riding near the curb in the same direction as traffic; (3) riding in less trafficked areas; (4) walking across busy intersections; (5) avoiding riding double or stunting; (6) using extra caution at driveways; (7) wearing helmets, especially on mopeds; (8)

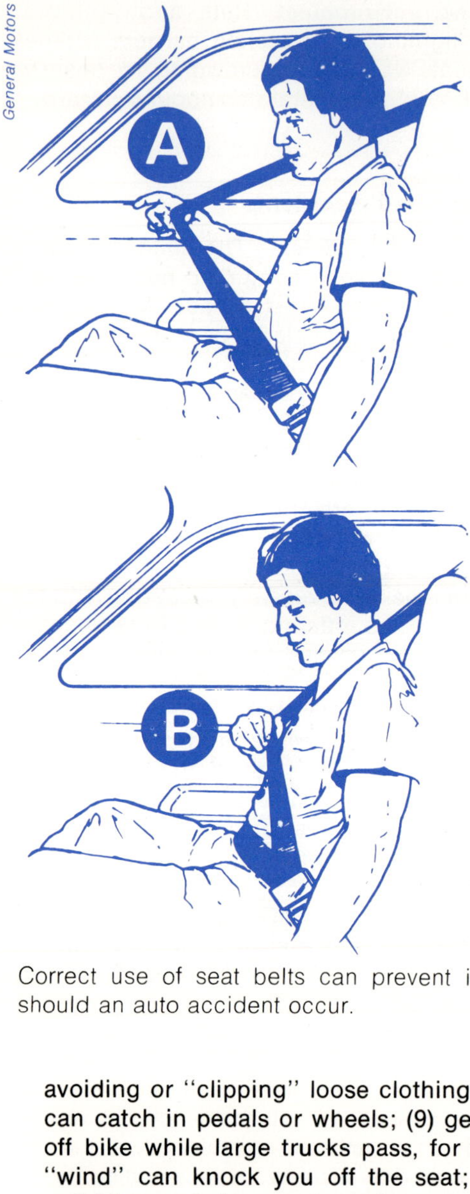

Correct use of seat belts can prevent injury should an auto accident occur.

avoiding or "clipping" loose clothing that can catch in pedals or wheels; (9) getting off bike while large trucks pass, for their "wind" can knock you off the seat; (10) watching out for sewer grates or other obstructions; (11) using retroreflective trim on clothing, or special flashlights strapped to legs and arms at night.

- *The safe bikeway* Bicycle paths are still the exception in the United States, but federal and local efforts have been aimed at improving and increasing bikeways. Bikers can help their cause by reporting potholes and other hazards to local highway authorities and by pressuring legislators to provide additional bikeway funds.

Motorcycle safety The National Safety Council considers the growing number of motorcycle accidents an "epidemic." The reasons are many: (1) Though the National Highway Safety Bureau requires states to set up motorcycle safety programs that include examination and licensing of operators, mandatory safety helmets and eye protection, inspection, and rearview mirrors, many do not adhere to such standards. (2) Because the motorcycle is seen by many as a plaything rather than the high-powered vehicle it is, many riders receive no instruction in its operation. (3) Some riders fail to adhere to traffic laws. (4) It is difficult for car or truck drivers to see a motorcycle coming up from the right rear. (5) The motorcycle is unstable, making a pebble a lethal, tumble-causing agent. (6) Risk of injury is high because drivers and passengers are not enclosed; the risk is even greater when protective gear is not worn.

Safety on two feet Pedestrian fatalities account for 1 of every 5 highway deaths, with children the most frequent victims. This toll can be reduced by cooperative efforts of parents (setting good examples, supervising young children, and teaching safety rules), drivers (who can be alert for small children), the community (which can provide supervised recreational areas to keep children off the streets, and lights or crossing guards at perilous intersections), and vehicle designers and manufacturers (who can design cars without sharp chrome ornaments and bumpers that increase injury). Similar efforts, including provision of safer and better-lighted walking and jogging paths, will help protect all pedestrians.

Hitchhiking It's cheap. It's convenient. It's interesting. It's ecologically sound. It can also

Why Some People Don't Buckle Up

- "The belts will trap me if my car starts to burn or ends up in the water somewhere." Fewer than 0.5 percent of all accidents involve fire or submersion in water. Even in those cases a belt is an asset, because it is likely to keep you from being knocked unconscious, making escape possible. Unbuckling tákes no more than a fraction of a second.
- "I'd rather be thrown clear of an accident than be stuck in the car." Then you will increase your risk of death 9 times. Between 5000 and 6000 persons each year die as a result of being thrown from an auto during a collision.
- "When I buckle up, I'm saying that I expect to have an accident, that I'm not, or the person I'm with is not, a good driver." Studies show that good drivers are more likely to buckle up than poorer ones. Putting a belt on says, "I take my driving seriously, but I realize there are others who don't." Like insurance, it is used "just in case."
- "Seat belts can cause injuries." True. In some very violent accidents, they have been known to cause bone bruises or internal injuries. In most cases this is because the belt was not worn correctly. It is also true that in almost every instance, the injuries were less severe than the injuries that would have occurred without belts.
- "I don't need the belt when driving slowly near home." The National Safety Council reports that more than half of all automobile deaths and two-thirds of injuries occur at speeds of 30 mph or less. Death can even occur at 12 mph. In addition, a majority of car accidents occur within 25 miles of home.
- "Maybe they save lives; but they are restrictive and uncomfortable." They *are* restrictive, to keep auto occupants from hurtling against dangerous surfaces such as windshields and steering wheels. But they also reduce driver fatigue and eliminate the necessity to brake on every sharp turn. Regular wearers swear they are uncomfortable *without* belts.
- "They might restrict the driver trying to avoid an accident." Trying to avoid an accident usually means staying behind the wheel and maintaining control of the auto. This is easiest when wearing a seat belt. For example: You are sideswiped by another car and knocked out of your seat, losing control of your car, which then continues into a fatal head-on collision. With a belt on, you would have been involved only in the minor sideswipe; no second accident would have occurred.
- "It's just a pain in the neck to keep buckling and unbuckling." In one study, this reason was given by 70 percent of nonusers or partial users; but psychologists involved in the study suspected that the real reasons for nonuse were deeper. A careful driver will take a minute to adjust rear- and side-view mirrors, to adjust the seat to a comfortable distance from the wheel. Buckling up takes less time than either. Regular use makes the action so automatic that regular users report no bother at all.

be frightening, dangerous, and even deadly. Whether or not to hitchhike is a major decision that thousands of young people make each day. While they may be well aware of the benefits, they rarely consider the risks of this once neighborly, now extremely chancy practice.

Police estimate that only 1 to 2 percent of unpleasant incidents are reported, and so accurate statistics on the uncertainties to which hitchhikers are exposed are rare. Horror stories, however, are common. There was the 19-year-old woman who accepted a lift from three young men in New Jersey, expect-

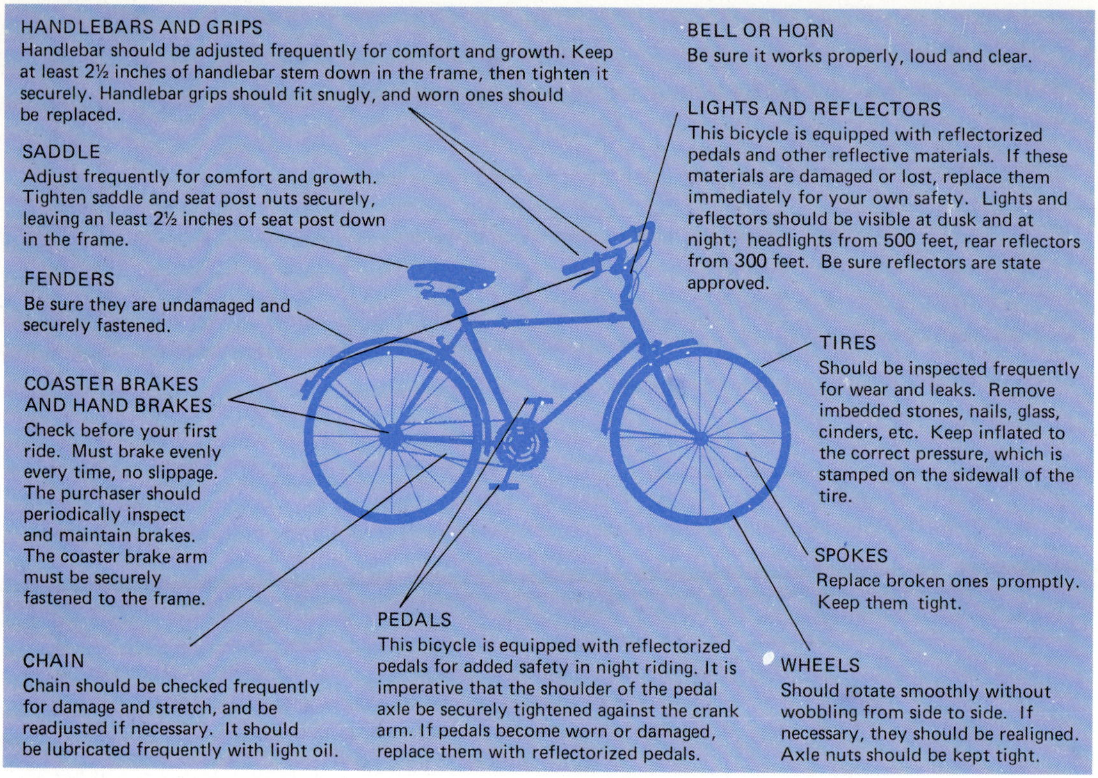

FIGURE 11.3 Buying and maintaining a safe bicycle. If purchasing a bike, be sure it meets Federal Safety Standards, which include seat and stern clamps, chain guards, and wide-angled reflectors. [*Bicycle Institute of America*, "Pedal Primer."]

ing a ride across the bridge to New York City. Instead they drove to a motel, where they gagged and repeatedly raped her. She was lucky; she escaped with her life. Less fortunate was the 18-year-old woman student who disappeared from campus after accepting a ride with a stranger, and whose decomposed body was found in a surburban sewage plant 2 years later. Male hitchhikers are less susceptible to sexual and physical assault, but a number of incidents document that they are far from immune. Hitchhikers face other hazards if the obliging driver is intoxicated or stoned, not the least of which is an automobile accident. Long-distance thumbers also risk assault or robbery by other hitchhikers, and being stranded in out-of-the-way places.

The villain's shoe may also be on another foot. Drivers offering lifts to strangers are subject to assault and robbery. They risk accident by stopping on a busy highway, and arrest if the passengers they pick up happen to be carrying drugs. Some have had money extorted by young girls threatening to call the police and cry rape unless they hand over all their money.

One way to reduce the trauma of hitchhiking is to end hitchhiking entirely. Suggested steps toward that end include: (1) teaching children of the dangers of accepting lifts at an early age (about 10); (2) making public transportation available to young people at student rates or free; (3) enforcing existing antihitching laws; (4) passing new laws that make both hitchhiker and driver liable (a Colorado law specifies 10 days in jail for first-time hitchers and a fine for the driver); (5) encouraging parents to see that their children have the money they need for transportation to work, school, and recreation. But a hitchhiking mentality has hardened in many young people, and legislation will not easily erase it.

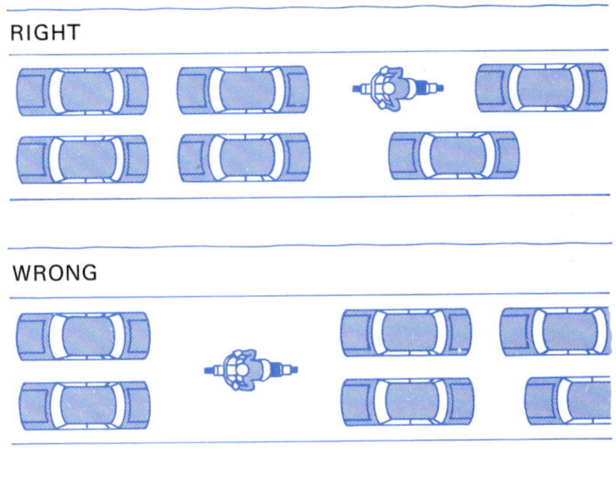

FIGURE 11.4 A motorcycle should be maintained in the same position in the lane of traffic as a car. If it is too far to one or the other side of the lane, an automobile driver might try to squeeze into the spot. A motorcycle near the middle of the lane is most visible to other drivers.

EMERGENCY CARE: REDUCING INJURY AFTER ACCIDENT

In the rugged Cascade mountain range of the state of Washington, a 20-year-old woman took a curve too fast. Her car rolled over, trapping her inside. When the local doctor, new in town, arrived with his medical bag, there was nothing he could do but watch her die. He had no winch to lift the car off her, no cutting tools, no specialized emergency equipment to sustain her life. During the 90 minutes that he waited for a tow truck, the physician vowed to set up a full-scale rescue team, complete with well-equipped ambulance—a vow he later kept.

A National Priority

What happened to the young Washington woman was not unusual. The inadequacy of emergency care, the third prong in the effort to reduce trauma, is nationwide. In 1971, 40 percent of trauma patients handled by ambulance crews in the United States received no medical attention until they reached the hospital, despite the fact that treatment during the first few post-injury minutes can make the difference between life and death. In many situations in traffic-clogged cities, but especially in isolated areas, getting an ambulance quickly to the scene may be a serious problem. Death from injuries is four times more likely to occur in a rural area than if the same accident occurred in a metropolis.

Since many of the annual deaths and much crippling and disability resulting from trauma could be prevented by better emergency care, Congress passed the Emergency Medical Services Systems Act in 1973. Some steps being taken to improve emergency care are:

- *Better trauma training* Emergency medical technician (EMT) training for thousands who ride ambulances professionally or as volunteers, lessons in basic resuscitation techniques (CPR), and emergency treatment for lay people
- *Dispersing emergency vehicles widely* Putting an emergency vehicle and crew just minutes away from anywhere in town
- *Two-way communications systems* Permitting the ambulance attendant to describe the patient's condition to a physician who can then advise on treatment, or using telemetry equipment to transmit the victim's vital signs directly
- *Helicopter services* Speeding accident victims from isolated locations and hurrying physicians to the site of serious crashes
- *Mobile intensive care units* Providing ICUs for immediate treatment of cardiac patients, newborns (especially premature babies), and the critically injured

St. Vincent's Hospital and Medical Center of New York

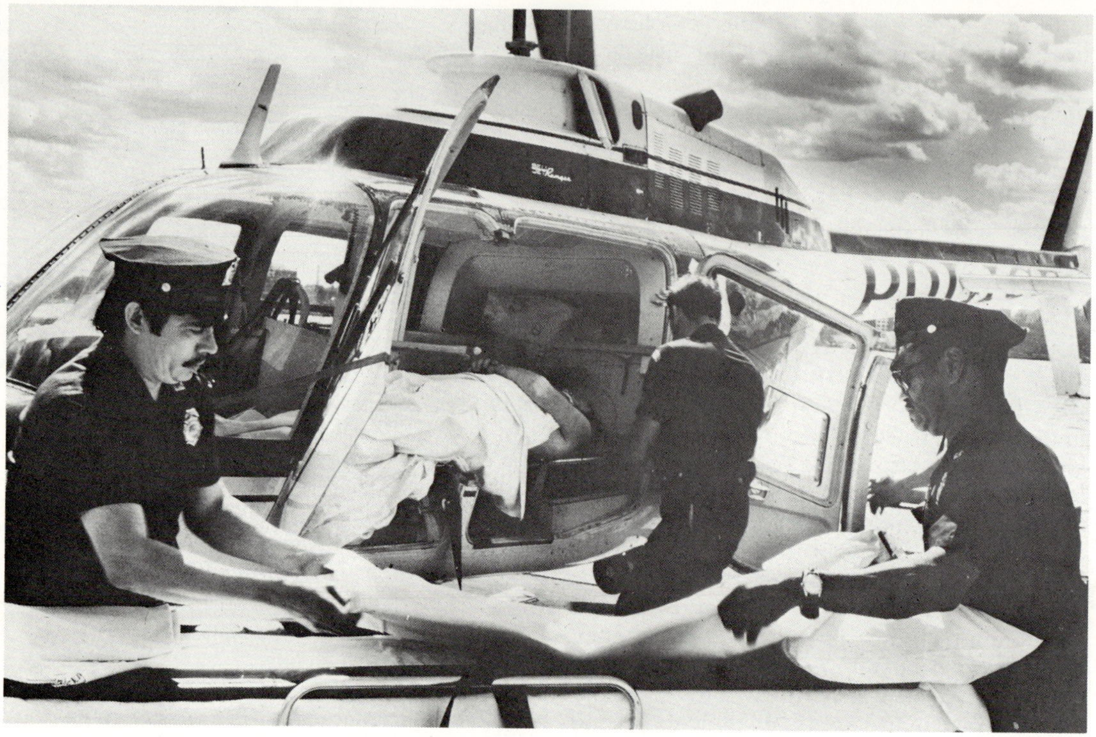

Helicopter rescue services are part of a nationwide effort to upgrade emergency medical care, especially for those in isolated locations.

- *Rescue squads* Providing equipment to cut away wreckage at the scene of an accident in order to free passengers for faster medical care

What Can You Do in an Emergency?

Recently, a young man was dragged from his family's backyard swimming pool, unconscious and with no pulse. His swimming companion ran for help and the emergency squad was called. Friends and family gathered around the boy's still body. No one knew what to do. By the time help arrived, it was too late. The youth was buried two days before his high school graduation day.

Clearly, the most important things we can do in an emergency must be learned before the emergency occurs. Had friends or family of the young man been qualified in cardiopulmonary resuscitation—a method that can be learned in about 3 hours and is taught in many Red Cross headquarters, community colleges, and high schools, as well as hospitals—he might well be in college today. Figure 11.5 demonstrates CPR techniques for use with children. CPR for adults is shown in Figure 10.8.

The "café coronary" is another common emergency for which most people are unprepared. In most cases, the victim has been drinking, talking, laughing during a meal. A chunk of meat or other food lodges in the throat. The victim cannot speak (which distinguishes him or her from a heart attack victim), and if the air passages are completely blocked, will be dead in 4 to 5 minutes. Figure 11.6 shows how to execute the recommended

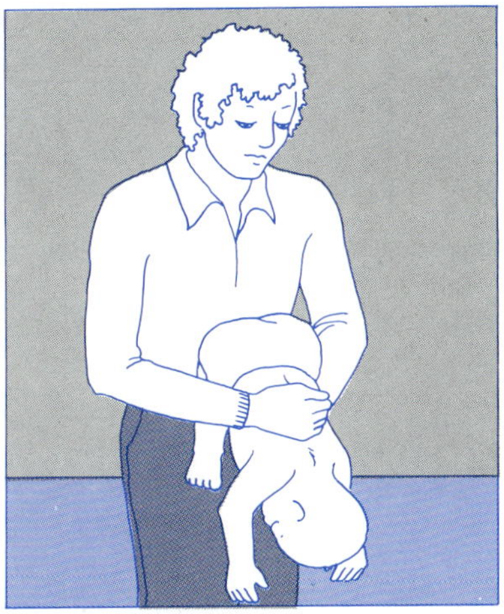

Airway technique

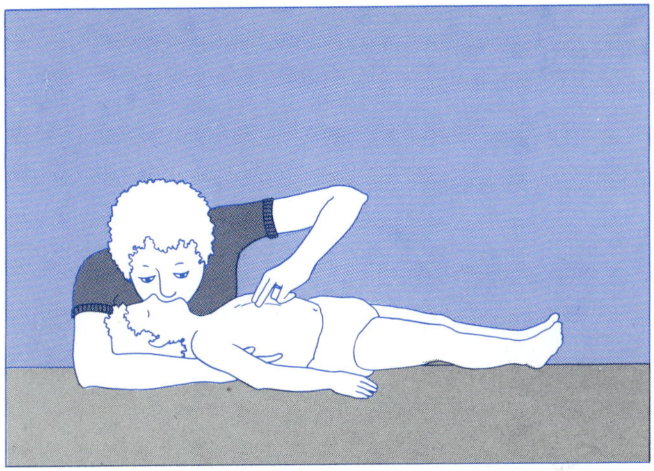

CPR technique

FIGURE 11.5 Rescue techniques for infants and children who are not breathing or whose hearts have stopped beating. Be gentle and use care in applying these procedures, in order to avoid further injury.

To clear food or an object from the airway, turn the child upside down over one arm (jackknife position), and deliver blows to the back between the shoulder blades. If breathing does not resume, begin CPR rescue breathing.

For rescue breathing, place the victim on his or her back. Clear the mouth of any obstructions with your fingers. Then cradle the child's head in your arm. Avoid exaggerating the backward tilt of the head since an infant's neck is so pliable that too much force could block breathing passages instead of opening them. Do not pinch the nose as in adult CPR; instead, cover the child's mouth and nose with your mouth, forming a tight seal. Give four small breaths 3 seconds apart. Check the pulse; if none is felt, begin compressions. If the heart is beating, continue giving 20 small breaths per minute until spontaneous breathing resumes.

For both small children and infants, use only one hand for compression; the other hand should be under the patient for firm back support. For infants, place the tips of index and middle fingers at mid-sternum (the midpoint of the breastbone) and compress the sternum toward the backbone about 1/2 to 3/4 inch in 80 to 100 short, quick thrusts per minute. Intersperse with a gentle puff of air between every five compressions. For children, use the heel of one hand to compress the mid-sternum between 3/4 and 1 1/2 inches, 80 to 100 times per minute, with breaths after every five compressions. Discontinue compressions when heartbeat is restored. Continue rescue breathing until the child is breathing naturally. [*Adapted from International Group Plans, Inc., Office of Consumer Affairs (copyrighted).*]

Heimlich maneuver that could save the estimated 2500 to 3900 Americans who die of café coronaries each year.

Table 11.4 gives some of the basic emergency treatments you might want to master. Better still is taking a first aid or emergency techniques course where learning is through doing. Such a course might be arranged through your health class, or through the college administration.

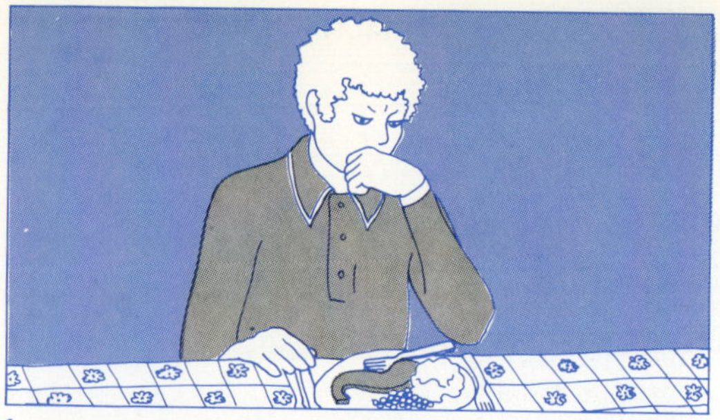

1 Partial blockage: The individual is coughing and can speak. Encourage him to cough up the piece of food.

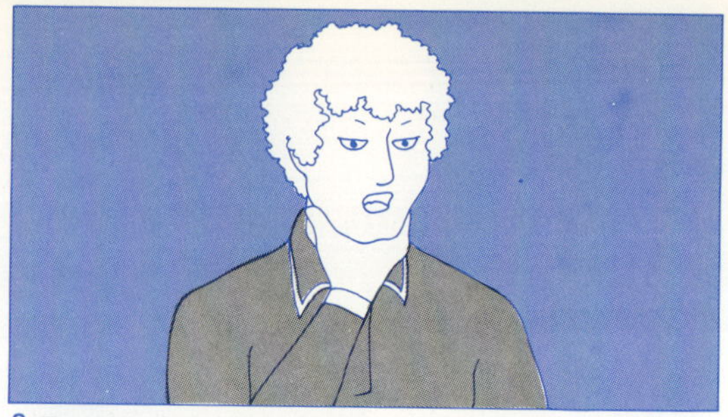

2 Total blockage: The victim cannot speak or breathe; he looks alarmed; he grasps at his throat. He begins to turn blue and finally collapses into unconsciousness.

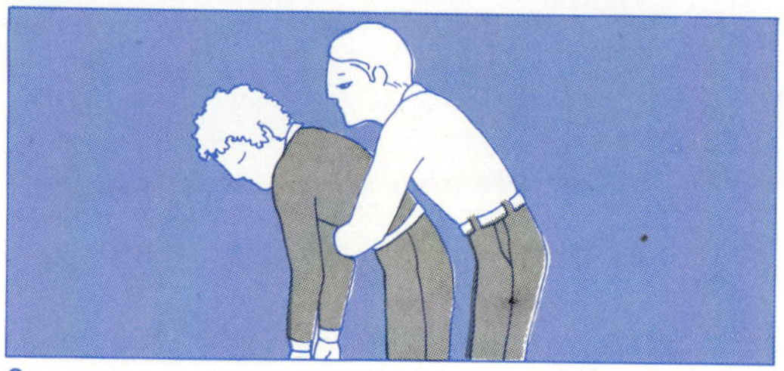

3 At first sign of choking, stand behind the victim and wrap your arms around his waist.

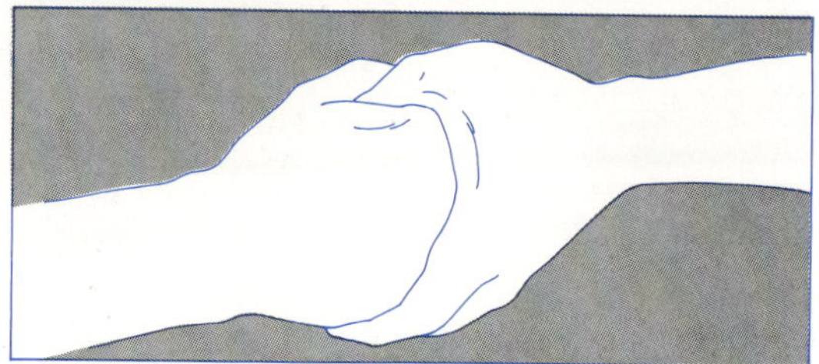

4 Place the thumb side of your fist against the victim's abdomen, slightly above the navel and below the rib cage. Grasp the fist with your other hand and press into the victim's abdomen with a quick upward thrust. Repeat several times, if necessary. The same procedure can be performed with a seated victim.

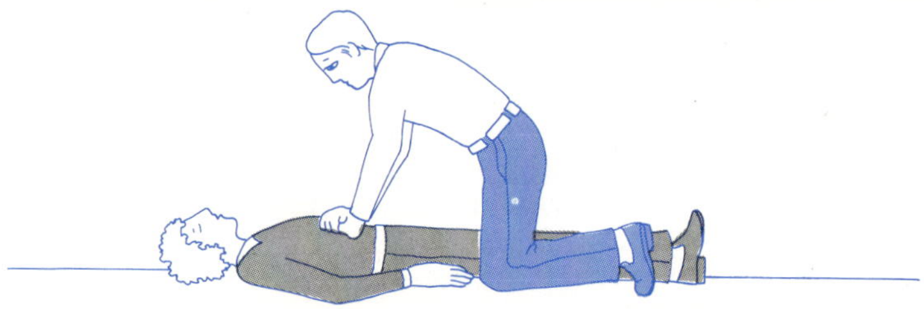

5 If the victim has collapsed to the floor: With the victim lying on his back, sit astride his hips. With one of your hands on top of the other, place the heel of your bottom hand on the abdomen slightly above the navel and below the rib cage. Press into the abdomen with a quick upward thrust. Repeat if necessary.

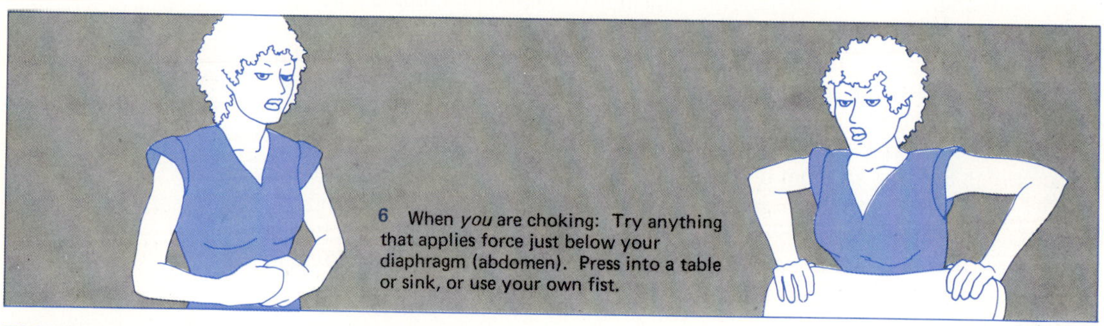

6 When *you* are choking: Try anything that applies force just below your diaphragm (abdomen). Press into a table or sink, or use your own fist.

FIGURE 11.6 The Heimlich maneuver for rescuing the choking victim. Should a piece of food lodge in the throat, blocking airways, the individual will die of strangulation in 4 or 5 minutes, unless the food is dislodged. The recommended rescue procedure is shown here. The victim should be seen by a physician immediately after the rescue.

TABLE 11.4 Basic emergency care

INJURY	TREATMENT	FOLLOW-UP	SEEK MEDICAL CARE
Asphyxiation (breathing has ceased)	Get patient to fresh air; give rescue breathing as shown in Fig. 10.8. Continue until breathing resumes (this may take hours) or help arrives.	Patient should rest at least 1 hour following resumption of natural breathing.	In any case.
Back or neck injury	*Do not move* unless patient is in immediate danger from fire, traffic, etc. Loosen clothes, make comfortable; prop rolled-up clothes or blankets around neck area to prevent movement.	Do not raise head to give patient a drink. If moving is urgent, try to find board, door, or other flat surface on which to transport patient. Have several persons help to roll patient, keeping head and spinal column in line, onto makeshift stretcher. Bind to stretcher with sweaters, belts, etc.	Immediately; emergency squad.
Bites, animal	Wash wound with soap under water, for 5 minutes.	Find and confine animal for rabies tests.	In any case.
Broken bones, fractures	Apply ice or cold compresses* for 30 minutes; do not move; give aspirin for pain; stop bleeding in open breaks.	If moving is absolutely necessary, splint injury.	Immediately.
Bruises	Apply ice, cold compresses*; rest and elevate injured part if possible.	After 24 hours, apply heat for pain.	If severe or disabling.
Burns:			
Mild, first-degree (redness, pain, swelling)	Put under cold, running water, or apply ice or cold soaks for 1 hour; begin immediately.	Wash gently with soap and water; apply medicated ointment; cover with clean non-stick gauze dressing.	Only if large area of body is affected.
Moderate, second-degree (as above plus blisters)	Treat as for first-degree burns.		If 10% or more of body is affected; if patient is under 14 or over 64; if pain persists.

Note: Also seek immediate emergency help for any of the following symptoms: prolonged convulsions; symptoms of heart attack (see Fig. 10.7); loss of consciousness from known or unknown cause; sudden, unexplained, and unexpected severe pain in chest, abdomen, head, or back; loss of large amounts of blood in vomitus, diarrhea, or urine, or from vagina; sudden behavior changes—confusion, violence, loss of memory, and so on; extremely high fever or extremely low temperature (see p. 78).

*See Appendix.

TABLE 11.4 ***(Continued)***

INJURY	TREATMENT	FOLLOW-UP	SEEK MEDICAL CARE
Severe, third-degree (deep layers of skin involved; skin blackened, charred)	Remove burned clothing; apply sterile dressing or cover with clean sheet; do not wash; treat for shock if necessary.	Give fluids if patient is conscious.	Immediately.
Chemical	Wash long and thoroughly with water (shower is good for large burns).		Immediately except in very small, mild injuries.
Choking on food or foreign object	Heimlich maneuver (Fig. 11.6) if patient cannot breathe.		In any case in which Heimlich maneuver is used.
Cuts and wounds	Wash with soap under warm water for 5 minutes; apply pressure with sterile compress or clean cloth until bleeding stops; use ice or cold water if bleeding is not a problem. If pressure on wound does not stop bleeding, apply additional pressure to major artery leading to area. Use tourniquets only as last resort in life-threatening bleeding.	Apply antibacterial ointment and dress with sterile gauze; keep dry, covered, protected for 1 week.	If cut is more than 1 inch long and gapes open; if bleeding persists; if there is fever; if there is increasing pain, or if red streaks radiate from wound; if patient is unable to move joint below wound; if wound is a "dirty," outdoor injury, especially puncture type.
Electric shocks	Turn off power if possible. Do not touch victim until contact is broken; use wooden pole, rope, or dry cloth to rescue. If breathing has stopped, use CPR (Figs 10.8 and 11.5).		In any case.
Foreign bodies embedded (splinters, etc.)	Sterilize needle and tweezers over flame or in boiling water; wash area around splinter and numb it a bit with ice cube; free splinter by probing with needle and remove with tweezers.	Wash area with soap and water; apply dressing if needed; change as needed; apply hot soaks* 3 times daily.	If foreign body is deeply embedded; was dirty or from out-of-doors; if swelling, red streaks, fever, increasing pain, or swollen lymph glands near site are present.
Frostbite (tingling, numbness; pain, purpleness; burning, itching; no sensation, dead white)	Do *not* rub. Immerse in warm, not hot, water (103–107°F).	Give tea, coffee, aspirin; no smoking; after thawing, raise and lower part rhythmically.	In all cases except very minor frostbite.

INJURY	TREATMENT	FOLLOW-UP	SEEK MEDICAL CARE
Head injuries:			
Conscious patient	Keep patient flat on back; do not move; do not allow to walk around	Observe for 24 hours for danger signs: dizziness, grogginess, nausea, vomiting; double vision, dilated pupils; loss of fluid from ears, nose, mouth; coma; severe headache.	If any danger signs appear.
Unconscious patient	Loosen clothing; keep airways clear; place patient on side; do not slap to revive.	Try to find cause: drugs, alcohol, head injury, etc.	Immediately; emergency squad.
Heat exhaustion (fatigue, faintness, clammy perspiration, weak pulse and breathing, brief loss of consciousness)	Remove victim to cool place; put in reclining position; remove or loosen clothing; cool body with wet cloths, fans, etc.; revive with spirits of ammonia	Give salt solution or salt tablets if conscious; salt solution enema if not; give cool, sweet drinks (e.g., iced coffee with sugar)	If patient does not revive quickly, feels ill.
Heatstroke, sunstroke (high fever, 105°F and over; collapse in hot weather)	Cool patient immediately: in tub of cold water with ice added; with wet sheets; using fans; etc.	Keep semireclining	Immediate emergency medical care.
Insect stings and bites, bees, wasps	For bee sting, remove venom sac by scraping gently; wash with soap and water and apply meat tenderizer;* treat with antidote if patient is allergic.		Immediately if patient is allergic or if shock or severe swelling anywhere in body or breathing difficulties are present.
Poisonous	Keep patient quiet; keep affected part below heart level; place a constricting band* 2 to 4 inches above wound; apply ice wrapped in cloth. Remove band after 30 minutes.		Immediately.
Nosebleeds	Apply pressure to nostrils by pressing together with thumb and forefinger for 5 minutes; repeat if bleeding continues.	Keep patient quiet, sitting, leaning forward; avoid blowing nose, laughing.	If bleeding is not controlled after 3 tries; if nose is deformed by injury; if there is difficulty in breathing; if nosebleed occurs frequently; in high blood pressure.

TABLE 11.4 *(Continued)*

INJURY	TREATMENT	FOLLOW-UP	SEEK MEDICAL CARE
Poison ivy, oak, sumac exposure	Wash site immediately; continue for 5 to 10 minutes; change and wash clothing.	Calamine lotion, hot and cold compresses,* antihistamines can help relieve itching.	If discomfort is severe and rash widespread.
Poisoning (also see Chap. 18 on treating drug emergency)	Feed large quantities of water or milk; induce vomiting (with finger, liquids, or emetic, e.g., syrup of ipecac) *except* when poison is acid or caustic, or has a kerosene, gasoline, or benzene type base. Place vomiting patient on stomach with head hanging over basin at end of bed. Give antidote if known (check container), or universal antidote if possible; if not available, feed milk, beaten raw egg whites in water, or a thin mixture of flour and water. Do *not* give milk or other fatty substances if phosphorus poisoning is suspected.	*Universal antidote:* 2 tablespoons activated charcoal, 1 tablespoon tannic acid, 1 tablespoon magnesium oxide mixed in ½ glass water. *Homemade universal antidote:* 2 tablespoons finely crushed burnt toast fed to patient followed by 1 tablespoon very strong tea, 1 tablespoon milk of magnesia mixed in ½ glass water.	Call poison control center immediately, or hospital or physician.
Serious multiple injury	Follow these procedures: (1) Clear airways; check breathing; give CPR if necessary. (2) Stop major bleeding with pressure compresses. (3) Treat for shock if necessary. (4) Make patient comfortable: loosen clothing; cover lightly; put blanket beneath patient; raise feet unless there is head injury or heart attack.	Do not move unless absolutely urgent; splint possible fractures before moving. Give fluids to conscious patient: orange juice, or special drink.*	Immediately; emergency squad.

INJURY	TREATMENT	FOLLOW-UP	SEEK MEDICAL CARE
Shock (pale, bluish, cold, clammy skin; weak, fast pulse and breathing; weakness; thirst; nausea)	Place on back, feet elevated (unless there is head injury or heart attack); cover lightly but do *not* apply heat; reassure patient; if patient is conscious and not vomiting, feed special drink,* strong coffee, tea, or orange juice.	Medical care will include replacement of body fluids and glucose and salts.	Immediately.
Snakebite	If mild symptoms (swelling, burning, sweating, nausea) occur, apply constricting band.* If severe symptoms (pain, severe swelling, vomiting, difficulties with breathing, vision, speech, weakness, paralysis, convulsions) occur, clean wound with soap and water. Sterilize knife or razor over open flame, and make shallow vertical incision over each fang mark—½ inch long and just into skin. Suck out venom with suction cup or your mouth, if you have no open sores. (Do not swallow.) Continue for 30 minutes. If swelling reaches band, add another 2 to 4 inches higher.	Get away from snake; it can bite again. Keep affected part below heart level. Carry patient, if possible. Do not treat if medical help can be reached within 1 hour and no symptoms are evident. (If snake is poisonous, there will be fang marks at wound. Try to identify snake or take dead snake to E.R.)	As soon as possible.
Sprains, ankles, wrists (pain, swelling, blueness)	Apply ice or cold compresses* for 1 hour; elevate and immobilize for 24 hours; wrap in cold, wet towel.	Hot soaks (15 minutes, 3 times daily) and massage speed healing after first 24 hours.	Because of difficulty in evaluation of sprains (especially of ankle), they should be seen by a doctor.

LOOKING BACK

REVIEWING CONCEPTS IN CHAPTER 11

- Trauma, or injury, is the fourth major cause of death in the United States; it is the No.1 killer of those between 1 and 38 years of age.
- As with disease, a variety of factors contribute to injury: a susceptible host, a causative agent, a mode of transmission, and environmental factors.
- Though accidents can never be completely eliminated, both the individual and the community can do much to reduce their number and severity.
- Injury can be prevented by forestalling the accident that causes injury, or by reducing the risk of injury should an accident occur; injury can be minimized by providing immediate, high-quality care and treatment for the injured.
- Accidents can be prevented by controlling the various accident risk factors—at work, at play, at home, on the road.
- Emergency care in many rural and center city areas of the United States is inadequate, but federal and local efforts to improve it are under way.
- Knowledge among laypeople of simple rescue techniques, such as CPR and Heimlich's maneuver, and of basic first aid can do much to reduce injury and death from accidents.

12 WHEN ILLNESS STRIKES

WHAT'S AHEAD IN CHAPTER 12 When is the best time to select a family physician? What kinds of information might you want to know about a physician before making such a selection? How safe is surgery? Can its risks be reduced by intelligent choices on the part of the health consumer? How? How prevalent is chronic illness? In what ways may it affect the family stricken by it? How can these effects be minimized? What is the lot, today, of those who have been disabled by illness, injury, or birth defect? What steps can be taken to improve this lot by the community? By individuals?

It is nice to know what makes your heart tick or your lungs expand, which microorganisms cause disease, and what factors contribute most to accidents. But what do you do when the ticking speeds up alarmingly or the chest hurts, when a virus strikes or a friend sprains an ankle? Usually, the first thing we do is locate a doctor. But that is sometimes easier said than arranged, unless you already have a personal physician. To demonstrate the difficulty of obtaining medical care at certain times and places, Dr. Keith Sehnert made a bet with a doctor friend who believed the problem was greatly exaggerated (Sehnert and Eisenberg):

> "Pick up the phone," I challenged, "and say you're a newcomer in town with a sick four-year-old. I'll bet you can spend the entire evening on the telephone and not get a firm commitment from a doctor to see your child—not just tonight, but tomorrow." To Bill, that sounded like easy

Erika Stone/Peter Arnold

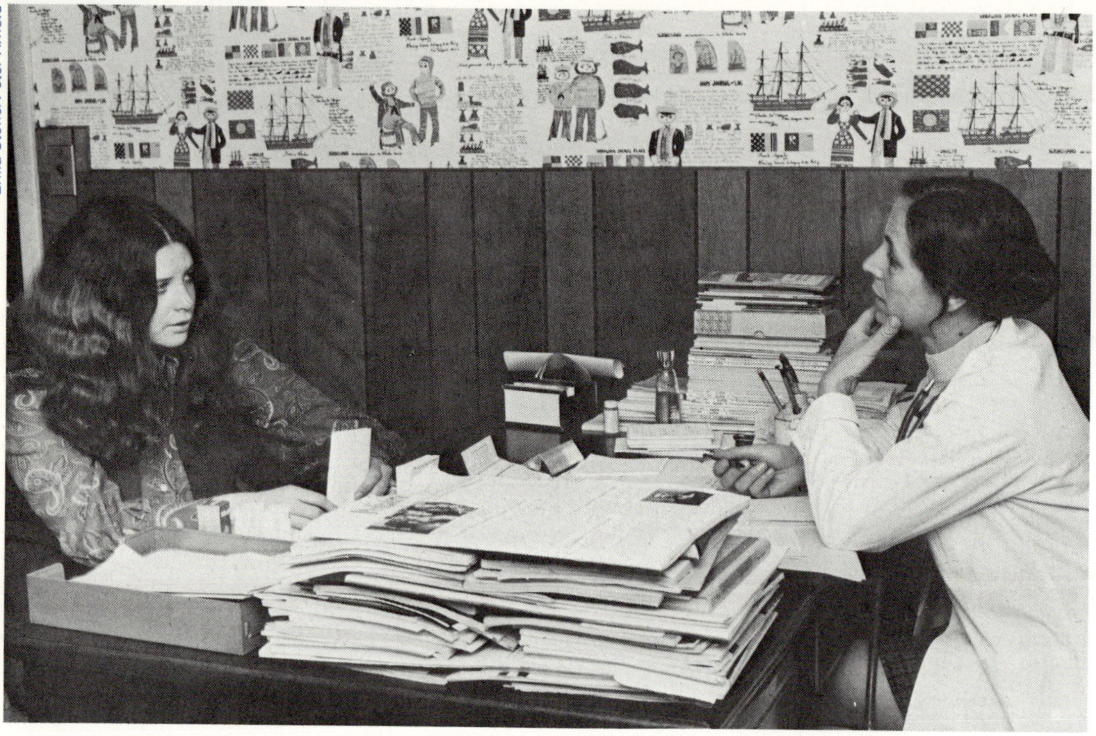

The selection of a physician is a major health decision. It is best done before illness strikes.

money. He riffled through the Yellow Pages and began calling. He spoke to private physicians. He argued with answering services. He called hospital emergency rooms. At the end of the evening, he opened his billfold and reluctantly handed me a well-earned $10 bill. (p. 85)

It is clear from this experiment, and from the experiences of the 1 in 5 Americans who move every year, that the time to find a doctor is *before* an emergency occurs.

CHOOSING A PHYSICIAN

The selection of a physician is a major health decision. As in most decision making, if one knows the right questions and where to look for information, finding answers is easier.

What Type of Doctor Do I Need?

Most people prefer and need a doctor who can provide *primary care*: regular checkups, care of routine illnesses, the first examination for serious illness or injury, referral when necessary, and follow-up of specialists' care. In the first half of this century, primary care was provided by the *general practitioner* (sometimes called the G.P.), who had gone into practice after four years of medical school and, often, a year of hospital internship. During the 1950s and 1960s, the provision of primary care came to be shared with three specialty groups: the *pediatrician* for child care, the *internist*, a specialist in internal medicine, for adult care; and the *obstetrician-gynecologist* for care of the pregnant woman before, during, and after childbirth, and for treatment of disorders of the female reproductive system. In the mid-1960s, a new primary care specialty arose: the *family physician*.

Though they treat the whole family as did the general practitioner, family physicians are more highly trained. Family physician training includes a three-year residency that covers internal medicine, obstetrics and gynecology, pediatrics, minor surgery, and psychiatry in addition to supervised experience in the treatment of patients in a family practice clinic.

Most United States physicians are medical doctors (M.D.s), but about 15 percent are osteopaths (D.O.s). Though originally emphasizing skeletal manipulation, osteopathy's view of disease and treatment is now closely aligned with that of orthodox medicine. Osteopaths can now join the AMA and have unlimited practice privileges in 42 states and the District of Columbia.

Getting a Doctor's Name

Once you know the kind of physician you want, there are several sources you can consult for specific names:

- *A consumer medical directory*, if your community has one, which can often provide names plus such information as average waiting time, fees, time allotted for each patient, whether or not house calls are made, when payment is due, whether Medicaid patients are accepted
- *The local Medical Society*, which will provide the names of two or three physicians, but no information about them
- *The American Medical Association Directory*, found in hospitals and some public libraries, which lists physicians geographically, along with their ages, training, specialties, type of practice, and other information
- *Your present physician*, who may be able to provide a recommendation in a new community
- *Neighbors*, especially in the health field (ask why they like a particular doctor)
- *A hospital or local medical college*

Is this Doctor the One for You?

Once you have the name of a likely prospect, it is time to find out more. Arrange for a 10 to 15 minute appointment, even if it is necessary to pay for the doctor's time. Try to get these questions answered:

- *What are the doctor's fees?* For office visits, house calls? Is payment due immediately, or at the end of the month? How are charges for extras figured—shots, lab fees, x-rays? Is there a charge for telephone consultation?
- *What are the doctor's credentials?* Does he or she have board certification earned by completion of three to five years of residency training in a specialty area, plus two years of specialty practice, plus achieving passing scores on written and oral exams in the field? What about hospital affiliation? A physician who is not affiliated with a hospital is unlikely to be able to provide complete care. Is the hospital accredited?
- *Is the physician involved in continuing medical education?* Reading scientific (not political or economic) journals, attending seminars and lectures, participating in a continuing education program sponsored by the AMA or a specific specialty help a physician keep up to date. Certificates are often awarded for such participation.
- *What kind of office organization does the physican have?* Is it a solo office, with just one doctor? The advantage is you always get to see the same doctor; the disadvantage, you have no one familiar with your case to turn to when the doctor is sick, on vacation, or unavailable. If it is a partnership, do you like both physicians? If a group practice, do patients see the same family doctor each visit, or any doctor at random? Does the physician have an efficient and friendly staff? Does he or she

WHO'S WHO IN HEALTH CARE
Medical Specialists

- *Anesthesiologists* Administer necessary anesthetic drugs during surgery or diagnosis.
- *Colon and rectal surgeons* Diagnose and treat disorders and diseases of the lower digestive tract.
- *Dermatologists* Diagnose and treat diseases of the skin.
- *Family practitioners** Provide total health care needs for patient and family, coordinating work of any needed specialists.
- *Internists** Diagnose and treat disorders and diseases of the internal organs.
- *Neurologists* Diagnose and surgically treat disorders of the brain, spinal cord, and nervous system.
- *Obstetrician-gynecologists** Diagnose and treat disorders of the female reproductive organs; provide care for pregnant women before, during, and after delivery.
- *Ophthalmologists* Diagnose and medically or surgically treat diseases or defects of the eyes.
- *Orthopedists* Diagnose and medically or surgically treat diseases, fractures, and deformities of the bones and joints.
- *Otolaryngologists* Diagnose and treat diseases of the ears, nose, and throat.
- *Pathologists* Study and evaluate changes in organs, tissues, and cells, as well as alterations in body chemistry.
- *Pediatricians** Provide care of the well child as well as diagnosis and treatment of diseases of children.
- *Plastic surgeons* Surgically correct, repair, or restore deformed or mutilated parts of the body; surgically improve facial or body features.
- *Psychiatrists* Diagnose and treat emotional disorders, mental disorders, and organic diseases affecting the nervous system.
- *Public health specialists* Work toward prevention of disease and promotion of health through epidemiological studies and public health measures.
- *Radiologists* Diagnose and treat disease through the use of radiant energy, including x-rays, radium, and cobalt.
- *Specialists in physical medicine and rehabilitation* Diagnose and treat, by physical procedures, disease or injury, with emphasis on the restoration of function to those disabled by illness or disease.
- *Surgeons* Diagnose and treat disease, injury, or deformity by manual or operative procedures.
- *Thoracic surgeons* Diagnose and surgically treat diseases involving the heart, lungs, or large blood vessels within the chest.
- *Urologists* Diagnose and treat diseases and disorders of the kidney, bladder, ureters and urethra, and the male reproductive organs.

*Usually provide primary care, and are the first doctors that patients contact in the case of illness or injury.

employ a team of nurses, physicians' assistants, social workers, and so on? Some patients like the team approach, others are uncomfortable with it.

- *How available is the physician?* Does the doctor make house calls (only 1 in 4 still does), accept telephone calls? Are office hours convenient for you? How long must one wait for an appointment? What about emergencies on weekends, evenings, days off? Is there someone else on call when the physician is unavailable? Will he or she meet patients in the emergency room when necessary?

- *Are you comfortable with the physician's personality?* Some patients like the informal, easy going, first-name type of relationship. Others prefer the starchy authoritarian physician. Some patients want a doctor who tells them everything in detail, explaining thoroughly; others a father figure who pats them on the head, hands them a prescription, and assures them, "Everything is fine."
- *What about philosophy?* Do the doctor's ideas match yours on such issues as vitamins and nutrition, preventive medicine, patient education, tranquilizers, use of antibiotics, diet pills, breast-feeding, natural childbirth, and so on?

When a Specialist or Second Opinion Is Needed

There are times when the primary physician believes a consultation with a secondary physician—a general surgeon, for example, when hernia or gallbladder surgery seems needed—would be useful. The referral could be to a tertiary, or third level, physician who specializes even more narrowly, a heart or brain surgeon, for example.

Some people go directly to a specialist (an allergist for hay fever or a dermatologist for acne) but this often leads to fragmented care. Your personal physician does not know what the specialist is doing and vice versa.

WHEN SURGERY IS NEEDED

Every year, an estimated 18 million Americans go "under the knife" (Brody, *c*). That a close friend or relative will be operated upon at some time is almost inevitable. Still, other than what we see on TV medical dramas, most of us know very little about what happens in an operating room, or about the components of an intelligent decision about elective surgery. About 80 percent of all surgery is elective; no life-threatening emergency is involved, and the patient could live without the operation, though perhaps less comfortably or happily. Crucial questions for the health consumer to ask are listed below.

Is It Dangerous?

Every surgical procedure involves some risk which must be weighed against benefits. Is the danger of death from surgery less than the danger of death from the illness or injury? Is relief from the discomfort or disability caused by the illness worth the slight risk of death or further injury from surgery? The answers in every case will vary. But in every case it is important to know the alternatives to surgery.

The risk of complications from surgery differ for each type of operation. Though the average for all surgeries is 1 death for every 72 operations, it is almost negligible for hemorrhoidectomy, about 1 in 5000 for tonsilectomies, and 1 in 70 for gallbladder removal. These are averages and vary greatly depending upon the hospital and the physician.

Who Should Do the Surgery?

An estimated 94,000 physicians perform surgery on a full- or part-time basis, but only 52,000 of these are specially trained and fully certified by a specialty board. Another 12,000 are residents in surgical training programs who operate under close supervision of qualified surgeons. The remainder, some 30,000, perform surgery without special credentials, though many have had some surgical training (Zuidema). Studies show that physicians without certification are responsible for the greatest number of unnecessary operations, though soaring malpractice insurance premiums have led many of these doctors to discontinue that most risk-fraught component of

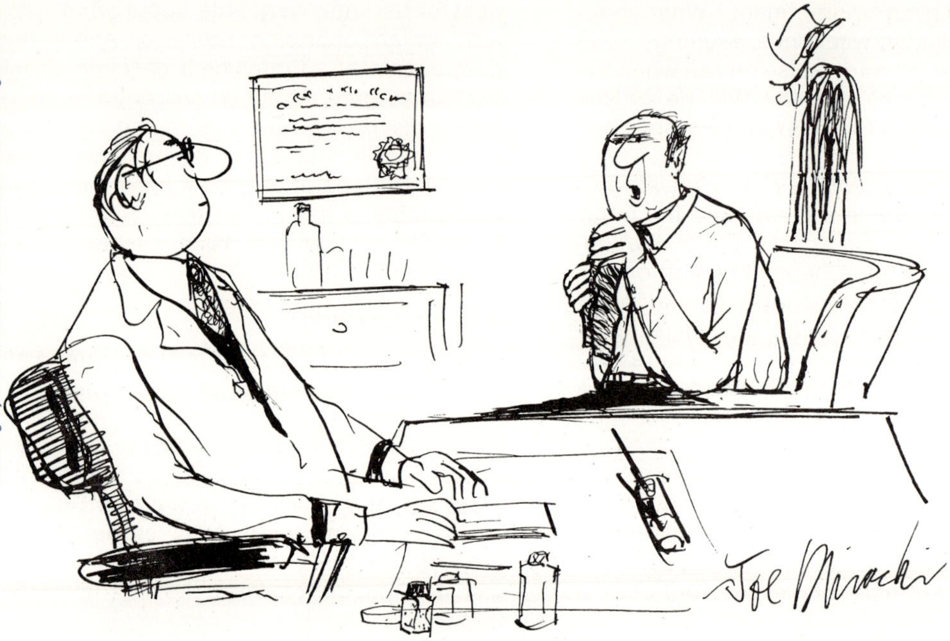

"Well, which is it this time? Something I have to live with or something I have to live without?"

their practices. It is possible to check the basic credentials and training of surgeons (and other specialists) in the *Directory of Medical Specialists*, found in hospitals and some general libraries.

Who Makes the Decision?

Ultimately, the patient or the next of kin makes the decision whether to have surgery or not. No physician can operate without "informed consent," written permission which follows thorough doctor-patient or doctor-family discussion of the procedure, its possible risks, and alternatives to surgery. The final decision usually leans heavily upon the physician's advice, and the great majority of surgeons are ethical and skillful, but some persons prefer to consult a second physician before deciding.

Is Surgery Necessary?

In some types of surgery, where symptoms are vague and time is a critical factor (appendectomy, for example), it is virtually impossible to be certain of the need to operate. In others, a competent surgeon's diagnosis can be expected to be accurate. Yet it has been estimated that 2 million of the 18 million operations performed in the United States annually are unnecessary (Denenberg, *b*). Some find that figure too high, others believe it conservatively low. There is general agreement, though, that some surgery is performed unnecessarily (Lavin and Bucek). Many reasons have been suggested:

- *Physician incompetence* Some physicians exercise poor judgment, use outdated diagnostic techniques, and perform "routine" operations, such as tonsillectomies, out of habit.

- *Fee-for-service medicine* The physician is encouraged to do more (and more major) surgery, because the patient or the insurance company pays for each operation. (On the other hand, it has been suggested that some physicians in prepaid groups, who are *not* paid by the operation, tend to leave some necessary surgery undone.)
- *An oversupply of surgeons and hospital beds* Parkinson's Law can be applied to the health care system: Patient admissions for surgery expand to fill beds, operating suites, and surgeons' time.
- *Lack of hospital controls* In some smaller hospitals, particularly those privately owned, any physician can perform surgery even without the necessary qualifications. (The increase in malpractice suits has, however, accelerated a trend toward stricter requirements and regulation.)
- *Patient insistence* It has been said that Americans take a "fix-it" approach to everything including health, that they are "operation-happy," that they pressure physicians into performing surgery. Lavin and Bucek quote Dr. John P. Bunker, author of *The Anesthesiologist and the Surgeon*, as follows: "We've oversold the product, and the patients themselves are calling the tune, even though they don't really know enough to do so. We knuckle under, because if we don't, they'll go to another doctor who will. . . ." (p. 70)

Is a Second Opinion Needed?

A patient can avoid unnecessary surgery by exploring alternatives, understanding risks, and seeking a second, or even a third, opinion. Seeking an opinion from another physician, one who will *not* be performing the surgery, may be recommended by your surgeon and may even by required by your health insurance group. Though use of the second opinion reduces the number of operations, it is not absolutely certain that this reduction is beneficial in the long run. Studies are under way to determine whether patients who do not have surgery get better or worse, whether they require more extensive medical care, whether the quality of their lives suffers, and whether they eventually need surgery anyway.

What Kind of Anesthesia Will Be Used?

Anesthetics have come a long way since whiskey and "biting the bullet" were prevalent. Modern anesthesia—tailored to patient, type of surgery, physician preference, and experience and training of the anesthetist—can totally eliminate the discomfort and pain

Is surgery necessary? Before making the decision to proceed with surgery, the intelligent health care consumer will consider a number of factors, including risks versus benefits and the qualifications of the surgeon, will seek a second opinion if possible, and will explore alternatives.

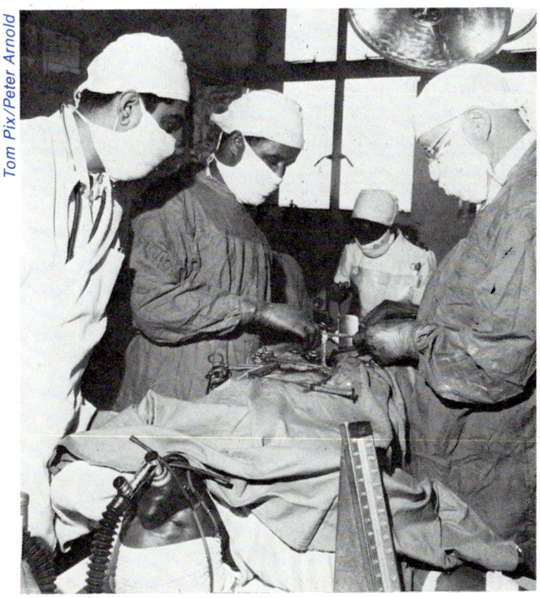

Tom Pix/Peter Arnold

CONSUMER HEALTH TIP

Deciding about Elective Cosmetic Surgery

A decision to undergo cosmetic surgery should not be taken lightly. The potential candidate should first consider some important questions:

1 *Do I consider the desire to change the way God made us somehow sinful?* If you feel this way and do not modify your feelings, then plastic surgery may leave you with guilt feelings.
2 *Is the idea entirely my own, or is it being pushed on me by family and friends?* Undergoing cosmetic surgery can be traumatic when personal motivation is not strong.
3 *Do I expect cosmetic surgery to change my life, solve all my problems, in effect, make me a new person?* Persons whose self-confidence has suffered because of their appearance often get a tremendous lift from the surgery. But surgery will not solve deep social, emotional, or marital problems, and there is often a great letdown when it does not solve them. Psychological counseling prior to cosmetic surgery is often helpful.
4 *Do I expect cosmetic surgery to turn me into a beauty?* Occasionally, results are quite dramatic, but generally the most that can be hoped for is an improvement in appearance.
5 *Am I aware that plastic surgery is a serious medical procedure, not a beauty salon treatment?* There may be pain, discomfort, or occasional complications, and results may not be fully apparent for as much as a year.
6 *Are those closest to me—parents, spouse, boy or girl friend—in favor of the surgery?* Such support makes any procedure easier and is worth trying to win.
7 *Have I selected a physician who is qualified in the field of cosmetic surgery?* The results of dealing with an unqualified or unscrupulous practitioner can be disastrous.

of most surgery. Anesthetics can be classified as: (1) *local*, such as the novocaine used by dentists to numb the gums; (2) *spinal*, injection of an anesthetic into the spinal fluid; (3) *inhalant*, breathed in, such as ether ("gas"), putting the patient to sleep; and (4) intravenous, pentothal injected into a vein, which makes the patient oblivious to what is happening. Sometimes a combination of anesthetics is used. When the patient's condition does not permit local or general anesthesia, hypnosis or acupuncture (which is not effective for all patients or all types of surgery) is sometimes employed.

Where Should Surgery Take Place?

Results are generally better at accredited hospitals, those affiliated with medical schools, or teaching hospitals. For less commonly performed operations, a major medical center may be the best place. Some minor surgery (removal of a cyst, for example) can be performed safely and easily in the physician's office. Other uncomplicated procedures may be performed at a hospital or surgical center on an outpatient basis; the surgery is done, and the patient rests briefly and then goes home the same day. Office and outpatient surgery greatly reduce costs. In recognition of this, many health insurance policies now pay benefits for such procedures.

How Can the Patient Be Reassured?

It is so normal for someone about to undergo surgery to be frightened that, in fact, absence of anxiety is a danger sign. Such patients are likely to be most distraught if something goes wrong later. But excessive fear can also be dangerous. It can be kept within bounds by being certain the surgeon is highly qualified, the hospital accredited, and the need for surgery verified by a second opinion. The patient whose physician has explained exactly what to expect at each step of the way, and how much pain and discomfort to expect afterwards, will endure the experience more easily than an uninformed patient. Some patients need to be assured that they will not awaken in mid-surgery, or blurt out deep, dark secrets while under anesthesia.

CHRONIC AND CATASTROPHIC ILLNESS

In most of your college classes, there are several people with chronic illnesses, some as minor as hay fever, others as serious as diabetes, asthma, or arthritis. A U.S. Public Health Service study has shown that during a two-year period, nearly 50 percent of the civilian population not in institutions suffered from one or more chronic illnesses. Many of these illnesses were in no way disabling. In 1974 chronic ills kept 3.3 percent of the population from all major activities (school, work, housework, etc.) and hampered another 6 percent in carrying out these activities.

Living with chronic illness poses a variety of problems for both individual and family, including: control of symptoms, learning where to turn for help with various health needs, handling of a medical crisis when it arises, dealing with the social isolation that special health problems may lead to, learning to alter lifestyles, and learning to interact with one another and with others outside the family under new conditions.

Some illnesses are so economically and emotionally draining that they are called *catastrophic illnesses.* In this category are chronic hereditary illnesses (hemophilia), serious injuries (severe burns or brain trauma), and failure of a body organ (the heart or kidneys). The most common catastrophic illness in the United States, however, is cancer. Unlike heart diseases, which often bring instant death, cancer is usually a long, drawn-out illness. Thus, cancer is a good example of what happens when catastrophic illness strikes.

The Financial Burden of Catastrophic Illness

Most Americans feel reasonably secure about health costs. Some 92 percent possess some form of health insurance, or are covered by Medicaid or Medicare, nationally funded medical insurance for the poor and elderly. But should serious long-term illness strike, most will find their insurance does not cover the bills. One study found that middle-income families caring for an advanced cancer patient at home can be reduced to poverty in less than two years (Cancer Care, *b*).

In many instances, the patient's spouse is forced into early retirement to care for the patient full-time, further worsening the economic crunch. Life savings are depleted, future plans abandoned, careers changed, homes and other assets lost, families saddled with long-term debt, jobs or promotion opportunities lost. Adult sons and daughters are forced to cancel or postpone college plans and take jobs to help pay medical bills. Families report cutbacks in food, clothing, and health care for both adults and children, and elimination of dental care, children's summer camps, vacations, and recreation. Proposed legislation to help families cope with catastrophic illness may eventually ease such painful financial burdens.

The Emotional and Personal Costs of Catastrophic Illnesses

"A living hell" is the way one member of a family hit by cancer put it. A "time of horror and helplessness," said another. These are not unusual reactions. In the castrophic illness study, 76 of the 115 families reported difficult emotional, psychological, and adjustment problems. Children were confused and

TABLE 12.1 Unanticipated costs in catastrophic illness shatter family finances

COSTS USUALLY ANTICIPATED AND PARTIALLY COVERED BY INSURANCE	COSTS USUALLY NOT ANTICIPATED AND NOT COVERED BY INSURANCE	
Doctor	Social work counseling	Child care
Hospital	Medical homemaker	Extended care facility
Drugs	Housekeeper	Personal care of patient
Burial	Dentist	Home attendant
	Special diets	Domestic equipment
	Special clothing	Patient laundry
	Nurse	Laboratory tests
	Blood transfusions	Patient transportation
	Psychiatric treatment	Special treatment
	Modifications of dwelling	Other patient care
	Nursing home	Food for home help

Source: *The Impact, Costs and Consequences of Catastrophic Illness on Patients and Families:* A Report of a Social Research Study of Selected Families Stricken by Advanced Cancer. Copyright 1973 by the National Cancer Foundation, Inc., and Cancer Care, Inc.

frightened and became insecure about their lives and relationships with others. Some acted out; others withdrew. Schoolwork suffered. In some instances, there were extreme reactions: delinquency, alcohol or drug abuse, compulsive behavior, bedwetting, psychosomatic and psychiatric illnesses. Studies of families in which a child has died show that in the absence of supportive programs, marital difficulties, divorce rates, and problems with other children soared.

Illness does not have to be fatal to be destructive. Many families have been torn asunder by the strain of caring for a retarded, disabled, or chronically or acutely ill child, or of institutionalizing such a child when they cannot cope. When a child's illness is hereditary, there is usually guilt on the parents' part, and sometimes there are angry recriminations from the child. Even when heredity and neglect are not factors, parents tend to blame themselves and each other for a child's serious illness. Relationships between parents and children change. Parents often become more loving and indulgent toward the sick child, or less often, they become resentful and uncaring. Other children are often given short shrift, and they respond with resentment and then with guilt about being resentful. The sick child may learn to manipulate the guilt and concern of parents and siblings to get even more favored treatment. Some teenage diabetics, for example, will purposely neglect diet or insulin shots when they do not get their way.

Many of the same mechanisms operate when an adult is the patient. A cycle of resentment, guilt, fear, love, and hate sets in, and help is often needed.

REHABILITATION

In the past, people maimed by injury or illness, deformed at birth, brain-damaged, blind, or without hearing were often relegated to dark attics or cellars. Even in the enlightened twentieth century, many individuals with mental or physical disabilities have been "filed away" in nursing homes or state or private institutions.

Today, with the coming of age of the health specialty of rehabilitative medicine, such

WHERE TO FIND HELP

When Catastrophic Illness Strikes

Cancer Care, Inc., a voluntary agency that is a branch of the National Cancer Foundation, is probably unique among national disease-centered organizations in offering some financial aid and housekeeping services as well as information and counsel to families hit by catastrophic illness. The parent organizations of national groups such as Muscular Dystrophy, Cerebral Palsy, American Heart Association, and the March of Dimes are largely research- and information-oriented, but local chapters can often direct patients and their families to local private (e.g., Community Service Councils) or public (e.g., Medicaid) avenues of help and can advise on sources of treatment. Too, local chapters and hospital social service departments can frequently refer families to self-help, help-each-other groups that offer valuable shared psychological support.

In such self-help groups diabetic teenagers may talk out their problems concerning diet, sports, fitting in with peers, and college plans. Parents of children born with cleft palates may discuss feeding problems, kinds of surgery, handling of neighbors who gawk. Women who have had a breast removed may talk with those about to undergo, or recovering from, such surgery about the practical problems of prosthesis fitting, physical therapy, and wearing a bathing suit, and about the more difficult challenges of emotional acceptance of the mastectomy by the woman, her husband, boyfriend, family.

warehousing is changing. Where good medicine is practiced, rehabilitation of the maimed and disabled has become an integral part of medical care. The goal of rehabilitation is important not only in human terms, but in terms of national resources. It has been estimated that 51.1 million Americans, about half of them under the age of 65, are disabled in some way, and that number is growing. A good rehabilitation program extends into every aspect of the patient's life and includes the following points.

Bringing Back the Ability to Function

Physical and speech therapy The road back to use of limbs, voice, or hands following injury or illness may be slow and painful. But great strides are being made in helping those disabled through stroke, birth defect, or injury to train or retrain themselves in tasks simple to the rest of us: walking and talking, picking up a spoon or reading a daily newspaper, basic self-care.

Prosthetics to replace the real thing When an arm or leg has been amputated or an eye or breast removed, replacements called *prosthetics* are substituted. Such replacement of human limbs and other parts has come a long way since Peter Pan battled Captain Hook. Artificial arms and legs today have a nearly real look, and function well enough to carry out many tasks through electrical impulses. Glass eyes, on the other hand, look genuine but are sightless, although scientists are working on a false eye that may make some vision possible.

A breast prosthesis is often a form specially designed to match the natural breast, worn in a special bra, with a totally natural look when worn beneath clothing. Sometimes, when the tumor removed is a very small one in early stages, plastic surgery can be used to rebuild the breast with silicone implants. This can greatly ease the agony of breast surgery, especially in young women.

Mechanical aids Many mechanical aids

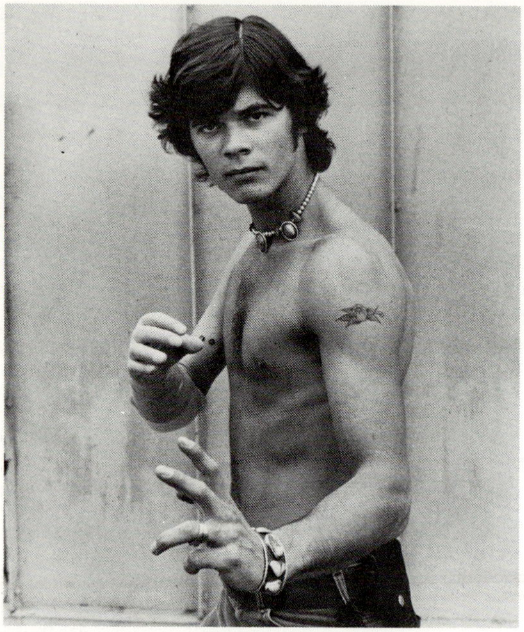

James Collison, © 1978/Time Magazine

Great strides are being made toward helping the disabled regain the ability to function.

make it possible for the disabled to function. Scores of specially designed wheelchairs permit almost every paraplegic (a person who has no use of the legs) to get around, special automobile equipment allows many to drive, telephones can be altered for the hard of hearing, and electronic canes can help the blind to "see" where they are going.

Making It Back into the World

Often the restrictions the disabled meet in the world are more handicapping than the disabilities themselves. The chief problems faced include the following.

Relations with others and self-concept The two are intimately linked. In an article on "crip lib," clinical social worker Peter Leech, himself confined to a wheelchair since a bout with polio, is quoted on the social conditioning that affects the handicapped:

> We are assaulted daily with a set of standards: A beautiful body clothed in a certain kind of clothes . . . and enjoying relationships and activities of a very certain kind. . . . Clearly, the persistence of these ideas . . . bears directly on the difficulty faced by one who becomes permanently damaged. The individual's self-concept is shattered. As a result, the person participates in the societal view that he or she is "in-valid," dependent, asexual—generally ineffective, noncontributory, and unacceptable. (p. 23)

Leech theorizes that this social conditioning affects the way disabled people are treated by others. For example, most of us avoid staring at the disabled to such an extent that we simply ignore them or do not see them. Says Leech:

> People say to me: "I can't look at you because I might call attention to the fact that you're disabled." Well, isn't that absurd? Who knows better than I that I have to live with a disability? Really, though, I don't think it's that we don't want to embarrass the other person. I think it's that we don't want to be embarrassed ourselves. People with disabilities remind us of our own vulnerable places and make us hurt a little bit. . . . (p. 23)

Adjustment to a life of disability may be as difficult as adjustment to dying:

> I had lost the power of speech, that marvelous gift that separates men from the animals. Gone. Totally gone. I felt my head start to turn toward the wall. It was a feeling I experienced off and on for days, weeks, and months. Turn to the wall, away from life, toward blankness and death. The void of the wall, with its blank face expressionless and empty like an idiot's mind or a blind man's sockets, held comfort.
>
> A patient who had a laryngectomy, removal of the larynx or voice box (Searcy, p. 35)

In effect, the attitude of others toward the disabled person becomes a second handicap sometimes worse than the first. Deaf persons are often assumed to be retarded, as are those with cerebral palsy and epilepsy. Those who cannot walk are deemed to be weak and helpless. Nearly all handicapped people are believed to be without sexuality. None of these suppositions is true. With encouragement and opportunity, there is almost nothing the physically disabled cannot accomplish. And even the mentally handicapped—the retarded, the brain-damaged—can often be guided to productive lives.

Disabled persons look for caring and respect from family and friends, not pity. They want the kind of aid that will help them toward independence: "Install a ramp so I can get in and out of the house by myself, instead of carrying me down the steps every time I want to go out." "Treat me like everyone else—allow me to do the most I am capable of!" That is how Danny Thompson, a shortstop with the Texas Rangers, felt when he continued to play baseball while being treated for chronic leukemia. One day he made two errors and the fans booed him loudly. Said Danny: "That was super. I didn't want people saying, 'Oh, he's got leukemia, he can make errors.' They booed the hell out of me and I loved it. I knew they were accepting me as a ball player" (D. Anderson, p. V,5).

Employment Though employer attitudes toward the handicapped have improved since World War II, when many disabled soldiers returned from battle looking fruitlessly for work, only 1 of every 3 blind persons, 1 of 7 cerebral palsy victims, 47 percent of paraplegics, and 25 percent of epileptics were employed in 1973. Yet 80 percent or more are employable.

Unemployment, depriving the disabled of the chance to be independent, can be devastating. One young man with a master's degree in clinical social work, turned down for job after job because of a major disability, gave up, turned to drink, and ended up in a nursing home a beaten man. New federal and state laws, however, now extend to the disabled the protection already given to other minorities in the labor force. These laws may well benefit employers themselves, because studies have shown that the disabled make better than average employees, with fewer accidents, lower absentee rates, and strong determination to succeed. In a DuPont study, supervisors rated 96 percent of handicapped workers average or above on safety performance, 91 percent average or higher on job performance, and 79 percent average or better in attendance (Garner).

Today, federal law requires public school systems to provide programs for children with physical, emotional, and intellectual disabilities.

Ira Wyman

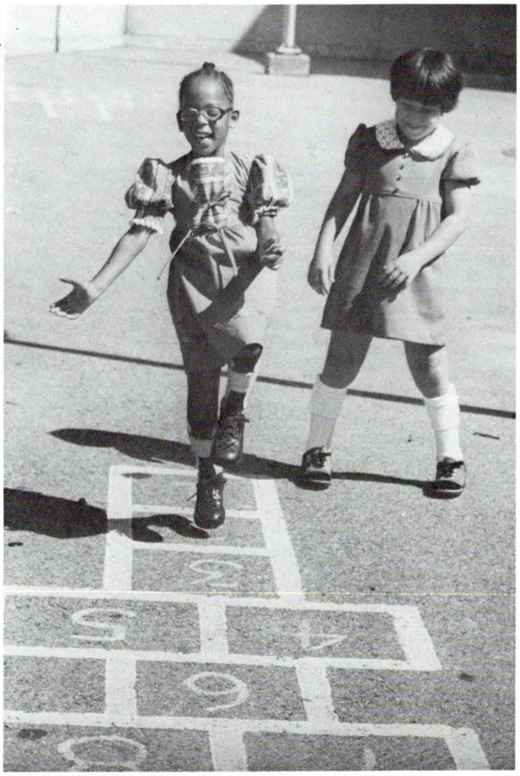

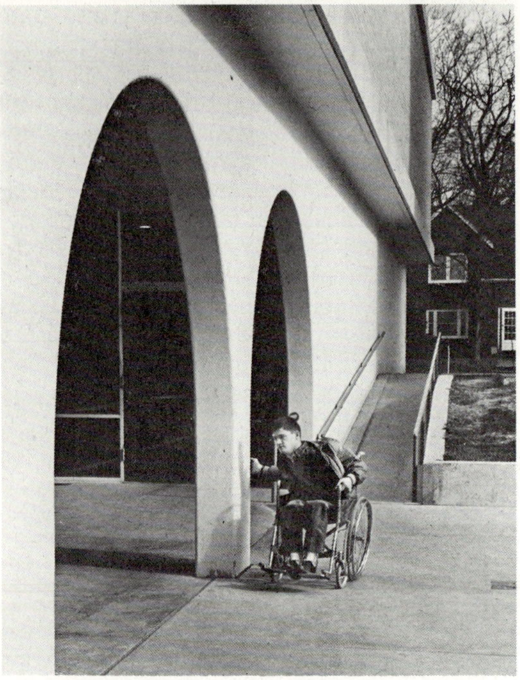

George W. Gardner

Many colleges have removed environmental barriers, literally opening their doors to disabled students. But person-to-person barriers often still exist.

Education Until the mid-twentieth century, lack of education was an added handicap for disabled persons. Today, federal law requires public school systems to provide programs for children with physical, emotional, and intellectual disabilities, in regular classes when possible. Some private schools, such as the Perkins Institute for the Blind and the Blind/Deaf and the Lexington School for the Deaf, provide excellent specialized education. But many private and public institutions offer little more than custodial care, neglecting education, recreation, and socialization.

Many colleges and universities, slowly following the lead of the University of Illinois in 1949, have opened their doors to the handicapped, literally widening doorways and making other physical changes in dorms and classroom buildings. In 1978, the University of California, once charged with not admitting handicapped students, had 900 self-identified disabled students enrolled.

Recreation and travel Work and education fortify self-respect, but the opportunity to participate in recreation and travel provides fun as well as the chance for the disabled to feel "like everyone else." The blind now ski; wheelchair athletes compete in basketball, throw the discus, and lift weights; the deaf compete in their own World Games; the retarded have their own annual national Olympics. Some colleges and schools are developing physical education programs for the handicapped, instead of simply excusing them from physical education classes as in the past.

Travel has opened up, too, allowing the blind, the mentally retarded, and the wheelchair-bound to float in the gondolas of Venice, view Paris from the Eiffel Tower, ride elephants in India. Many travel agencies, hotels, and airlines are cooperating to make this possible.

Community Responsibility toward the Disabled

How can society enable the nation's tens of millions of handicapped to enter life's mainstream? Several steps are possible:

The development of rehabilitation centers Staffed with experts to deal with the multiple problems of the handicapped (physical, psychological, social, economic), such centers can provide follow-up when patients leave the centers, so that adjustment to "the real world" can be made more smoothly. Adult rehabilitation centers are now functioning in some places; and the most successful have handicapped persons on the staff.

Removing environmental barricades Try brushing your teeth, shooting a basket, or drinking from a water fountain while sitting in

Most architectural barriers I've learned to take in stride.
Those steps, those curbs, those revolving doors that make me stay outside.
But if I get to heaven and sent before the gate,
Will St. Peter say our doors are 20 inches wide, your wheelchair 28.

A multiple sclerosis patient, in Laufer, p. 1B

a chair. Or try getting to all your classes for a day blindfolded. If you do, you will better appreciate why special alterations have been legislated in many communities (reserved parking spaces, washrooms with wide stalls and railings, ramps, etc.), toppling some of the physical barriers that have so long stood in the way of the handicapped. Home attendant programs, providing help with personal care, have knocked down the barriers that kept disabled people from living independently instead of in institutions.

The New Militancy

"An entire social movement arose over the question of where certain people must sit when they ride the bus. I can't even get on the bus." This feeling, expressed by a wheelchair traveler, is behind the new militancy of such organizations as PUSH (People United for Self Help) and WARPATH (World Association to Remove Prejudice Against the Handicapped). The disabled have filed lawsuits, staged demonstrations, and pressured local and federal legislators to pass rehabilitation legislation (Downey).

Some self-help groups focus on children. Closer Look[1] provides information on services and legal rights of disabled children. Some groups focus on students. The federally funded Physically Disabled Student Program, for example, established in 1970 at the University of California, offers counseling and referral services to individual students that have cut red tape, lowered drop-out rates, and helped students raise grades and enjoy both a higher standard of health and a higher degree of activity and mobility. The program has now expanded out into the community as the Center for Independent Living.

[1]For information, write: Closer Look, P. O. Box 1492, Washington, DC 22013.

LOOKING BACK

REVIEWING CONCEPTS IN CHAPTER 12

- Finding a physician in an emergency is difficult, and so the search for a personal physician should take place before an emergency occurs. The consumer-patient should not hesitate to ask the doctor questions about his or her background, type of practice, fees, and so on. Personality and philosophy should also be considered.
- Surgery affects nearly everyone at some time or other, either directly or through a friend or relative. The risks entailed by surgery can be reduced by good diagnosis, an experienced and well-trained surgeon, and a well-equipped and well-staffed hospital. A second opinion can often avert unnecessary surgery.
- Chronic illness can range from relatively harmless hay fever to very serious diabetes, asthma, arthritis, and cancer.

- Some chronic illnesses can have a catastrophic effect on patients and their families, both financially (health insurance benefits often do not cover the costs) and emotionally. Self-help groups and other forms of counseling often ease these burdens.
- Rehabilitation has, in modern medicine, replaced warehousing of the physically and mentally disabled.
- Rehabilitative therapy, prosthetics, and mechanical aids often permit the disabled to be fully or partially self-sufficient. Often the hardest handicaps to overcome are the attitudes of others, the discrimination in education and employment. Many associations of the handicapped have sprung up to combat this discrimination.

13
DEATH AND DYING

WHAT'S AHEAD IN CHAPTER 13 What are the attitudes toward death and dying among your family and friends? In the larger community? Are attitudes changing? How do relatives and friends respond? In what ways is the family of the dying person affected? How can the effects of a long deathwatch be made less damaging? Can death be made easier, more comfortable, even meaningful, for patient and family? How? Should the dying person be told the truth? How can friends best help those in mourning? How is life defined? Death? What is brain death? Do individuals in various incurable states of suffering have an inalienable right to death? What must be considered in a decision to allow a patient to die, rather than to sustain him or her by extraordinary means, when there is no hope of meaningful life or when death is imminent anyway?

All but gone are the days when several generations of an extended family lived under the same roof. Then, when an elderly, or young, family member died, it happened at home, and everyone shared the grieving. Today, children are sheltered from death, often kept away from funerals, wakes, burials. Death is sterile even to adults, because dying usually takes place in a hospital, in an impersonal and mechanized way. The constant exposure to violent death on TV and in movies estranges us even further by increasing the unreality of death. The television victim will return next Thursday at 8 P.M. in another role.

It is no wonder that attitudes toward death in our society are confused and uneasy. It has been suggested that until recently death was in approximately the same position as sex was 50 years ago; it went on all the time, but nobody talked about it. Times have changed. Death has become a major topic, not only of conversation but of study, in colleges, universities, medical schools, and law schools.

ATTITUDES TOWARD DEATH AND DYING

When Marcel Proust lay on his deathbed, he suddenly ordered a servant to bring him a chapter from a manuscript which described the death agony of one of his characters. Explained Proust: "I have several retouchings to make here, now that I find myself in the same predicament."

Our feelings about death, unless we have had a close brush with it, are usually similarly fuzzy. No matter what our attitudes may be in a hypothetical discussion, they may suddenly become quite different when death approaches us or someone very close to us.

Attitudes among Health Professionals

The image of the physician as lifesaver is a mystique as comforting to physicians as it is to their patients. When they cannot save a life, and that happens often enough, doctors may feel cheated, resentful, defeated. They often erect a defense against death. The dying person becomes a nonperson. Visits by the physician may be few and perfunctory. Bedside manner becomes abrupt, conversation and explanations almost nonexistent. The attitude usually spreads to other hospital personnel, who find death equally difficult to confront. Nurses hardly ever drop in, food trays go undelivered and pain shots unadministered. Many patients report: "It's like I'm dead already."

Recently, however, the medical community, prodded by dying patients themselves or by their survivors, has taken note of the problem. Courses are being taught in hospitals and medical schools; conferences convene; specialists are trained in the field of death and dying: *thanatology (thana* = death + *ology* = study). Physicians and other medical personnel are coming to realize that they must do more than save lives; they must also comfort those whose lives they cannot save.

Attitudes of the Dying Patient

Dr. Elisabeth Kübler-Ross (*b*), an authority on death and dying, concluded, from a study of 500 patients over a span of 4 years at the University of Chicago, that patients who are told they have a fatal illness go through five stages: *denial* ("It can't be true; there must be some mistake!"); *anger* ("Why did it happen to me, dammit!"); *bargaining* ("God, if you let me live, I promise to be a good person, to go to church every Sunday."); *depression* ("I don't want to see anyone, I don't want to eat—just leave me alone."); and finally, *acceptance* ("I'm OK now . . . I'm at peace . . . I'm ready.") But Dr. Kübler-Ross warns that these stages may blur into one another; sometimes a patient slips back to an earlier stage instead of moving forward. Some authorities have criticized Kübler-Ross's position that patients move through all these stages and reach acceptance. Roy Branson, Ph.D., professor of bioethics, suggests that people who are dying prematurely have a right to be angry and that we cannot "force the dying to accept the unacceptable."

Sometimes the problem is sidestepped. Family, friends, doctors, nurses all pretend that the terminal patient is going to get well. But few patients are fooled. Feeling pretense will make things easier on their loved ones, they may participate in the game. But with feelings bottled up, visits with family are strained and uncomfortable. This is particularly frightening to the child patient. The illness seems so terrible that even those closest, the mother and father, avoid discussing it. Older patients are unable to put their business and personal lives in order, to say their goodbyes. Several studies have shown that most people would rather know the truth than agonize in uncertainty. Most psychiatrists now recommend that, except in unusual situations, the patient should be told the truth (Hackett, *c*).

Attitudes of Family and Friends

Often family and friends go through stages similar to those experienced by the dying patient. Dr. Kübler-Ross described a woman, standing outside the room where her child lay dying, who looked as though she were about to erupt:

> I asked, "Do you feel like screaming?"
>
> "Do you have a screaming room in the hospital?"
>
> "No, but we have a chapel."
>
> Then she really gave it to me: "In a chapel you have to be quiet and pray. I want to scream and yell at God, 'Why did you let this happen to my baby? Why did you let this happen to me?' " (*b*, p. 30)

This woman was obviously in the anger stage. Sometimes those facing the death of a loved one are unable to release their anger, and they withdraw instead. One woman, whose 11-year-old daughter was dying of leukemia, went to bed and stayed there, rejecting food, talking to no one, ignoring her other children. Her youngest child, craving his mother's attention, curled up at the foot of the bed and refused to leave. Finally, the mother had to be hospitalized, leaving the husband to serve as both father and mother to his dying daughter and two sons.

The critical illness of a spouse can be equally traumatic. John, 24, was teaching physical education and working toward his master's degree. Mary, 21, worked as a secretary to save money for the family they hoped soon to begin. Their world fell apart when John learned that he had incurable cancer. He lost confidence in himself, resented his dependence on Mary. Torn by grief, guilty about resenting her young husband's imminent "abandonment," anxious about her future, Mary began to experience psychosomatic pains in her head and chest. Bickering and bitterness replaced love.

Without help from compassionate medical personnel, from self-help groups of the type mentioned in Chapter 12, or from organizations such as Cancer Care (which assisted and counseled the two families described above), the survivors often become victims as well.

THE OCCASION OF DYING

Along with the current recognition that attitudes toward death need redefining is the realization that death is an occasion of special significance in the life cycle, one which requires special attention as to where, how, and with whom it will occur.

Where Death Takes Place

For some, there is no choice. Death is sudden. For many, however, dying becomes a long, drawn-out process. And where one spends one's last days on earth may be of considerable psychological importance. Those who remain in a hospital may have their lives prolonged by the latest in life support equipment and medical care. Those who die at home die in familiar surroundings, among loved ones, without the well-intentioned torments of heroic, short-term, life-prolonging measures. Some patients and their families prefer the first approach, others the second. Factors that must often be considered include:

1 *Financial resources* Sometimes hospital insurance benefits run out; and taking the patient home to die will relieve survivors of heavy future debt.

2 *Emotional and physical strain on family* Caring for a terminal patient at home can be difficult and demanding, and may be too taxing a family burden.

Linda Bartlett/Woodfin Camp & Assoc.

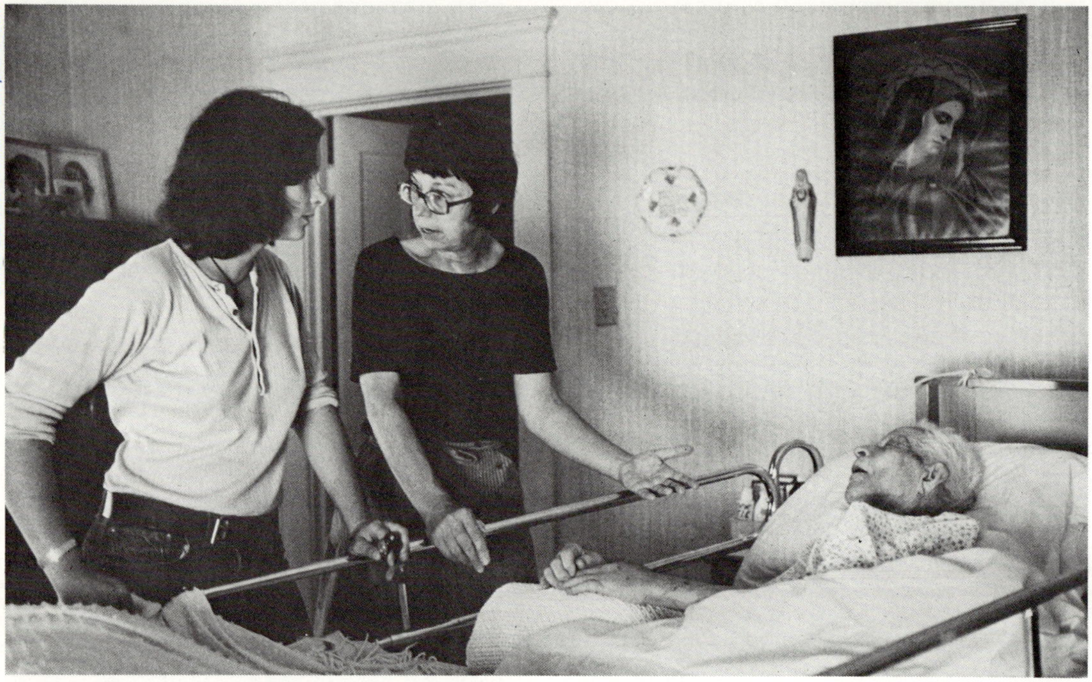

Linda Bartlett/Woodfin Camp & Assoc.

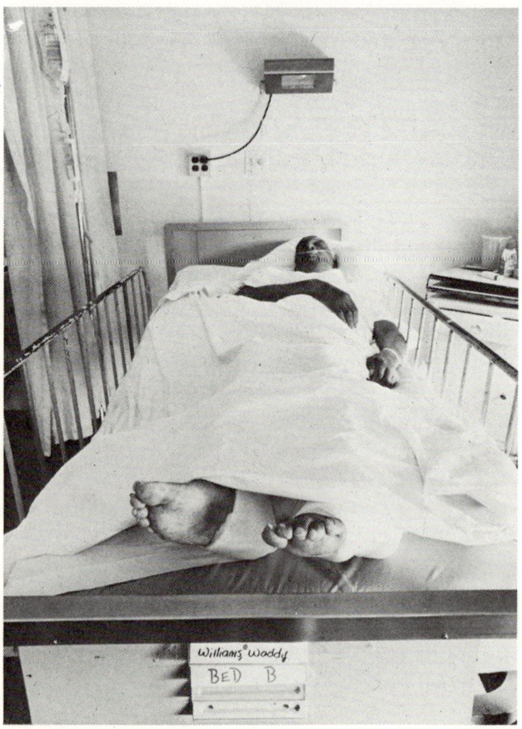

An important decision for terminally ill patients and their families involves the choice between care at home in familiar surroundings and treatment in a hospital, where sophisticated medical equipment is available.

3 *Space and facilities at home* Many small homes are unsuited to full medical care; nursing and equipment costs to convert a bedroom into a hospital room may be high.

4 *The patient's wishes* Some prefer to be alone; some may not want to be a burden or may not want to be remembered in their terminal condition; others may feel more in control of their final hours at home; may want to be surrounded by family and loved ones.

5 *The attitudes of family and patient toward use of extraordinary tactics for preserving life* Some prefer to die without the indignity of being hooked up to machines.

6 *The patient's condition* For those who are comatose, the surroundings make little difference.

One woman, Caroline Driver, whose husband was dying, wanted to have the best of medical care without sacrificing homelike environment. With grudging consent from hospital authorities, she moved into her husband's private hospital room and turned it into "home":

> I kept colorful bedspreads on both our beds and brought in four thick throw rugs for the floor. We lined one wall with photographs of the children playing, singing, being alive and free as we had taught them to be. Books began to pile up on the windowsill. The scratchy hospital radio gave way to our own FM-stereo from home. We even laid in some good white wine, kept it cool on top of the air-conditioner, and drank it from heirloom blue wine glasses from home. (p. 83)

Mrs. Driver brought her children in to visit, despite hospital rules. She cooked meals in an electric frypan (cooking by family members is common in Asian and African hospitals) and even threw a couple of parties. Not many people are forceful enough to do what Caroline Driver did. But development of hospices for the terminally ill in the United States, modeled after St. Christopher's Hospice in London, may offer a middle ground for those unwilling or unable to have the dying patient at home, yet disturbed by the impersonality of the typical hospital or nursing home. The hospice usually offers medical and nursing care to minimize pain and discomfort, but does not attempt to extend life mechanically. The atmosphere is relaxed and more homelike, with family members encouraged to visit and assist with nursing care. An embryonic "hospice at home" movement in the United States teams professionals and volunteers to offer nursing, psychological, and even household help to dying patients and their families.

The Role of Others at the Time of Death

Hospitals run on schedules. So while anxious family members sit on waiting room couches or at home, many persons die alone. But it does not have to be that way, says psychiatrist Thomas Hackett (*c*), who has treated many dying patients. He suggests the revival of the old-fashioned deathwatch, in which relatives and friends take turns staying at the patient's side around the clock, so that someone familiar is always close. If death seems imminent, other family members can be summoned. Hackett recalls one instance in which a gentle lady in her eighties lay dying after a massive stroke:

> Her large and loving family assembled on the late December day when her declining temperature and waning pulse had signaled that the end was near. Linking hands, with the snow falling outside the window, they sang Christmas carols for

"Seth died as we had often talked about—cuddled in our arms before a blazing fire in utter quiet and peace. We have such good feelings about the peace of that moment that it has been immeasurably easier to deal with this reality."

Seth, who died of leukemia when he was 19 months old, was part of a National Cancer Institute project designed to assist families who would prefer to care for their dying children at home. Though a nurse is on call 24 hours a day and a physician is available for consultation, the parents become the "primary care givers" for their child. The average cost of home care for 16 such children who died at home was $945. Comparable terminal care in a hospital would have cost $12,225. Ironically, many insurance policies cover the hospital costs but not home care, though sometimes its expenses can be negotiated for in advance. Project Director Dr. Ida Marie Martinson has found that the home care approach leaves parents better able to cope with and less guilty about the death of their child. (Brody, *d*, p. 20:3) her. At some point in the singing, she quietly died. [The memory of such an] appropriate and touching episode . . . is a wonderful solace. (p. 141)

Relating to the terminally ill Both close family and casual acquaintances often find it difficult to behave naturally with someone they know is dying. Yet the dying have a need for normal treatment. Hackett cautions against both "kid gloves" and the "premature burial" that deprives the patient of much-needed emotional support. Most patients want to discuss "what will happen when . . ." and family and friends unwilling to discuss these questions do them a disservice.

Involvement in patient care Involving the family in patient care not only assures better care in busy hospitals, but may also relieve the helpless feeling of many who must sit by and watch a loved one die. Support can be much more than emotional. Family members can help with feeding and other aspects of daily care, and can be trained in basic relaxation techniques, massage, and hypnotherapy to relieve anxiety and pain. Family participation can be dramatically effective. Dr. Hackett tells of a young woman with massive body burns who was considered a terminal case. Her husband, trained by a physician to hypnotize her, relieved her pain by 80 percent and contributed to her unexpected recovery.

Visualizing Death

What happens at the moment of death? No one knows for sure. Fear of death is thus fear of the unknown. Many patients fear that it will be painful, that it will be preceded by extreme disfiguration, loss of speech, or a vegetative state. Others have difficulty coming to terms with the idea of a world without them, of the disappearance of self (Glaser and Strauss). A major question unasked by many is, "Is there an afterlife?"

Dr. Kübler-Ross (*c*) proposes that her studies of patients who have clinically "died" and been resuscitated prove that there is. A typical report of such a patient is described by Dr. Kübler-Ross:

> The patient saw a nurse come in, take a look at her, and dash out. *Then she floated out of her body.* She floated a few feet above her body and watched her corpse in the bed. She was surprised at how pale she looked. She had this beautiful feeling of peace and equanimity. Then she watched the resuscitation team come in, and she described to me in minute detail who came into the room, what they did to her body, who behaved how. . . . She had no vital signs—no heartbeat, no blood pressure, no respiration. She had this urgent need to tell them to relax, take it easy, let go. . . . When she regained [consciousness], she was again lying in her hospital bed. (p. 68)

Other patients reported being met by an important next of kin who had died earlier, or by a religious figure such as Jesus or Mary. But though Dr. Kübler-Ross has come to believe that these are actual examples of what death is like, many scientists and others remain unconvinced by her evidence. More research will obviously be needed before it can be said with scientific certainty what happens after death.

GRIEF AND MOURNING

After death, grieving and mourning by survivors follow. Where death was expected and protracted, the mourning may have begun much earlier, and so grieving after death is less intense. Grieving after the death of a loved one is not only normal but necessary. The person who neither cries nor expresses some anger is the one most likely to run into trouble. Hackett suggests danger signs that indicate abnormal grief:

- *When grief is unduly prolonged* Normal grief usually lasts 4 to 12 weeks, but may exceed that for the death of a young child.

Eve Arnold/Magnum

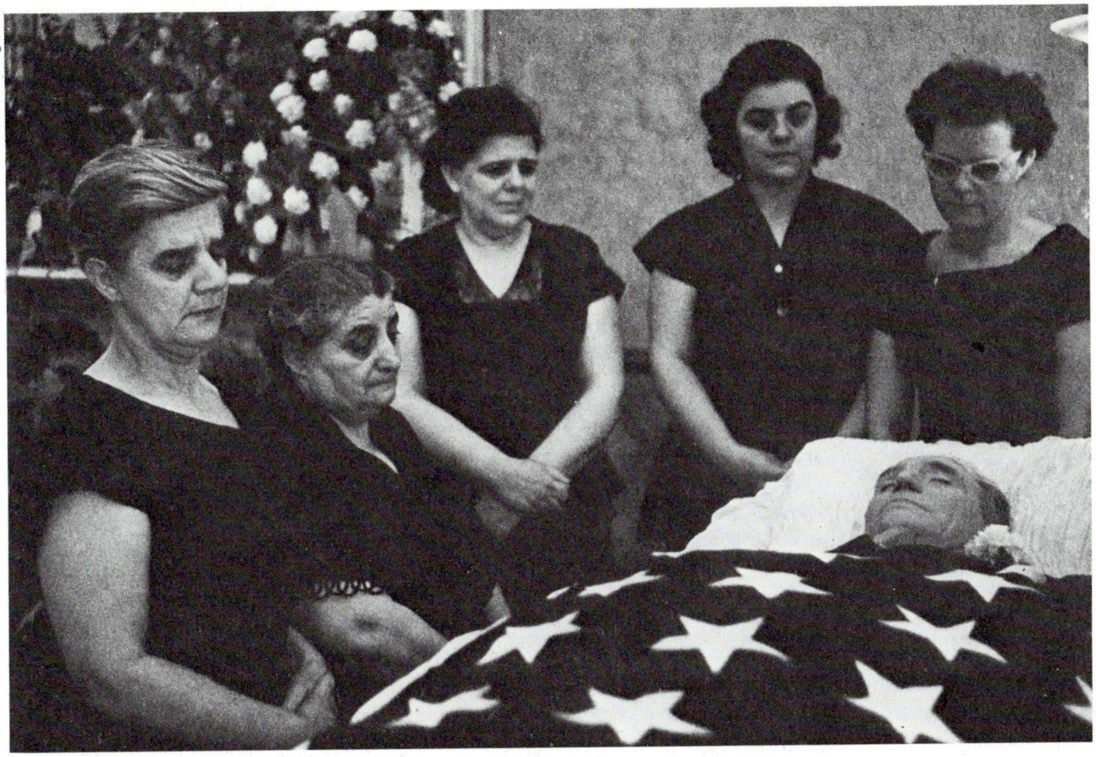

Grieving after the death of a loved one is not only normal but necessary.

- *When the death is denied* This occurs most often when death takes place far from home (during wartime, in an accident abroad) and the body is not viewed by the family, or during a catastrophe (earthquake or flood) when the body is not recovered.
- *When the bereaved exhibits false euphoria* Friends are shocked to see a person who has suffered a great loss bubbling with good humor. But this abnormal reaction is a form of denial, often followed by deep depression when the effort to deny finally crumbles.
- *When the person overreacts to someone else's troubles* Sometimes, for example, a mother registers little apparent emotion at the death of a child, but for years afterward cries uncontrollably whenever she hears of a child dying. The tears she sheds are, in fact, for her own lost child.
- *When the bereaved develops a symptom of the deceased* If a parent dies of a heart attack, the adult child may fear having a similar attack. Sometimes this fear evolves into an unhealthy hypochondria.
- *When the patient turns melancholy at certain times of the year* Sometimes the sorrow is unconsciously related to the time of death of a loved one, sometimes to an annual celebration formerly enjoyed with the deceased.

Persons exhibiting these symptoms should seek help from family physician, clergyman, counselor, or psychiatrist. During a normal period of grief, the best thing a friend can do is help the mourner grieve. Urging the bereaved to "keep a stiff upper lip" or "be brave" may lead to an unhealthful bottling up of emotion. Explains Hackett, "Unexpressed grief, like money in the bank, gathers interest with the passing of time" (*b*, pp. 97, 101).

THE RIGHT TO DIE

We take for granted the right to live, and our Constitution affirms it. But how absolute is that right? In an age when we can mechanically prolong life almost indefinitely, is there also a right to die? Do individuals on death's threshold, in great pain, or totally detached from the world, have the right to death? To understand the issues, we must first look at life and death.

Life and Death

What is life? Some see life as the opposite of death. Some describe both life and death as points along a biological line: we begin at life and end at death. Still others see life in terms of its positive attributes: Does a person have the ability to know, to sense what is happening, to relate to others? Some go still further and speak of a sense of personhood and dignity, and of the ability to enjoy life as essential to being truly alive.

Just what enjoying life means, of course, varies from one person to another. To some it means work, play, and love in all their fullness and nothing less; to others it may be enough to recognize a beloved wife sitting at a bedside, or to appreciate the difference between light and dark, heat and cold.

When is death? There are four commonly accepted entryways to death: heart, lungs, kidneys, brain. When any one of these organs ceases to function, death comes. In the past, when a person stopped breathing or had no pulse, death was declared to have occurred. But today we can keep the heart and lungs, and even the kidneys, operational almost indefinitely with the use of respirators, heart/lung machines, dialysis, pacemakers, and the like. Only the activities of the brain cannot be mechanically duplicated. Thus many physicians have come to believe that death should be announced at the moment of "brain death." Harvard University has developed these criteria for brain death: lack of spontaneous respiration; no response to pain (as when pricked with a pin); fixed, dilated pupils with no eye movement or blinking; no reflexes; a flat electroencephelogram (reading of brain waves) on separate tests 24 hours apart. Several states have adopted brain death as the official criterion for death; several others have legislation pending; a few have rejected the concept.

Between life and death Somewhere along the line between life and death, there is a gray area not easily defined, except perhaps as "living death" or "more dead than alive." In this category are persons in long-term incurable coma—people like Karen Anne Quinlan, whose case became known worldwide when in 1975 her parents sued to have her removed from a respirator and other apparatus so she could "die with dignity." In this category, too, are children born with severe brain damage, who "live" and die without ever having had a human relationship, without knowing, communicating, loving.

Mercy Killing

Euthanasia, or "mercy killing," probably as old as the Greek name it bears, has taken on new dimensions in our technological society. There are two basic forms of euthanasia: *passive*, allowing a person who is hopelessly ill and suffering to die painlessly by making no attempts to prolong life; and *active*, administering a fatal dose of a drug, or "pulling the plug" to hasten death. According to a Louis Harris poll (*b*), a substantial majority of Americans support passive euthanasia and a slightly smaller majority favor "pulling the

Opinions on Euthanasia

Between her wanting to die and her death, a terrible thing happened to her, to her husband, and to everyone who loved her. She became someone else, someone bereft of all the qualities that had made her what she was. I don't think she and those she left behind should have been thus robbed for the sake of mere biological continuance. . . . The place for a person to become a nonperson is not a hospital bed but a grave.

Tom Gallagher, writing on the death of his sister, p. 152

My sister suffered through three years of a particularly dreadful form of skin cancer which caused intense pain, drastically altered her appearance and, gradually, eroded her entire personality. Many times, visiting her at the hospital or at home, I felt that she might be better off dead, despite the grievous loss it would mean to me. She knew the nature of her illness; she knew that it was incurable. Yet, even the day before she died, . . . she asked me for her hand mirror and held it up while I brushed her hair. "Oh, dear," she sighed, "look how my hair is falling out. I'll have to arrange for scalp treatments soon." Drugs which would have ended her life were in her own medicine chest, but it was evidently *her* judgment to live as long as possible. Should I have substituted *my* judgment for hers?

. . . To me the concept of dignity-in-dying is inextricably bound up with moral and legal concepts which seek to preserve and protect the preciousness of life. Dignity can be attained by means which owe nothing to euthansia or to any other means of intervention, but everything to the inner spirit and inner strength of the individual.

Terry Morris, writing about her sister's death and in opposition to euthanasia, pp. 149–150

I've had to make a distinction between a semblance of life and life that can be considered meaningful.

One of my present patients suffered a severe stroke. . . . It's doubtful that he will ever come out of the deep coma. . . . But his wife comes to his bedside every day. She wants to have him alongside her until the last possible moment. His life remains meaningful to her, and therefore I must fight to preserve it.

The circumstances are different with another stroke victim. His condition had slowly deteriorated for 12 years before the stroke—after a bad fall . . . and his wife had devoted every day of those years to nursing him. When he recovered consciousness from his stroke, he told me he had nothing to live for. I talked this over with his wife and she agreed there would be no value to him or to her in keeping him under oxygen and applying other measures that might have kept him alive but helpless for an unpredictable time. We simply transferred him from the hospital to a nursing home, where he soon died peacefully.

Walter Sackett, Jr., M.D., crusader for death with dignity, p. 93

I've declined to accept a role as executioner and have acted instead on the opposing principle [to the "right to die"]—"the patient's right to live." . . . [The patient's] wish to die . . . is often due more to severe depression than to a truly terminal condition. In the face of such a possibility, is the doctor to abandon his traditional mission and let the patient prescribe the ultimate treatment? Clinging to hope is our best insurance against overlooking a cure that actually exists or may be discovered. . . . If we accept the thesis that one individual can decide whether to prolong another's life, then the way is open to arbitrary decisions about every aspect of human existence.

Franklin H. Epstein, M.D., professor of medicine at Harvard Medical School, p. 97

plug," removing all life support services, for the hopelessly ill. When is euthanasia most commonly considered?

Defective newborns Every year, some 200,000 babies are born in the United States with serious defects. Many die in spite of anything medical science can do. Recently physicians have admitted that many more die (estimates range from 2000 to 80,000 annually) because medical care has been withheld. This is most often done when the prognosis for a meaningful life appears hopeless. Of course, this is a tricky decision, since physicians cannot always predict when treatment will save an infant for a happy, useful life, or when such treatment will keep a child only technically "alive."

Saving infants with serious hereditary disorders poses further questions. What about the boy with hemophilia who survives to adulthood thanks to hundreds of blood transfusions and costly medication, marries, fathers a daughter who carries the disease to her four sons? Or the girl with PKU (phenylketonuria) who reaches adulthood without becoming retarded because of modern diagnosis and treatment, but who has three retarded children of her own because of her elevated blood phenylalanine levels?

Human "vegetables" They cannot walk, talk, think, swallow. Whether the person is a newborn or an 80-year-old, the questions are the same. Is this life? Should it continue? Some believe not. When the daughter of Queen Elizabeth's cousin deteriorated to that state—brain three-quarters destroyed, totally blind and deaf, fed through a tube in the nose—the mother fed some barbituarates in milk through the tube, drop by drop, then wrapped the child gently in a blanket and allowed her to die peacefully.

The hopeless, the dying The question here is, do we really know when a case is hopeless? Everyone has heard stories of miraculous recoveries. The parents of 4-year-old Laurie were told that their comatose child was dying, and perhaps they should just let her go quietly. But they insisted treatment be continued; a new drug was tried, and after 39 terrible days, little Laurie rallied, then recovered entirely. A British youth critically injured in an automobile accident, prognosis hopeless, today holds a job as an airline reservations clerk and gets about successfully in a wheelchair.

These are rare exceptions. Should life for all "hopeless" patients be prolonged and nurtured indefinitely on the one-in-a-million chance that their miracle, too, will happen?

The suffering To some, a life of pain is worse than death. A young veteran whose facial nerves, damaged in a heroic effort to save a helicopter pilot in Vietnam, caused him excruciating pain finally ended his misery in suicide. A father of young children, who was blind and also suffered from diabetes, thyroid disease, and kidney disorder, took himself off a kidney dialysis machine that kept him alive because he preferred certain death to certain agony.

Who Should Decide?

A JAMA editorial stated in 1974:

> The cessation of the employment of extraordinary means to prolong the life of the body when there is irrefutable evidence that biological death is imminent is the decision of the patient and/or his immediate family. The advice and judgment of the physician should be freely available to the patient and/or his immediate family. (O'Donnell, p. 501)[1]

When patients are alert enough to make such decisions, most would agree they should, but not without physican input. A person wracked with pain may "want to die," but the physician may know that the pain is

[1]A 1977 Massachusetts court decision, among others, ruled the decision should be made by the courts.

TO MY FAMILY, MY PHYSICIAN, MY LAWYER, MY CLERGYMAN
TO ANY MEDICAL FACILITY IN WHOSE CARE I HAPPEN TO BE
TO ANY INDIVIDUAL WHO MAY BECOME RESPONSIBLE FOR MY HEALTH, WELFARE OR AFFAIRS

Death is as much a reality as birth, growth, maturity and old age—it is the one certainty of life. If the time comes when I, ____________________________ can no longer take part in decisions for my own future, let this statement stand as an expression of my wishes, while I am still of sound mind.

If the situation should arise in which there is no reasonable expectation of my recovery from physical or mental disability, I request that I be allowed to die and not be kept alive by artificial means or "heroic measures". I do not fear death itself as much as the indignities of deterioration, dependence and hopeless pain. I, therefore, ask that medication be mercifully administered to me to alleviate suffering even though this may hasten the moment of death.

This request is made after careful consideration. I hope you who care for me will feel morally bound to follow its mandate. I recognize that this appears to place a heavy responsibility upon you, but it is with the intention of relieving you of such responsibility and of placing it upon myself in accordance with my strong convictions, that this statement is made.

Signed ____________________

Date ____________________

Witness ____________________

Witness ____________________

Copies of this request have been given to ____________________

FIGURE 13.1 The Living Will. A living will is available from CONCERN FOR DYING, 250 West 57th Street, New York, NY 10019. [*Reprinted with permission of CONCERN FOR DYING.*]

temporary, and the patient will recover. When the patient is an unconscious or incompetent adult or child, the question becomes more difficult still. Thousands of adults have avoided finding themselves at some future time in a position where they cannot themselves make such a decision by making a "living will." The document states that these persons, if terminally ill, do not wish to have their lives prolonged by extraordinary means (See Figure 13.1).

Though advocates in at least 20 states have tried, only in California has legislation been passed defining the right to die. The California law, like the living will, puts the ultimate decision in the hands of the patient; but it can only be signed by someone already incurably ill, and it must be signed before two witnesses, neither of whom can be a relative or beneficiary of the patient, a physician, or a member of the hospital staff. The law frees the physician of any liability in a death resulting from the request and forbids insurance companies to withhold life insurance payments by classifying such deaths as suicide. The removal of life supports can only be carried out under this law when "incurable injury, disease or illness certified to be a terminal condition by two physicians" is present, where "the application of life-sustaining procedures would serve only to artificially prolong the moment of . . . death," and where "death is imminent whether or not life-sustaining procedures are utilized."

Guidelines for Euthanasia

At present; there are no formal guidelines to help persons who are faced with a decision on euthanasia, especially when the patient is unable to share in that decision. Richard A. McCormick of the Kennedy Center for Bioethics at Georgetown University suggests that needed guidelines should be neither too narrow nor too broad:

> A guideline is not a sliderule that makes the decision. It is far less than that. But it is far more than the concrete decision of the parents and physician, however seriously and conscientiously this is made. It is more like a light in a room, a light that allows the individual objects to be seen in the fullness of their context. (p. 173)

Many considerations come into play. These include some we have already discussed (the quality of life that will be available to the patient and the chance for recovery) as well as compassion for the misery of the patient, the emotional strain on all the persons involved, the financial burden on families and the community (a respirator can cost $500 a day, costs in a premature baby nursery can run as much as $30,000 per infant), loss of resources and finances that could benefit others in the community or the family, and the possible long-term effects on the family.

The Ethical Consequences of Euthanasia

Does an easy acceptance of euthanasia lead to too easy an acceptance of taking a life? Does it lead to an attitude like that of the Nazis, who killed the handicapped, the senile, and others deemed unfit to live? Will it lead to cutting lives short because of the costs, or for earlier inheritance?

Will, on the other hand, a rejection of euthanasia and an all-out effort to preserve life, any kind of life, lead to a crippling of nature's plan for natural selection? Instead of the natural weeding-out process that keeps a species strong, there could be a perpetuation of genetic defects. Will such defects become prevalent, even widespread?

These are not easy questions to answer, but they must be asked. And they must be explored if individuals and the community are to make sound and informed decisions about the extension and termination of life.

LOOKING BACK

REVIEWING CONCEPTS IN CHAPTER 13

- After years of being hidden away in sterile hospital rooms, death has become a subject of discussion. The aim is to ease the experience of dying, both for the patient and for his or her loved ones.
- It has been suggested that patients who know they are going to die go through five stages: denial, anger, bargaining, depression, and acceptance. The idea is controversial.
- Loved ones, too, go through a crisis. Without supportive therapy, families awaiting a death often collapse under the strain.
- Where death should take place is often a major issue today, for both financial and emotional reasons.
- Dying patients usually suspect the truth and, most often, want to know. They want to be treated honestly and normally.
- Grief and mourning are normal and necessary. Absence of mourning or unduly prolonged mourning may signal emotional problems.
- There are many ways to determine death. Brain death is an increasingly accepted criterion.
- The ability of medical science to prolong life, sometimes almost indefinitely, has led to the question of the right of the individual to "death with dignity."
- Many physicians and laypeople support the concept of allowing a patient to die when there is no hope of meaningful life. Others oppose this position.
- In making such a decision, many considerations, both personal and social, come into play.

IV

DRUGS: BOON OR BANE?

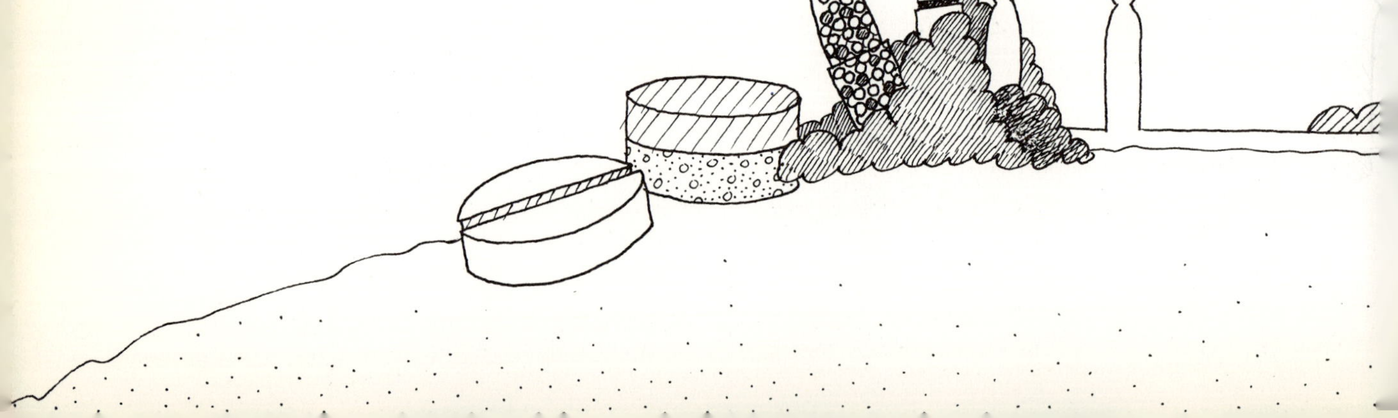

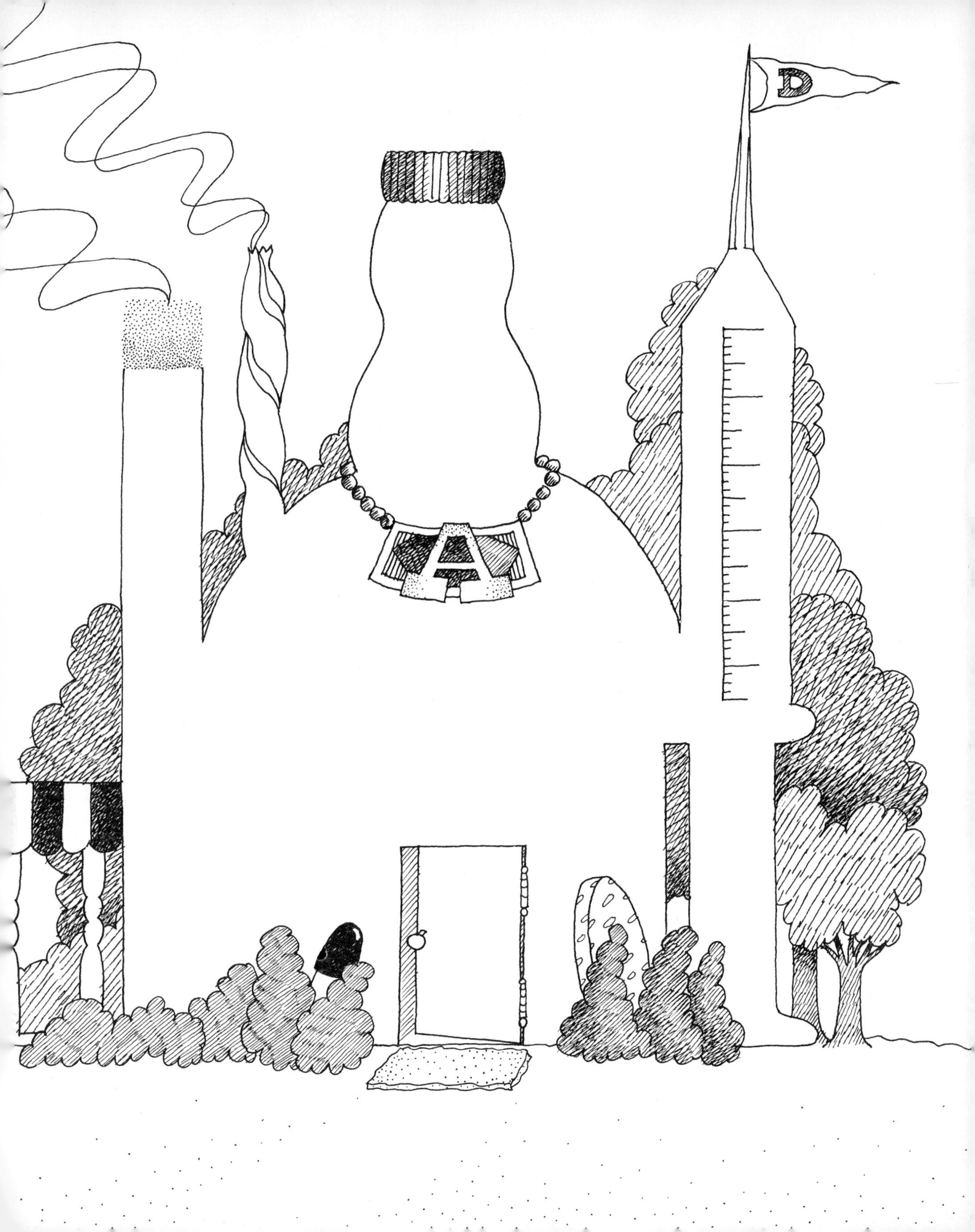
D
A

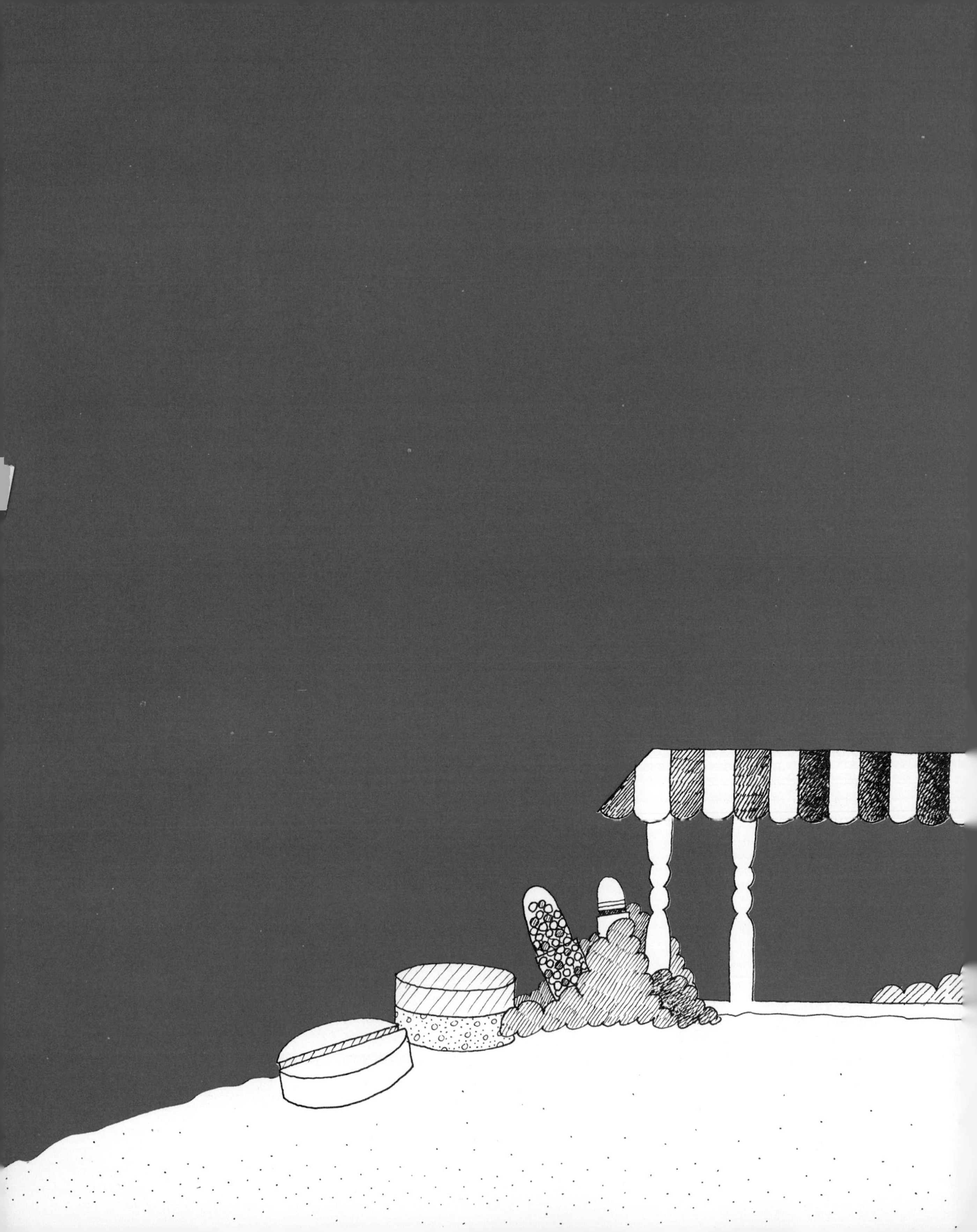

14 DRUGS AND THEIR SAFE USE

WHAT'S AHEAD IN CHAPTER 14 What roles do drugs play in human lives? Is their role positive or negative? Is there such a thing as a "safe" drug? What factors determine an individual's response to a particular drug? What kinds of bad or "adverse" reactions to drugs are common? How is the risk-benefit theory employed in drug-use decisions? How might a physician or a layperson "misuse" drugs? How do "natural" and "synthetic" drugs compare? Who has the responsibility for wise use of drugs for medical purposes? How does an informed consumer make decisions about buying nonprescription drugs? What questions should you ask the prescribing doctor about medications you are to take? What is the best policy when it comes to stocking a medicine chest in the home or dormitory? What safety rules for taking drugs reduce risks? How can the pharmacist help to make drug use safer?

Ancient peoples had no Food and Drug Administration to tell them which of their drugs were safe and which were not. Drug use was mostly trial and a great deal of error. They sampled ground snakeskins, flowers, animal entrails, herbs, roots, leaves, fermented fruits and grains, and other natural substances in potions and poultices, hoping to cure or control physical and mental illnesses, or to comfort the sick when cure seemed impossi-

Half the modern drugs could well be thrown out the window, except that the birds might eat them.
Martin H. Fischer (1879–1962)

ble. If a patient died or recovered, they could not be sure whether it was because of the drug or in spite of it.

FRIENDS AND FOES

These ancient users of drugs discovered that drugs could be blight as well as blessing. Moderns have found the same thing. Dana L. Farnsworth, M.D., chairman of the nonprofit organization, Medicine in the Public Interest, writes:

> The use of drugs will always be accompanied by some dangers, but the ideal goal is learning how to use them as safely as possible, keeping the risk factors low. . . . [Then] their contribution to the relief of human suffering is incalculable. (*d*, p. 5)

Advances in pharmacology have already eased human suffering immensely, reducing death and pain from a wide range of diseases—from polio to pneumonia, high blood pressure to asthma, cancer to mental illness. But the advent of "new and better" medications has not been without cost: There are published estimates of 60,000 to 140,000 annual deaths in the United States from adverse drug reactions (ADRs). While these are thought by many scientists to be exaggerated statistical miscalculations, many deaths from the use and misuse of drugs do occur daily.

The reason is that *no* biologically active substance (no substance that affects living things) is entirely safe. All reach toxic (harmful, but not necessarily deadly) levels at some point. Many cause allergic reactions and other side effects. Even the "common everyday aspirin," consumed by Americans at the rate of more than 120 million five-grain doses a day, can be hazardous.

Aspirin causes an allergic reaction in about 1 in every 10,000 people. It can aggravate some forms of asthma and can increase the risk of excessive bleeding during childbirth, in persons with ulcers, and in some others. Recent evidence indicates it may interfere with the body's defenses against disease, contribute to infertility in males, prolong labor (putting newborns at greater risk), and even increase the spread of cold germs.

When we realize that a drug taken as casually as aspirin presents risks, when we examine the small-print list of possible side effects in a typical medical journal advertisement, when we recognize that it has been estimated that from 6000 to 14,000 people[1] in the United States die each year from an allergic reation to some form of the "wonder drug" penicillin, it becomes clear that drugs must be handled with care as well as appreciation.

Factors Influencing Drug Effects

Chemically, you are not the same person today you were yesterday or will be tomorrow; your reaction to a drug may differ from one day to the next. As many as 32 different factors can influence that reaction, including: *age* (the very young and the elderly are most susceptible to adverse drug reactions), *size and weight* (a tablet prescribed for a 110-pound woman might be ineffective for her 210-pound husband), *race* (alcohol acts differently on different racial groups), *nutritional status, sex, physical condition, allergy proneness, sensitivity*, and any *tolerance* that has been developed to particular drugs. *Pregnancy* may also be a factor in drug response, as will *other drugs or medications* that are being taken.

[1]The Pharmaceutical Manufacturers Association estimates 6000 to 10,000 deaths a year. Other estimates range up to 14,000 (Edelson).

Ken Heyman

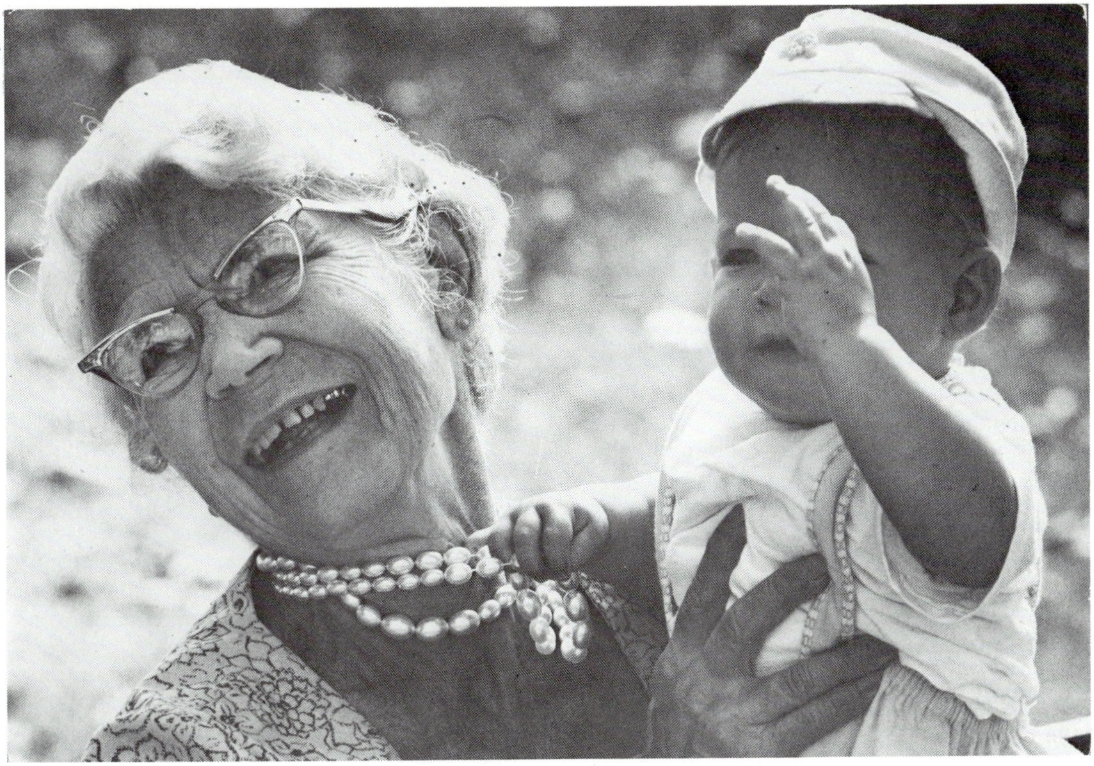

Age is an important factor in drug response. The very young and the elderly are most susceptible to adverse reactions.

Perhaps most significant of all are *mood and expectation.* Some investigators have found that almost 1 of every 3 persons given a placebo (a medication with no active ingredients) for pain enjoys relief (Bonica). It is much the same with psychoactive drugs, those that affect the mind. Reese Jones experimented with experienced marijuana smokers in their usual setting, with lights, music, and fellowship just right. The only variation was the "marijuana," which was a substitute with no active ingredients. Unaware, the smokers enjoyed the experience, reported their usual highs, and, on a scale of 0 to 100, rated the placebo pot only a few points lower than they rated average marijuana.

The drug itself—its *potency or strength, age, quality,* and *purity*—also affects how people will react to it. So do the *time of day* the drug is taken and *how it is administered.* (See Figure 14.1.) Some drugs work best on an empty stomach; others following food; still others, like aspirin, must be taken with a full glass of liquid. Some react badly with certain foods.

It is easy to see, then, that drug use must be individualized to fit patient, illness, and drug. Passing pills around or using someone else's medication can be hazardous. There is risk, too, in failure to follow the doctor's instructions: doubling the prescribed dose or discontinuing it earlier than instructed (for example, before an antibiotic has a chance to finish off target bacteria).

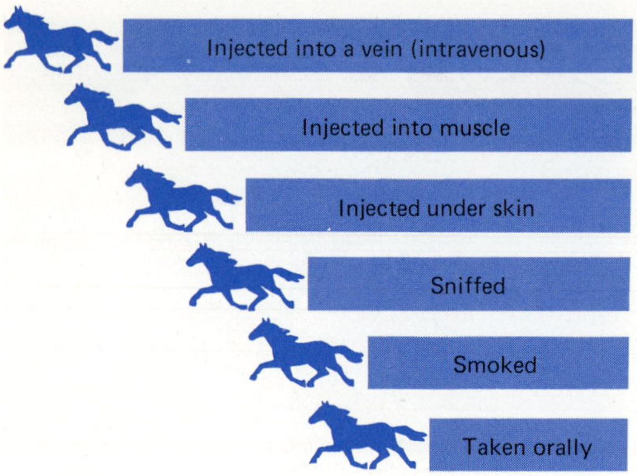

FIGURE 14.1 Relative speed with which drugs enter the bloodstream. The actual time varies depending upon the drug and other factors.

Adverse Drug Reactions

Toxic reactions A harmful reaction is often due to an exaggeration of the known and desired action of a drug. Barbiturates are meant to depress the central nervous system. An overdose could depress it too much and cause unconsciousness, even coma and death. A toxic reaction may also occur from repeated small doses of a drug with slow detoxification qualities; the body cannot break down the substance as quickly as it is ingested, and thus it accumulates in the system. There is currently a debate among medical authorities about whether marijuana is such a drug. Arsenic definitely is. Murder mystery fans are familiar with the plot in which the villain slowly poisons a wealthy aunt by stirring minute amounts of arsenic into her bedtime hot chocolate.

Side effects Drugs rarely have only one action. An antihistamine taken for hay fever may also cause drowsiness. Most drugs produce such side effects, but they are often so mild they go unnoticed. If they are severe, the dosage may be reduced or another drug substituted. Any physical or psychological symptom that appears concurrently with the use of a drug should be reported to a physician.

Allergic reactions Sometimes the body overreacts in defense against a drug to which it has been sensitized earlier. This allergic response is not dose-related and may occur within minutes of contact or be delayed for 7 to 14 days. Symptoms often disappear when the drug is discontinued, though in the case of long-acting or time-release medications they may hang on. (See Table 14.1.)

Adverse reactions of unknown origin The mechanisms triggering 30 to 40 percent of all ADRs are unknown. The AMA and the Food and Drug Administration (FDA) are cooperating to obtain more data through a drug reaction early warning system. If many doctors or hospitals suddenly report a particular adverse reaction with a drug, a pattern can be spotted quickly.

Polypharmacy When two or more drugs are administered to a patient at the same time, they may have an *antagonistic* effect, blocking each other out (1 + 1 = 0). Or they could

TABLE 14.1 Allergic reactions to drugs

REACTION	SYMPTOMS
Anaphylaxis	Reddening, labored breathing, shock, occasionally death
Serum sickness	Hivelike eruptions, swelling, enlarged lymph nodes, joint pain, fever, weakness
Contact dermatitis	Eczema or inflammation of the skin resulting from contact with drug or medication
Other reactions	Asthma, fever, liver damage, inflammation of heart muscle, other coronary effects

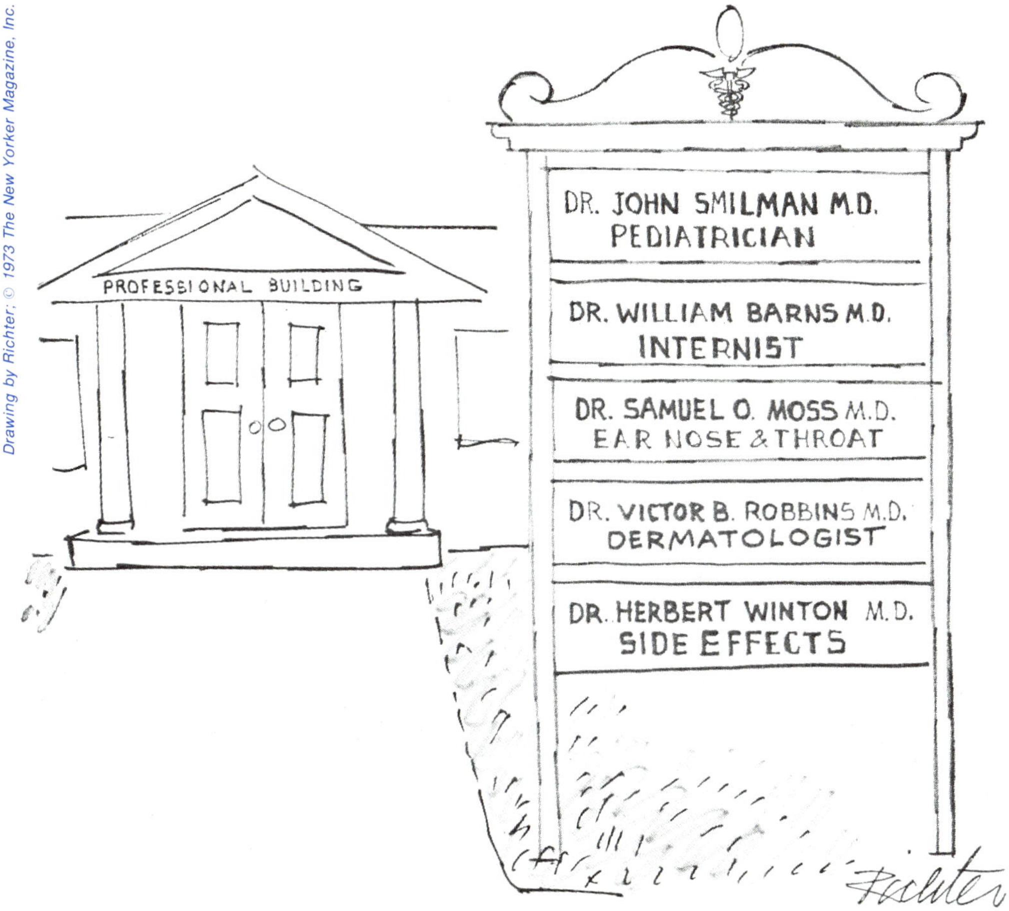
PROFESSIONAL BUILDING
DR. JOHN SMILMAN M.D.
PEDIATRICIAN
DR. WILLIAM BARNS M.D.
INTERNIST
DR. SAMUEL O. MOSS M.D.
EAR NOSE & THROAT
DR. VICTOR B. ROBBINS M.D.
DERMATOLOGIST
DR. HERBERT WINTON M.D.
SIDE EFFECTS
Richter

have a *potentiating synergistic* effect, an effect stronger than either one alone would produce (1 + 1 = 3). Certain drugs, each relatively safe in moderate doses, can become lethal when combined—sleeping pills and alcohol, for example.

Psychological drug reactions Subtle or very obvious personality changes (depression, hyperactivity, aggressiveness) may occur temporarily even with the use of drugs that are not basically psychoactive (mind-affecting). Severe psychological symptoms should be reported to the physician. Physical or psychological dependence (discussed under drug abuse in Chapter 15) is a distinct danger accompanying use of psychoactive drugs.

Drugs can also cause a paradoxical or reverse reaction in some individuals. Many hyperactive children, for example, are calmed rather than stimulated by amphetamines.

USING DRUGS SAFELY

The possible adverse effects of drugs so alarm some people that they adamantly refuse to take them—even an aspirin for headache or penicillin for strep throat. They take almost a moral position: Drugs are bad. At the other extreme are those who believe a little pill will solve any problem, cure anything. They take drugs for a sniffle, to stay awake, or to fall asleep. But there is another way to think about drugs: weighing risk against benefit.

The Risk-Benefit Theory

Are the risks of a particular drug (and you have seen there are risks with *every* drug, including aspirin) worth the benefits of using it? This question is asked by the physician prescribing tetracycline (a drug that can cause diarrhea and other side effects) for acne and by the cancer specialist prescribing methotrexate (a drug so strong it can kill the patient) for cancer. It is asked by the health-activated layperson who is considering taking an aspirin, smoking a cigarette or a joint, having another drink, or using somebody else's sleeping pills.

Steps can, of course, be taken to increase benefits and reduce risks. The physician prescribing lithium for a depressed patient reduces the risks by carefully monitoring the response to the drug, and enhances the benefits by giving the patient psychotherapy along with the drug. A person who decides to use a recreational drug may decrease the risks by using one that is legal, by limiting dosage, and by not driving while under the influence of the drug.

The use of hexachlorophene is an excellent example of the careful weighing of benefit versus risk. An antigerm cleansing agent, it had been used in hospitals for many years to prevent deadly staphylococcal and other infections. Then came reports linking it to possible brain tissue damage in infants. A strict curtailment of use was ordered by the FDA in September 1972. That, however, brought a sixfold increase in the incidence of staph epidemics in hospital nurseries, some resulting in infant deaths. The risk of hexachlorophene use was high, but so was the benefit. Officials sought to alter the balance. They reduced the risk by working out a sensible compromise: a modified-use plan which caused no apparent damage to infants, but blocked staph epidemics.

Use and Misuse

If we follow risk-benefit theory, we can say there are times when drugs *must* be used (when benefit clearly outweighs risk), times when they *probably should not* be used (when benefits appear smaller than risk), and times when they *should definitely not* be used (when risk is considerable and the benefit small or nonexistent). Of course, because of the limits of our knowledge, there are times when physician and patient must take a calculated gamble.

Sometimes intelligent decision making is not employed. A drug is prescribed for the convenience of the physician or patient, or to placate a patient who "wants something." The result may be the *misuse* of drugs. Using drugs to mask symptoms so that they go unnoticed and untreated (for example, using a hemorrhoid preparation for rectal bleeding instead of seeing a doctor about what might be a serious condition) is another form of misuse. So is *overuse*. Studies indicate that 49 percent of patients who see their physicians for colds are given antibiotics (Simmons and Stolley).[2] Yet these drugs have *no effect on the cold virus*, or any other virus, and the potential for allergic reactions (an estimated 15 percent of the population are allergic) and other adverse responses to them is great. In addition, overuse has led to the development of strains of microbes resistant to the drugs and to a disruption of the microbiological environment that can have serious consequences.

Natural versus Synthetic Drugs

Some assume that "natural" drugs and medicines, such as herbs, roots, teas, and their derivatives, are safe to take, while "synthetic"

[2]A culture of exudate from throat or nose will tell whether infection has progressed to bacterial and antibiotics are needed.

medications are less beneficial, even dangerous. There is no truth to this assumption. Synthetic penicillin produced in the laboratory is identical down to the last atom, to "natural" penicillin extracted from a mold. Natural and synthetic vitamin C are likewise identical. In some instances, however, the natural form of a drug is contaminated by extraneous substances that can produce unwanted side effects. The purer, synthetic form may thus be safer.

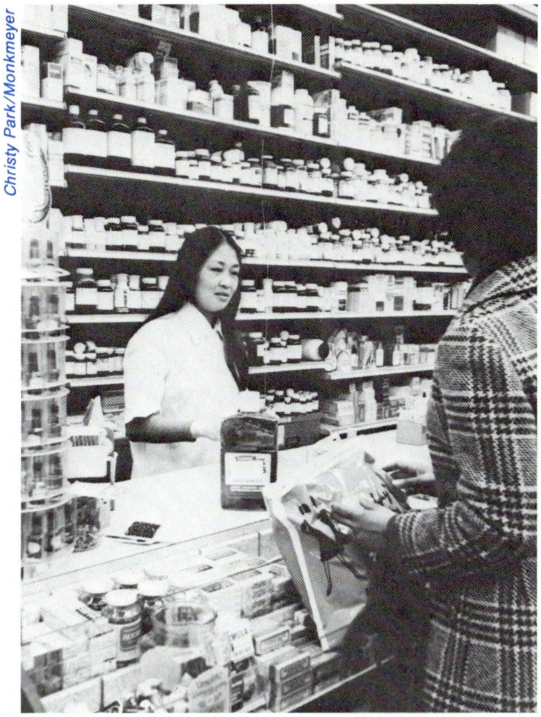

Christy Park/Monkmeyer

Activated health consumers see themselves as ultimately responsible for their own bodies and well-being, and thus for the safe use of the wide variety of medications and other pharmaceuticals available.

Whose Responsibility?

In the use of recreational and nonprescription drugs, the individual assumes full personal responsibility, within limits drawn by FDA and government legislation. With prescribed drugs, the division of responsibility is not so sharply defined. Legally, liability is the physician's and the drug company's. But activated health consumers see themselves as ultimately responsible for their own bodies and well-being. They know the names, purposes, and effects of any drugs they are taking; keep track of adverse reactions; inform physicians about such reactions and about other drugs they are taking; and may even refuse to take a particular medication because of possible side effects.

DRUGS AND THE HEALTH CONSUMER

Americans spent $9.6 billion on tranquilizers, antibiotics, birth control pills, and other prescription drugs in 1977, more than double what was spent in 1963. They bought $4.4 billion worth of pain relievers, antiacids, cold tablets, and other packaged nonprescription medications (Drug Topics). Often they did not know enough about the products to weigh risk against benefit.

The Drug Persuaders

The Council on Economic Priorities estimates that, in 1972, the drug industry dispensed about $1 billion on promotion to persuade physicians and institutions to buy their products. Much of that went to "detail men," making rounds of doctors' offices in a person-to-person sales effort. Hundreds of millions more are spent annually to advertise over-the-counter (OTC) drugs to the public, often in a style that has been likened by *Consumer's Union* to that of the medicine show huckster peddling snake oil.

When ads are blatantly dishonest or misleading, the FTC will demand they be withdrawn and sometimes will insist upon "correction" ads. But the message has already been spread and believed. A 1972 FDA survey found 38 percent of respondents naively believed that advertisements about medications

The Bettmann Archive

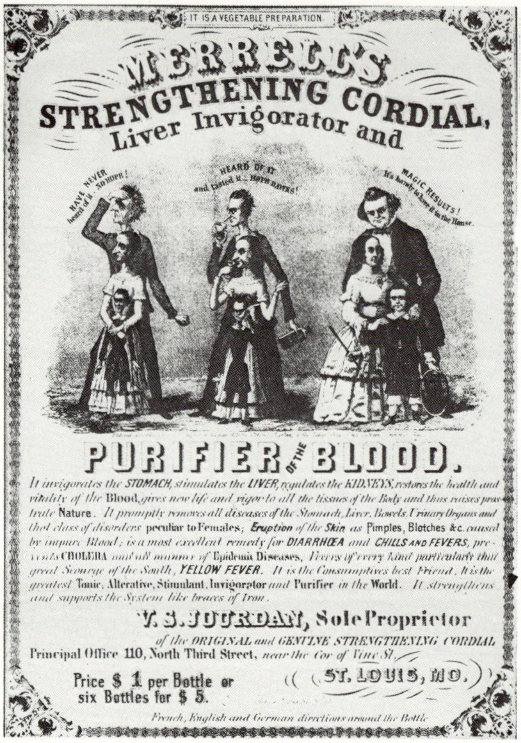

The Bettman Archive

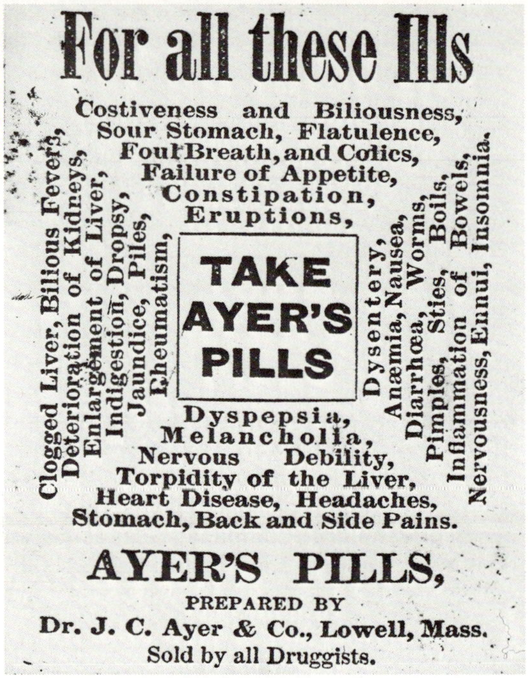

Unlike nineteenth-century advertisements for drugs, modern advertising is subject to FDA monitoring; however, the health consumer cannot rely on sales pitches alone for accurate information on drugs and their use.

and health aids "must be true or they wouldn't be allowed to say them." Some health advertising skillfully walks the FDA tightrope. It takes an alert health consumer to recognize this sly "weasel-wording." For example, how would you evaluate such lines as: "Tests showed no product performed better than product X" or "Product Y may help to relieve the itching and burning temporarily" or "Wonder drug! Increases energy! Improves sexuality! Extends lifespan! Improves learning!"?

Advertising is a subtle form of health education. Every TV viewer knows where the sinuses are located and how they "drain," and how aspirin dissolves in the stomach. But because advertising aims more at selling than telling, it is a highly unreliable form of education. Intelligent health consumers will turn instead to their own physicians, well-informed pharmacists, authoritative books and magazine articles, and increasingly available health education courses, in schools, hospitals, doctors' offices, medical groups, and community centers, for their health information.

Buying Nonprescription Drugs

Drugs which may be sold OTC without a prescription, also called *proprietary drugs*, are generally less potent than prescription drugs; some, in fact, are too weak to be effective (Dretchen). They can be purchased

HEALTH CONSUMER TIP

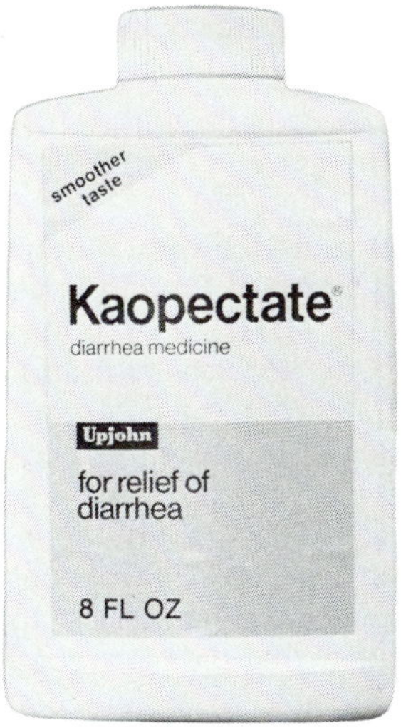

KAOPECTATE

The appropriate dose should be taken after each bowel movement, or as required — When to take medication

Dosage for relief of diarrhea:
Adults -- 4 to 8 tablespoonfuls etc. — How much to take

Shake well before each use
Protect from freezing
Store at room temperature
Keep all medications out of the reach of children — Care and storage information

Expires Aug. 1, 1980 — Do not use after this date

SINUTAB

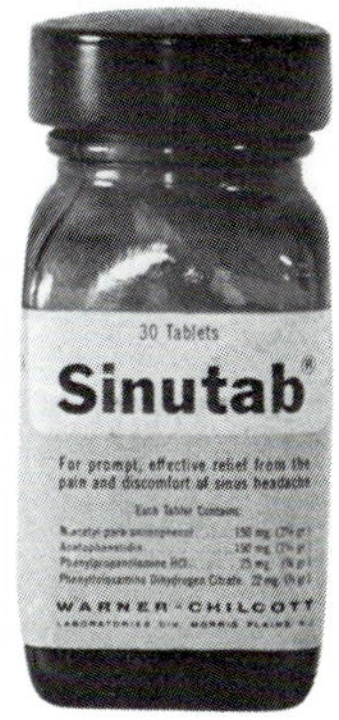

Warning: Not to be taken by persons with thyroid disease, high blood pressure, or diabetes except on medical advice. — Warnings about who should not use preparation

If drowsiness occurs, do not drive or operate machinery. — Warnings about possible side effects

If symptoms persist for more than ten days consult your physician. — Limits on self-medicating

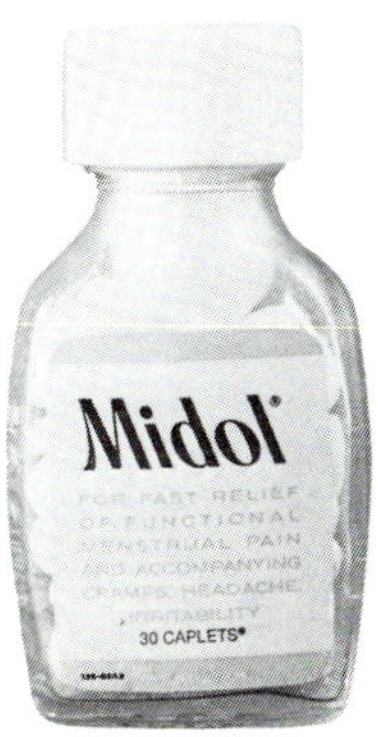

MIDOL

Each tablet contains: aspirin 454 mg cinnamedrine hydrochloride 14.9 mg, and caffeine 32.4 mg — Check label for ingredients to which you may be allergic or sensitive (e.g., aspirin or caffeine)

FIGURE 14.2 What medicine labels can tell you.

without a prescription because they are also potentially less harmful. But, like any foreign substance entering the body, they are not totally harmless. Loopholes in drug laws have allowed many products that have not been proven to be both safe[3] and effective to remain on the market, though efforts are now under way to eliminate such products.

Until these efforts succeed, the consumer will continue to face a bewildering display of products making dramatic and conflicting claims. Many authorities suggest ignoring the alluring promises and trying simple, reliable home remedies for minor ills first: hot saltwater gargles for sore throats; steam inhalation for a cough; hot soup or tea with honey and lemon for upper respiratory infections; a brief rice and banana diet for diarrhea; and prunes and bran for constipation (see Appendix). If medication seems necessary, start with the simplest; the fewer ingredients in a medication, the fewer chances for adverse drug reaction.

Buying Prescription Drugs

A prescription drug is one dispensed by a licensed pharmacist on order of a licensed practitioner for a clinically justified purpose, ideally with full patient understanding of risk-benefit potential. Until the mid-1970s, the medical-pharmaceutical mystique made prescription drugs probably the only major consumer product on the market for which there was no convenient way to comparison-shop. Most states prohibited all advertising, or even listing, of prescription drug prices. These often varied dramatically from store to store. Consumers were obliged to purchase the brand-name drug prescribed by their physicians, even if a comparable and less expensive one was available.

Today, however, laws are changing in many states. Price advertising is permitted, and in some states, price posting in drugstores is mandatory, permitting the consumer to compare before buying. The much more complex subject of brand-name drugs, compared with generics of lesser cost, is still somewhat cloudy. To understand it, it is important to know what is meant by generic drugs.

Generic versus trade-name drugs When a giant pharmaceutical firm like Squibb develops and patents a drug, the new product is assigned a generic name to classify it and a trade name to market it. When the company's exclusive 14-year manufacturing rights on its patented formula expire, smaller drug firms hasten to produce chemical copies, apparently identical in almost every way except high price—which is possible because the small firms have had a free ride on costly research, development, and promotion costs.

On the surface, the issue seems simple. Consumers ought to be able to purchase the less costly generic product. But, in reality, two drugs that appear identical chemically will not necessarily work exactly the same way on a patient. At least 32 manufacturing variables can affect a drug's disintegration and dissolution and thus how available it is (its bioavailability) to the patient (Leeson). Until government testing guarantees the *bioequivalency*, as well as the chemical equivalency of competing generic and trade-name drugs, the consumer must depend upon his or her physician to recommend "the least expensive, fully effective" drug, be it generic or trade name. The pharmacist may be helpful, too.

Federal Drug Control

Which drugs we can buy over the counter, which by prescription only, and which ones we cannot buy at all, as well as the safety and purity of those we can buy, are controlled by federal legislation. It was not always thus.

Around the turn of the century, there were no controls. Patent medicines generously spiked with opiates were freely sold in pharmacies. Many unsuspecting users became

[3]It must be remembered that even "safe" drugs can cause side effects and allergic responses.

Ralph Morse

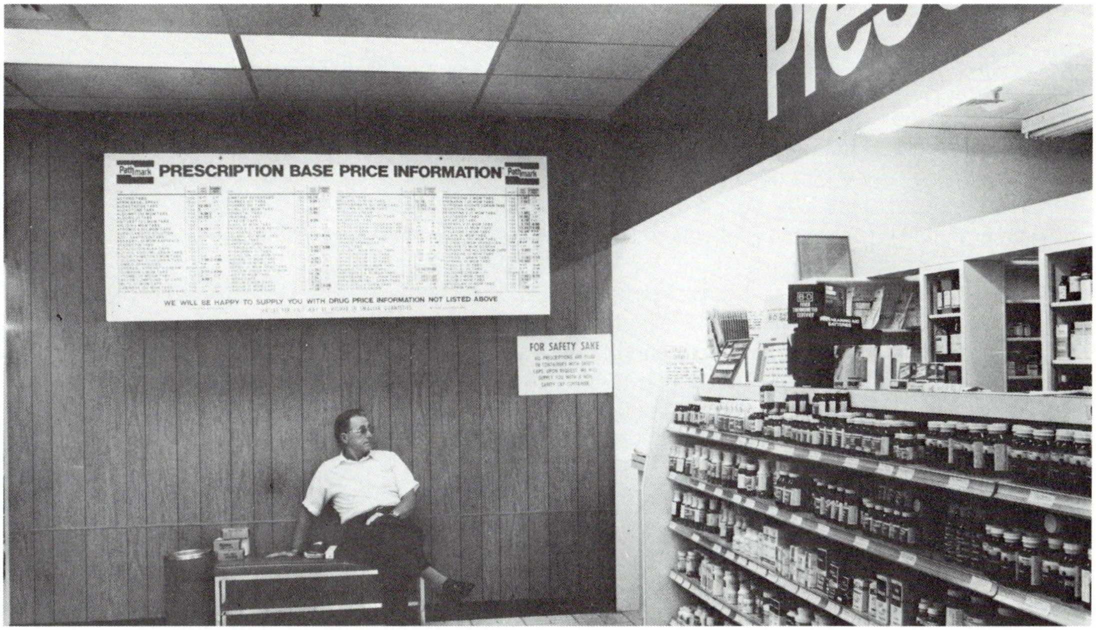
PRESCRIPTION BASE PRICE INFORMATION
WE WILL BE HAPPY TO SUPPLY YOU WITH DRUG PRICE INFORMATION NOT LISTED ABOVE
FOR SAFETY SAKE

Price advertising is permitted in many states. In some, price posting in drugstores is mandatory, permitting the consumer to compare before buying.

addicted. This led to the first Pure Food and Drug Act in 1906 which required listing of opiates on labels. Later amendments called for listing of quantities and for standards of purity and identity. By 1914, international distress over the opium trade spawned the Harrison Narcotic Act, requiring registration and taxation of persons who produced, imported, or dealt in opium or coca leaves.[4] Patent medicines containing small amounts of the drugs were exempted and physicians' prescription privileges were protected.

Later, however, the right of a physician to prescribe a prohibited drug was denied. Drug legislation, in an effort to counteract abuses, became stricter. But prohibitive laws and harsh penalties—for possession, not for addiction, after the Supreme Court decision that addiction is an illness, not a crime—did not end abuse, as you will see in Chapter 15.

[4]A technical error; cocaine is a stimulant, not a narcotic.

Today's crazy-quilt collection of laws governing the use or prohibition of many kinds of drugs is indicative of the confusion in our society over drug use. The laws often have little to do with the danger to public health of the individual drugs. Caffeine, a stimulant, is freely available in a variety of beverages and OTC preparations, though it is hazardous in large doses. Alcohol, our major drug abuse problem, is regulated and licensed and readily obtainable by adults. In some states alcohol intoxication is a crime. Highly addictive heroin is not legally available, and possession and sale are rigidly forbidden, but intoxication is not a crime. Tobacco, a lethal drug, is licensed, subsidized, and taxed by the government, with no penalties for use, sale to adults, or possession, as long as taxes are paid.[5] Marijuana is not legally available but is used

[5]Tobacco is further protected by being exempted from hazardous substances acts.

HEALTH CONSUMER TIP

Questions to Ask the Prescribing Doctor

- What is the generic name of the drug and what is it supposed to do?
- Will it react adversely with other drugs, e.g., aspirin, alcohol?
- Are there any common side effects? Any serious ones I should report?
- When and how often should I take the medication? Before or after meals? With juice, milk, water?
- Will it make me drowsy? Can I drive after taking it?
- How soon can I expect results? When should I call if I don't feel better?
- How long should I continue the medication? Can I refill the prescription?
- If it is for long-term use, can I buy it in bulk?
- Will it have an adverse reaction on any medical conditions, such as allergies, pregnancy, high blood pressure, diabetes?

Put the doctor's directions in writing or ask the pharmacist to put them on the label.

widely; penalties for its use vary from state to state, from nominal fines to lengthy prison terms. Except for alcohol, tobacco, and caffeine, all drugs are federally regulated under the schedule shown in Table 14.2.

Two federal agencies are primarily concerned with drug control: the Food and Drug Administration, which regulates drug use, safety, and effectiveness and the Drug Enforcement Agency (DEA), which deals with drug abuse.

THE MEDICINE CHEST

Most of us have our medicine chests jammed with a Hungarian goulash of tablets and liquids, unguents and ointments, with labels dimmed by time and humidity. There is, however, no need for such a collection. Even in the event of an atomic war or a pharmacists' strike, most of these pharmaceuticals will have become either totally ineffective with age, or (like tetracyclines, which become deadly after long storage) even dangerous.

That is not to say that an empty medicine chest is best. Properly used, medications have an important place in health care. Just what makes a well-stocked medicine chest varies according to personal and physician philosophy, family or individual health problems, and the distance from or availability of a doctor and/or druggist. A suggested list appears in Table 14.3.

Using Medicine Safely

We can greatly reduce the risks in using drugs if we know and follow the rules for safe use:

1 Use only fresh medications. Flush unlabeled preparations, those whose freshness date has passed,[6] and any that seem to be deteriorating (aspirin that smells like vinegar, liquids or ointments that have debris floating in them) down the toilet, minus their containers.

2 Follow directions exactly (when, how much, how often) whether they come from the doctor or the label.

3 Never use a medication prescribed for

[6]Look for and purchase OTC products that have expiration dates as required by the FDA. When buying prescription drugs, ask the pharmacist to put the expiration date on the label.

TABLE 14.2 Schedules of controlled substances

DRUG CHARACTERISTICS	EXAMPLES
SCHEDULE I	
High potential for abuse. No currently accepted medical use in U.S. Lack of accepted safety.	Heroin Nonmedically useful opiates, e.g., Phenoperidine, Dextrorphan Nonmedically useful opium derivatives, e.g., codeine-N-oxide LSD Mescaline Peyote Marijuana Psilocybin Tetrahydrocannabinols
SCHEDULE II	
High potential for abuse. Currently accepted medical use, or use with severe restrictions. Abuse may lead to severe psychological or physical dependence.	Opium Medically useful derivatives of opium Coca leaves and derivatives including cocaine Amphetamines Some barbiturates Methadone
SCHEDULE III	
Potential for abuse less than in schedules I and II. Currently accepted medical use in U.S. Abuse may lead to moderate or low physical or psychological dependence.	Derivatives of barbituric acid not listed elsewhere: Glutethimide, Chlorhexadol Preparations containing limited quantities of narcotic drugs such as codeine
SCHEDULE IV	
Low potential for abuse relative to schedule III. Currently accepted medical use in U.S. Abuse may lead to limited psychological or physical dependence relative to schedule III.	Barbital Chloral hydrate Meprobamate Phenobarbital
SCHEDULE V	
Low potential for abuse relative to schedule IV. Currently accepted medical use in U.S. Abuse may lead to limited physical or psychological dependence relative to schedule IV.	Preparations containing limited, specified quantities of narcotic drugs, or stimulants, or depressants diluted in compound with other substances that reduce or eliminate the potential for abuse of these substances

Source: Public Law 91-513.

HEALTH CONSUMER TIP

TABLE 14.3 What you should know about stocking the medicine chest*

TYPE OF DRUG	PURPOSE	COMMENTS
Analgesic-antipyretic (aspirin or, if you are sensitive to aspirin, an acetominophen such as Tylenol)	Relieve pain, headache; reduce fever	Take with full glass of water; do not exceed recommended dosage; do not take without medical advice if you are pregnant, have an ulcer, or are taking other drugs.
Antacid (Di-Gel, Maalox)	Relieve heartburn and simple indigestion	Buy the simplest preparation; do not use frequently; avoid sodium bicarbonate if you are on a low-salt diet.
Antiseptic Alcohol	Cleanse area *around* wounds, splinters, etc.; back rubs; cleanse thermometer, etc.	Use soap and water *on* wounds.
Neosporin ointment	Treat abrasions and skin infections	See a doctor if there is no improvement.
Laxative (Senokot granules)	Relieve constipation	Use only if natural methods (bran, bulk, prunes, exercise) have failed.
Antipruretic (Calamine lotion, Caladryl)	Relieve itching, poison ivy, insect bites, etc.	
Antidiarrheal preparation (a kaolin-pectin combination such as Kaopectate, Parepectolin,† Lomotil)	Cure diarrhea	Wait 6–8 hours before using unless your physician says to take immediately.
Decongestant (nasal spray or drops such as Neosynephrine or tablets such as Ornex or Sinutab-II)	Relieve stuffiness of common cold, sinusitis	Do not use drops or sprays for more than 2 days.
Antihistamine (Sudafed, Benadryl, ChlorTrimeton)	Relieve allergy symptoms	Do not drive or operate machinery following use of this medication.
Emetic (syrup of ipecac)	Induce vomiting	Use in treating poison victims (except when vomiting would be dangerous, as when poison is caustic).
Antiemetic (Emetrol)	Prevent vomiting	

FIRST-AID AND SICKROOM EQUIPMENT

Adhesive bandages (bandaids)	Electric vaporizer or steam inhalator
Roll bandages	Penlight for viewing throat
Sterile gauze pads (nonstick)	Otoscope (if you have been trained in ear examination in class or by physician)
Elastic bandages for sprains	Blood pressure cuff (if you have been trained in its use)
Adhesive tape	Stethoscope (if you have been trained in its use)
Scissors to cut tape	Disposable wooden tongue depressors
Tweezers with fine point for removing splinters	First-aid manual (see Table 11.4)
Ice bag, for immediate treatment of joint or muscle injury and bruises	Telephone numbers of doctor, hospital, emergency squad
Electric heating pad or hot water bottle	
Thermometer (rectal type for young children)	
Enema equipment or disposable enema kits	

*A locked cabinet out of reach of children in a bedroom or other low-moisture area.
†You may be asked to sign a registry at the pharmacy.

someone else, and never let anyone else use yours.

4 Never take medicine in the dark or when you are drowsy; check the label before and after you have taken the dose.

5 If you are taking a nonprescription medicine for an illness that does not clear up within a few days, or if a prescription drug does not seem effective, consult your physician.

6 Do not discontinue a prescription without your doctor's approval, especially antibiotics, which usually must be finished to the last pill even when symptoms clear up earlier.

7 If any new symptoms develop after you have begun taking a medicine, tell your physician. Change in dosage or in the drug itself may be necessary.

8 If, for some reason, you do not fill a prescription or take a medication prescribed, let your doctor know.

How the Pharmacist Can Help

Many persons like to have a regular family pharmacist much as they have a regular family physician. Such pharmacists keep individual drug profiles, required in a few states, and can often catch potential problems, as when drugs that might interact badly have been prescribed by two different doctors. Although no substitute for a physician when illness strikes, a good pharmacist can answer questions about medications—dating, when to take, storage, possible side effects—and recommend nonprescription preparations.

LOOKING BACK

REVIEWING CONCEPTS IN CHAPTER 14

- Wisely used, drugs are of great benefit to humankind; carelessly used, they can bring distress and disaster.
- No drug or other biologically active substance can be considered entirely safe.
- Drug reactions vary from person to person and time to time, depending on such factors as age, size, health, and mood.
- Adverse or bad reactions to drugs can result from an exaggeration of the desired action (toxic reaction), from other (side) effects of the drug, from allergic reaction, from mixing of drugs (polypharmacy), or from unknown causes.
- Wise use of drugs depends upon weighing risk versus benefit.
- Using drugs when risks outweigh benefits, when they are unnecessary, or to mask serious symptoms that should be treated is misuse of drugs.
- There is no chemical difference between "natural" and "synthetic" drug preparations; sometimes synthetics are safer because they contain no impurities or contaminants.
- Patient and physician share responsibility for wise drug use.
- To derive the most benefit at the least risk from drug purchases, the consumer should learn to evaluate drug advertising.
- Nonprescription, or over-the-counter, drugs are often ineffective; home remedies may work as well or better. The safest OTC preparations are those with the fewest ingredients.

- Prescription drugs are sold by either a trade name or a generic name; generics are usually less expensive, but are not always as effective.
- Medicine chests should be located in a nonhumid part of the home, out of reach of children; outdated preparations should be discarded regularly; medications should not be shared, and should always be taken according to directions.
- The pharmacist can be a useful ally in answering puzzling questions about medications, their effects, expiration dates, and so on.

15
DRUG ABUSE: INSULT TO THE BODY

WHAT'S AHEAD IN CHAPTER 15 How does our own perspective affect the way in which we view drugs and drug abuse? What are the ways in which drug abuse is defined? Is it limited to one group or type of person? Is use of drugs for recreational or "fun" purposes new? What factors must be considered in a decision to use a particular drug for nonmedical purposes? How do societal attitudes contribute to the drug abuse problem? What kinds of personal motivations drive an individual to experiment with, or abuse, drugs? Is drug abuse a victimless crime that hurts only the abuser? In what ways does drug abuse affect society? Those around the abuser? The abuser? What kinds of dependencies on drugs are possible? Can drugs that are commonly abused be lumped into a single category? Do the differing effects of drugs have much to do with the way they are viewed in the community and treated under the law?

The words "drug abuse" conjure up different images in different people, for we each have our own perceptions of reality.

- A shop owner calls the police whenever teenagers congregate in front of her luncheonette. She is convinced they are "drug addicts." She drinks a dozen cups of coffee and smokes two packs of cigarettes during the day "to keep going." By evening, she can't stop "going," and so she takes something to help her sleep.
- A mother won't let her children visit friends whose father is an alcoholic. But she takes Darvon regularly for headaches and Librium when she's upset.

Kids are very different today,
I hear every mother say:
Mother needs something today
to calm her down.
And though she's not really ill,
There's a little yellow pill—

She goes running for the shelter
Of her mother's little helper,
And to help her on her way,
Gets her through her busy day. . . .

Doctor, please,
Some more of these;
Outside the door,
She took four more. . . .
The Rolling Stones (1966)

- A college student smokes pot on weekends. He thinks that people who use hard drugs are unwise. When reports suggest hazards in marijuana smoking, he ignores them, confident that his own experience refutes them.
- A state trooper often picks up students for possession of marijuana. When he goes off duty, he stops at his favorite pub for a couple of beers. He has a few more drinks with dinner "to unwind."
- A dedicated high school health education teacher sees drugs as a dread plague and details all their evils for her students. One of her students, who takes phenobarbital to prevent convulsions, thinks, "She didn't say how drugs can help people. If the kids find out I'm taking pheno, I'll die!"

Most of us are aware that drug problems exist—for someone else. We see drugs through our own egocentrically tinted glasses. This chapter offers a chance to remove those glasses and look at the facts: how the scientific community views drugs today, and how to evaluate these facts and make intelligent decisions about drug use by employing risk-benefit theory.

WHAT IS DRUG ABUSE?

There is no single generally accepted definition of drug abuse, a form of human behavior that apparently goes back thousands of years. A Manual for Law Enforcement Officers describes three forms: (1) *consumption, without medical authorization*, of medically useful drugs capable of altering mood and behavior, (2) use of a mood-altering drug for *a purpose other than that for which it was prescribed*, and (3) use of a mood-altering drug that has *no legitimate medical application.*

Drug abuse authority Dr. Joel Fort defines drug abuse in terms of its effect on the user, as chronic excessive use that definitely impairs social or vocational adjustment or health. A government guideline for drug abuse education defines abuse in terms of social norms, as that which interferes with community-accepted standards of economic, social, psychological, or physical well-being. Dana Farnsworth (*b*), M.D., includes as abusers physicians who prescribe dangerous drugs without being fully aware of their effects, prescribe a strong drug when it is not needed, or allow a patient to take a drug indefinitely without follow-up, as well as patients who demand an antibiotic every time they get a cold.

DRUG ABUSE AND DECISION MAKING

Every year, millions of Americans make decisions to use drugs nonmedically, to improve performance, on social occasions, for religious purposes, for mind altering. And the numbers continue to grow, particularly among the young. As decision makers, these users usually fall into three categories: (1) Those who have thought the question through and have decided that benefits as they see them outweigh risks; their values play an important part in their decisions. (2) Those who have not considered risk versus

Mimi Forsyth/Monkmeyer

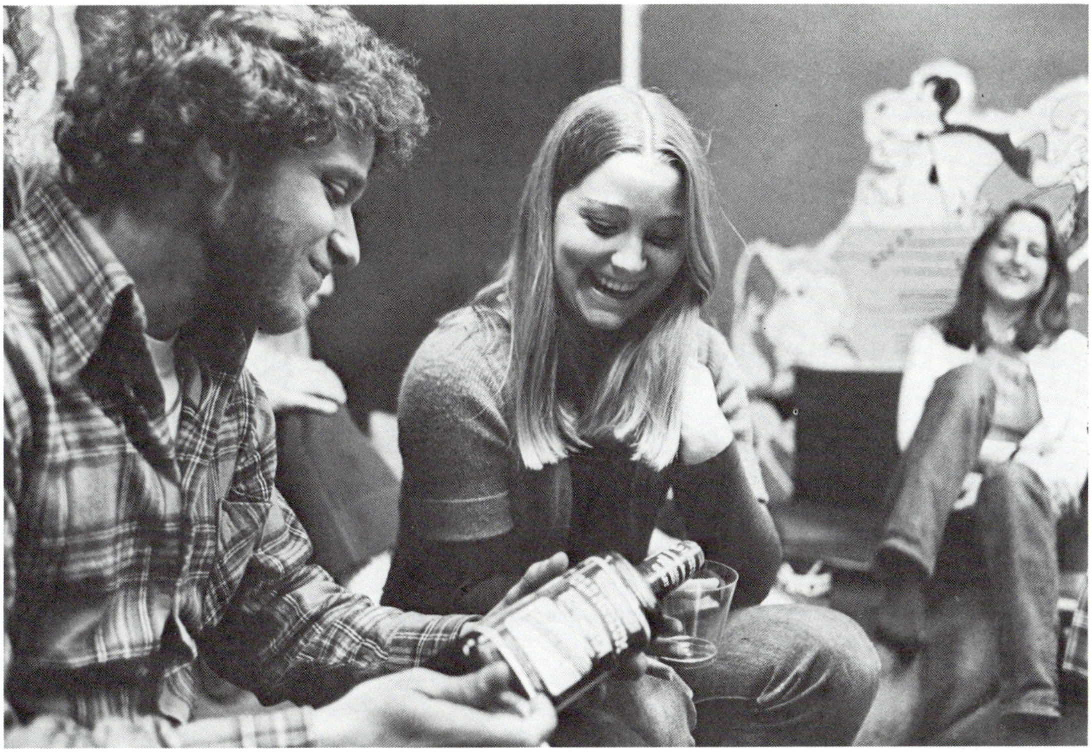

In making decisions about recreational drug use, a variety of factors should be considered, including legality, physical and psychological effects, purpose, and personal values.

benefit but have simply drifted into drug abuse without much forethought; if challenged, however, they can readily rationalize a benefit. (3) Those who have attempted to weigh risk against benefit but have incorrect or insufficient information on which to base their decisions.

A book like this can offer correct and adequate information. It can suggest factors that might be considered in decision making. But it cannot make decisions. Decisions must be made by individuals applying their personal values to these factors, which include: (1) *expected benefits*; (2) *personal needs*; (3) *community needs*; (4) *legality of the drug* (penalties for use, if illegal); (5) *physical effects* (short- and long-term); (6) *psychological effects* (short- and long-term); (7) *effects on life, family, work, school* (positive and negative); (8) *future consequences* (good and bad); (9) *purpose of use* (is it to avoid coping with problems?); (10) *financial cost of long-term use*; (11) *hazards* (when driving, operating machinery, etc.); (12) *effects on present or future children*.

INFLUENCES LEADING TO DRUG ABUSE

Attitudes and Values

An impressive armamentarium of drugs and other pharmaceuticals has been developed in

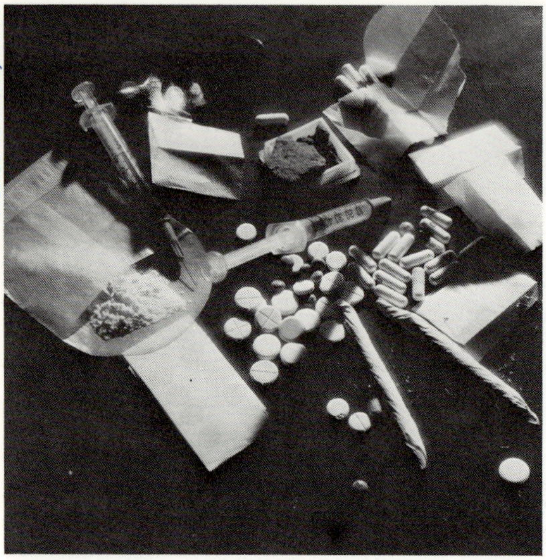

Fred De Van/Nancy Palmer

An impressive armamentarium of drugs and other pharmaceuticals has been developed in our society, but we have not simultaneously developed a suitable system of values and attitudes governing the use of these products.

our society, but we have not simultaneously developed a suitable system of values and attitudes governing the use of such products. Yet values and attitudes have a major influence on whether or not people abuse drugs.

How do attitudes develop? Gilbert Guerin, Ph.D., describes a typical 12-year-old who has had injections to prevent and cure illnesses; who has swallowed (by direction of parents and physicians) countless medications and pills; who has watched TV commercials offering instant drug cures; who has seen adults consume alcohol, coffee, cigarettes, and tranquilizers when tense; and who, when he has trouble falling asleep, is handed an aspirin. Comments Dr. Guerin:

> If there had not been a drug available, the mother may have rubbed the boy's back to soothe him, or . . . discussed with him what was really bothering him . . . suggested other devices to fall asleep, for example, counting sheep, or using pleasant thoughts to overcome unpleasant thoughts. (p. 81)

When pills are doled out automatically, children learn neither critical and evaluative attitudes toward drugs nor alternatives to drug use. Influenced by parents who think of pills as problem solvers and by advertising promoting quick relief, children develop faith in the power of drugs. In the view of Farnsworth (*b*), far from being a sign of rebellion against society and establishment, drug abuse often represents an acceptance of early training and propaganda.

Personal Motivation for Drug Abuse

In 1747, Lord Chesterfield wrote to his son:

> I always naturally hated drinking; and yet I have often drunk, with disgust at the time attended by great sickness the next day, only because I then considered drinking as a necessary qualification for a fine gentleman and a Man of Pleasure.

Chesterfield's motivation is clear. But what are the motivations of contemporary drug abusers, including many who, like Chesterfield, get no pleasure from drug use? Researchers such as Graham Blaine, Norman J. Levy, Leon Wurmser, and Farnsworth have suggested a number of common motivations:

- *Escape* Drug users often want to escape from the pressures of school, job, family; from responsibility, from doing something they really don't want to do (going to college, staying home with a baby); from fear of not being able to live up to their own expectations or those of others; or from an inability to "feel," to respond to the world around them.
- *Rebellion* Some need to rebel against the establishment, parents, school, society in general, or what they consider the hypocrisy of drug laws.
- *Getting even* Some want to take revenge on parents or others.

There have always been almost as many reasons for drug abuse as there are abusers, as seen in this quote about tobacco use in England in 1667:

> . . . One smokes because it enables him to see better, another because it disperses water in the brain, a third to ease his toothache, a fourth to stop the singing in his ears, a fifth will tell you that it makes him sleep, a sixth that it quenches his thirst, a seventh that it neutralizes the bad effects of too much water-drinking, an eighth that it expels evil humours, a ninth smokes to pass the time and a tenth because he doesn't want to be unsociable.

- *Substitute for sexual experience* Some people, especially males, whose sex lives are not satisfactory, use drugs as a substitute.
- *Experimentation* Sometimes drug users feel they have found a way of saying, "I'm not afraid, I'm invincible; nothing can happen to me," of winning a badge of courage that is difficult to achieve in a society they believe to be devoid of the challenges and excitement of new frontiers.
- *Self-destruction* Drug use can be a form of risk taking that says, "I don't care what happens to me!"

Middle-class youth want to escape from boredom, lack of challenge:

When you get
So bored
You begin to see
The Blankness
And you
Drink, take drugs,
Or get married.
You do something like that
You need something to label you
To pretend
You are Something
For some Reason.

Nancy Ernst, high school student, "Long Winter," in Divoky, p. 230

Poverty youth want to escape the misery and hopelessness of their lives:

They [the boys] have to make it for themselves 'cause most of them don't have fathers. . . . It's a lonely feeling 'cause a lot of times you want to lean on somebody; you need somebody that could try and talk to you and tell you certain things. The problems that I have I can't, you know, express them to my mother 'cause a lot of times she don't understand it.

Ghetto youth, in Goro, p. 84

Many young people want to escape from pressures:

All I heard was how I had to make it—make grades, make a team, make a good reputation, make this, make that. I hated it, every minute of it, because none of it was for me. It was all for my parents. I escaped through drugs.

Former drug user, age 20, in "Pursuit of High," p. 54

Drugs and Sports

When an athlete wins a meet, but is later disqualified for drug use, news reports usually imply that he or she won because of the drugs. This enhances a misleading drug mystique. No mention is made of losers who may also have used drugs, but who lost anyway. Such news reports are also unfair in that they penalize and stigmatize the winners for using drugs but leave losers unnoticed. Often losers are not even tested.

There is, however, firm evidence that drugs like amphetamines and anabolic steroids (with or without protein tablets) do *not* improve performance beyond the placebo effect for those who believe they will help. Use of pharmacological aids may, in fact, be dangerous, especially for the poorly conditioned athlete. They have led, in some cases, to permanent injury and death. According to the National Collegiate Athletic Association, the only way to make a muscle larger and stronger is to work it and overload it. Training and hard work, and these alone, are the ingredients of success in athletics.

Dr. Kenneth Clarke, authority on drugs and sports, sees drug use, especially since it has been sensationalized via drug testing at the Olympics, as a threat to sports: "Everything, even the ethical considerations are forgotten in the necessity to win."

- *Peer group identification* The young who have still not answered the question "Who am I?" and thus have difficulty separating self from group may find a sense of belonging when they use drugs. For adults still unsure of themselves, the social sharing of marijuana joints, pills, or a bottle of wine also brings a feeling of closeness. For hard-core addicts, the drug culture camaraderie often becomes more important than life itself.
- *Curiosity and kicks* Some users are thrill seekers searching for immediate gratification and pleasure. (Ironically, among the apparent effects of prolonged heavy drug use is the inability to gain normal pleasure from sex, food, friends, work.)
- *Self-discovery, consciousness expansion* These motives are most common among users of hallucinogens and marijuana, who believe that these substances can spur creativity, heighten aesthetic response, provide a rapturous semispiritual high, and allow exploration of submerged places of the mind. (There is no evidence that such inner safaris have allowed more than a few to achieve golden consciousness.)
- *Finding identity* The addict's feeling that drugs make him or her a "somebody" has been expressed this way: "*You* are a teacher. *You* are a cop. *You* are a parent, a man, a woman, a citizen, a voter, a landlord, a housewife. *Me,* I'm a junkie." (Chein, p. 76)
- *Personality improvement* Some people use drugs to reduce inhibitions, to try to improve communications and interperson-

Dr. Dana Farnsworth contends that drugs do not enhance creativity:

> The great philosophical theories are developed, but they are not written down; the great paintings are envisioned but no paint is applied to canvas; everything draws to a halt. . . . Psychoactive drugs rarely increase awareness of the world; they are much more likely to contract people's lives, negate conflict, and deal with stress by dissolving it rather than meeting it with fully human and creative awareness. (*b*, pp. 34–44)

. . . After I got high I made sure I ran into people who would see just how high I was. "Boy, was he stoned!" they would say about me, which I thought was great for my image.

An 18-year-old male, in "Pursuit of High," p. 54

al relations, to end loneliness, to cure emotional hangups, or to enhance sexual desire or performance. (While changes may appear to occur during the high, they are gone when the user comes down.)

Drug use, particularly compulsive use of hard drugs, often stems from deep psychological problems. Such abusers often come from problem families and their drug taking is frequently a disillusioned and angry response to the absence of true parental concern and guidance and/or an imitation of parents' immature behavior, often involving drug use.

Moving from Experimentation to Abuse

The transition from casual drug user to serious abuser is seldom planned. Most persons are certain that "It can never happen to me." Yet it often does. The crossover may occur when interaction between drug effects and personality causes a loss of control over drug use or when the use of drugs becomes a means of "solving" or avoiding life's problems. Casual users may decide that they wish to experience more often the pleasant state of euphoria offered by the drug they are using. They are not hooked, but they are on their way. Others get high on amphetamines and need barbiturates to come down. They ride a cycle of uppers and downers that is likely to end in barbiturate dependency.

Sometimes drug abuse stems not from inner need or pleasure hunting, but from medical treatment. Continued use of painkillers or psychoactive drugs for physical or mental illness, especially when the patient increases the dosage or physician supervision is lax, can lead to drug dependency and abuse.

Motivations for Abstaining from Drugs

Motivations for not using drugs are as varied as those for using them. But according to a survey of students at a California high school, the major reason is "I don't need them." In other words, "Life is fine," "I'm happy," "I turn on in other ways." Another major reason is concern for physical or mental health or athletic condition.

EFFECTS OF DRUG ABUSE

How Drug Abuse Affects Society

Most drug abusers do not intend to harm society and, in fact, drug abuse is classifed as a *victimless* crime. Yet costs to society are high: for support of those who "drop out" because of drugs; for rehabilitation of drug

Sometimes, as in the case of former First Lady Betty Ford, drug abuse stems not from inner need or pleasure seeking, but from continued use of painkillers in medical treatment, which can lead to dependency.

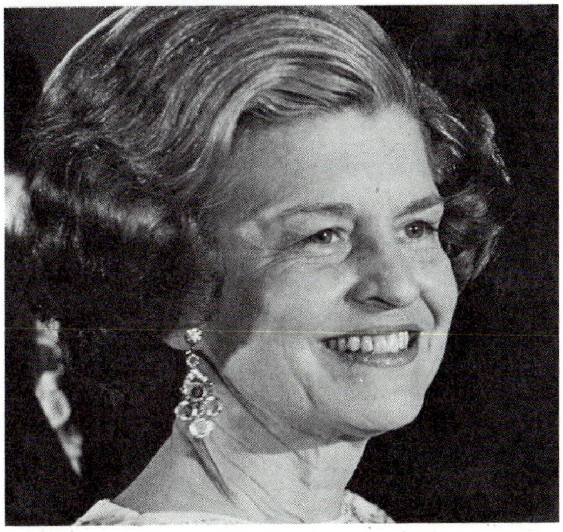

Ray Ellis/Photo Researchers

Bob Combs/Photo Researchers

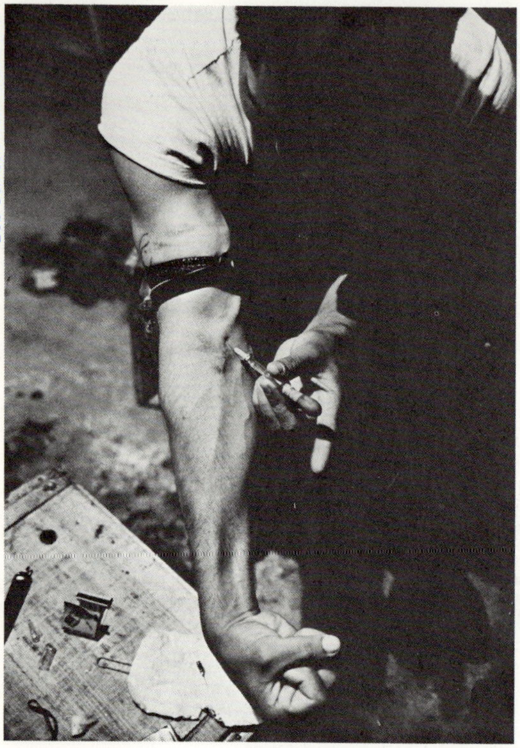

While drug abuse is classified as a victimless crime, the costs to society are high.

abusers; for apprehending, trying, and imprisoning those driven by crime to support their habits or by a drug-induced loss of inhibitions. Even more costly is the increase in violence, both physical and to the human spirit, ranging from prostitution to murder, as well as the increase of wealth and power of the international crime syndicates that merchandise illegal drugs.

There are human costs as well: loss of productive workdays; illness and death; accidents and injury to users and those with whom they come in contact; psychological, emotional, and financial damage to friends, families, marriages, and children of drug abusers; jobs lost, talent wasted, hearts broken.

How Drug Abuse Affects the Individual

The risks of drug abuse are many, including: imprisonment and a criminal record or a fine when the drug is illegal; damage to physical health (and sometimes death) from the drug itself or from malnutrition and venereal disease which are common among users; emotional breakdown because of dependence on or effects of drugs; interference with mental, emotional, intellectual, or physical maturation when the user is young; estrangement from families, jobs, school, friends; entrapment in an underground culture from which it may be difficult to escape.

Drug abusers also risk being used and abused by others, especially pushers, and may be forced into burglary or streetwalking in order to pay for their habits. Possibly the greatest risk, often unrecognized, is the potential loss of freedom. Though many begin dabbling in drugs "to find freedom," they often find, too late, that they have built themselves a prison. Who is less free than the person who will trudge through a blizzard to buy a pack of cigarettes, who cannot face a problem or challenge without a drink, or who must inject heroin every day just to avoid the dreaded withdrawal symptoms?

DRUG DEPENDENCY

Drug abuse can lead to a drug habit: a need to take drugs that is physical, psychological, or both. Because so little is known about the mechanisms that cause this need or dependency, definitions have continued to change over the past several years. Presently, most scientists believe there are two basic types of dependencies, but there are probably many variations within each category and considerable overlap.

Psychological dependence Some people develop a psychological need for a drug or other substance quickly; others may never develop such a need. Over a period of time, psychological dependency can become very strong, a very hard-to-break habit. When a drug on which a person is psychologically dependent is discontinued, there are no physical withdrawal symptoms, but the psychic misery can be considerable.

Physical dependence Physical dependence usually develops more gradually than psychological dependence. Its presence is generally signaled by:

1 *Tolerance* A weakened response to the same dose of a drug on repeated usage, or the need for increasingly larger doses to produce the same effects. Thus, drug-dependent people find they must take more and more of the drug in order to experience its effects.
2 *Abstinence syndrome* Withdrawal symptoms, or a pattern of physical symptoms that occurs upon abrupt withdrawal of a substance which a person has been using regularly and to which the body has become accustomed. This leads to a vicious circle: The person must continue taking the drug, even when pleasant effects are no longer achieved, in order to continue normal functioning and avoid withdrawal symptoms.

DRUGS OF ABUSE

Drugs of abuse vary greatly both in natural properties and actions, and in the way society views them. They are generally put in the same category, just as the pistol and the cannon are both classified as guns, but they vary considerably in impact and should not be lumped together by anyone using or considering using them. Some drugs of abuse are relatively harmless in small doses, for example, alcohol. Others, such as LSD, can be dangerous in low doses, even on first use. Those widely used, such as alcohol and tobacco, present a greater public health problem than less used drugs, such as heroin. Some sort of dependence is a major hazard in the abuse of most drugs, though the extent of dependence varies with the drug and the individual using it.

Assessing drugs is not easy. Benefits are often more readily apparent than risks. When heroin was first introduced, it was not only believed to be nonaddictive, but was hailed as a "cure" for morphine addiction. It was perceived as "heroic," thus the name. At other times, however, dangers seem greater than they really are. When coffee was first brewed, fear of its hazards was so great that the beverage was banned in Mohammedan Arabia and harsh penalities were imposed for its use.

When tobacco arrived in Europe, it was both praised for its supposed therapeutic effects and damned for its damnable ones; 400 years later, scientists determined its real hazards sufficiently to justify printed warnings on cigarette packages. Alcohol has been avidly consumed since before the invention of the bottle. Yet some of the most serious consequences of heavy drinking were not recognized until this century.

The most abused drugs are those that are directly or indirectly psychoactive. Often masquerading as body chemicals, they are able to alter mood and behavior in ways that are not yet fully understood. Used widely, under medical direction, some of these drugs

The sufferer is tremulous and loses his self-command; he is subject to fits of agitation and depression. He has a haggarde appearance . . . as with other agents, a renewed dose of the poison gives temporary relief, but at the cost of future misery.

A turn-of-the-century description of a coffee addict, Gillie, p. 75

can be used to blunt severe anxieties and depression, though not enough to eliminate entirely the normal highs and lows of life that differentiate us from robots or zombies.

Scientific knowledge about each drug presented here is the most current available. But it is subject to change as more information is learned in the future. However, what we know in general about all drugs will not change: *No* drug is safe for all peoples at all times. All have some risks. These risks must be weighed against benefits.

This chapter will focus on the opiates, sedatives, stimulants, and hallucinogens, the major characteristics of which can be seen in Table 15.2. Chapter 16 will deal with alcohol and marijuana, and Chapter 17 with tobacco.

The Depressant Drugs

Depressants (substances which depress the central nervous system), also called sedatives, hypnotics, or "downers," are misused and abused by people of all ages. In this

TABLE 15.1 Drugs most commonly named in drug emergencies in United States emergency rooms* May 1976 to April 1977

RANK	DRUG	ESTIMATED CASES
1	Diazepam (Valium)	54,400
2	Alcohol in combination†	47,400
3	Aspirin	17,600
4	Heroin	17,000
5	Flurazepam (Dalmane)	11,500
6	D-propoxyphene (Darvon)	10,800
7	Chlordiazepoxide (Librium)	9,300
8	Phenobarbital	7,700
9	Amitriptyline (Elavil)	7,500
10	Secobarbital, Amobarbital (Seconal)	7,400
11	Tuinal (sedative)	7,300
12	Chlorpromazine (Thorazine)	6,100
13	Marijuana	5,700
14	Methaqualone	5,500
15‡	Thioridazine (Mellaril)	5,300
15‡	Dilantin	5,300
17	Ethchlorvynol (Placydil)	5,000
18	Acetaminophen (Tylenol, Datril)	4,700
19	Methadone	4,500
20	PCP	4,100
21	Doxepin (Sinequan)	3,300
22	Meprobamate (Miltown, etc.)	3,200
23	Pentobarbital (Nembutal)	2,900
24	Codeine	2,700
25	Glutethimide (Doradin)	2,000

*Drug-related deaths are most frequently reported for: alcohol in combination, heroin, D-propoxyphene, diazepam, secobarbital, amitryptaline, pentobarbital, Tuinal, phenobarbital, codeine, and aspirin.

†Alcohol is included in this reporting system only when involved in a medical emergency with another drug.

‡Tied for fifteenth place.

Source: Drug Enforcement Administration, project DAWN V (Drug Abuse Warning Network).

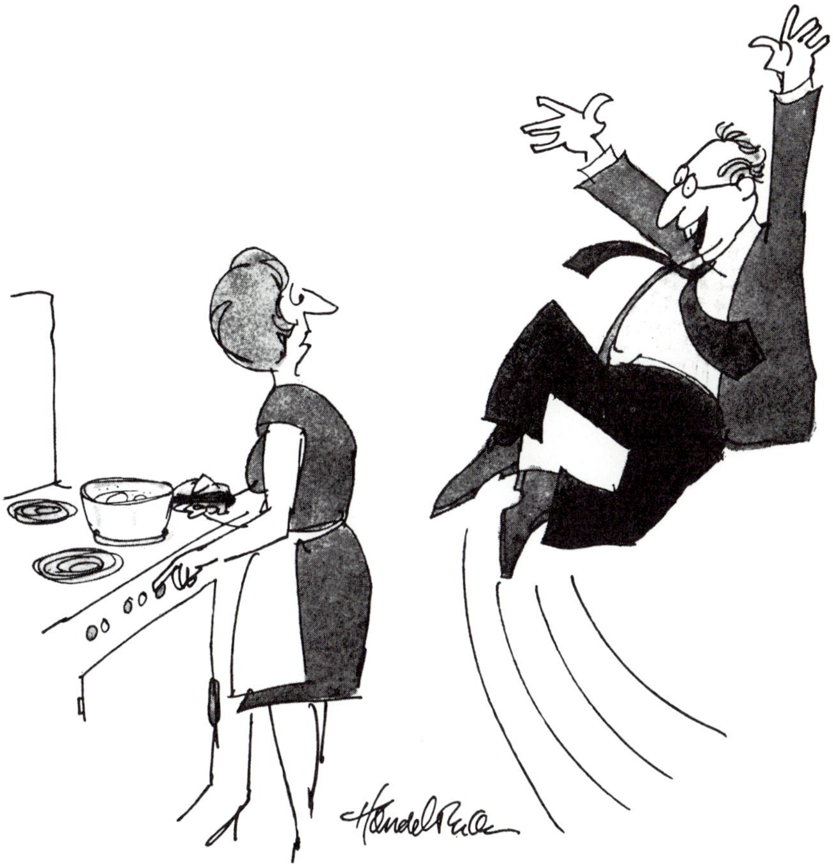

"Your eggs will be ready in a minute. Meanwhile, take a mood stabilizer."

category are tranquilizers, barbiturates, several nonbarbiturate sedatives, and alcohol. Some are obtained legally, others illegally. Many over-30 sedative abusers are introduced to the drugs in small prescribed doses by their physicians. When they have difficulty coping, they increase the dosage without consulting their doctors and become dependent.[1] Most younger abusers obtain depressants through illegal channels.

[1]The problem is particularly serious among women. The National Institute of Drug Abuse estimates that 2 million American females are dependent upon prescription drugs.

Tranquilizers The daily consumption of millions of doses of tranquilizers makes them the most used controlled drug in the United States. The tranquilizer Valium is the No. 1 prescription drug in the country and the No. 1 drug of abuse (Dupont, *a*). Although tranquilizers may be used to treat nausea, and to relieve muscular tension, they are primarily prescribed to reduce the physical (psychosomatic ailments such as colitis, asthma, and ulcers) and psychological effects of tension and stress. Prolonged and excessive use may result in dependence.

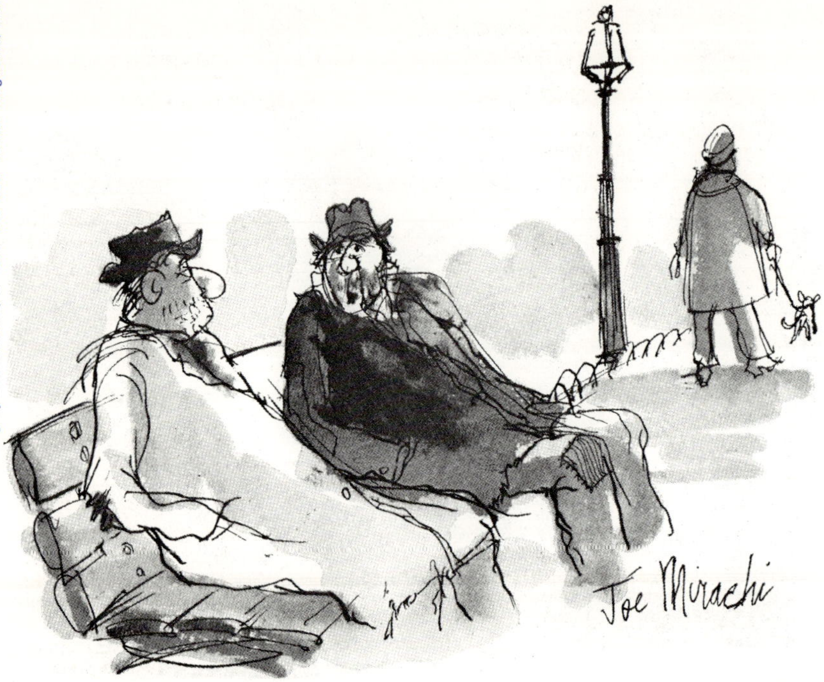

"Do you have anything on you for the relief of simple nervous tension?"

Unlike barbiturates, tranquilizers sedate only when very large amounts are taken. But they can temporarily mask anxiety, removing the cutting edge of a disturbing emotion without entirely eliminating it. Use of tranquilizers on a more than occasional basis has been criticized fiercely by some ("It's a crutch!") and defended by others ("A crutch allows people to walk without putting full weight on a painful injury; a tranquilizer allows people to function without putting full weight on a painful emotional problem"). Steady use of tranquilizers to substitute for positive coping devices, however, is generally agreed to be harmful (see "Coping," Chapter 2).

Barbiturates In small therapeutic doses, these derivatives of barbituric acid have a calming effect. Larger doses cause sleep; very large doses cause coma and even death. Some users have a temporary feeling of excitement similar to alcohol intoxication before depression sets in. Secobarbital (Seconal), pentobarbital (Nembutal), and amobarbital (Amytal) are among the most commonly abused of the barbiturates.

Barbiturate addiction, which can result from as little as 600 milligrams per day over a long period, is most similar to alcohol dependence. Both types of abusers exhibit violent and aggressive tendencies and paranoid behavior, as well as lack of control. Withdrawal from either without proper medical supervision can be fatal.

Because an overdose is deadly, barbiturates are the drug of choice in 1 out of 3 intentional suicides. They are also involved in many accidental deaths. Some of these occur when barbiturates are taken with alcohol, dangerously multiplying their depressant effects. Others occur when victims have taken a couple of pills in order to sleep. When the pills fail to work, they take two more. Later, still sleepless, but now groggy, they forget how many they have taken and swallow another dose. This barbiturate confusion continues until unconsciousness and, often, death occur.

Methaqualone A synthetic nonbarbiturate sedative originally believed to be safe and nonaddictive, methaqualone was prescribed freely when introduced in 1963. By the time reports of overdose, dependence, and toxic reactions began to accumulate, many people were already hooked on it.

Methaqualone has been touted as an aphrodisiac or love drug, because users tend to feel more relaxed, receptive, and uninhibited, but there is no scientific evidence it increases either sexual pleasure or performance. With larger doses, especially in combination with alcohol, a stupor takes over, and intercourse may be impossible. When used with wine (called "luding out") an ataxia, or loss of control, with "pins and needles" in fingertips, lips, and tongue may lead to falling and other accidents.

Other sedatives, too, are abused, including chloral hydrate, Placydil, and glutethimide. Effects of these can be seen in Table 15.2.

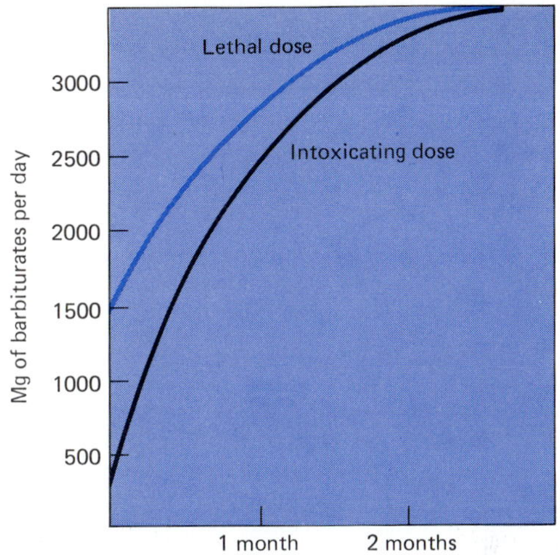

FIGURE 15.1 Tolerance and toxicity in barbiturate use. With the daily use of barbiturates, tolerance develops, and larger and larger doses are needed to achieve an effect. The lethal dose (the dose that can be fatal) rises more slowly. Thus, during the second or third month of use the two doses become dangerously close. [*Adapted from U.S. DHEW, t.*]

Stimulants

Drugs that stimulate the central nervous system are abused by the student who wants to stay up all night studying for finals, the weary truck driver determined to log another 200 miles, the homemaker who needs a lift to get through a long day of dirty dishes and crying children. But attempts to drive our bodies beyond capacity often fail. The student may successfully stay up all night, but her responses may be so deadened that she writes gibberish on her exam. The truck jockey may become so tired that he "sees" an elephant crossing the road and jacknifes while swerving to avoid it. The homemaker may get through the day, but the drugs may mask a serious physical or psychological problem crying for attention. All become victims of a misleading feeling of confidence or power generated by the drug.

Stimulant drugs include the nicotine in tobacco, discussed in Chapter 17, and cocaine, amphetamines, and caffeine.

Cocaine The most powerful stimulant and antifatigue agent known, cocaine was first isolated from the leaves of the erythroxylon coca plant in 1869, but did not win a following medically or recreationally until Sigmund Freud enthusiastically endorsed it for its exhilarating effects and for treating morphine and alcohol addiction. Freud apparently used cocaine himself in small doses on an irregular basis for a few years, until a friend he treated for morphine addiction deteriorated into a pathetic victim of cocaine dependency.

Today, despite its high price ($2800 per

TABLE 15.2 Major drugs of abuse

DRUG	SCHEDULE*	BRAND NAMES OFTEN PRESCRIBED	MEDICAL USES	DEPENDENCE POTENTIAL	
				PHYSICAL	PSYCHOLOGICAL
NARCOTICS					
Opium	II	Dover's powder, paregoric	Analgesic, antidiarrheal	High	High
Morphine	II	Morphine	Analgesic	High	High
Codeine	II, III, V	Codeine	Analgesic, antitussive	Moderate	Moderate
Heroin	I	None	None	High	High
Meperidine (pethidine)	II	Demerol, Pethadol	Analgesic	High	High
Methadone	II	Dolophine, Methadone, Methadose	Analgesic, heroin substitute	High	High
Other narcotics	I, II, III, V	Dilaudid, Leritine, Numorphan, Percodan	Analgesic, antidiarrheal, antitussive	High	High
DEPRESSANTS					
Chloral hydrate	IV	Noctec, Somnos	Hypnotic	Moderate	Moderate
Barbiturates	II, III, IV	Amytal, Butisol, Nembutal, Phenobarbital, Seconal, Tuinal	Anesthetic, anticonvulsant, sedation, sleep	High	High
Glutethimide	III	Doriden	Sedation, sleep	High	High
Methaqualone	II	Optimil, Parest, Quaalude, Somnafac, Sopor	Sedation, sleep	High	High
Tranquilizers	IV	Equanil, Librium, Miltown, Serax, Tranxene, Valium	Antianxiety, muscle relaxant, sedation	Moderate	Moderate
Other depressants	III, IV	Clonopin, Dalmane, Dormate, Noludar, Placydil, Valmid	Antianxiety, sedation, sleep	Possible	Possible
STIMULANTS					
Cocaine†	II	Cocaine	Local anesthetic	Possible	High
Amphetamines	II, III	Benzedrine, Biphetamine, Desoxyn, Dexedrine	Hyperkinesis, narcolepsy, weight control	Possible	High
Phanmetrazine	II	Preludin	Weight control	Possible	High
Methylphenidate	II	Ritalin	Hyperkinesis	Possible	High
Other stimulants	III, IV	Bacarate, Cylert, Didrex, Ionamin, Plegine, Pondimin, Pre-Sate, Sanorex, Voranil	Weight control	Possible	Possible
HALLUCINOGENS					
LSD	I	None	None	None	Degree unknown
Mescaline	I	None	None	None	Degree unknown
Psilocybin-Psilocin	I	None	None	None	Degree unknown
MDA	I	None	None	None	Degree unknown
PCP‡	III	Sernylan	Veterinary anesthetic	None	Degree unknown
Other hallucinogens	I	None	None	None	Degree unknown
CANNABIS					
Marijuana	I	None	None	Degree unknown	Moderate
Hashish	I	None	None	Degree unknown	Moderate
Hashish oil	I	None	None	Degree unknown	Moderate

*Scheduling classifications vary for individual drugs since controlled substances are often sold in combination with other medicinal ingredients.
†Designated a narcotic under the Controlled Substances Act. ‡Designated a depressant under the Controlled Substances Act.
Source: Drugs of Abuse, pp. 16–17.

TOLERANCE	DURATION OF EFFECTS, IN HOURS	USUAL METHOD OF ADMINISTRATION	CLUES TO USE		
			POSSIBLE EFFECTS	EFFECTS OF OVERDOSE	WITHDRAWAL SYNDROME
			NARCOTICS		
Yes	3–6	Oral, smoked	Euphoria, drowsiness, respiratory depression, constricted pupils, nausea, nodding, loss of appetite, sweet-eating jags, scratching	Slow and shallow breathing, clammy skin, convulsions, coma, possible death	Watery eyes, runny nose, yawning, loss of appetite, irritability, tremors, panic, chills and sweating, cramps, nausea
Yes	3–6	Injected, smoked			
Yes	3–6	Oral, injected			
Yes	3–6	Injected, sniffed			
Yes	3–6	Oral, injected			
Yes	12–24	Oral, injected			
Yes	3–6	Oral, injected			
			DEPRESSANTS		
Probable	5–8	Oral	Slurred speech, staggering, disorientation, drunken behavior without odor of alcohol, sleepiness, difficulty concentrating	Shallow respiration, cold and clammy skin, dilated pupils, weak and rapid pulse, coma, possible death	Anxiety, insomnia, tremors, delirium, convulsions, possible death
Yes	1–16	Oral, injected			
Yes	4–8	Oral			
Yes	4–8	Oral			
Yes	4–8	Oral			
Yes	4–8	Oral			
			STIMULANTS		
Yes	2	Injected, sniffed	Increased alertness, excitation, euphoria, dilated pupils, increased pulse rate and blood pressure, insomnia, loss of appetite	Agitation, increase in body temperature, hallucinations, convulsions, possible death	Apathy, long periods of sleep, irritability, depression, disorientation
Yes	2–4	Oral, injected			
Yes	2–4	Oral			
Yes	2–4	Oral			
Yes	2–4	Oral			
			HALLUCINOGENS		
Yes	Variable	Oral	Illusions and hallucinations (with exception of MDA); poor perception of time and distance; increase in blood pressure, heart rate, and blood sugar levels	Longer, more intense "trip" episodes, psychosis, possible death	Withdrawal syndrome not reported
Yes	Variable	Oral, injected			
Yes	Variable	Oral			
Yes	Variable	Oral, injected, sniffed			
Yes	Variable	Oral, injected, smoked			
Yes	Variable	Oral, injected, sniffed			
			CANNABIS		
Yes	2–4	Oral, smoked	Euphoria, relaxed inhibitions, increased appetite, disoriented behavior, possibly dilated pupils, bloodshot eyes	Fatigue, paranoia, possible psychosis	Insomnia, hyperactivity, and decreased appetite reported in a limited number of individuals
Yes	2–4	Oral, smoked			
Yes	2–4	Oral, smoked			

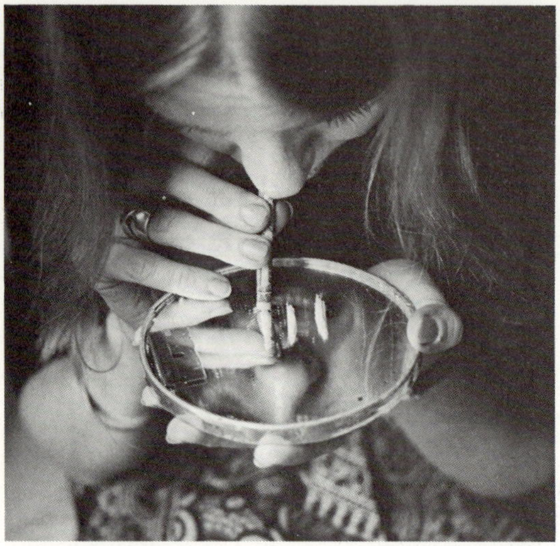

Charles Gatewood

In spite of the high price and potential danger, cocaine use has increased dramatically in the past decade.

ounce), cocaine use is up dramatically—700 percent between 1970 and 1975. Its roots are deeper in middle- and upper-class groups than are heroin's. Abusers have been found in high schools and colleges, and reportedly it has been served "as if it were cheese dip" at elegant Beverly Hills parties.[2] The 1977 federal report on cocaine calls the drug the most "self-reinforcing" of all abused drugs, meaning experimenters are most likely to want to repeat use because they enjoy it. (Experimental animals self-inject to the point of death.)

Users are indifferent to pain and believe they are experiencing greatly increased muscular strength and mental capacity, with potentially disastrous results. At heavy dosages euphoria may be mixed with suspicion and anxiety, sleeplessness, and depression, and may progress to ataxic syndrome, which is similar to amphetamine psychosis. Ataxic syndrome is characterized by delusions of persecution (paranoia) and hallucinations that may turn to violence in self-defense against the user's supposed persecutors. In rare instances, death may occur.

[2]One result of cocaine use is holes in the nasal septums of some chronic cocaine sniffers, leading stars among them.

Amphetamines Though for several decades amphetamines were widely used medically, particularly for weight control, they were reevaluated in the 1970s because of their potential for abuse as well as their apparent lack of effectiveness in treating either physical or psychological ills. The question was raised: Do the benefits of amphetamine use outweigh the risks? For the most part, the answer was no. The drugs were reclassified as schedule II (very high abuse, restricted medical use), and quotas were set to limit production. Amphetamines were virtually banned in some states and prescribing by physicians dropped dramatically.

It has been suggested that people abuse amphetamines simply because they want to "feel better"—less anxious or unhappy, more energetic or capable, or more responsive. At first, amphetamines help: The users do feel better. But after a short while they find themselves on a roller coaster. Every time they go up, they come down. And they can't stop.

There are three typical forms of abuse:

- Intermittent or consistent use of small doses to achieve an immediate aim, such as increasing alertness or reducing fatigue, that becomes a way of coping.
- Chronic moderate doses that lead to tolerance and then to a need for ever-larger doses to spur the body on, to meet school deadlines, lose 30 pounds for bikini season, be "up" for a series of job interviews. Eventually, distortion of thinking processes occurs.
- Chronic high doses, administered intravenously ("speeding"), cause such serious mental (amphetamine psychosis) and physical damage that "speed freaks" rarely can continue the habit for more than two years. They may withdraw from the drug or switch to another, or the old highway warning may become their epitaph: "Speed kills."

Caffeine Some people respond to caffeine's stimulant action with shakiness, nervousness, excitement, more "go" power. Others feel a paradoxical calming effect. In small doses, caffeine may be safe for some people, off limits for others. Moderate use stimulates the cerebral cortex, producing rapid and clearer reaction time. Very large doses affect heart rate and rhythm, blood vessel diameter, circulation and blood pressure, urination, and other physiological functions and may be implicated in ulcer formation and damage to the fetus during pregnancy.

Excessive use (5 cups of coffee a day or more) can lead to chronic poisoning: restlessness, headaches, disturbed sleep, heart irregularities, digestive tract irritation, and diarrhea. More than 1 gram a day (over 7 cups of coffee) can lead to mild delirium in some people; 10 grams can be a fatal dose. A typical cup of brewed coffee has 100 to 150 milligrams of caffeine; instant coffee, 86 to 99 milligrams; tea, 65 to 75 milligrams. Cola drinks run about 40 to 60 milligrams per glass, and many medications, including Anacin, Pre-Mens, and APC, contain caffeine. Diluting coffee and tea with milk and taking them with or after meals helps to reduce the impact of caffeine.

Heavy coffee drinkers appear to have a higher death rate from all causes than nondrinkers, possibly because they are often heavy smokers as well. Decaffeinated coffees and "uncolas" offer alternatives to caffeine consumption.

Hallucinogens

Because the effects of hallucinogens are not fully understood, none are legally licensed for medical use in human beings in the United States except by medical research facilities. As a result, most are processed in clandestine labs and sold in nonstandardized, often contaminated, sometimes "hit-or-missynthesized" forms, frequently mislabeled or misrepresented. Many "mescaline" pills purchased from different street sources have, for example, been found to contain not the faintest trace of that drug.

A mixed bag of effects that include pseudohallucinations or "visions" are brought on by hallucinogens. Effects are influenced by the user's mood and feelings, health, expectations, and the setting. Experimenters are more likely to have a bad trip when they take hallucinogens in a sterile hospital setting than when they take the drugs in warm, friendly surroundings. Because of the variability of drug quality and strength and of individual differences, it is impossible to predict just how a user will respond at any given time (see Table 15.2).

LSD Lysergic acid diethylamide, or "acid," is made from lysergic acid, found in a fungus that affects rye grains and in laboratory-synthesized diethylamide. It is so potent that an amount equal to two aspirin tablets would power 6500 "trips" of 8 to 16 hours each. Like other hallucinogens, LSD is most often taken to achieve mind expansion, mystical experience, or enhanced creativity. These benefits, however, have not been confirmed scientifically.

Use of LSD may have other psychological effects, including suicidal or violent behavior, and long- or short-term psychoses resembling schizophrenia, that may persist for weeks or months following withdrawal from the drug. Distorted perception has caused users to walk out windows, "fly" down stairs, drive cars up trees. Flashback, in which the user's psychedelic trip or its symptoms recur long after the drug has worn off, is not uncommon among LSD users.

Mescaline The primary active ingredient of the peyote cactus, mescaline is available on the street in both natural and synthetic forms. It is often contaminated with other substances such as amphetamines, STP, PCP, insulin, barbiturates, or physostigmine. Alone or contaminated, it can be very toxic.

Its use by the American Indian Church, however, is an example of how responsible

Kal Muller/Woodfin Camp

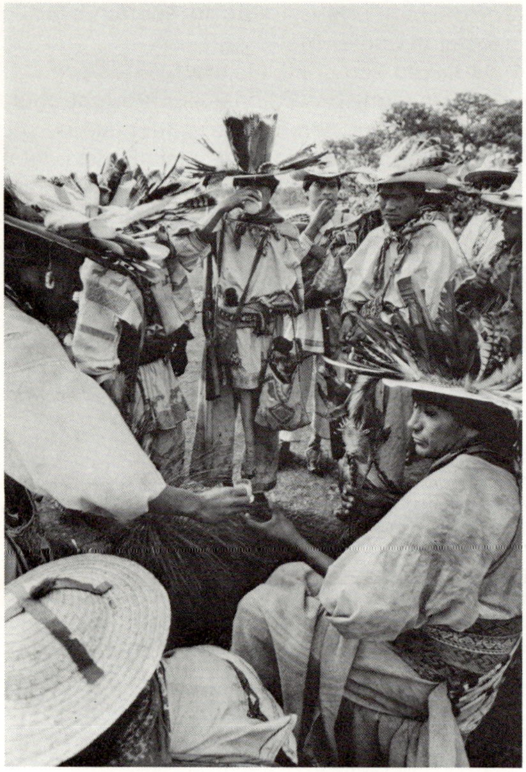

Use of peyote by Huichole Indians of Mexico is an example of how responsible drug use can eliminate many of the negative effects of mind-altering substances.

drug use, integrated into the fabric of a society, can alter the drug's effects. Church members take the drug in a family setting with experienced leaders. They strive for a totally nonvisual, nonhallucinatory experience that concentrates on "higher things" and on keeping family and group together.

Phencyclidine Also known as the *PeaCe Pill* (PCP) or angel dust, this drug has been banned for human use and is available legally only as an animal tranquilizer. In spite of its bizarre and dangerous effects (violent behavior, psychosis, convulsions, even coma at high doses), its use is booming. Most often it is combined with marijuana or peddled to unsuspecting buyers under other names.

Other hallucinogens Psilocybin and psilocin are the active ingredients found in several species of mushrooms and, not surprisingly, these hallucinogens are called "mushrooms" on the street. They fall between LSD and mescaline and in potency have effects similar to LSD. *Nutmeg*, in large quantities, and European *morning glory seeds* are also reported to cause hallucinogenic effects.

Opiates or Narcotics

Although other drugs are sometimes legally classified as narcotics, scientists apply the term only to opiates: (1) opium (the dried juice of unripe pods of the opium poppy); (2) its constituents (e.g., morphine, codeine); (3) its derivatives (semisynthetic heroin); (4) synthetic drugs with chemical compositions similar to natural opiates (Demerol, methadone). About 90 percent of all narcotic abuse involves the use of heroin, though the problem rises and falls with such factors as availability.

Heroin abuse If the first experience with heroin, which often occurs out of casual curiosity or thrill seeking, is pleasurable (and it often is not), the experimenter may wish for an encore. Since dependence does not develop immediately, the new user becomes certain "It can't happen to me." But it does, gradually. First there is psychological dependence. Then, usually after about two average "bags" a day for two weeks, comes physical dependence. The user is hooked.

Some authorities believe there is another level of heroin dependence which is more difficult to cure: "craving," an abnormal willingness to take any step to fulfill the desire for the drug regardless of consequences, coupled with a stubborn unwillingness to accept a substitute (Ashley). A few occasional users,

But one thing I'm certain of . . . was that the addiction that followed was predictable. . . . I knew this; I was absolutely convinced that drugs were the one thing I couldn't handle—that they rendered me powerless over my acts. . . . I can only marvel at this, and wonder. A strong death-wish? An inability to assimilate success? The uncontrolled anger and rebellion of my earlier years? . . . Who knows? Least of all I.

Excerpted from a letter from an addict who resumed drug use following a long abstinence, Geis, p. 130

it seems, fail to develop any physical dependence.

Effects of long-term use Occasional examples of individuals who have lived productive lives while heroin-dependent, without visible signs of physical or mental deterioration, are sometimes presented as evidence that heroin is not harmful. But most of these extremely rare individuals have taken maintenance doses of the drug—levels high enough to prevent withdrawal symptoms but too low to produce a euphoric high. And they had no difficulty either obtaining or paying for their heroin.

In our society, however, where heroin is illegal and extremely expensive, addicts do not fare so well. With their next fix their only goal, they often neglect personal appearance, health, jobs, and families. They may appear "doped," out of it, disinterested in sex and food. In this state, they are rarely violent or antisocial, but as withdrawal begins and desperation mounts, they may be willing to do anything (scrounge, steal, prostitute themselves) for a fix.

Some authorities believe heroin should be provided to addicts legally and at low cost through government agencies. Most do not agree that this would solve the heroin problem. All recognize, however, that under our present system heroin addicts can expect to live 15 to 20 years less than the average person; to suffer from disease and malnutrition, from degradation and ostracism; and to become involved in crime.

Overdose The OD, or overdose, is a serious heroin hazard. Most street heroin is diluted (cut) so much that individual doses of actual heroin are small. Should heroin users happen unknowingly upon a bag that is pure or only slightly cut, they risk death from overdose. There were 1700 estimated heroin-related deaths in the United States between May 1976 and April 1977. New York City medical examiner Milton Halpern suggested that some of these deaths are related to an overwhelming shock reaction due to sensitivity to the injected material rather than an overdose. Others may be due to the use of other drugs, such as alcohol, with the heroin.

Solvents and Inhalants

Solvents and inhalants, abused substances not classified as drugs, may be called "kid stuff," but they can be deadly. Children and adolescents are the most frequent abusers of: *glue fumes*, which produce dizziness, stupor, vomiting, and unconsciousness; *lighter fluid fumes*, which can induce euphoria and, on sustained use, unconsciousness; *gasoline*, which does likewise, but is more toxic; and *ether*, which is not easily available but is used to achieve euphoric release.

The most dangerous effects of solvent inhalation are psychotic behavior and death from suffocation. It can also cause damage to kidneys, liver, heart, blood, and nervous system, and severe anemia in persons with sickle-cell disease (Chapter 23), depending upon the substance abused.

LOOKING BACK

REVIEWING CONCEPTS IN CHAPTER 15

- Most of us are aware that drug problems exist—for somebody else. Yet abuse of drugs is much more widespread than is often realized.
- Drug abuse may be defined in many ways, but basically it means the use of drugs to alter mood and behavior without medical authorization, especially when physical, psychological, or sociological damage occurs.
- Drugs have been used recreationally since earliest times.
- Many factors, in addition to medical information about a drug and its effects, need to be considered when making a decision about drug use.
- Society's wide acceptance of pills and nostrums as problem solvers contributes to the development of drug abuse.
- Strong personal motivation based on a variety of needs (e.g., to escape, to rebel, to experiment, to get even, to get kicks, to identify with peers, to discover self and meaning in life, to improve oneself) contributes to drug experimentation.
- Those who become chronic drug abusers frequently have additional psychiatric problems, often stemming from family difficulties.
- Drug abuse, often called a victimless crime, actually takes a great toll on society as well as on individuals.
- Often drug abuse leads to either psychological or physical dependence. If the latter, withdrawal symptoms occur when the drug is discontinued.
- Drugs of abuse vary widely in the effects they have on the individual and in the way they are viewed and legislated by society.

16

ALCOHOL AND MARIJUANA: THE TWENTIETH CENTURY'S SOCIAL DRUGS

WHAT'S AHEAD IN CHAPTER 16 What are the similarities between alcohol and marijuana, the two most-used social drugs in the United States today? What are the differences? What are the short-term effects of each on the user? The long-term effects? Does dose make a difference? What is the effect of combining drinking and/or smoking marijuana with driving? What is the impact of these drugs and their abuse on society? Does the legal status of each reflect its impact? What is problem drinking? Alcoholism? Are drinking problems limited to a particular segment of the population? How has it been suggested we go about changing present attitudes toward alcohol in the United States in order to make drinking safer? What are the arguments for and against legalization, or decriminalization, of marijuana? Will such legislation eliminate the problem of marijuana abuse?

During the 1960s, alcohol and marijuana were symbols of the conflict between the young and their elders. Parents drank liquor; their children smoked grass. By the mid-1970s, the scene had changed. Large numbers of the young were turning to alcohol, and many older people were experimenting with marijuana.

The two drugs have much in common. Both are used for much the same purposes: to increase sociability, to relax, to reduce inhibitions, and to become pleasantly intoxicated. Abuse patterns appear similar, too. About 9 percent of Americans are heavy drinkers (L. Harris); estimates for heavy marijuana use are about 10 percent of those who try it (Yolles).

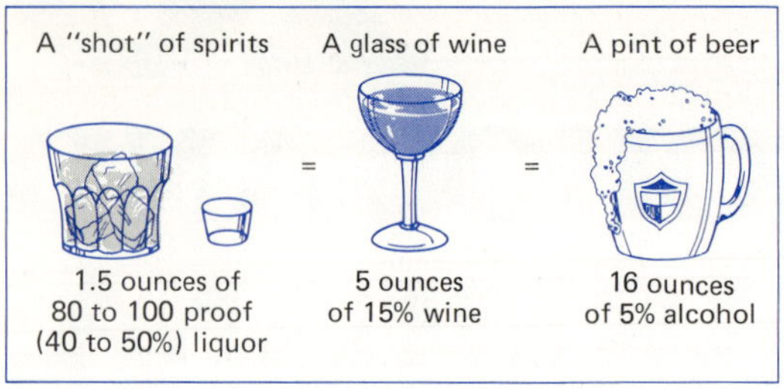
A "shot" of spirits
A glass of wine
A pint of beer
=
=
1.5 ounces of
80 to 100 proof
(40 to 50%) liquor
5 ounces
of 15% wine
16 ounces
of 5% alcohol

FIGURE 16.1 Alcoholic equivalents.

But alcohol and marijuana are treated very differently in our society. Alcohol is deeply entrenched in Western culture, dating back to at least biblical times. Attempts to outlaw its use through Prohibition, ratified in 1919 and realistically but reluctantly repealed in 1933, were unsuccessful. However, when marijuana was outlawed by the Marijuana Tax Act in 1937, there was barely a ripple of protest. Not until use became widespread, particularly among middle-class youth, were voices raised against its prohibition. Even in 1976, when an estimated 1 in 7 Americans had tried marijuana, majority opinion did not appear to favor removing all restrictions on the drug.

The similarities between alcohol and marijuana are used as arguments both by those who favor retaining antimarijuana laws and by those who want to see them liberalized. The former point to the disastrous impact alcohol has had on our society and ask: Do we want to repeat the tragedy? The latter declare it is unfair to allow alcohol to be sold legally and to outlaw marijuana. As you read this chapter, you might consider how the use of intelligent decision making can aid individuals and the community in dealing with these major drugs.

WHAT IS ALCOHOL?

The major chemical ingredient in beer, wines, and distilled liquors is a natural substance, known as *ethyl alcohol* or *ethanol*, formed by fermentation (a metabolic process) of sugar with yeast cells. Ethanol differs from *methyl* or *wood* alcohol, used in antifreeze and fuels and highly toxic even in small doses, and from *isopropyl alcohol*, the equally toxic main ingredient in most rubbing alcohols. Ethanol is colorless and flammable, and can cause intoxication and a wide variety of other effects on the body. As a drug, it is a depressant.

The various alcoholic beverages are produced from different sources of sugars: wine from grapes, berries, or other fruits; beer from malted (germinated) barley; whiskey from malted grains; vodka from grains, fruits, or vegetables (especially potatoes); and rum from molasses. "Hard" liquor (such as whiskey, scotch, gin, vodka) is further concentrated through distillation, giving it a higher alcohol concentration. Alcohol content of beer and wine is usually listed by percentages, while the potency of hard liquor is indicated in "proof"—double the percentage. This sometimes confuses those trying to compare the wallop of a couple of cans of beer to that of a martini. (See Figure 16.1.)

Ethanol is sometimes classified as a food because it is metabolized, producing energy; 83 calories in an ounce of 100-proof whiskey, 150 in a 12-ounce can of beer. Unlike food, however, it has no nutritive value and does not need to be digested.

IMMEDIATE EFFECTS OF ALCOHOL

Alcohol affects nearly all body tissues—heart, blood vessels, digestive tract, liver, pancreas, endocrine glands, skin, and blood. Its most noticeable effect is as a depressant on the central nervous system, which is a surprise to many who associate it with a "lift." This lift, however, is not from stimulation, but from a relaxation of inhibitions. In general, low doses of alcohol may have a pleasant effect, high doses a detrimentally depressive one; one or two drinks may relieve stress, four or five increase it. As little as one drink can impair some functions, such as the ability to respond to a highway emergency or solve a complex problem.

Only moments after alcohol is ingested, it can be found in all tissues, organs, and secretions of the body. About 20 percent of each sip is absorbed directly into the bloodstream from the mouth and stomach; the rest only a bit more slowly through the intestinal tract. The effects, particularly on the the brain, are almost immediate.

As with other drugs, reactions to alcohol are individualized. Some people maintain that just "a whiff" of hard liquor sends them reeling. Others claim "a hollow leg," the ability to take in unlimited quantities without getting drunk. These reactions depend on a number of factors:

- *Heredity*
- *Personality, size, gender* The outgoing extrovert, the small person, the female are all more likely to become intoxicated quickly than the introvert, the large person, the male.
- *Mood and setting* A drink taken when tired or under stress has more impact than one taken when comfortable and happy.
- *Expectation* If you expect to "feel" one drink, you will.
- *Previous exposure*
- *Type of beverage* Straight liquor has the strongest, most immediate impact; wines and beers, because they are diluted with other substances, are absorbed less rapidly.
- *Accompanying mixers or food* Water or juice dilutes and slows absorption of alcohol, carbonated beverage accelerates it,[1] and food taken with or before alcohol allows for slower and more even absorption.
- *Speed of consumption* Gulped drinks produce almost immediate effects, sipped ones more gradual effects.

[1]The carbon dioxide bubbles tickle the pyloric valve, causing it to open wide its entrance to the stomach.

The more rapid the absorption of alcohol, the more rapidly the blood alcohol concentration (BAC) rises. A person experiencing a happy high from one or two drinks may take several more in an attempt to keep the feeling from wearing off. But as more drinks go down, BACs go up, and effects become less pleasant (see Table 16.1).

ALCOHOL AND HEALTH

Although heavy drinking reduces life expectancy by 10 to 12 years (Chafetz, *b*), light to moderate drinking appears to have no serious negative effects on health. Just when someone reaches the threshold above which martini becomes menace is difficult to pinpoint. But a nineteenth-century British physician, Francis Anstie, devised guidelines still in use. Moderate drinking, according to Anstie's Law, means consumption of no more than 1½ ounces of absolute alcohol per day. This means three 1-ounce shots of whiskey, half a bottle of table wine, or four glasses of beer, taken with food in a relaxed atmosphere. Those who regularly exceed Anstie's ceiling risk many health problems.

Physical Effects of Alcohol

The liver Alcohol causes a scarring or fibrous hardening of the liver that interferes with its functioning. This alcoholic cirrhosis is the fourth leading cause of death for men 25 to 65 living in major United States cities. Though cirrhosis is associated with "falling-down-drunks" in the minds of most people, the disease may develop over a 20-year period in someone who nevers gets drunk, but has a couple of martinis at lunch, a couple more before dinner, wine at table, and brandy as a nightcap.

The brain The mechanism of how ethyl alcohol affects the brain is as uncertain as how it induces drunkenness or sleep. Possibly it

TABLE 16.1 Effects of varying amounts of alcohol on a 150-pound person within 1 hour

NUMBER OF DRINKS	BLOOD ALCOHOL LEVELS	BEHAVIOR, SUBJECTIVE FEELINGS, AND EFFECTS ON BODY	BOGEN'S PROGRESSION
None			Dull and dignified
1	Not measurable	Pleasant relaxation; slight changes in mind and behavior (these may be learned).	Dashing and debonair
2 (2 cocktails, 2–3 cans beer, 2 glasses wine)	0.05	Release from tensions, inhibitions; sleepiness in some; thought, judgment, restraint affected.	Dangerous and devilish
5	0.10*	Voluntary motor actions of arms, hands, legs become clumsy; speech slurred.	Dizzy and disturbing
8	0.20	All motor activity impaired; person staggers easily; easily angered; emotionally unstable; garrulous, aggressive, excited; may weep uncontrollably; drunk.	Disgusting and disheveled Delirious and disoriented
11–12	0.30	Deep areas of the brain now depressed; confusion; if lucky, the person will pass out or be in stupor and be unable to continue drinking.	Drunk
Additional	0.40	Coma; depressing of brain centers that regulate breathing and heartbeat.	Dead drunk
Still more	0.50	Death (1000 deaths each year directly attributable).	Dead

*The legal definition of "drunk" in many states.
Source: U.S. DHEW, *I,* pp. 37, 38; Bogen, p. 136.

interferes with brain function by blocking essential molecular processes. Long-term use appears to cause pronounced brain damage (Jones and Parsons). The consequences of such damage are seen in many long-time alcoholics: they exhibit poor judgment and inability to profit from experience or to sustain their actions long enough to work toward a goal.

The heart Latest evidence indicates that alcohol is *not* a significant factor in heart attack.[2] In fact, moderate alcohol use is associated in some studies with lower risk of heart attack, and quitting drinking appears to involve a higher risk. Researchers speculate that this unexpected statistic may be because those who quit are in poorer health generally; 25 percent are estimated to quit for health reasons.

[2]An exception may be the 12–15 percent of American men whose abnormally high blood fat (trigyceride) levels, associated with heart attack, are dramatically increased by alcohol (Mendelson and Mello).

There is considerable evidence, however, that alcohol does damage the heart *muscle*, leading to a condition known as *alcohlic cardiomyopathy*, which can be fatal. Heavy drinking also appears to cause deterioration of other muscles in the body.

The reproductive system Alcohol may loosen sexual inhibitions and even increase desire, but heavy doses often prevent successful completion of the sex act. Recent investigations indicate that long-term alcoholism in males may also lead to severe damage to the testicles, and sterility (Perper). In females, the effects of alcoholism on the reproductive system are most apparent during pregnancy. Infants born to heavy-drinking women (six drinks per day or more) suffer severe abnormalities labeled fetal alcohol syndrome (see Chapter 23). The infants may also suffer from physical dependence and withdrawal symptoms at birth. The recommended limit in pregnancy is two drinks per day.

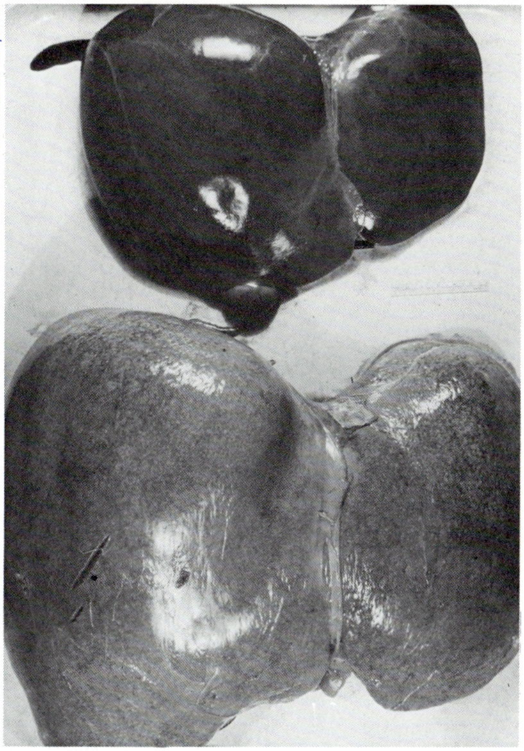

Dr. Milton Helpern

Normal liver and swollen, fatty liver, the result of prolonged use of alcohol.

Alcohol and Cancer

The link between smoking and cancer has received so much attention that most people remain unaware that both clinical and epidemiological studies have implicated the *excessive* use of alcohol, especially when combined with smoking, in the development of cancers of the mouth, pharynx, pancreas, and esophagus, as well as in development of primary cancers of the liver. The type of beverage consumed may also be a factor, as distilled liquors appear related to some kinds of cancer, beer to others.

Alcohol and Antisocial Behavior

Accidents Problem drinkers die more often in accidents than moderate or nondrinkers

MACDUFF What three things does drink especially provoke?

PORTER Marry Sir, nose-painting, sleep and urine. Lechery Sir, it provokes and it unprovokes; it provokes the desire, but it takes away the performance . . . therefore much drink may be said to be an equivocator with lechery . . . it sets him on and it takes him off; it persuades him and disheartens him; makes him stand to and not stand to; in conclusion, equivocates him in a sleep, and giving him the lie, leaves him.

Macbeth, Act II, Scene 3

TABLE 16.2 The relationship between cancer at various sites and the use of alcohol and tobacco

	RELATIONSHIP TO USE OF	
SITE	ALCOHOL	TOBACCO
Hypopharynx	Very strong	Very strong
Larynx	Very strong	Very strong
Esophagus	Very strong	Strong
Lung		Very strong
Oropharynx	Strong	Very strong
Tongue	Very strong	Strong
Oral cavity	Strong	Very strong
Lips		Strong
Bladder; other urinary cancers		Strong

Source: U.S. DHEW, *bb,* p. 54, from Flamant et al.

and, too often, they take others with them. Alcohol is related to 1 of every 3 sudden and unexpected deaths in young adults, to 1 in 3 suicides, to nearly half the drownings of persons over 14, to 8 out of 10 after-dark snowmobile accidents, and to a large proportion of deaths by fire (U.S. DHEW, *bb*).

In nearly 1 of every 2 automobile accidents in which someone died, the driver had an illegally high blood alcohol concentration,

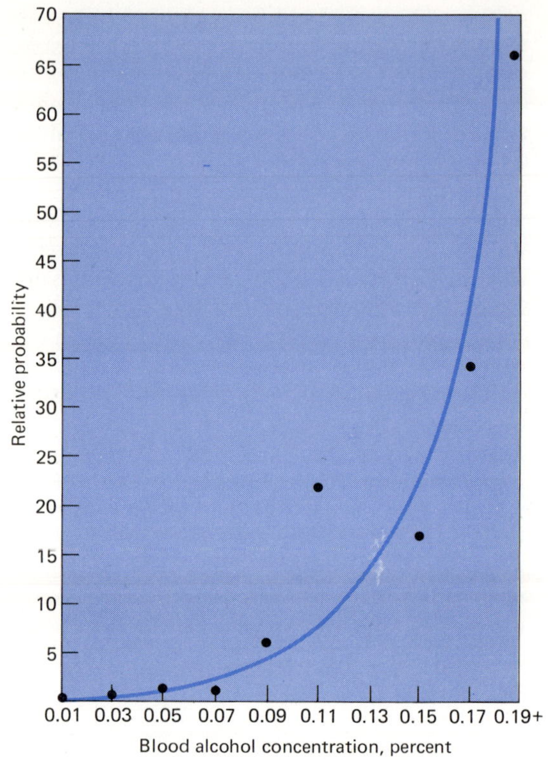

FIGURE 16.2 Relative probability of being responsible for a fatal crash in relation to blood alcohol concentration. [*Adapted from Perrine et al.*]

TABLE 16.3 Dose-related risk of oral cancer with exposure to alcohol and tobacco

AMOUNT OF PURE ALCOHOL PER DAY	CIGARETTES PER DAY			
	0	FEWER THAN 20	20–39	MORE THAN 40
None	1.00*	1.52	1.43	2.43
Less than 0.4 ounce	1.40	1.67	3.18	3.25
0.4–1.5 ounces	1.60	4.36	4.46	8.21
More than 1.5 ounces	2.33	4.13	9.59	15.50

*Relative risk for person who neither smokes nor drinks is 1.00.
Source: U.S. DHEW, *bb,* p. 55, from Rothman and Keller.

usually above 0.10 percent. That means the average 180-pound male driver had probably downed five or more drinks in the hour before getting into the car. Even smaller doses significantly alter driving performance and lead to accidents. Studies in which drivers took measured doses of alcohol and drove automobile simulators in the laboratory show clearly that, as BACs rose, response time slowed, clumsiness increased, inhibitions dissolved, and judgment was lost. Alcohol also contributes to pedestrian accidents. About one-third of adult pedestrians killed by autos have BACs of 0.10 percent or higher, often making them the guilty party in the accident (Waller).

Crime Being high on heroin is not a crime, but until very recently, 2 million Americans were arrested annually for being high on alcohol. Recent acceptance of alcoholism as a disease rather than a crime has prompted more than half the states thus far to pass legislation decriminalizing drunkenness and opening doors to hospital treatment wards instead of jail "drunk tanks."

Although alcohol apparently does not generate antisocial behavior, it may intensify and complicate it. Alcohol can also remove the inhibitions that keep most of us from engaging in antisocial behavior. Alcohol is related to one-half the homicides and violent crimes committed in the United States, and one-half of all imprisoned felons have alcohol-related problems. At one treatment center, 35 percent of convicted rapists were found to be alcoholics, and 50 percent had been drinking prior to committing the offense (Rada).

Breathalyzers, used increasingly by law enforcement officers, make it possible to determine a driver's level of intoxication by measuring the percentage of alcohol in the blood.

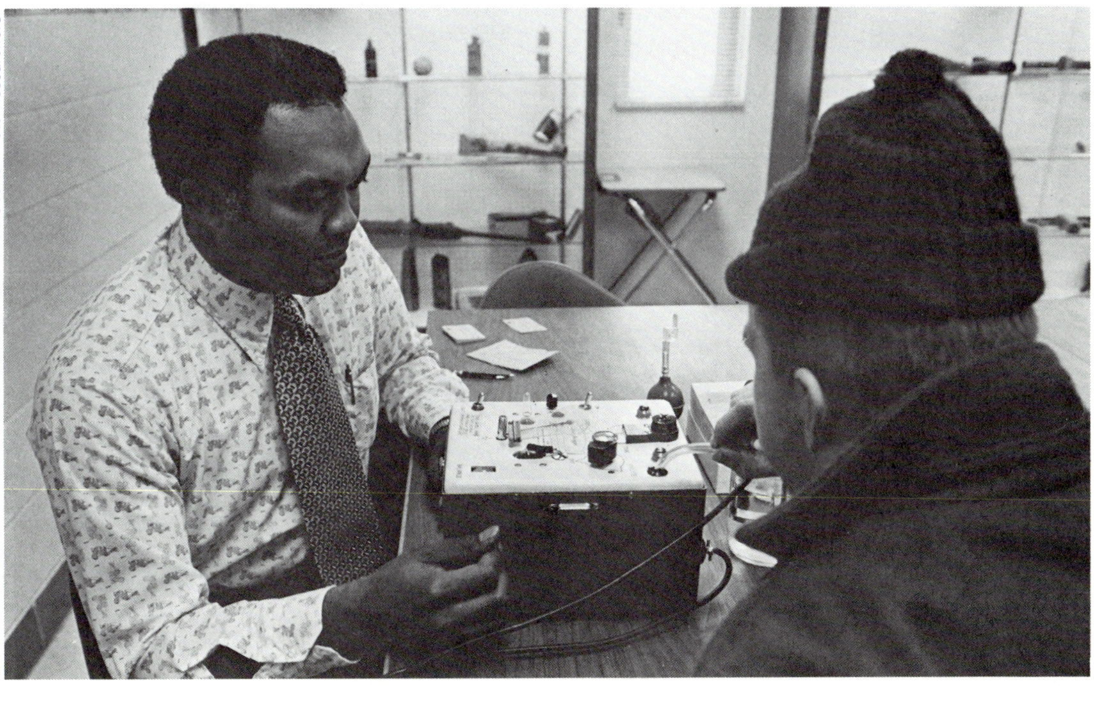

Bruce Roberts/Photo Researchers

PROBLEM DRINKING

In 1785, Dr. Benjamin Rush, Surgeon General of the Continental Army, called intemperate use of distilled spirits a "disease and an addiction," and estimated that 4000 deaths in America's population of 6 million were due to alcohol. The problem is with us still.

Problem drinking might be categorized as any use of alcohol that leads to physical damage, psychological difficulties, problems in functioning, irresponsible behavior, or loss of time from work, school, or other responsibilities. This would include the heavy drinker who daily consumes large quantities of alcohol without ever being noticeably drunk, the weekend drinker who becomes intoxicated and abusive, the partygoer who drinks and drives, and the compulsive drinker or alcoholic.

Unkempt, unshaven gutter winos make up fewer than 5 percent of problem drinkers in the United States. The others are found in every socioeconomic group, at every educational level, in every career or job category. Of the 10 million Americans believed to be problem drinkers, some 20 percent live in inner cities, another 40 percent are blue-collar workers, and 30 percent are middle class. More than 5 percent stand on the highest rungs of the socioeconomic ladder (Kissin). The top rungs have more drinkers but fewer problem drinkers than the bottom. Problem drinking has become so serious a concern on

While most associate problem drinking with Skid Row derelicts, alcohol-related problems are found in every socioeconomic group.

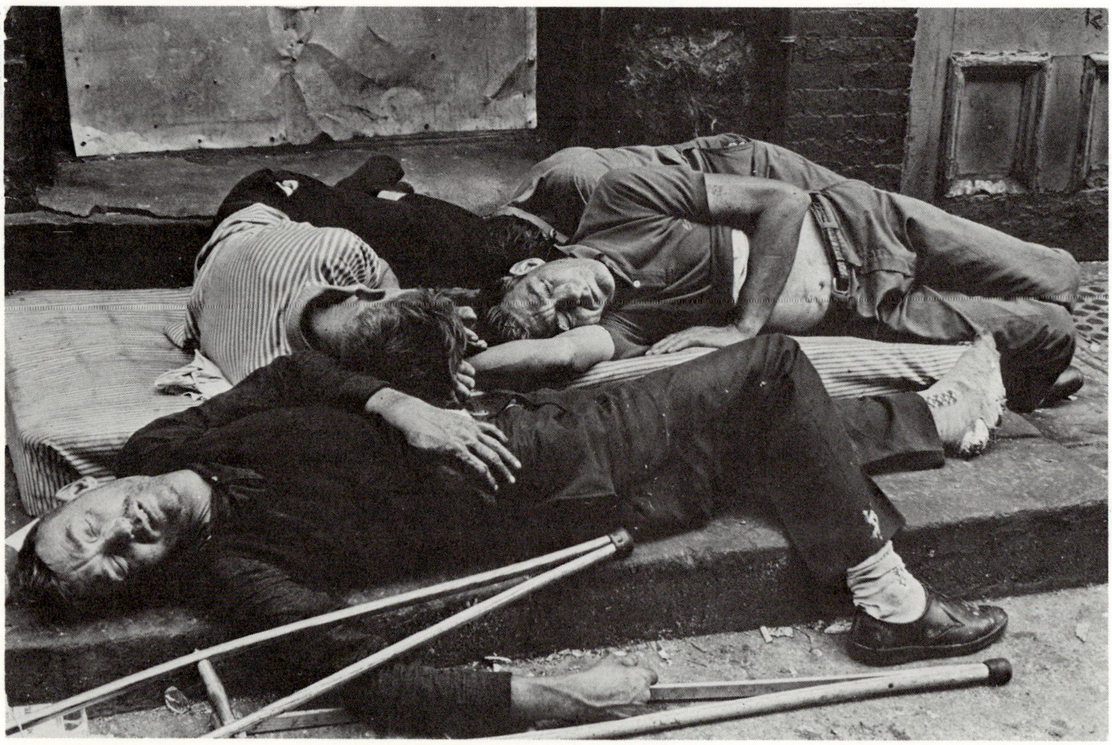

Hella Hammid/Photo Researchers

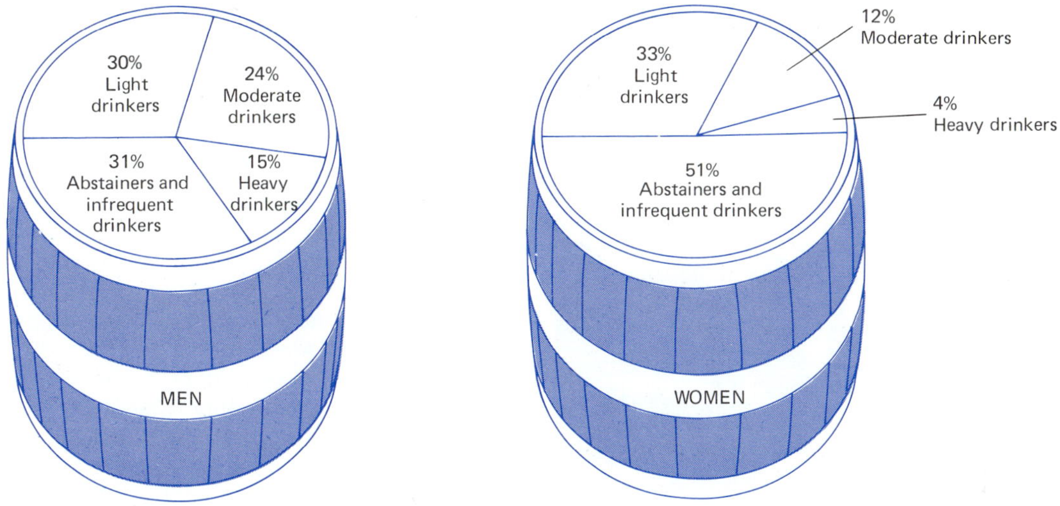

FIGURE 16.3 Percentage and types of drinkers by sex, United States, 1972–1974. *Abstainers and infrequent drinkers* drink less than once a month or not at all. *Drinkers* drink once a month or more. Light drinkers drink at most 0.22 ounce absolute alcohol per day. Moderate drinkers drink 0.22 to 1.0 ounce per day. Heavier drinkers drink 1.0 or more ounces per day. [*Adapted from U.S. DHEW, bb, p. 11.*]

college campuses that some schools have instituted alcohol education programs.

The percentage of women with drinking problems is believed to have doubled since World War II (National Council on Alcoholism), and women now make up one-third of alcoholics (Chafetz, *b*). Where alcohol problems are most common in men in their twenties, women are more likely to have such difficulties in their thirties and forties.

Teenage Drinking

Drinking patterns are often set in high school. Thus the growing use of alcohol by adolescents and even preadolescents and the high rate of misuse and abuse are of increasing concern. An estimated 1.3 million teenagers and preteens drink to excess. Though casual drinking is found among all groups of teenagers, problem drinking is found more often among students who also engage in other types of deviant behavior, who value and expect achievement less and esteem independence more than nondrinkers, and who are more tolerant of deviant behavior in others. Girls with drinking problems are likely to have parent problems (Jessor and Jessor).

Alcohol, most often in the form of beer or sweet wines, is the most-used drug among adolescents. Marijuana is second. Most marijuana users also use alcohol (92 percent), but only about 1 of every 3 alcohol users also uses marijuana. Boys drink more than girls, though drinking is increasing among girls. One theory about the growing popularity of alcohol suggests that teenagers in the 1970s became less rebellious and thus elected alcohol, the drug of the Establishment. Alcohol is also cheaper than other drugs. Another factor frequently blamed is parental permissiveness. While teenagers from permissive homes are

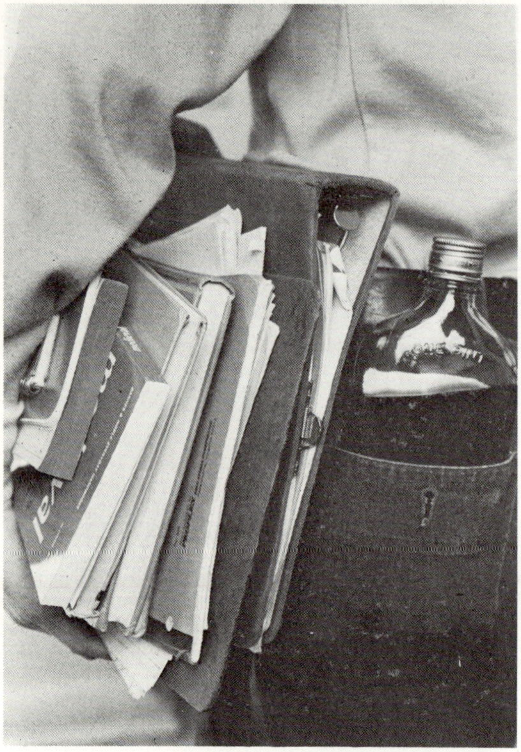

Use of alcohol by adolescents and even preadolescents has been growing steadily, and the high rate of misuse and abuse is of increasing concern.

more apt to drink than those from homes that forbid alcohol, there are indications that the latter, when they drink, are more apt to have drinking problems (Globetti).

Public laws that do not permit a gradual introduction to drinking may also influence drinking patterns. Some young people, suddenly legally free to drink at 18 (or 19 or 21), may have trouble handling alcohol. Others, still under age, find the legal taboo makes drinking more attractive: It represents maturity because it is considered *bad* for children, *good* for adults. Restrictive laws also often influence young people to drink where adults are not present, most often at night in the worst possible place, automobiles.

The Alcoholic

Alcoholism is not a moral weakness, but rather a serious lifelong disease that can be controlled by eliminating alcohol, but cannot be cured. Actually, it may prove to be several diseases with similar symptoms but differing causes. Some of these diseases, or a predisposition to them, may be transmitted genetically from parent to child. Others may be environmentally caused. Children of alcoholic parents are more likely to become alcoholics than others. Alcoholism may also be "contagious," caught as part of a lifestyle from friends or the community. Scientists as yet can only speculate why some people become alcoholics, while others, with similar pressures, heredity, environment, and exposure to alcohol, do not. It has been suggested that alcoholism is a complex disease that is one part psychological, one part physical, one part sociological, and one part alcohol.

Physical dependence, signs of tolerance, severe withdrawal symptoms, and an inability to abstain from the drug distinguish the alcoholic from the problem drinker. The alcoholic drinks compulsively and feels powerless to stop. An occasional, very susceptible person is in trouble with the first drink, but most cases of alcoholism develop over a period of 5 to 10 years of heavy drinking. Changes are so gradual that close friends and family, or even the developing alcoholics themselves may not be aware of them (M. Block). Drinking patterns may not appear to differ from those of the typical heavy drinker, but there are clues or symptoms that indicate trouble (see the sidebar on page 368).

THE NONDRINKER

It is difficult to swim against the tide, and yet 31 percent of men and 51 percent of women either abstain or drink less frequently than once a month. There are fewer abstainers at younger ages, when experimentation is going on, and more at middle age and beyond. But at every age, there are many who say "no" to

June had her first drink at age 8 when an adult handed her a drink at a party. The woman found it amusing to see such a small girl drink. Says June, "I was drinking sloe gin and taking pills regularly when I was nine." She got barbiturates from a friend whose mother worked in a pharmacy.

Liquor wasn't hard to get either: "Booze was simple to buy. You just wait outside a liquor store and see a nice older gentleman or a young guy and you ask him to buy a six-pack because you are having a party."

Like many child alcoholics, June is the daughter of an alcoholic. She remembers: "I was 5 years old and taking care of her, and I never brought friends home. [Later in my childhood] I would get drunk, mostly on weekends. I knew I had a problem, but I didn't want to identify myself as an alcoholic because I didn't want to be what my mother was." (Adapted from Trout, p. 22)

alcohol. Psychiatrist Morris Chafetz, former director of the National Institute on Alcohol Abuse and Alcoholism (NIAAA), believes that these abstainers need reinforcement, that they need to become less defensive about their position and less antagonistic toward those who drink.

A decision not to drink may be based on the hard facts about alcohol's effects on the body, or it may be based on a variety of other personal reasons, including: religious or family convictions; a dislike for the taste of liquor; a distrust of the high that accompanies it; or a lack of need for a drug in order to feel high, happy, and sociable. Some people also choose to be light drinkers or occasional nondrinkers, particularly when they are tired, depressed, or ill; have a heavy work schedule the next day; have to drive home; or are counting calories, taking other drugs (especially barbiturates or other depressants), or just do not feel like drinking. No reasons need

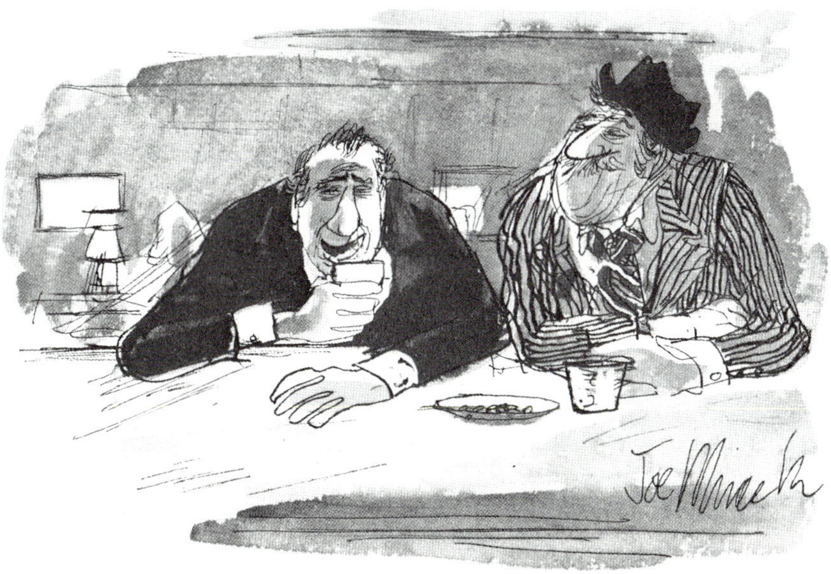

"And another thing about a Martini—it's low in tar and nicotine."

WHEN TO SEEK HELP

Signs of Alcoholism*

Early stages

- Occasional heavy drinking following a disappointment, a quarrel, or a distressing incident, or when under pressure
- Drinking alone
- Ability to handle more liquor than previously, or more than associates can handle
- Lapse of memory on a "morning after" (a "blackout") even though one did not "pass out"
- Taking extra drinks secretly; gulping drinks
- A feeling of discomfort when alcohol is not served or not available
- Occasional feelings of guilt about drinking

Middle stages

- Feelings of annoyance when others discuss one's drinking habits
- Increase in frequency of blackouts
- A desire to continue drinking after others have had enough
- Regret when sober for things done or said while drinking
- Unsuccessful attempts made to control or cut down on drinking
- Avoidance of family or close friends while drinking
- Increase in number of financial and work (or school) problems; absenteeism, especially after weekends
- A feeling of being treated unfairly, when there is no good reason for the feeling
- Irregular and inadequate diet when drinking
- Drinking in the morning to relieve occasional "shakes" or hangovers

Late or final stages

- Getting drunk more quickly on less alcohol
- Long periods of drunkenness, often lasting several days
- Depression and doubts about the worth of life
- Alcohol-related accidents or arrests
- Seeing things that are not there or having feelings of terror after some drinking bouts
- Neglect of eating, health, appearance; inability to function without drinking; constant tremors or nervousness relieved only by alcohol; severe deterioration of health, and of family, work, and other relationships
- Physical complaints: nerve pain, muscle weakness, redness in palms, nausea, loss of appetite.

*These vary from person to person; the presence of even a few of them can indicate a problem.
Source: Adapted from National Council on Alcoholism.

be given to a host, hostess, or friend who offers an unwanted drink. A simple "no, thank you," clear and firm, should be enough. A person who tries to insist that someone else take a drink is, in effect, pushing drugs.

TOWARD A NEW ALCOHOL ETHIC

- The hero in a TV drama returns home after a long day and heads straight for the whiskey closet. On a soap opera, an alcoholic goes through a shaking, crying, praying withdrawal. On a comedy show, the audience howls as an entertainer plays a funny drunk.
- A recession closes down the only grocery store in a small upstate New York town, but its two bars continue to flourish.
- Teenagers are caught drinking beer in the high school parking lot during a dance. Their parents breathe sighs of relief that it was only beer, not pot or "hard stuff."

Attitudes and behavior relating to alcohol use in the United States are confusing and erratic, and drinking patterns reflect the confusion. We laugh at the drunk, but condemn the drunk driver. We do not recognize drunkenness as drug overdose and resolutely turn our backs on the fact that alcohol is *the* major drug problem in the United States.

Prohibition, which began in 1919, was an attempt to eliminate the problem, and it failed. Are there other approaches that can reduce the damage to individuals and to society caused by alcohol misuse? There may be some clues to be found in societies with low incidence of problem drinking. In such cultures, drinking is integrated into the fabric of life; there is substantial agreement about the values, norms, and practices that regulate alcohol use; and drinking is subordinated to family, religious, recreational, and other pursuits, rather than used as the prime attraction of a social activity.

In the United States, on the other hand, our cultural melting pot contains an international goulash of mores, customs, beliefs, and values relating to alcohol. There are Mormons and some Protestants who consider drinking immoral, French and Italian Americans to whom a meal without wine is not a meal, traditional Jews who use alcohol for religious purposes but frown on drunkenness, members of a half-dozen ethnic groups who view heavy drinking as manly, and native Americans whose culture was alcohol-free until the white man came bearing firewater and disaster. Social activities often revolve around drinking: the cocktail party, the bar, the saloon, the pub, the commuter train bar car. Adults ask friends to "drop by for a drink," not for conversation. Teenagers go out "drinking," not to have fun or see friends.

Can this situation be changed? Apparently, yes. Drunkenness was a problem among ancient Hebrews. Yet temperate drinking became the established norm among Jews when their national culture was reformed around 525–350 B.C.E. In this century, both France and Denmark have reduced per capita consumption of alcohol in response to campaigns calling for moderate drinking.

In 1974, the NIAAA started a national program that attempted to educate Americans toward accepting the following attitudes:

- Alcohol is a drug.
- Alcohol can be physically, psychologically, and socially beneficial in small doses, but used irresponsibly it can be dangerous, even life-threatening.
- Drunkenness indicates weakness or disease; it should not be viewed as positive social behavior.
- Alcoholism is a treatable disease.
- The decision to drink or not to drink should be a personal one. Those who choose not to drink and those who choose to drink must come to respect each other's decisions.
- Those who choose to drink have a respon-

Ken Heyman

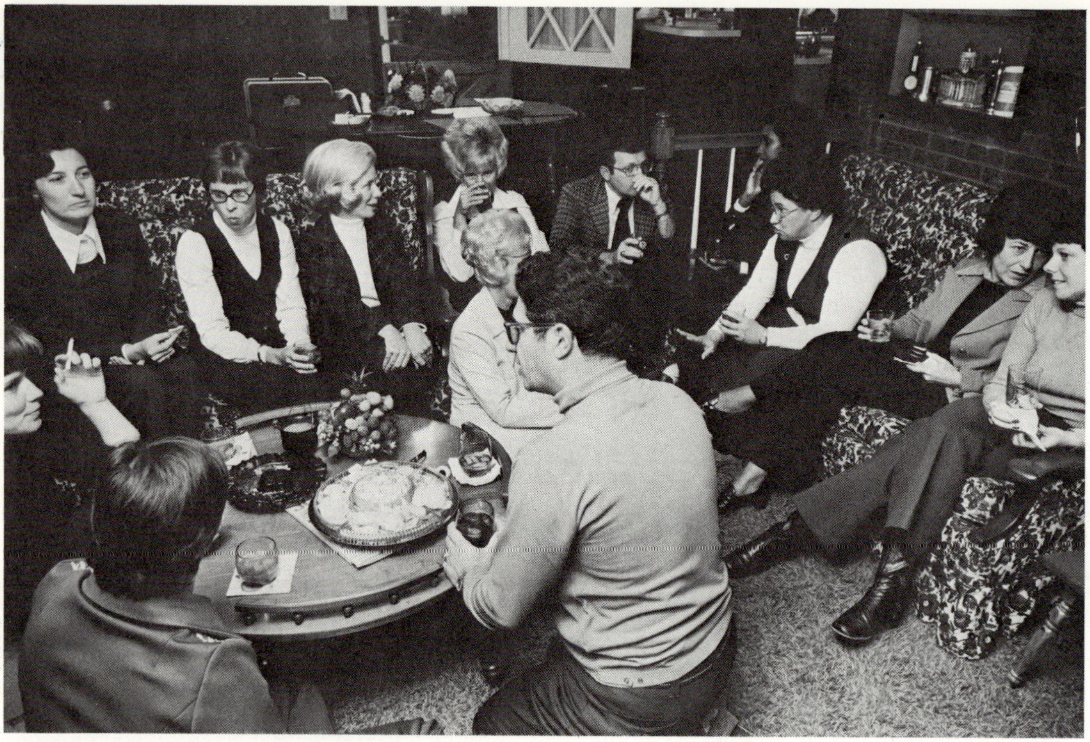

Social activities often revolve around drinking.

sibility not to destroy themselves, their families, or their relationships with society. Responsible drinking includes: avoiding overdose and resultant drunkenness; not using alcohol to solve problems or to relieve depression or other psychological difficulties; sipping, not gulping drinks; not drinking before driving or operating machinery.

- Servers of drinks, too, have a responsibility.[3] They can serve alcohol only with food; measure drinks with care rather than overgenerosity; mix distilled liquors with water, juices, etc., to dilute the strength; refuse to sell or serve drinks to those already intoxicated, and not push drinks on reluctant guests; offer alternatives such as soft drinks and juices; not insist on "freshening" drinks. Hosts and hostesses should see that coffee is served and the bar is closed a good hour or more before the end of a party. They can offer transportation or overnight accommodations to intoxicated guests.
- New and alternative recreational settings need to be developed in which drinking is a coincidental factor, rather than the main reason for people frequenting them. Bars and cocktail parties that serve only alcoholic beverages should be eliminated.

[3]California courts have ruled that hosts or bar operators who serve alcohol to obviously intoxicated persons can be held legally liable if these persons later injure others, as in an automobile accident.

MARIJUANA

In a 1930s film, a young man arrested for smoking marijuana is brought into court, a raving lunatic. The district attorney, convinced that the young man is "hopelessly and incurably insane—a condition caused by the drug marijuana to which he was addicted," recommends that he be placed in an institution for the criminally insane for the rest of his natural life. A narrator then proclaims, "Yes, that happened right here. To your neighbors. It is not too much to say that in your hands lies the possibility of averting other tragedies like it. We must work untiringly so that our children are obliged to learn the truth. Because it is only through knowledge that we can safely protect. The next tragedy may be that of your daughter . . . or your son . . . or yours . . . or yours . . . or yours."

This melodramatic filmscript, used in the "war against marijuana" at a time when misinformation about the drug was circulated as fact, helped to spread inaccurate early impressions of marijuana. Today the film is being used as propaganda once more—this time by promarijuana forces to show how old-fashioned and ridiculous the antimarijuana faction is. These uses of an obviously contrived film demonstrate the way in which opposing sides in the marijuana dispute have let bias for or against the drug color their actions and thinking. Neither side has been willing to look at marijuana objectively, as they might look at antibiotics or aspirin.

Some of the confusion about what marijuana *is* stems from the confusion about what it is not. Due to its long-time listing on federal statutes alongside narcotics like heroin, many people incorrectly assumed (as the film described above dramatized) that marijuana, too, was an addictive "menace to society." When popular experimentation began, users woke up the morning after to find their brains had not rotted and they had not gone mad. Thus they lost faith in the accuracy of Establishment drug information.

Marijuana is the popular name for a hemp plant scientifically classified as *cannabis*. When inhaled in smoking or eaten, the resinous flowering tops and leaves of the plant can intoxicate. Quality and effectiveness vary with strain, climate, and other conditions. Hashish, used in the same way as marijuana, is a highly concentrated form of resinous material from the same plant, but it produces effects that are much more complex and pronounced, as well as potentially more hazardous. The major ingredient in both drugs is delta-9-tetrahydrocannabinol (Δ-9-THC), but there are other active ingredients as well.

Like other drugs bought illegally, marijuana is not always delivered as represented. A report by the Department of Health, Education, and Welfare (DHEW) described an evaluation of 36 samples sold as "high-quality marijuana." Only 64 percent contained any marijuana at all; some samples were simply lawn grass clippings or hay. Many of those

Like other drugs bought illegally, marijuana is not always delivered as represented. It may be contaminated with other substances or may not be marijuana at all.

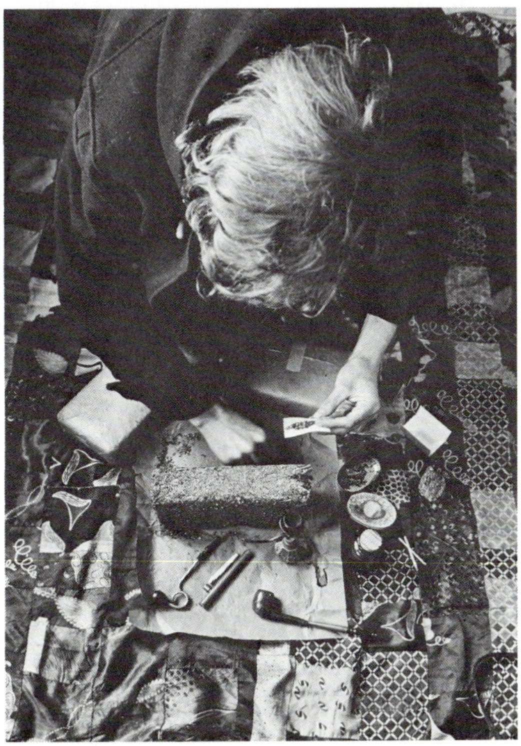

Bob Combs/Photo Researchers

that did contain marijuana were cut or contaminated with other substances, some highly dangerous. In 1978 shipments of Mexican marijuana were found to be contaminated with a toxic herbicide.

Marijuana does not fit strictly into any single drug category. It has some of the characteristics of hallucinogens and can be either stimulating or depressing, exaggerating the mood of the user. It has been suggested that it be considered an "intoxicant" similar to alcohol. But, unlike alcohol, marijuana has not been known to cause death in overdose—toxic levels appear to be extremely high.

MARIJUANA USE

The 1975 *Report to Congress on Marijuana and Health* indicates that nearly 1 in 5 American adults, 1 in 4 under 18, and 1 in 2 in the 18 to 25 age group had tried marijuana at least once (U.S. DHEW, *x*). Wide differences existed between geographic areas, with use highest in the West, lowest in the South. Use appears to be concentrated in the 18 to 25 age group, in which it is twice as common among males as among females, lowest among married men 20 to 30 years old, and highest among unmarried people living together.

A majority of marijuana experimenters do not become regular users, but daily or near-daily use is on the rise, particularly among young users. The myth that marijuana use automatically leads to heroin use has been debunked, but there is considerable evidence that marijuana users are more likely than nonusers to experiment with other drugs. Marijuana is a step in the standard pattern of the young drug abuser in the United States, following beer, wine, liquor, and cigarettes.

Reasons for use and nonuse of marijuana are similar to those for drug use and nonuse in general, discussed in Chapter 15. Like other serious drug abusers, heavy users of marijuana, who must be differentiated from occasional smokers, have often been found to have serious personality problems. They are often underachievers who do not work up to their mental capacity, display an air of self-neglect, general lassitude and indifference, and a lack of productivity. Hostility exhibited by many heavy users gives rise to the theory that they use marijuana to get relief from feelings of anger, resentment, frustration, and aggression, much as tranquilizers are used on the Establishment level.

Marijuana use often ceases when young people graduate from college, become socially isolated from other users, and constrained by jobs, marriage, and family (Brown et al.). College students may temporarily cease use when studying, or "under pressure, obligation, or responsibility" (Cheek et al.).

MARIJUANA AND HEALTH

Serious research on the implications of marijuana use for the American people was late in starting (1967–1968) and has often been hampered by a variety of problems: (1) lack of standardized natural and synthetic material for experimental use, (2) intense controversy surrounding the topic, (3) assorted legal and bureaucratic barriers to conducting research on an illegal substance, and (4) subjective feelings of investigators either for or against the drug.

In addition, there are two serious problems similar to those that hampered cigarette research earlier. First, rare or subtle effects do not show up unless very large numbers of people are studied over long periods. Few Americans have been heavy marijuana smokers for enough years for scientists to be able to gauge effects, and studies of foreign smokers are difficult to apply to American users because of differences in culture and other factors. It took 30 years and studies of tens of thousands of smokers to demonstrate that cigarette smoking caused lung cancer and was an important factor in heart disease. It may take that long to learn the full effects of marijuana. Second, most chronic, heavy users also use other drugs, and so it is difficult to tell just what is causing any adverse effects.

In spite of all the research difficulties, a good deal is being learned each year. Much of it is contradictory and, thus, inconclusive. Several areas of hazard are suggested, and it is clear that those who opt to use marijuana are, in effect, guinea pigs testing an experimental substance.

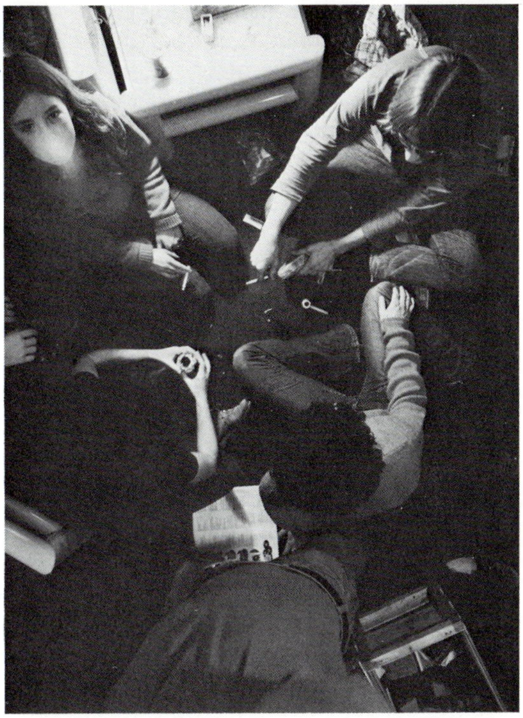

Tim Brown/Nancy Palmer

The effects of long-term use of marijuana are still not known. Users of the drug may consider themselves guinea pigs in the continuing research.

Immediate Effects of a Single Dose

Because marijuana is a natural substance, its quality and strength are unpredictable. Most cannabis grown in the United States is of relatively weak potency, but there has been a surge of higher-potency imports (and of hashish and hashish oil), increasing the risk of adverse effects. As with other drugs, outcome is also affected by mood, physical and mental condition, setting, and how the drug is administered. Eating raw marijuana can make people sick; injecting fermented marijuana can be fatal. Smoked marijuana is the easiest to control, for it is puffed until the desired high is reached.

Subjective reports of effects of marijuana Several studies have cast doubt on subjective reports of the effects of marijuana. One researcher found that, though his subjects claimed to be happier, friendlier, warmer, and less likely to be angry or defensive after using the drug, objective tests of their attitudes did not support these claims (Galanter et al.).

Several leading marijuana authorities question whether *any* effects actually occur at low dosages. Reese Jones suggests that the reason many first-time users report no reaction is that there is none. He believes that the effects described may really be based on long-term social learning rather than on the actual effects of the drug.

The effects most commonly reported at the usual social usage in the United States include: alteration of time and space perception; sense of euphoria, relaxation, well-being; loss of inhibition; dulling of attention; fragmentation of thought; impaired immediate memory; altered sense of identity; giggling; increased suggestibility. Marijuana appears to be a mood exaggerator, making the happy happier, the gloomy gloomier. Less commonly reported effects are dizziness, feelings of lightness, and nausea. At low doses, users appear to be able to "suppress the marijuana high" if the situation so demands.

At higher doses, the effects of marijuana use become more pronounced and may include thought distortions, disrupted sense of body, a sense of piecemeal unreality, visual

Marijuana Experience

. . . Grass gets you into yourself. It heightens whatever it is you really feel, and if you're with someone you don't like . . . the grass makes you really hate them. . . . And I really have touching, personal, mysterious experiences on it. An example? . . . Well, I was walking around the block, very high with a close friend one night, and suddenly he knelt down and put his arm around a fireplug. Well, you see, I found that touching, terribly significant. . . .

Woman weekend smoker, quoted in S. Blum, p. 58

Thoughts moved so fast it was as though someone was holding a deck of cards. . . . As each card dropped it held a thought that for the moment was extremely clear . . . yet instantly forgotten as another thought arrived. . . . Periodically I would become paranoid, filled with fear I was going insane, that I might be busted, that my friends might turn on me or that I might be physically harmed. When that happened the part of me that was a "monitor" would say, "It's cool, man. Everything's all right . . . it will pass . . . just relax and take it all in and enjoy it."

User reporting to Bloomquist, p. 157

. . . I feel as if I control my universe. I feel as if every beautiful thing I want is right here in my room. . . . I see beauty in myself, how sensitive I am. I can see into truths and look for and find the answer to them. Marijuana takes away fear and shyness. . . . I can see causes of my problems and can decide how to change things. There's nothing to fear. That is what you learn on pot.

Woman, 28 years old, quoted in Goode, pp. 81, 82

distortions, sometimes hallucinations and paranoid thinking, and less often, psychosis.

Effects on performance Like alcohol and several other drugs, even a single dose of cannabis can lead to a reduction in ability to operate an automobile or other machinery, or to perform complex unfamiliar tasks. Thus, driving under the influence of marijuana is definitely hazardous to health, even after the individual no longer feels high.

Bad trips Although most users find marijuana use pleasurable—or, at least, not unpleasant—the bad trip, or "bummer," does occur, possibly in about 6 percent of users (R. Blum). A bad trip can occur on first use, twentieth, or not at all, and it cannot be predicted in advance. Higher doses than normally taken may trigger one. The risk can be reduced by using the drug in comfortable surroundings, among friends, and only when in a good frame of mind.

There are many forms of bad trips: a panic reaction, irritation, fear of dying, disorientation, paranoia ("Everyone is out to get me!"). Users may also fear that the loss of identity and control they are experiencing will not end. With higher doses, or with hashish, hallucinations are possible. The worst kind of adverse reaction mimics a true psychotic state. Anyone who is uptight about using an illegal or dangerous drug, or who is not guided on first-time trips by experienced users, is a possible candidate for a panic reaction. For how to help someone down from a bad trip, see Chapter 18.

Flashback Flashback is commonly associated with LSD use, but it occurs in marijuana users, too, usually triggered by a stimulus that was present during an earlier trip. Bloomquist reports the case of a 16-year-old who told him:

> I was driving along a road when I suddenly noticed a red airplane warning light flashing in

> the distance. . . . Suddenly, man . . . wow, I was on the same trip I had been on three weeks ago. [There had been a flashing red light the night he had last smoked marijuana.] Trouble was, I was driving pretty fast at the time, and I noticed I was just sitting there with my foot on the accelerator and my hands in my lap enjoying the lights. It was all I could do to pull over and let the thing pass. (p. 141)

There are subjective reports, though no confirmation, that marijuana can trigger an LSD flashback. This would suggest that anyone who has experienced a bad trip on LSD should avoid using any hallucinogen, including marijuana.

Physical Effects of Chronic Marijuana Use

> While there is little evidence to suggest that there are deleterious physical effects arising from a single episode of use, or from infrequent use of marijuana, the issue of long-term, chronic use and its effects remains unresolved. It is generally conceded that there is no such thing as an entirely "safe" drug, and cannabis is not likely to be an exception. (U.S. DHEW, *x*, p. 15)

The question raised above in the third report to Congress on marijuana and health remains unresolved in the 1974 and 1975 reports, which neither give marijuana a clean bill of health, as some might hope, nor support the fear and irrationality expressed by others in discussing the drugs.

Since marijuana has some of the characteristics of both alcohol and tobacco, it may have some harmful effects in common with each of these drugs. An added cause for concern is the fact that THC, marijuana's major active ingredient, is fat-soluble, and thus is retained in the fatty organs such as brain and testes longer than most other drugs. No one knows what the effects of a long-term accumulation might be. Though there is much more to be learned about the effects of chronic marijuana use on the body, research has already pointed to several possible hazards and suggested areas for urgent study.

Marijuana and the respiratory system Since marijuana is most often smoked, it is not surprising that there are reports that heavy users are more likely than nonusers to have emphysema, pharyngitis (sore throat), and bronchitis, and to cough up excess lung secretions. Contrary to the belief of some smokers, the copious secretions are not "a clearing out of the lungs," but a sign of assault to and irritation of the tender tissues of the respiratory tract.

There is extensive disagreement on how damaging marijuana is to the respiratory system. But several researchers fear it may ultimately be established that cannabis is more damaging than tobacco because it is inhaled more deeply, forcing larger quantities of potent carcinogens into the lungs. Several recent studies lend support to this theory.

Marijuana and the reproductive system Earlier reports of chromosome damage have not been proved or disproved. More recent studies indicate that chronic marijuana use may interfere with the production of testosterone in males (Kolodney et al.). This raises some significant questions: (1) Does marijuana reduce fertility or lead to impotence? (There have been some reports of heavy users complaining of impotence and less frequent intercourse.) (2) Might it interfere with the sexual development of young users? (3) Might it lead to abnormal sexual development in a male fetus whose mother is a heavy user?

Since THC passes through the placenta to the fetus, use during pregnancy suggests other hazards. There have been reports of low-birth-weight babies among marijuana-smoking mothers, but whether other damage will show up later as a result of the THC stored in an infant's tissues is not known. Certainly it can be said that use of any drug not prescribed by a physician is unwise during pregnancy.

Marijuana and the cardiovascular system Some studies show pulse and heartbeat are speeded up, and ECGs (graphs of heart action) are significantly altered during the use of marijuana. Tachycardia, a very rapid heartbeat, is common in older experimenters and in those who have a panic reaction. Persons who have diagnosed cases of coronary artery disease experience pain sooner and after less exercise while smoking marijuana than while smoking a placebo (Aronow and Cassidy).

Other possible effects Suspected effects of marijuana on the immune system present both hazard (heavy use may weaken cellular immunity, increasing susceptibility to disease and infection) and hope (the drug might be potentially useful in lowering the body's resistance to and rejection of organ transplants). Possible adverse effects also include a diabeteslike response, a decrease in REM sleep (essential dream stage of sleep), damage to brain tissues, and interference with DNA and RNA synthesis. Each warrants further study.

Since marijuana stimulates appetite (the "munchies") in many people, regular use may also add to obesity problems, especially since the drug decreases control over one's actions.

Medical use of marijuana Some test results have shown cannabis, or THC, potentially useful in reducing the nausea and vomiting of cancer patients on drug therapy, in dilating the bronchial tubes of asthma patients, and in relieving the intraocular (*intra* = within + *ocular* = eye) pressure of glaucoma.

Effects of Chronic Marijuana Use on Mind and Performance

Studies of the effects of marijuana on behavior have been perplexingly contradictory. Several major studies—some on students in the United States, others on users in Jamaica, Greece, and Costa Rica—have shown no significant differences in work level, motivation, intellectual capacity, or mental illness between marijuana users and nonusers. On the other hand, there have been studies and individual clinical reports indicating serious psychological, intellectual, and motivational problems in heavy users. Psychiatrists Kolansky and Moore report:

> In the past decade, we have seen hundreds of patients suffering from psychiatric and neurological symptoms that resulted from cannabis use . . . we detailed the toxic psychological effects of cannabis use in 51 of our patients, all of whom demonstrated symptoms that simultaneously began with cannabis use and disappeared within 3–24 months after cessation of drug use. *Moreover, a correlation of the symptoms to the duration and frequency of smoking was established.* When these observations were coupled with the stereotyped nature of the symptoms seen, regardless of psychological predisposition, we presumed that with intensive cannabis use, biochemical and structural changes occurred in the central nervous system.
>
> All subjects clearly demonstrated *an early diminution in self-awareness and judgment, along with slowed thinking and shorter spans in concentration and attention.* We also reported a gradual development of "*goallessness,*" *blunted emotions, a counterfeit impression of calm and well-being, and a prevailing illusion of recently developed insight and emotional maturity.* (p. 923)

Similar findings, particularly memory loss, have been reported by other investigators as well as by individual users and physicians. University of California psychiatrist Dr. Harvey Powelson, who thought marijuana harmless in 1964, began in 1970 to become concerned about increasing effects of marijuana on students he was seeing at the Berkeley Health Service. In 1975, he contended that marijuana use seemed to interfere with students' ability to think, to function, to be in touch, and (in large doses over long periods) with all aspects of their lives. Individual effects vary because marijuana tends "to exaggerate whatever is pathological in people's thinking." He believes that, though at social doses there appears to be no effect on certain kinds of schoolwork (fairly complex abstract thinking), judgment about how well or poorly one is doing is affected.

Impairment of judgment may also carry over into users' evaluation of marijuana. This, along with a combination of wishful thinking and of defending an enjoyable habit, may help to explain why many users underreport negative effects (Galanter et al).

Amotivational syndrome For a long time, it was believed that heavy marijuana users show very little motivation to do anything constructive. Tests to verify or disprove the concept have been difficult to devise, and the question remains undecided.

Marijuana and sex It helps, and it hampers. Many people have reported enhancement of the sex act under the influence of marijuana. Marijuana also loosens inhibitions, much as alcohol does, making it easier for some to forget their hangups, and their convictions as well. In some cases, loosened inhibitions have led to promiscuity.

On the other hand, there have been some reported instances of impotence following marijuana use, as well as reports that sexual relations under the influence of marijuana can be "empty of meaning and love—a solo, instead of a duet."

Dependence

The 1930s caricature of the insane marijuana addict is certainly unrealistic, but whether or not marijuana causes some type of dependence is still not known. Research has shown that tolerance does develop, and withdrawal symptoms (sleep disturbance, irritability, hyperactivity, sweating, weight loss, etc.) have been reported upon withdrawal of chronic heavy doses. It is believed that these have not shown up in American users because of the relatively low doses and infrequent use typical currently in the United States (U.S. DHEW, *ff*).

Reverse tolerance with marijuana use, in which less and less rather than more and more of the drug appeared to be needed for the desired effect, has not been substantiated. It has been suggested that the reason many heavy users need less of the drug is that they have developed greater skill in reaching the desired high.

British researcher P. A. L. Chapple sees the question of physical dependence as one of semantic nitpicking. He pictures someone so dependent upon a drug's euphoric effect that he or she finds life empty and meaningless without it, and will go to any lengths to satisfy this expensive and illegal self-indulgence, despite erratic effects it may have on work performance. Chapple asks, "If this person is not addicted, what is his psychiatric state?" (p. 271).

The fact is, of course, that large numbers of people have been able to take marijuana without showing signs of dependence. Many have also dropped the habit with apparent ease. Others are certain they can stop any time they wish. (This certainty, however, is also present in people dependent upon other drugs, including alcohol.) Many do not wish to stop because the experience is pleasurable. Whether we will begin to see instances of physical dependence if use, marijuana potency, and dosages continue to grow in this country cannot be predicted.

MARIJUANA AND THE LAW

There are those who have long believed that the most serious hazards faced by marijuana users were not medical, but legal. And, indeed, in 1973, some 420,000 Americans were arrested for possession of marijuana (R. L. DuPont, *a*).

As marijuana arrests climbed, especially among middle-class youth, a cry arose for changes in marijuana laws. By 1977, many

Opinions on Marijuana and the Law

I . . . support the concept of . . . a non-criminal fine of a modest kind, something in the range of $25 to convey the message that marijuana use is prohibited behavior, but also not to threaten the young people with a criminal record or incarceration.

Robert L. DuPont, p. 8

It is possible to stop most drug addiction in the United States within a very short time. Simply make all drugs available and sell them at cost. Label each drug with a precise description of what effect—good and bad—the drug will have on whoever takes it.

Gore Vidal, p. 29

With alcohol firmly entrenched in the American way of life and with all the sorrow it brings, can we afford to legalize another habit that has at least equal, if not greater, potential of causing national harm?

Edward R. Bloomquist, p. 281

Driving the pot-smoker underground . . . also drives him nearer the hard-drug culture and the criminal world that feeds it. . . .

Tom Wicker, p. 39

All laws which can be violated without doing anyone any injury are laughed at. Nay, so far are they from doing anything to control the desires and passions of men that, on the contrary, they direct and incite men's thoughts the more towards . . . what is forbidden.

Baruch Spinoza (1632–1677)

If we should ever, in a wild moment, decide to legalize marijuana, I think we could sap the strength of a whole nation. Any disrespect for the law could be minor compared to the lack of drive, goals, and ambition that legalization could produce. I really think it could make the United States a second-rate nation.

Rossides, p. 27

states had passed some form of decriminalization law which replaced prison sentences for small quantities of marijuana with fines. Popular opinion was split on such decriminalization (43 percent for, 45 against), but a large majority opposed legalization (69 percent to 25) and almost as many opposed its use altogether (66 percent to 28).

Whatever the legal action, it is clear that laws will not provide all the answers. As we have seen with alcohol, neither strict prohibition of sale and use nor unrestricted sale and use can eliminate abuse of a popular drug. Open sale has not even eliminated the illicit tax-free alcohol black market of $700 million a year, nor the growing illegal sale of untaxed cigarettes.

It has been suggested that the sanest policy would be to treat marijuana like any drug about which little is known. Until safety is proven, sale should be prohibited. Those who use it should be lightly penalized, those who sell it more heavily punished. Scientific research should be encouraged to discover both the risks and possible benefits of use. If enough benefits were found, marijuana could be reclassified to schedule II (see Table 14.2) along with medically useful but controlled drugs such as morphine. If not, or if serious risks were found, the ban would continue.

LOOKING BACK

REVIEWING CONCEPTS IN CHAPTER 16

- Alcohol and marijuana, major social drugs in the United States, have much in common and are widely used and abused.
- Alcohol is the most widely abused drug in the country.
- Alcohol, absorbed directly into the bloodstream, with almost immediate effects, is a depressant drug. How it affects each individual depends upon sex, age, genetic makeup, and mood, and upon how, when, what, how much, and with what it is drunk.
- In moderate doses alcohol appears to have no serious negative effects, but in large doses it can be extremely harmful to the liver, heart and other muscles, brain, and reproductive system, and it is implicated in the development of many cancers.
- Problem drinking or alcohol abuse is a problem for 10 million Americans from teenage to old age, rich and poor, successful and unsuccessful. It contributes to antisocial behavior, accidents, and crime.
- The alcoholic differs from the problem drinker in being physically dependent upon the drug, powerless to stop drinking. Alcoholism is an illness.
- The nondrinker has the right to refuse a drink without embarrassment.
- Prohibition did not end the problems of alcohol abuse; the only way to achieve that goal may be development of a new alcohol ethic in the United States, an ethic that would subordinate alcohol to other pursuits rather than making it a center of activities.
- Attitudes about marijuana have often interfered with its being viewed objectively.
- Marijuana, hashish, and other derivatives of the cannabis plant come in widely varying potencies which yield widely varying responses.
- Experimenters are often nonconformists; chronic users are likely to have serious personality or coping problems.
- Because long-term effects of marijuana use are not known, users of the drug may consider themselves guinea pigs in the continuing research.
- At low doses, marijuana intoxication may be more "learned" than a result of the drug; at high doses, effects on thinking, inhibitions, and perceptions have been confirmed; at all doses, debilitating effects on performance, particularly driving, have been confirmed.
- A panic reaction or "bad trip" can occur to anyone (new or experienced user), especially when anxiety or increased dosage is involved.
- Research suggests that long-term, steady use may be related to damage of the respiratory system, lowering of male hormone levels, low-birth-weight babies, reduced cellular immunity, as well as changes in thinking and behavior.
- Physical dependence has been shown *only* at very high levels of use; psychological dependence is possible at lower dosages.
- Many states have decriminalized personal use of marijuana, a step supported by most Americans.

17 TOBACCO: WHEN HEALTH GOES UP IN SMOKE

WHAT'S AHEAD IN CHAPTER 17 What positive results could be expected from a major reduction in the use of tobacco in the United States? What are the trends in smoking today? Why? What elements in tobacco smoke make it hazardous? What are the short- and the long-term effects of smoking on the body? How do dose, style of smoking, use of filters, tar and nicotine levels, and duration of use influence these effects? Can users become dependent upon tobacco? How easy—or difficult—is quitting? Can risks be reduced for those who continue to smoke? What is the effect on nonsmokers of exposure to smoke in classrooms, restaurants, automobiles, at home, and so on? Do nonsmokers have a right to protect themselves? What can they do to assert this right?

We, all of us together, have it in our power to eliminate 11 million cases of chronic illness a year and 80 percent of this nation's lung cancer, to massively reduce deaths from heart attack, esophageal cancer, and fire; to greatly decrease incidence of peptic ulcers, mouth cancers, bronchitis, and emphysema; and to decrease the number of babies who are born dead or who die in infancy.

We do not have to spend billions on research or medical care facilities, nor do we need to train 100,000 new physicians. *All* we have to do is to eliminate smoking, a habit linked to more than 500,000 deaths a year. But this is easier said than done. Even as scientists discover new risks in smoking, an estimated 3000 to 6000 young people become smokers each day, and millions of others find quitting "impossible." Many feel coronaries or cancers only happen to "the other person." They block out cause-effect claims, prefer to draw comfort from the aunt or grandfather who smoked for 50 years or more with no visible impairment. Many smokers, however, are concerned. A DHEW survey found that 9 out of 10 smokers would quit if they could easily do so (U.S. DHEW, *dd*). A survey of some 55,000 college students found similarly that only 12 percent of female smokers and 13 percent of male smokers were unconcerned about the harmful effects of smoking. Nevertheless, almost one-quarter of the students surveyed had just begun smoking, in their freshman year.

TABLE 17.1 When students start smoking

SCHOOL YEAR AT ONSET OF SMOKING	PERCENTAGE
Before senior high school	18.35
During first two years of senior high	16.56
During third year of senior high	14.02
During fourth year of senior high	16.74
During first year of college	23.55
During second year of college	7.21
During third year of college	2.98
During fourth year of college	0.57

Source: Dilley, p. 232.

TOBACCO: A MIXED HISTORY

The natives of North and South America cultivated tobacco for medical and ceremonial (the "peace pipe") reasons long before Christopher Columbus's ship came in. In 1556, the tobacco leaf was introduced to Europe, where it won a mixed reception, and from there it spread like a weed to other parts of the world.

Some, like Jean Nicot, French ambassador to Lisbon, who won enduring fame when he lent his name to the *Nicotinium tabaccum* plant, believed that the leaves had useful medicinal purposes. Others praised tobacco for the pleasure it gave: "Tobacco, divine, rare, super excellent Tobacco . . . ," said Robert Burton (1577–1640). Many physicians, however, tendered no testimonials. Tobias Venner (1577–1660) warned: "Tobacco drieth the brain, dimmeth the sight . . . corrupteth the breath, induceth a trembling of the limbs, exciteth the windpipe, lungs and liver, annoyeth the milt, scorcheth the heart, and causeth the blood to be adjusted."

Contemporary debates on marijuana sound much the same, except for the modern language. It is devoutly to be hoped that modern scientific procedures will resolve the marijuana controversy in less than the 400 years it took to settle the debate over tobacco.

For centuries, tobacco was consumed mostly in the forms of cigars, chewing leaf, pipe tobacco, and snuff for sniffing and sneezing. Cigarettes, tobacco wrapped in paper, were invented in Brazil in the eighteenth century, and in the 1870s the first cigarette-rolling machinery was built. Cigarette smoking caught on quickly, and in 1880, 1.3 billion cigarettes were consumed in the United States, about a pack per person per year. By the 1920s, production had increased nearly twentyfold, and by the 1930s, some scientists had begun to suspect that cigarettes were "coffin nails." One reason was the steady and rapid increase in the incidence of lung cancer, which coincided with the billowing growth of cigarette smoke (see Figure 17.1).

The Surgeon General's Report and Federal Regulation

Still, people were far from persuaded that this pleasurable habit could endanger health. Then studies by the American Cancer Society, begun in 1949, and by other research groups found extensive suggestive evidence linking cigarette smoking to premature death and cancer. On Jan. 11, 1964, after a review of thousands of previous research reports and studies and consultations with 175 experts, a

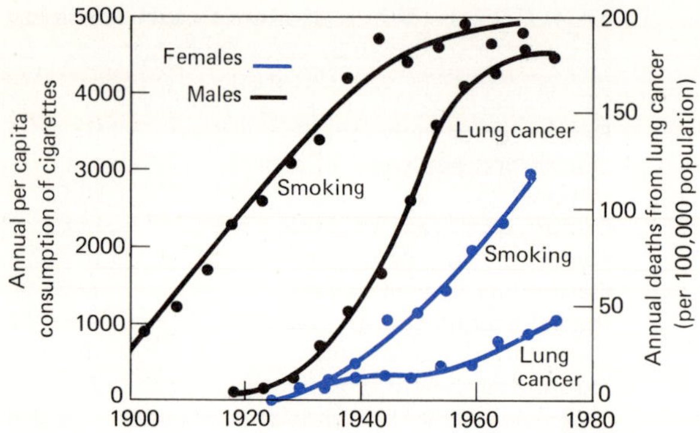

FIGURE 17.1 Cigarette smoking and lung cancer. The growth of the incidence of lung cancer closely parallels the growth in the consumption of cigarettes, as can be seen in this graph of data collected in England and Wales. The more than 20-year gap between the two represents the period of time it usually takes for cancer to develop in cigarette smokers. The picture is much the same in the United States and elsewhere. [*Data from Cairns, p. 72.*]

committee appointed by the U.S. Surgeon General concluded that "cigarette smoking is a health hazard of sufficient importance in the United States to warrant remedial action."

In 1965, under heavy political pressure, Congress passed the first national law requiring all cigarette packages sold in the United States to bear a warning. Four years later, the FTC began making public the tar and nicotine contents of branded cigarettes, and the Public Health Cigarette Smoking Act of 1970 outlawed all cigarette advertising on radio and TV. It also strengthened the cigarette label to: "Warning: The Surgeon General has determined that cigarette smoking is dangerous to your health," and ordered it to appear in newspaper and magazine ads.

Smoking Trends Today

As evidence mounted, millions of Americans quit smoking (18 million by 1975, including half of all physicians who smoked). But cigarette sales, after a short dip, continued to rise as the population grew and as young people, particularly low-achieving dropouts and females,[1] took up smoking in increasing numbers. However, in 1977 Dr. Daniel Horn (*b*), director of the National Clearing House for Smoking and Health, stated that statistics suggested that the upward trend had leveled off and that the growth of the cigarette habit had been halted.

WHAT'S IN A SMOKE?

We shudder at talk of chemical warfare. Yet every day millions of Americans bombard themselves and their neighbors with some of the most dangerous poisonous gases and chemicals known to humankind.

Active Ingredients in Tobacco Smoke

The gases Concentrations of carbon mon-

[1]In one major study, researchers found that 33 percent of college women and only 23 percent of college men smoked (Wechsler).

oxide (CO), a major air pollutant, appear in cigarette smoke at about 400 times the safe industrial exposure. Hydrogen cyanide, a powerful poison, is found at about 160 times the "safe" concentration.

The chemical compounds The tars in cigarette smoke are actually a sticky condensed form of more than 200 chemicals that make up the millions, even billions, of tiny particles in the particulate matter in every cubic centimeter of smoke. These chemicals, many toxic, include:

- At least ten hydrocarbons known to produce cancer in animals
- Cocarcinogens that act with other chemicals to stimulate cancer growth (see Chapter 10)
- Irritants that cause coughing and other respiratory distress and are probably responsible for the deterioration of lung tissue which results in emphysema
- Chemicals that act to paralyze the cilia (hairlike projections) which protect the respiratory tract from foreign substances

Nicotine This oily, colorless substance, sold as an insecticide, is so powerful a poison that just one drop will kill a person in seconds. The average nicotine content of a cigarette (an average of 1.1 milligrams, with a range from 0.5 to 2.5 milligrams) is well below the lethal level, but can still have many deleterious effects on the body.

Variations in Intake

How much the smoker absorbs of the gases and chemicals in tobacco smoke varies with smoking style. One smoker may puff on a

Herb Taylor/Editorial Photocolor Archives

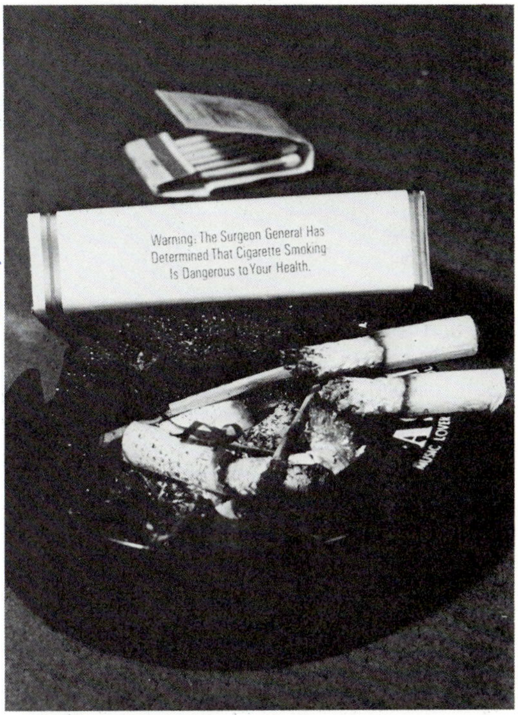

In 1965, under heavy political pressure, Congress passed the first national law requiring a printed warning on all cigarette packages sold in the United States.

George W. Gardner

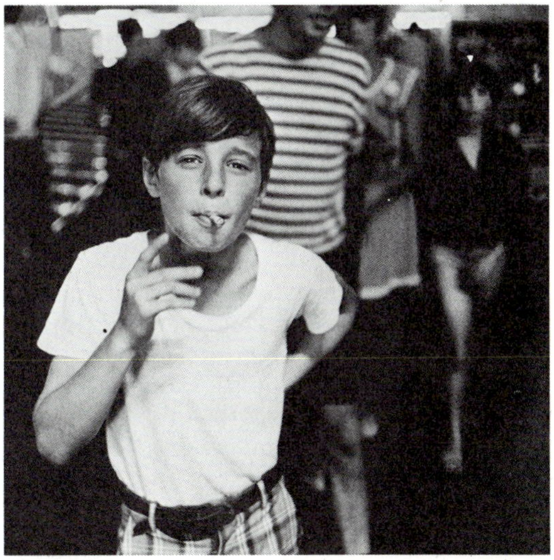

Despite mounting evidence about the dangers of smoking, cigarette sales in the 1970s continued to climb as the population increased and thousands of teenagers became new smokers each week.

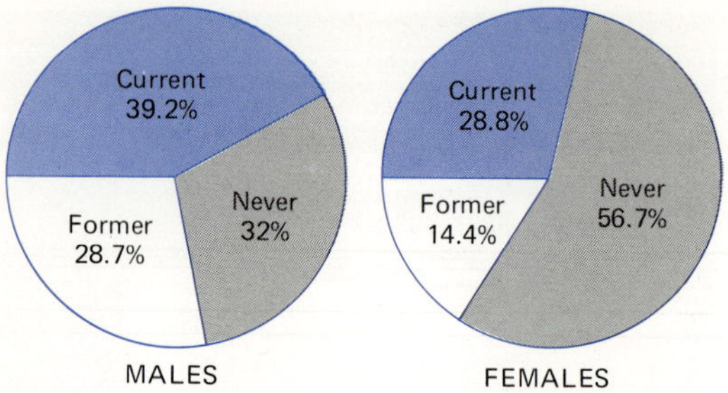

FIGURE 17.2 Current smokers, former smokers, and people who have never smoked, United States, 1975. Subjects considered were 20 years of age and older. The male population was 66.1 million, female 72.7 million. [*Data from U.S. DHEW, dd, p. 1.*]

cigarette 3 or 4 times, half a second each time and with relatively light force, and then discard it. Another may take as many as 20 pulls of 4 seconds each, inhaling with considerable force, smoking down to a 1/2-inch butt. Obviously, the quantity of gases and tars they absorb will differ. Since the cigarette acts as a filter while it is burning, the frugal smoker who goes down to a stub takes in considerably more contaminants than the one who smokes only the first half. Pipe and cigar smokers ingest considerably less because they rarely inhale.

TOBACCO AND HEALTH

Short-term Effects

The classic portrait of the farm boy smoking his first cigarette behind the barn and getting sick is actually a case of mild nicotine poisoning. The symptoms may include dizziness, faintness, quickened pulse, increased blood pressure and heart rate, drop in skin temperature (cause of cold, clammy skin), contraction of peripheral blood vessels, and in some, nausea, vomiting, and diarrhea. The symptoms are usually mild and last about half an hour, after which the smoker may again light up. Tolerance usually develops quickly, and most of these symptoms disappear.

Mood changes Many people smoke for the lift they get from nicotine, for relief from fatigue, or paradoxically, for relaxation, tranquilization, and a lessening of feelings of anxiety and aggression. But these effects are short-lived and usually replaced by more fatigue, more depression, more hostility and aggressiveness. To keep the desired effects from departing, the smoker lights another cigarette and the cycle continues.

Physical effects of regular smoking Quite well established scientifically, physical effects include: the well-known smoker's cough; shortness of breath feared by athletes and caused by concentrations of carbon monoxide in the blood and lowered oxygen supplies; loss of appetite and dulled taste buds, often considered pluses by weight-conscious smokers; bad taste and foul breath; sluggishness and reduced stamina; and slowed digestion.

TABLE 17.2 How smoking affects life expectancy Estimated years of life at various ages for males in the United States, by daily cigarette consumption

AGE	NEVER SMOKED REGUALRLY	NUMBER OF CIGARETTES SMOKED PER DAY			
		1–9	10–19	20–39	40 AND OVER
25	48.6	44.0	43.1	42.4	40.3
30	43.9	39.3	38.4	37.8	35.8
35	39.2	34.7	33.8	33.2	31.3
40	34.5	30.2	29.3	28.7	26.9
45	30.0	25.9	25.0	24.4	23.0
50	25.6	21.8	21.0	20.5	19.3
60	17.6	14.5	14.1	13.7	13.2

Source: American Cancer Society, *a*, p. 20, from Hammond.

I'll never forget when I was 12 or 13, and not a smoker yet, but I took a cigarette out of my mother's purse . . . and walked down the street with it lit, but not smoking it, just lit, and I experienced a distinct, even at that age, erotic excitement of having this symbol of manhood or adulthood in my hand.

William Styron, twentieth-century author, in Lear, p. 18

He that will refuse to take a pipe of *Tobacco* among his fellows . . . is accounted peevish and no good company.

James I of England (1566–1625), in *A Counter-Blaste to Tobacco*

Downing the body's defenses Cigarette smoke prepares for more serious attacks on the body by first paralyzing and later totally destroying the hairlike cilia that line the respiratory tract to expel foreign particles. With this protective mechanism out of order, particles in cigarette smoke and in other pollutants, as well as infectious organisms, find easy access to the lungs, increasing the incidence of respiratory and lung diseases.

Long-term Health Effects

As a group, cigarette smokers, especially those who start early in life and inhale, are 30 to 80 percent more likely to die at a given time than are nonsmokers. In most instances, the risk is dose-related; the more cigarettes smoked, the greater the excess mortality. The mortality rate of pipe and cigar smokers and those who quit smoking cigarettes approaches that of nonsmokers. But for heavy pipe or cigar smokers, and for smokers who inhale, the mortality rate is 20 to 40 percent greater than that of nonsmokers. Women smokers have a mortality rate greater than that of nonsmoking women, but less than that of male smokers.

Smoking also increases disability. It is estimated that smoking is responsible for 11 million cases of chronic illness a year in the United States, for 77 million extra personal days lost from work, for 88 million more days in bed, and for 306 million more days in restricted activity (U.S. DHEW, *v*).

The use of lower tar and nicotine content cigarettes lowers risk of many diseases slightly. Air pollution and exposure to pollutants on the job increase risks. Major smoking-linked diseases include the following.

Lung cancer Cancer of the lung is the leading cause of cancer death in men, and the incidence of the disease is rising rapidly among women. It is among the most difficult cancers to cure: Only 6 out of 100 victims survive five years after diagnosis. Epidemiological evidence places the blame for most cases of lung cancer squarely on cigarette smoking. The rise in incidence has closely paralleled the rise in smoking. Laboratory work adds further substantiation. Cigarette tars painted on mice cause cancer. And lung tumors, some cancerous, have been produced in the laboratory in beagles who "smoked" 9 cigarettes a day for 875 days. Though not every beagle or every human who smokes gets lung cancer, it appears that no one escapes the lung-damaging effects of tobacco entirely. All heavy-smoking beagles developed tumors, and autopsies done on human smokers have shown lung damage in every one.

Heart and circulatory diseases Smoking is believed to increase fatty deposits in blood vessels and the thickening of small arteries in various organs, and it may contribute to clotting of blood. Nicotine also speeds heartbeat, increasing the heart's need for oxygen supplies. At the same time, carbon monoxide in the smoke reduces oxygen in the blood, and diminished lung capacity further cuts oxygen

American Cancer Society

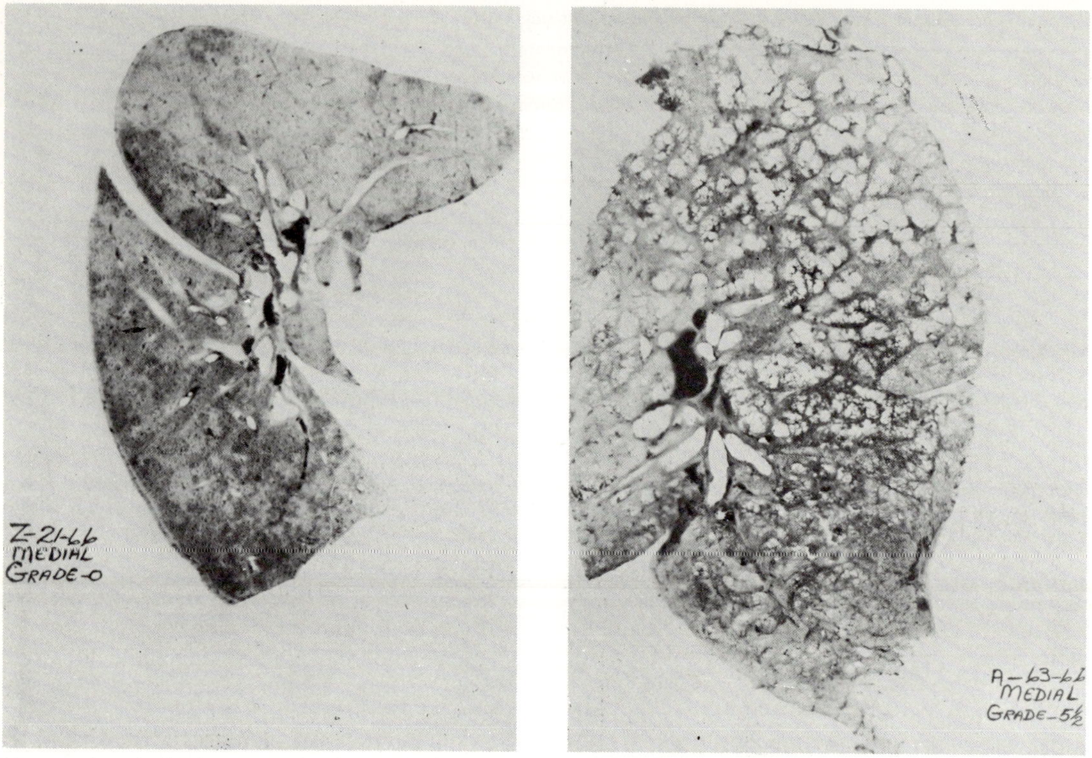

No smoker is immune to the lung-damaging effects of tobacco. The lung tissue of a heavy smoker (*right*) shows an abundance of greatly enlarged air sacs. The air sacs in normal lung tissue (*left*) are too fine to be visible.

supplies. So while the smoker's body demands more oxygen, it receives less.

These factors explain in part the more than 188,000 deaths from heart disease each year attributed to smoking and the increased risk of stroke in smokers. Quitting smoking, however, decreases the risk of death from heart attack sharply within 1 year's time; in 10 years or so, the risk drops almost to the nonsmoker level.

Of course, several other factors have been identified as significantly related to heart attack (see Chapter 10), but cigarette smoking is the most influential. A smoker with just one other major factor is 70 percent more likely to have coronary artery disease than the nonsmoker. If smoking and all other major factors are present, the risk soars to 300 times that of the nonsmoker. Smoking combined with the use of the oral contraceptive also multiplies risk, especially in women 40 to 44.

Chronic bronchitis and emphysema Deaths from pulmonary emphysema and chronic bronchitis, referred to in tandem as COBD, or chronic obstructive broncho-pulmonary disease, have soared 1100 percent from 1945 to 1968. Chronic bronchitis, in which there are chronic or recurrent excessive mucus secretions in the bronchial tree, is almost as common among teenage smokers as among adults. The two most obvious symptoms of this are a chronic cough and excessive sputum, which may be either clear or full of pus from lung infection. As the condition progresses, the air passages become narrower and narrower, making breathing more difficult.

Pulmonary emphysema, which disables 1 out of 14 wage earners, is a disease in which the walls of the tiny air sacs in the lung, through which air is absorbed into the body, are progressively destroyed, offering less "wall space" or total surface for the absorption of oxygen. Normal adults expend about 5 percent of their energy in breathing; people

FIGURE 17.3 How smoking and other causes of chronic obstructive pulmonary disease (COBD) hamper normal breathing. [*Adapted from* Patient Care, *b, p. 119.*]

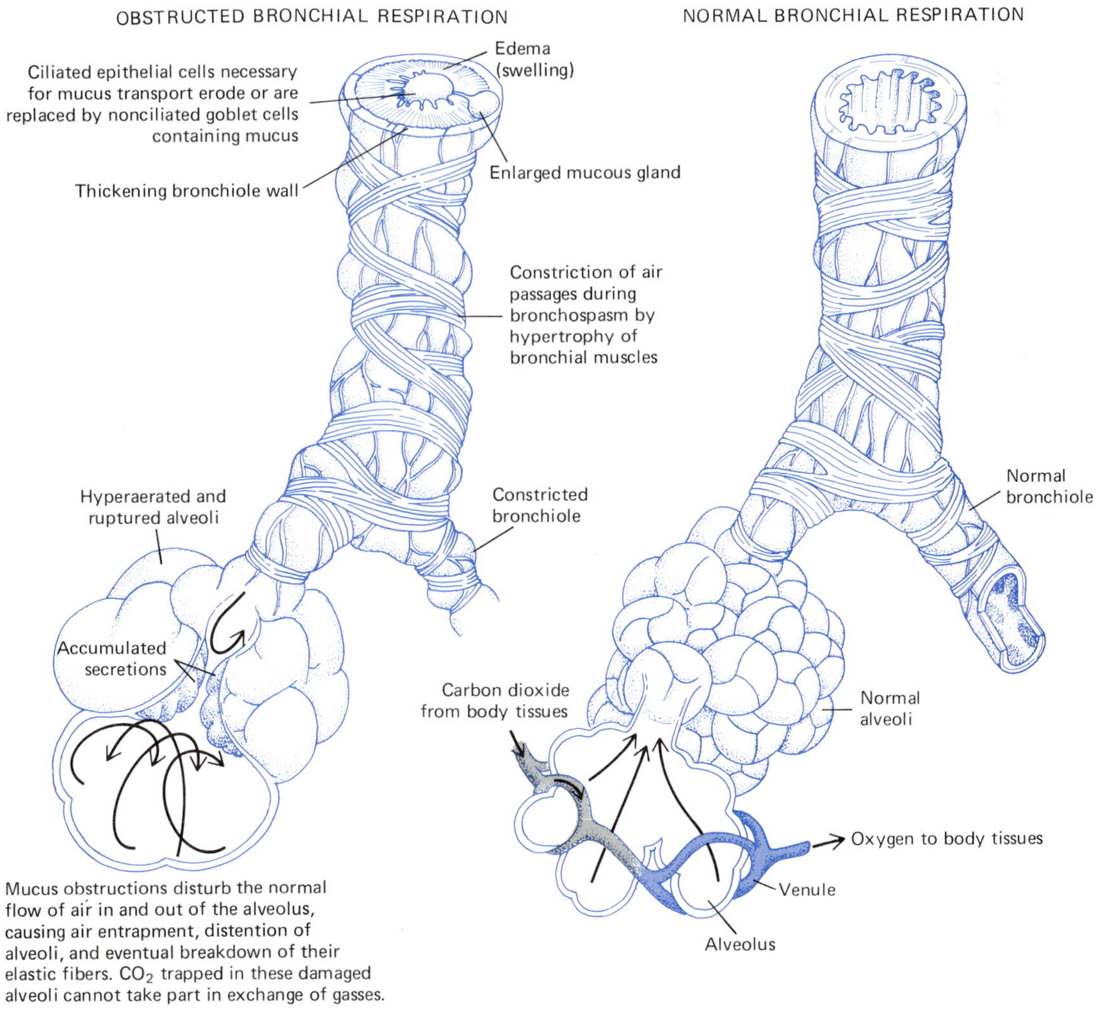

TABLE 17.3 Dose-related incidence of COBD

CIGARETTES SMOKED PER DAY	PERCENTAGE	RESULT
One pack	13.1	No emphysema
	11.7	Advanced diseases
More than one pack	0.3	No emphysema
	19.2	Advanced diseases
None	90	No emphysema
	0	Advanced diseases

Source: Adapted from American Cancer Society, *a,* p. 41, from Auerbach et al.

with advanced emphysema use up to 80 percent of their strength to breathe.

COBD is apparently reversible in young patients with mild to moderate severe obstructions *who stop smoking.* When damage is advanced, some easing of coughing and breathlessness is possible with skillful therapy.

Other cancers Cigarette, pipe, and cigar smokers have four times as many cancers of the lip, tongue, floor of the mouth, palate, and other mouth areas as nonsmokers. Pipe smokers are most susceptible to cancer of the lip because of the intense heat and pressure of the pipe stem, which is often held tightly in the mouth for long periods. (Smoking is related, too, to a variety of noncancerous diseases of the mouth, including tooth loss and periodontal disease.) Risks of cancer of the larynx, bladder, kidneys, and esophagus are all multiplied for the smoker. In the case of esophageal cancer, the risk escalates even more when alcohol is involved (see Tables 16.2 and 16.3).

Ulcers The belief that smoking calms nerves and improves digestion is discounted by the strong association that has been shown between ulcers and smoking. To add injury to insult, smoking also appears to reduce the effectiveness of treatment and to slow ulcer healing.

Effects on Pregnancy and Progeny

Low birth weight, a serious survival risk in newborns, is more related to the mother's smoking during pregnancy than to any other factor. Studies have also found a significantly higher proportion of spontaneous abortions (miscarriages) and of stillbirths (babies born dead), as well as of babies who die in the first month of life or are victims of sudden infant death, among women who smoke during pregnancy than in nonsmoking mothers. However, it appears that if the mother quits by the fourth month of pregnancy, the baby's chances are almost normal. One follow-up study of children whose mothers continued to smoke found that, at age 7, the children were shorter in stature, were relatively retarded in reading ability, and rated lower in social adjustment than children of nonsmokers (N. R. Butler et al.).

The evidence is as yet inconclusive, but there are even indications that smoking while nursing a baby may be hazardous. It appears possible that smoking may diminish the milk supply, that nicotine passes into the breast milk and is ingested by the infant, and that (as animal experiments have shown) nitrosamines, which are known to cause cancer, also pass through the milk to the child.

Smoking and Fires

The cigarette is not finished doing its damage when the smoker is finished with it. Tossed carelessly into a wastebasket, dropped onto the bedclothes by a drowsy smoker, crushed in a paper plate at a party, the cigarette continues to kill. In 1975, the National Fire Protection Association estimated that more than 137,800 fires were related to smoking.

Tobacco and Sex Appeal

Cigarette ads make smoking appear the almost exclusive province of the Beautiful People. And many youngsters, especially girls, begin smoking in order to "look glamorous." But there is nothing glamorous about the nicotine stains cigarettes eventually leave on teeth and fingertips. Nor is stale cigarette breath appealing.

Many researchers are convinced that tobacco can do more harm to one's sexuality than diminish attractiveness. Dr. Alton Ochsner, M.D., a smoking research pioneer, pointed out the cause-and-effect relationship between smoking and lung cancer 28 years before the Surgeon General's report. He now reveals evidence linking cigarette smoking to sexual inadequacy, and he is supported by the many ex-smokers reporting revitalized and improved sex lives after quitting. Other researchers are finding that men who smoke heavily may have low sperm counts, and that what sperm they have may be sluggish. In several cases, attempts to conceive a child were unsuccessful until the men stopped smoking.

TOWARD A NONSMOKING SOCIETY

Tobacco Dependence

> When the defeated people of Germany were deprived of tobacco by post-World War II shortages, a majority of habitual smokers preferred to do without food . . . rather than forgo tobacco . . . smokers were still willing to barter food rations for tobacco . . . cigarette butts were picked up out of the street dirt by people who, on their own statements, would in other circumstances have felt disgust at such conduct. Smokers also condescended to beg for tobacco. . . . (Arntzen, p. 425)

Obviously some people crave tobacco above all other pleasures. There is no agreement about whether the reason is psychological dependency alone or physiological dependency as well. Part of the answer hinges on whether or not withdrawal syndrome, one of the prime indications of physical dependency, is present. Some authorities claim it is not. Dr. Ernest Wynder, cancer specialist and president of the American Health Foundation, which has done much work in helping people quit smoking, says: "Of course, there are physiological effects. You get pulsings—little pulsating releases of adrenalin, and undoubtedly these reinforce the habit. But that doesn't make it an addiction. . . . When you stop smoking, you don't collapse" (p. 18).

Psychopharmacologist Jerome Jaffe, past director of the National Special Action Office for Drug Abuse Prevention, disagrees:

> Millions of people are out of control and obviously killing themselves. That doesn't sound like a habit to me. By most measures nicotine is less addicting than heroin or the barbiturates or alcohol. But each drug that reproduces body adaptation is followed by its own set of body disruptions when it's stopped. It's not the d.t.'s, but it's *not nothing.* (p. 19)

Many who have quit smoking—once or many times—have reported such body disruptions. And a 1966 study found that a majority of smokers deprived of their drug experienced some kind of withdrawal symptoms.

Murray E. Jarvik, U.C.L.A. psychopharmacologist, who has done much of the classic work on nicotine, believes the evidence of addiction is not conclusive because the psychological dependency is so great it overshadows the physical dependency. Studies have also shown that when smokers do not get their accustomed dose of nicotine (as in low-nicotine cigarettes), they tend to smoke more in order to get it. With high-nicotine

TAXIDRIVER Jesus, I'm suffering, let me tell you. I'm trying to quit smoking.

PASSENGER Ah, how long ago did you quit?

DRIVER Twenty minutes ago.

Reported by Lear, p. 90

TABLE 17.4 Why I smoke

Here are some statements made by people to describe what they get out of smoking cigarettes. How *often* do you feel this way when smoking them? Circle one number for each statement. *Important: Answer every question.*

STATEMENT	ALWAYS	FREQUENTLY	OCCASIONALLY	SELDOM	NEVER
A I smoke cigarettes in order to keep myself from slowing down.	5	4	3	2	1
B Handling a cigarette is part of the enjoyment of smoking it.	5	4	3	2	1
C Smoking cigarettes is pleasant and relaxing.	5	4	3	2	1
D I light up a cigarette when I feel angry about something.	5	4	3	2	1
E When I have run out of cigarettes I find it almost unbearable until I can get them.	5	4	3	2	1
F I smoke cigarettes automatically without even being aware of it.	5	4	3	2	1
G I smoke cigarettes to stimulate me, to perk myself up.	5	4	3	2	1
H Part of the enjoyment of smoking a cigarette comes from the steps I take to light up.	5	4	3	2	1
I I find cigarettes pleasurable.	5	4	3	2	1
J When I feel uncomfortable or upset about something, I light up a cigarette.	5	4	3	2	1
K I am very much aware of the fact when I am not smoking a cigarette.	5	4	3	2	1
L I light up a cigarette without realizing I still have one burning in the ashtray.	5	4	3	2	1
M I smoke cigarettes to give me a "lift."	5	4	3	2	1
N When I smoke a cigarette, part of the enjoyment is watching the smoke as I exhale it.	5	4	3	2	1
O I want a cigarette most when I am comfortable and relaxed.	5	4	3	2	1

Source: Adapted from the Smoker's Self-Testing Kit, National Clearinghouse for Smoking and Health, Test 3.

STATEMENT	ALWAYS	FREQUENTLY	OCCASIONALLY	SELDOM	NEVER
P When I feel "blue" or want to take my mind off cares and worries, I smoke cigarettes.	5	4	3	2	1
Q I get a gnawing hunger for a cigarette when I haven't smoked for a while	5	4	3	2	1
R I've found a cigarette in my mouth and didn't remember putting it there.	5	4	3	2	1

HOW TO SCORE

1 Enter the numbers you have circled to the questions in the spaces below, putting the number you have circled to Question A over line A, to Question B over line B, etc.

2 Total the 3 scores on each line to get your totals. For example, the sum of your scores over lines A, G, and M gives you your score on Stimulation—lines B, H, and N gives the score on Handling, etc.

							TOTALS
___ A	+	___ G	+	___ M	=	___	I Stimulation
___ B	+	___ H	+	___ N	=	___	II Handling
___ C	+	___ I	+	___ O	=	___	III Pleasurable relaxation
___ D	+	___ J	+	___ P	=	___	IV Crutch: tension reduction
___ E	+	___ K	+	___ Q	=	___	V Craving: psychological addiction
___ F	+	___ L	+	___ R	=	___	VI Habit

The score for each test can vary from 3 to 15. A score of 3 to 7 is *low*, 8 to 10 is *moderate,* 11 to 15 is *high*.

cigarettes (or nicotine injections), smokers tend to cut back.

Breaking the Habit

Perhaps the classic tobacco addict was Sigmund Freud, father of psychoanalysis. At age 38, his physician urged him to quit smoking because of some heart irregularities. Freud described the withdrawal symptoms as "torture . . . beyond human power to bear."

Within seven weeks he was smoking again, and later attempts at quitting also failed. At age 67, he noted sores on his right palate and jaw that failed to heal. There followed 33 operations for cancer of the jaw and mouth in the next 16 years. His jaw was removed and replaced with an artificial one. Often he could not chew or speak, and pain was almost constant. He suffered heart pain (angina) directly related to the intake of nicotine. Repeated attempts to quit were useless. In spite of his agonies, Freud contined to smoke cigars until his death.

Many young people starting to smoke feel, "It won't happen to me." But statistics, and experiences like Freud's, suggest it will. The American Cancer Society states that a 20 to

It Is Possible to Quit Smoking

There are a great many ways to quit smoking. The best method to choose depends upon the smoker. Because smoking is a learned habit, one of the most widely recommended cessation techniques is a form of behavior modification that helps the smoker to unlearn the habit. It is similar in concept to the approach to weight reduction discussed in Chapter 5. The following approach is adapted from that recommended by the American Health Foundation, leader in preventive health care, research, and education.

Step 1 Understanding why you smoke Make a list of your reasons for smoking. Then take the "Why I Smoke" test in Table 17.4. The higher your score in a particular category, the stronger a source of satisfaction that category is for you. Once you understand these reasons, you will be able to substitute other satisfactions as you attempt to quit smoking.

Step 2 Motivation for quitting List your reasons for not quitting. They may include statements like "It's too late; the damage is already done," and "All those millions of people who smoke can't be wrong." Whatever your reasons, you should be able to find a counterargument for them in the accompanying text.

Now list your reasons for wanting to quit. Be as specific as you can and include all the future rewards you can expect from being a nonsmoker—physical, financial, social. Think about being able to set an example for your children now or someday. Think about how it will be when friends won't have to ask you to please smoke outside in the hall or blow the smoke in the other direction. Make a list of some small luxury items you would like to have. Convert their costs to "packs of cigarettes" and plan to save your daily cigarette money to purchase these items.

Step 3 Prepare yourself Imagine yourself a nonsmoker in situations where you would ordinarily reach for a cigarette. What can you do instead? Start thinking of smoking as a pure activity. Do nothing else when you smoke. Better still, connect smoking with discomfort by smoking only in uncomfortable places—the garage, for example.

Step 4 Select a way to quit There are two basic approaches: cold turkey and tapering.

Cold turkey:

- Select a memorable date for quitting (a birthday, Christmas, etc.). It should be relatively soon.
- Plan how you will handle the first 24 hours without cigarettes. Consider smoking an excess the day before.
- Put your list of reasons for quitting in a prominent place; you may need it for reinforcement.
- Make a bet with someone that you will be able to quit.
- Have something to keep in your hands (pencil, paper clip, beads, etc.) and something to put in your mouth (a toothpick, nonsugar candy or chewing gum, or an empty cigarette holder).
- When you feel the urge to smoke, take long deep breaths, with a pause between each. Hold the last breath while you strike a match. Exhale slowly, blowing out the match. Pretend it was a cigarette and crush it out.

Tapering:

- Keep a 24-hour smoking diary that lists the time of day of each cigarette, what you were doing at the moment you lit it, your feelings at the moment, and how badly you needed the cigarette. Rate each cigarette on a scale from 1 (extremely important, can't function without it) to 5 (least important, not really aware I want it, or know I could do without it). Also note how much of each cigarette you smoked.
- The next day, begin by cutting out the cigarettes you rated 5. Continue to keep a daily record of cigarettes smoked. You may achieve a rapid drop at first, and then may reach a plateau as you try to eliminate the important cigarettes. There may even be some setbacks, but don't let them discourage you.
- Find substitutes for smoking—munching on raw vegetables, popcorn, gum, cough drops, hard candy. But avoid high-calorie, high-sugar foods.
- Avoid the settings you smoke in most often; frequent places with "no smoking" rules.
- When you crave a cigarette, wait until three minutes have passed before you light it. During that time, try to substitute another activity. The craving may go away.
- Change your brand of cigarettes weekly so you don't become attached to one brand.
- Buy cigarettes by the pack, not the carton; don't buy a new pack until the old one is finished.
- Change the way you hold the cigarette, the way you puff.
- Keep cigarettes in a hard-to-get-at place; don't carry them around with you.
- Never carry a lighter or matches.
- Always ask: Do I need *this* cigarette? If the answer is yes, light up in front of the mirror.
- If you smoke with coffee, switch to another beverage. If you smoke alone, smoke with others. If you smoke after meals, leave the table when you finish eating. (Check your diary for clues.)
- Review your reasons for smoking and find substitutes to satisfy these needs. If you need something in your mouth, chew carrot sticks. If you need something in your hands, try jigsaw puzzles, knitting, needlepoint, model airplanes, etc. If you smoke to relieve tension, try relaxation exercises, yoga, meditation. If you smoke to relieve boredom, try exercise, reading, sports. If you need the deep breathing, try running. (Also see the section on alternative roads to high, Chapter 18.) Be sure your substitute is an improvement over smoking.
- Develop a nonsmoker image: Imagine yourself not smoking in varous situations; when offered a cigarette say, "I don't smoke."

Step 5 Staying off cigarettes List the situations in which you are most tempted to smoke. Then try to avoid or alter them until you feel secure. Avoid, too, people who try to get you to smoke. Recognize that you may slip. Many people do. Just remember that each cigarette you do take should be preceded by a conscious decision. If you do slip, don't be discouraged. Get right back on the cessation program. Take one day at a time and keep the goal of you as a nonsmoker always in mind.

For further help

- National Clearing House on Smoking and Health, Center for Disease Control, U.S. DHEW, Atlanta, GA 30333
- American Health Foundation, 1370 Avenue of the Americas, New York, NY 10019
- American Cancer Society, 777 Third Avenue., New York, NY 10017 (or local office)
- American Lung Association, 1740 Broadway, New York, NY 10019
- Action on Smoking and Health (ASH), 2000 H Street, N.W., Washington, DC 20006
- Group Against Smoking and Pollution (GASP), P.O. Box 682, College Park, MD 20740

25 percent "cure rate" is par for every smoking cessation method they know. Of every 100 who try to quit, 25 quickly fail. Another 50 waver and wander, on again, off again, never quite making it all the way, and only about 25 succeed.

Women appear to have more difficulty quitting than men, possibly because smoking helps them cope, keeps weight down, and projects a desired liberated image. In addition, women who began smoking years ago, before the habit was acceptable, made a much larger psychological investment in smoking than did men.

Motivation is the key Quitting is tough, it's true, but 18 million Americans have managed to break the cigarette habit. Motivation is central to success. Serious illness or the threat of it works for some, but not all. Some stop to please a loved one. For others, the best motivation is to encourage a spouse or child or friend to team with them in quitting. Others may want to quit because they recognize smoking as a dirty habit, offensive to others. Some may simply decide, "It's time for *me* to be in control. I don't want to be manipulated by some crushed weeds wrapped in paper or by the tobacco companies."

Alvin R. Jaffin, director of the therapy program of the American Health Foundation, believes that those who succeed do so because they decide that for them, suddenly, smoking is not a negotiable issue. Says Jaffin, "It's like what happens on the subway: You don't smoke and you don't die. But the minute you get to the steps, you're dying for a smoke. That's because smoking on subways is a nonnegotiable issue . . . "(p. 91).

Substituting other satisfying activities for smoking can be a successful way of cutting down on cigarettes or quitting "cold turkey."

American Cancer Society

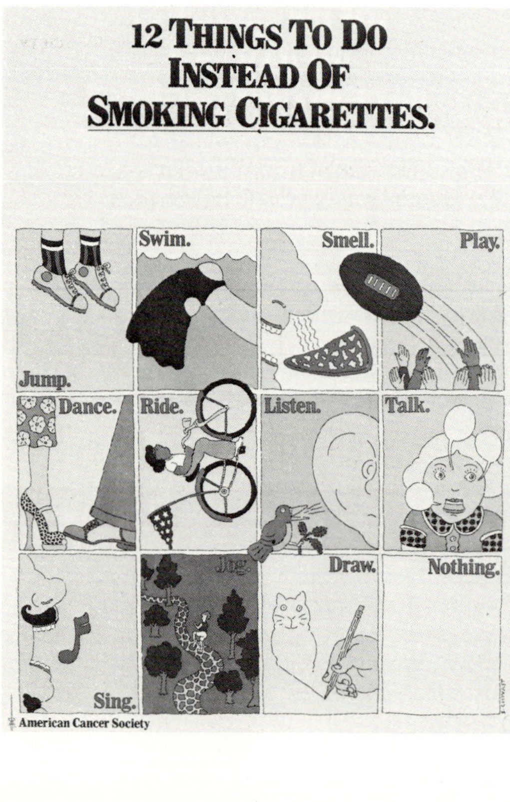

Ways of quitting Attitudes are more important than approach. An occasional backslide need not mean the end of the effort. Yet fear of failure keeps many from making the attempt. Approaches to quitting are as different as people who smoke. One woman, unsuccessful after many tries, saw the Dick Van Dyke film "Cold Turkey" and persuaded her hometown to do as the town in the movie did; everyone quit together, in mutual support and encouragement. Others have tried hypnosis, medication, psychotherapy, pacifiers, empty cigarette holders, even acupuncture (several West Coast doctors have reported success with ear staples). And tens of thousands have attended smoking cessation clinics, commercially sponsored or run by community groups, and have experienced both exhilarating success and discouraging failure.

For Those Who Cannot, or Will Not, Quit

The message is clear: "Unless you decide to quit, your problem isn't going to be smoking,

WHEN TO SEEK HELP

Danger Signs for Smokers

- Persistent cough
- Bloody sputum
- Vague chest pains
- Shortness of breath

your problem is going to be staying alive." For those who do not, or will not, get the message, there are a number of ways in which smoking hazards can be reduced (U.S. Dhew, *u*):

1 Choose a cigarette with less tar and nicotine; differences among brands can be considerable.
2 Don't smoke your cigarette all the way down. You get only 40 percent of the tar and nicotine from the first half, 60 percent from the last half.
3 Take fewer drags on each cigarette; you'll be cutting down and hardly notice it.
4 Inhale less often, less deeply; take short drags or just puff. Practice on a big cigar.
5 Smoke fewer cigarettes each day. Pick a time of day when you promise yourself not to smoke. Don't think of it as cutting down, just as postponing.
6 Use filter-tip cigarettes[2] or switch to cigars or a pipe.

Following these suggestions will not make smoking safe—just a little less dangerous.

The Nonsmoker Revolt

Nonsmokers used to be timid about asserting their rights. They either quietly tolerated a room fouled by tobacco smoke or discreetly left it. Now that silent majority—a majority because only 39.3 percent of males and 28.9 percent of females over 21 presently smoke—has decided that nonsmokers have rights. Supported by evidence on the dangers of passive smoking, organizations like ASH (Action on Smoking and Health) have launched a nationwide lobbying campaign against smoke-filled rooms. This effort is supported by 70 percent of nonsmoking Americans (U.S. DHEW, *dd*).

[2] Although filters slightly lower risk of lung disease, they may increase risk of heart disease.

Danger from passive smoking Being in a smoke-filled room has been called "passive smoking" because by breathing in contaminated air, the nonsmoker suffers many of the deleterious effects of smoking. Concentrations of harmful substances in such an enclosed space often equal or exceed legal limits for maximum air pollution. Cigar and pipe smokers and noninhaling cigarette puffers contribute more of these substances than do cigarette smokers who inhale most of the poisons into their own lungs. Passive smoking can be particularly harmful to heart patients, but many others (especially those with allergies) suffer nasal and eye irritation, coughing, sinusitis, headache, and wheezing when exposed to even moderate concentrations of smoke. In automobiles, where concentrations of carbon monoxide are already high, smoke can bring levels up high enough to interfere with driving ability, or even put the driver to sleep at the wheel. Children, especially infants, who live with adult smokers suffer increased heart and blood pressure rates and respiratory illnesses, including pneumonia and bronchitis.

Reducing risk Since concentrations of toxic chemicals from smoke are worst in enclosed places, the nonsmoker can reduce risks by requesting that windows in the room or automobile be kept open when others are smoking. Exhaust fans can help by drawing out stale air. The seating of smokers and nonsmokers in separate parts of a meeting room or classroom cuts risks, too. Since smoke from pipes and cigars is most hazardous to others, nonsmokers might request that they not be used in public places. Sharp restric-

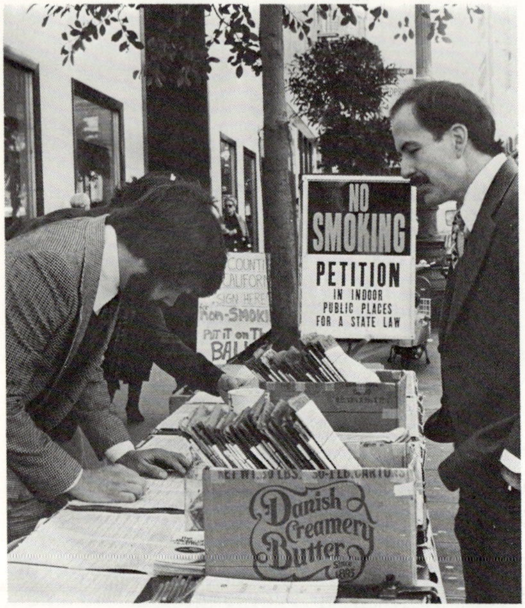
NO SMOKING
PETITION
IN INDOOR
PUBLIC PLACES
FOR A STATE LAW
Danish Creamery Butter
Christine Jakobs

With growing pressure from nonsmokers, legislation banning or limiting smoking in public places is on the increase.

tions on smoking are, of course, the best solution of all.

Bans on Smoking

A campaign for clean inner air is being waged by nonsmokers in private homes and public places. Some colleges have banned smoking in classrooms. Some people have posted "Thank you for not smoking" or "If you must smoke, don't exhale" signs in their homes. One restaurant started with a 35-seat nonsmoking section and now reports that half the 800 diners served daily are requesting "no smoking" space. A beautician who set up nonsmoking days has found them to be very popular with patrons. And several entertainers ask nightclubbers to stop smoking during their acts.

The Civil Aeronautics Board has made nonsmoking areas mandatory on commercial airliners and has banned cigars and pipes entirely. A majority of states and many localities have banned or limited smoking in public places: elevators, supermarkets, public meetings, hospitals, concert halls. But these bans have been difficult to enforce. And the smokers' lobby, generously financed by tobacco interests, has frequently managed to defeat antismoking laws.

The clean air campaign may benefit smokers in the long run. As they find themselves asked to sit in the rear of the bus or plane, to move to another car in the train, or not to smoke in a friend's home or a restaurant, some may well decide that smoking is not worth the effort, and may join the unhooked generation.

A smoker and a non-smoker cannot be equally free in the same railway carriage.
George Bernard Shaw

LOOKING BACK

REVIEWING CONCEPTS IN CHAPTER 17

- Reducing tobacco use is one of the best preventive medicine measures available to us.
- The percentage of cigarette smokers in the United States has been reduced since the hazards of tobacco became known, but thousands of new smokers take up the habit daily. The greatest percentage increase has been for adolescent girls.
- Though tobacco has been used in the West for more than 400 years, evidence of its dangers did not become apparent until cigarette smoking became widespread in the 1930s.
- Tobacco smoke is made up of some of the most hazardous poison gases and chemicals known.
- The amounts of poisonous gases and chemicals absorbed by the smoker depend on the type of cigarette smoked and on smoking style.
- There is disagreement about whether or not tobacco causes physical dependence, but there is little disagreement that it can lead to a habit that is difficult to break.
- The new smoker usually quickly develops tolerance to the effects of nicotine poisoning; increased doses are needed to achieve the same effect.
- Tobacco smoke has a variety of immediate and long-term effects on the body, leading to a reduced lifespan and increased disability for the heavy cigarette smoker.
- The best-known effects are on lungs and respiratory system, and heart and vascular system. Smoking is also a major factor in fatal fires and may contribute to automobile accidents.
- To stop smoking is difficult, but more than 18 million Americans have managed it. Motivation with reinforcement is the key.
- Persons unable to quit as yet can reduce risks slightly by modifying their smoking styles.
- Nonsmokers, a majority in American society, are now taking steps to protect themselves from the hazards of other people's smoking.

18 HELP FOR THE DRUG ABUSER AND THE POTENTIAL ABUSER

WHAT'S AHEAD IN CHAPTER 18 Is it "interfering" to try to help a friend with a drug problem without being asked? Or do we have a responsibility to try to help? How can a layperson help someone having a "bad trip" or an adverse drug reaction? What kinds of reactions need immediate medical attention? What elements are usually necessary for an individual to successfully "kick" a drug habit? What approaches are often used? Is there one best way? What is the role of rehabilitation programs in reestablishing of self-confidence and self-respect, and in replacing drug activity with alternatives? What are the advantages and disadvantages of methadone maintenance? How does heroin maintenance, often used in Britain, differ? What are the "alternative roads to high" that can replace dependence on chemicals for stimulation?

- Jim is drunk, but wants to drive home from the party.
- Brooke chain smokes. Even her rasping cough does not deter her.
- Ned started smoking grass on weekends. Now he smokes daily, and it has begun interfering with his classwork.
- Monica takes uppers to get her through the day and downers to sleep at night. Only her husband knows.

What is the responsibility of friends and family in these situations? Is it presumptuous to take Jim's keys and drive him home? Is it rude to remind Brooke of what cigarettes are doing to her or to try to get Ned to cut back on his marijuana use? Is it disloyal for Monica's husband to "go behind her back" and speak to a physician about her drug use?

These are important questions faced by millions of Americans of all ages every day.

Their responses will have a profound effect on drug abuse in our society. For those who decide to try to help, even at the risk of imperiling a relationship, it is important to know the kinds of treatments available, as well as how to treat a drug emergency. Perhaps even more important is knowing the alternatives to drug abuse that can prevent problems from developing.

RECOGNIZING DRUG ABUSE

The infrequent experimenter and the occasional recreational user of drugs are probably no cause for concern. But the individual who uses drugs as a way of solving problems, to fill deep emotional needs, or as a way of life is. What other signs point to a drug problem?

There may be symptoms associated with the use of specific drugs: restlessness, nervousness, talkativeness (amphetamines), appearing drunk with no smell of alcohol (barbiturates), pinpoint pupils and craving for sweets (new heroin addict), or any of the other clues listed in Table 15.2. Or more general signs may be noted: personality changes; lack of interest in personal appearance, school, or work; confusion and loss of memory; lack of appetite; red or runny eyes; problems with sleep or digestion. These could signal physical or mental illness rather than drug problems. Either way, they warn that help is needed. It is not always necessary to look for symptoms. Some abusers use their drugs in front of others, or leave pills, powders, or apparatus around or offer them to friends.

Other than friendship and support, there are two kinds of help a drug abuser may need. One is emergency treatment for an adverse reaction or for withdrawal symptoms; the other is long-term help in "kicking the habit."

EMERGENCY TREATMENT

Indications of acute adverse drug reaction—any *unexpected* response to a drug, or any expected response that lasts unusually long—vary with the drug, the individual, and the setting (see Table 15.1). Some symptoms indicate a bad trip that can be handled by a friend; others warn of a life-and-death situation demanding immediate medical care.

Handling a Bad Trip

Since there is no predicting a bad trip or panic reaction, experienced marijuana and hallucinogenic drug users rarely trip alone. It is recommended that the solo user who feels a bad trip coming on immediately call a friend; even talking on the phone can help.

Reassurance is what the person on a bad trip, or on a flashback of a bad trip, needs most. He (we will use the masculine pronoun here for convenience) may feel he is going to lose control and never come back. Friends need to assure him that this feeling will pass, that he is not going insane. They can help him reassemble reality by repeating his name, where he is, and with whom, and by talking and encouraging him to talk. It can be helpful to change the environment in which the trip took place, adjusting lights or sound, for example. Distracting the panicky tripper with an intricate picture, a piece of gossip, or a TV show may be useful. *Other drugs should not be given.*

The trip down may not be steady. The person may drift in and out of reality for a while. If the trip shows no signs of letting up at all, or seems to be getting worse, or if the patient becomes violent or difficult to handle, medical help should be sought. In severe cases, psychiatric treatment or hospitalization may be necessary.

Handling Drug Emergencies

As a general rule, it is recommended that immediate medical care be sought for a person who is unconscious, violent, having convulsions, vomiting uncontrollably, has a very high or very low body temperature, or is having trouble breathing, or if incoherent,

SELF-CARE

Treatment of Drug Emergencies

- Keep the patient quiet, comfortable, lightly covered.
- If the patient is drowsy, try to keep him or her walking.
- Turn a vomiting patient on his stomach; if not vomiting, turn him on his side with head extended.
- Try to keep airways clear; wipe vomitus or other secretions from nose, mouth, and throat.
- Administer *no* other drugs.
- If the drug was swallowed, try to induce vomiting; if the patient is conscious, try to reduce absorption of the drug by feeding milk or water.
- If the drug was injected, put ice packs on the site of the injection to try to stem the flow of the drug through the body. Cold water or compresses (see Appendix) may be substituted.
- If respiration is less than 10 breaths a minute, give CPR, steps 1 and 3 (Figure 10.8).
- *If the patient goes into convulsions (violent jerking and twitching)*, place cushion, arm, or foot under his head and otherwise restrain him, if necessary, to prevent injury. Put a padded tongue depressor or other blunt object in his mouth to keep him from biting his tongue. *Do not* induce vomiting.
- *If the patient goes into shock (pale or bluish, cold, clammy skin; weak, fast pulse and breathing; weakness; thirst; nausea)*, treat for shock as shown in Table 11.4.
- *If fever is very high or very low*, treat as shown in Chapter 4, page 79.
- *For individual drug reactions:*
  Amphetamines Keep room dark.
  Narcotics If the patient is awake, feed black, strong coffee; keep patient warm.
  Cocaine If the drug was sniffed, wash mucous membranes of the patient's nose with salt water or plain water.
  Depressants Give CPR (see Figure 10.8).
- *If the patient is violent*, restrain him if you can safely do so, to protect him and others. Do not slap the patient. Stay calm. If the patient is extremely violent (common with PCP), get out of the room and lock the door behind you.

psychotic, or violent behavior continues beyond the usual duration of the drug's effects. Sometimes help is not sought because of fear of getting a friend into trouble or being embarrassed because the drug used is illegal. But the alternative may be a very sick or very dead friend.

While waiting for medical aid, there are several things that can be done, as shown in the self-care sidebar. It is recommended that whatever drug the patient was using be taken to the hospital with him. The victim's clothing and the room should be checked for such clues as an empty bottle or the stub of a marijuana cigarette. This is especially important if the drug was bought on the street because street drugs are so often mislabeled or contain contaminants. If the patient used several drugs, including alcohol, the doctor should know that, too.

Drug Withdrawal

Withdrawal symptoms can range from mild to deadly, depending on the drug, how long it has been used, and the individual's response. Except for withdrawal from tobacco, drug withdrawal should usually take place under the direction of a physician. The most common symptoms of withdrawal for each drug are listed in Table 15.2. Until medical help is reached, the patient should be kept as calm and comfortable as possible, with symptoms treated as for other drug emergencies.

LONG-TERM TREATMENT

Kicking the Habit

Many of us have a picture of the drug user "kicking the habit," which we have drawn chiefly from old movie melodramas. Cut off from the drug, the user is forcibly restrained and endures an agonizing period of retching, shaking, screaming, kicking (hence, "kicking the habit"), and other tortured hours of crisis. If the kicker is a "bad apple" or lacking in will power, a return to drugs is likely. The "good egg" heaves a sigh of relief at having regained freedom and continues to stay clean through renewed self-discipline. There are a great many distortions in that familiar picture.

First, successful treatment of a drug habit can rarely be forced. Success is most likely when the patient really wants to quit, and occasionally, even that is not enough. Sometimes it takes a trauma—loss of job, school failure, threat of divorce, hitting bottom—to prompt a desire to quit.

Second, there can indeed be much psychic misery for the *psychologically dependent* person who gives up drugs. But not everyone with a drug habit experiences withdrawal symptoms. These are reserved for the user who is *physically dependent.*

Third, though withdrawal symptoms can be agonizing, and with some drugs dangerous to the point of death, they are sometimes much milder than antidrug "horror" films (with the best of motives and intentions) portray them.

Fourth, morality or goodness is not involved in drug abuse. Drug abuse is an illness. The person dependent on a drug has lost control and needs help to regain it, not scorn and punishment.

Finally, motivation and withdrawal of the drug are only the first steps in treatment of the drug abuser. The real goals are twofold: (1) rehabilitation that leads to or reestablishes personal confidence and self-respect, that helps an individual to be self-sufficient, to be productive, to find a job; and (2) helping the former abuser to find fulfilling alternatives to drug abuse.

There seems to be no foolproof, all-purpose method by which these goals can be successfully met for every abuser. As participants suggested at the American Psychiatric Association conference on drug abuse in 1975, treatment must be individualized, tailored to the patient, the drug, the circumstances. The person who has tried to give up drugs and failed is not doomed to a life of dependence. When one antibiotic does not work on an infection, the physician tries another. Similarly, another form of therapy, another type of facility or therapist, or simply one more try may kick the drug habit.

Chances of Success

Most drug dependency can be treated, though "cure" is not often a word applied to the results. A person who has a tendency to drug dependency retains it for a lifetime. An alcoholic who has been on the wagon for years but unwittingly takes a cough medicine containing alcohol may lapse back into a binge. Getting back on that wagon may be easier than the first time, but the reaction of the chemical-starved tissues is a reminder that the problem has not gone away. Some persons move from one dependency to another—off heroin and onto alcohol, for example. That is why the development of nonchemical routes to high (discussed later in this chapter) and of coping mechanisms (discussed in Chapter 2) are important aspects of treatment.

Heroin addiction may be the most difficult form of drug abuse to treat, though some bestow that distinction on tobacco. Reports

Arnold Hinton/Nancy Palmer

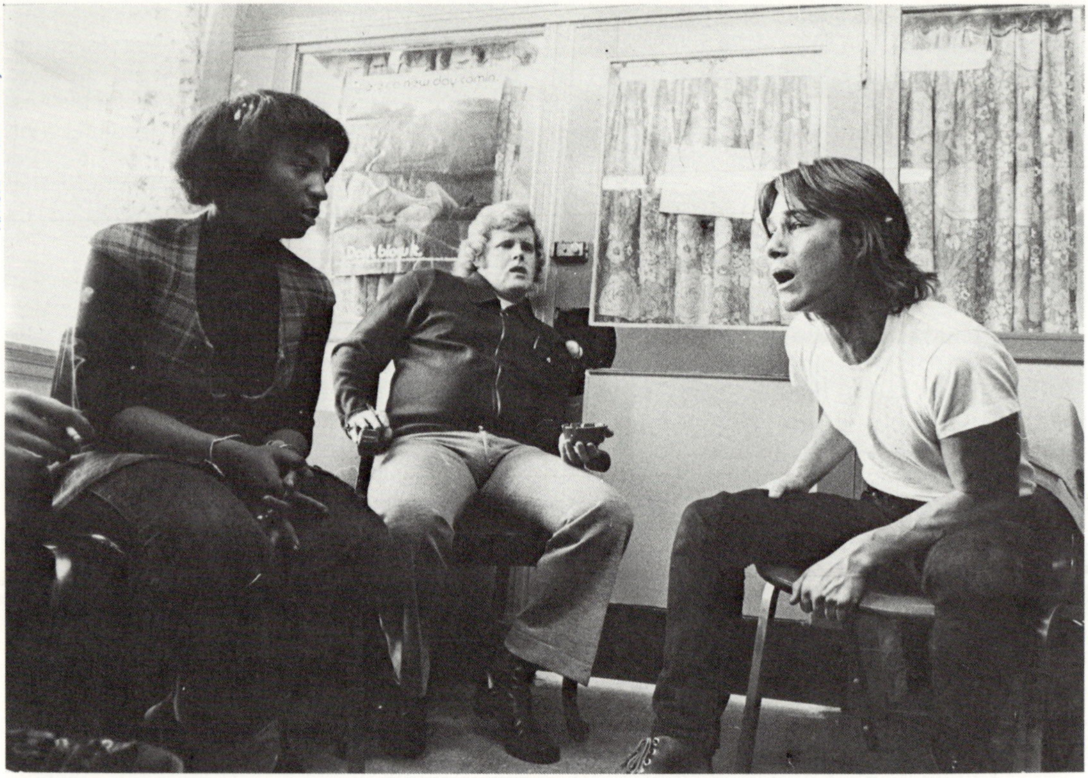

A variety of services, including group counseling and meditation sessions, are offered in drug treatment facilities.

of success rates for those physically dependent on heroin fluctuate widely, depending on many factors, from 10 to 95 percent. Some young addicts may be easy to wean from the habit because they are not truly dependent; the street heroin they have been using is too diluted to really hook them. Some long-time addicts become easier to treat when they reach their forties. Dr. Donald Louria speculates that this is because they used heroin as teenagers to relieve feelings of sexual inadequacy or aggression, and as the sex drive was reduced with age, so was the need for heroin.

Some believe that a heroin dependency is a lifetime "monkey on the back," that the dependent person will always crave the drug. They urge that young people who consider dabbling with heroin be warned of this possibility (Brecher).

Treatment Centers for Drug Abusers

There are some 3150 drug abuse treatment clinics in the United States. Some treat the hard-core heroin junkie, others middle-class men and women dependent on "pills"; still others deal with the alcoholic, the chronic marijuana user, or the multidrug abuser. Some treat anyone with any drug problem. Some facilities are funded by the federal government, others by local communities, religious groups, medical societies, or private donors. Staffs may be volunteer or paid, or a combination. Many include ex-addicts. In all

WHERE TO GET HELP

Alcohol and Drug Problems

Mental health facilities, school counseling services, physicians, or clerics can direct individuals in need of help to the appropriate source of assistance. Check your local phone book for AA and Alanon groups; see your physician or clergyman; or call a community mental health center or your school's psychological counseling service. Or contact any of the following organizations:

- National Clearinghouse for Alcohol Information
  Box 2345
  Rockville, MD 20852

- Alcoholics Anonymous
  P.O. Box 459, Grand Central Station
  New York, NY 10010

- Alanon Family Groups
  115 East 23rd Street
  New York, NY 10010

- National Council on Alcoholism, Inc.
  2 Park Avenue South
  New York, NY 10016

- Veterans Administration
  Alcohol and Drug Dependent Service
  810 Vermont Avenue, N.W.
  Washington, DC 20420

- National Clearinghouse for Drug Abuse Information
  P.O. Box 1080
  Washington, D.C. 20013
  (Request National Directory of Drug Abuse Treatment Programs)

- National Coordinating Council on Drug Abuse Education and Information
  1211 Connecticut Avenue, N.W.
  Washington, DC 20036

- STASH (Student Association for the Study of Hallucinogens)
  638 Pleasant Street
  Beloit, WI 53511

facilities, confidentiality is respected. Persons in treatment are not turned over to law enforcement officials. Many centers treat those remanded to them by the courts.

All treatment centers offer one or more of the following services, and a few offer all of them: drug-free and/or chemical detoxification, individual psychotherapy, group therapy, crisis intervention in emergencies, counseling (family, educational, religious), sensi-

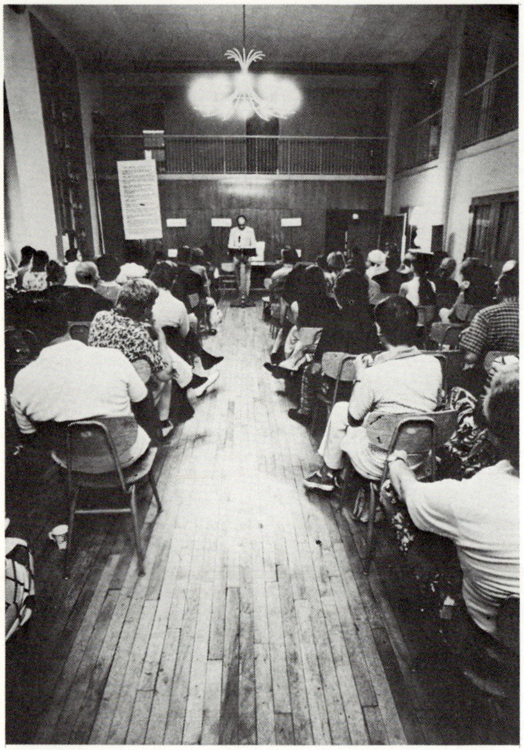
Alcoholics Anonymous

Alcoholics Anonymous groups have had remarkable success in rehabilitating people with drinking problems.

tivity training, meditation and awareness groups, social services, medical and surgical treatment, legal intervention when needed, job training and placement, and supervised work. Most refer patients elsewhere for services they cannot provide. Some treatment centers have received a great deal of attention because of their specialized approaches—among them, the therapeutic communities treating narcotic and other drug abusers, and Alcoholics Anonymous.

Therapeutic communities Summed up one addict: "If you can't be born into a family that cares for you, you have to make one." That, in effect, is what treatment centers like Daytop Village, Phoenix House, and Synanon attempt to do. But it is a very tightly supervised family, with strict discipline and strong peer group pressure. The goal is a life totally free of nonmedical drugs. Some communities work toward a gradual return to the community outside after a one- or two-year period in residence. Others are based on longer associations, possibly lifetime.

Therapeutic communities were at first hailed as *the* solution to the drug problem. But it soon became apparent that those who actually returned to their former lives and remained drug-free were painfully few. A Ford Foundation study noted a low 5 percent success rate. Whether specific programs are more successful will remain uncertain until better evaluation procedures are developed.

Some critics have condemned the rigid, peer-run discipline in many communities. They point out that drug addicts are often people who have not learned how to run their lives successfully and declare that a highly structured community where they have little opportunity to make decisions of their own is not likely to improve their abilities to cope independently. Supporters retort that dependence on a community is better than dependence on drugs. Whatever their weaknesses, therapeutic communities have helped some drug abusers.

Alcoholics Anonymous AA is a community of sorts, too. But its members of all ages live at home while sharing their experiences ("My name is Charlie M., and I'm an alcoholic"), their strength, and their hope to solve the common problem of alcoholism. Unlike many other drug programs, AA excludes no one. Anyone who wants to stop drinking can join without cost, drawing support from the group but depending primarily on himself or herself and on a concept of a "higher power," stressed in AA's "12 steps," which begin with the admission that alcohol has made life unmanageable. Criticism or recriminations are out at AA meetings, but no one is allowed to forget a basic AA tenet: "Once an alcoholic, always an alcoholic." Confounding those who once sneered at them, AA groups have

Alateen and Alanon: Help for Families of Alcoholics

When I was little, my father began coming home late, very drunk and violent. He'd go after my sister, my brother, and my mother. I'd wake up in the middle of the night and hear yelling and screaming and my father throwing things. I felt different from other kids and so I kept to myself. I had no friends at all. I was a bookworm and compulsive eater. At age 11, I decided I was causing the problems in the family and decided to solve them all by jumping off the roof of our apartment building. Luckily a couple of teenagers saw me and held me back.

My elder sister recognized my need for help and dragged me, actually kicking and screaming, to an Alateen meeting. I walked into a room and there were all these young people smiling and laughing even though they had the same family problem I had. I couldn't believe it. It kept me coming. There were group discussions, free and open exchanges of ideas and experiences. We used the same steps and stages as AA. We ventilated resentments and I got an understanding of what was happening inside me.

My mother and sister were in the program, too, but it was six years before my father came around to AA. In the meantime, we came to accept him with his alcoholism, to stop fighting with him. Nobody can force or even encourage an alcoholic. It wasn't until he was about to lose his job that he was willing to face his problem. He's been alcohol-free for two years now. I still have some problems and still go to Alateen meetings—but I really believe that Alateen saved my life.

The daughter of an alcoholic

had remarkable success in rehabilitating people from all walks of life, of all ages. AA does not work for everyone. Some do better with psychiatric or medical treatment, and "drying out" in a hospital is often necessary at some stage, frequently in conjunction with the AA program.

Drug Therapies for Drug Abusers

Drugs have often been resorted to in treating drug abuse, and they have often failed. But many physicians find that drugs can get the patient through the critical withdrawal stage, or permit more gradual withdrawal. Currently, many authorities support the concept of using drugs to "maintain" heroin addicts.

Methadone maintenance History repeats. As heroin was once used as a "cure" for morphine addiction, so methadone was originally proclaimed a cure for heroin dependence. But both heroin and methadone proved to be as addicting as the drugs they were to replace. The use of methadone today is primarily to bring addicts back into society, to help them function more normally, not to get them off drugs altogether. Methadone reduces the craving for heroin and blocks its action if the addict decides to use it anyway. It is preferred to heroin because it has less of a depressant effect, interferes less with sexual desires, and can be taken orally. But it must be taken regularly, for as soon as it is stopped, the craving for heroin returns.

Methadone maintenance clinics with well-controlled programs claim a higher success rate than do any other treatment methods to date. Others counterclaim that such clinics accept only older and better-motivated patients who are good risks. A government survey of methadone and nonmethadone facilities found little difference in success rates.

Critics also point out that the long-term effects of methadone are unknown, that there is some evidence of a higher rate of premature and low-birth-weight babies among women on methadone maintenance, and that

Leo Choplin/Black Star

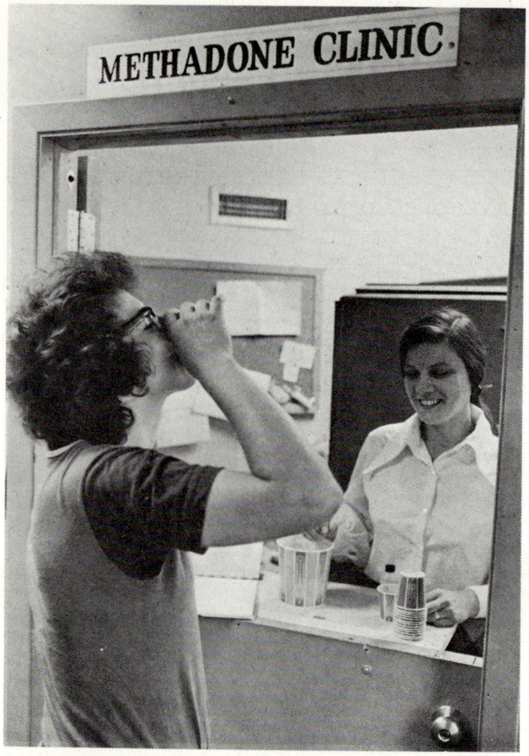

Methadone maintenance is designed to bring the addict back into society as a functioning and contributing member, but for many reasons it remains a controversial treatment.

many methadone patients use other drugs (especially alcohol, amphetamines, and barbiturates, all potentially more physically dangerous than heroin). Deaths resulting from methadone overdose have also begun to rise, and there were twice as many methadone overdose deaths as heroin overdose deaths in New York City in 1973. Most deaths were apparently among street users of illegal methadone rather than clinic patients, but much of the methadone used "leaked" from clinics. And deaths have been reported of children who got into their parents' supplies.

The methadone maintenance program has raised many serious questions: Is it moral to encourage and support lifelong dependence on drugs, even though legally administered? Is a dangerous precedent being set by giving the government such total control over people's lives? Will clinics eventually turn their patients into a cadre of obedient zombies? Are some of the clinics (as has been charged) "methadone supermarkets dispensing drugs for Medicaid payments," while failing to supply psychological and other services that might help their patients get off drugs completely?

In spite of the criticism, there is strong support for methadone maintenance programs. This is not surprising since, even if the program does not "cure" addicts, it appears to make them less dependent upon society, to bring many back to productive lives, and to remove them from the ranks of criminals, and it does all this at relatively low cost.

Heroin maintenance Some observers believe that methadone maintenance is not enough, particularly for the young heroin addict who is not ready to give up the heroin high. They point to the British system which for many years permitted free prescribing of heroin by physicians for treatment or maintenance of addicts. This system was modified in 1968, when it became clear that prescribed heroin was reaching the black market, where it was sold to nonaddicts, who, in turn, became hooked and went to the government for their legal fixes. Today's system permits prescription of rigidly monitored doses of heroin (or more often, methadone) at licensed clinics only.

Admirers of the British approach would like to see it emulated here. Others would like to go further and permit all drugs to be sold freely (under government supervision for safety and purity) over the counter without a prescription. They see this not as a medical problem, but one of civil rights (Geis).

Drug antagonists Several drug antagonists that can reverse and block the action of a drug in the body (nalorpine, naloxone, cyclazocine, and pentozocine among them) have recently been developed to counteract narcotics. They can be used to: (1) treat narcotics overdose by reversing the respiratory depression caused by narcotics; (2) diagnose addiction by bringing on withdrawal symptoms in addicts within minutes; (3) reduce pain.

Many researchers hold out hope that antagonists which block the euphoric "rush" heroin gives can eventually be developed to help in permanently withdrawing addicts from drugs. Detoxified addicts would be able to return to their former environments with less risk of relapsing to their old habits, fortified by continuing treatment to help them find new ways of coping.

Antagonists have also been explored for other drugs, including tobacco and alcohol. Those for tobacco have not been very successful. Antabuse (disulfiram), an alcohol antagonist, has not proved useful when used indiscriminately. But with selected patients, in an overall treatment program, the drug can give positive ego reinforcement, acting as a "chemical fence" to help alcoholics stay away from alcohol.

Nondrug Therapies

Every known approach to changing behavior has been tried on drug abusers, including the full range of psychotherapies outlined in Chapter 3. Even hypnosis and acupuncture have been attempted. When the method fits the patient and there is sufficient motivation, just about any method can claim some success.

ALTERNATIVE ROADS TO HIGH

In the early nineteenth century, Benjamin Waterhouse asked, "Cannot wisdom devise a plan of social intercourse, independent of the stimulus of the bottle?" Today physicians, educators, parents, drug abuse rehabilitation workers, and even drug abusers themselves are asking the same question. Are there not other ways of achieving the fleeting pleasures wrung from drugs without the torments, the risks to body and psyche, the hazards to community that are the companions of drug abuse?

The Need for Alternatives

Generally, people who abuse substances are in pursuit of something they lack or think they lack. Often they are simply pursuing happiness. But Stephen Chinlund, director of the Manhattan Community Rehabilitation Center in New York City, suggests that happiness cannot be directly pursued. It comes, he says, only as the incidental byproduct of other involvements—from the satisfaction of doing something well, or from giving ourselves to family and friends and sharing life with them, whatever happens, good or bad. Then, when we least expect it, we find ourselves overtaken by happiness (Messolonghites).

Drug abusers are searching for many other things: new experiences, involvement, exploration, adventure, excitement, connection with others, a sense of well-being, identity, self-understanding, and belongingness. These are things they have been unable to find in the nondrug society, perhaps because they have never been aware that there might be other options. They feel no sense of community, no vision of the future, no clear system of values. They turn to drugs for a *feeling* of being alive, but they get just the feeling, not the reality. And for those for whom being alive means despair, anxiety, hopelessness, or pain, drugs are used to dull the feeling of life, to turn it off, to find unreality.

Internist Richard Bates suggests that drugs offer no permanent help to these people, but rather are a block to emotional growth. They need, he says, the confidence born of facing fears, of conquering the unknown and the untried:

> People who learn in childhood to meet and overcome fears and problems find the challenges of getting into the swim of life so intoxi-

TABLE 18.1 Examples of alternative roads to high

WHEN THERE IS A NEED OR DESIRE FOR:	DRUGS MOST PROBABLY ABUSED	ALTERNATIVES THAT CAN BE SUBSTITUTED
	PHYSICAL	
Physical relaxation	Alcohol, tranquilizers, cannabis (marijuana, hash)	A variety of physical activities: relaxation exercises, "hatha" (physical) yoga; dance and movement training, outdoor work and play; physical recreation including competitive athletics (especially for fun), individual physical conditioning (jogging, biking, etc.), karate, judo, etc. Education in preventive medicine and positive health habits including diet and nutrition
Relief from pain, anticipation or prevention of sickness	Physician-prescribed drugs, over-the-counter drugs	
Increased physical energy; avoidance of fatigue	Stimulants	
	SENSORY	
Intensification and enrichment of sensory (sound, sight, touch, etc.) experience	Psychedelics, cannabis, sometimes others	Activities that increase sensory awareness; massage; visual exploration of nature; responsible sexuality (for adolescents, possible education in noncoital sex); music, art
Enhancement of sexual experience	Alcohol, cannabis, sometimes others	
	EMOTIONAL	
Psychological escape, release from emotional agony	Any, especially narcotics and alcohol	Various kinds of counseling; group therapy, individual therapy; psychodrama and role playing Effective education in personality development, values clarification, etc. Emotional awareness exercises (getting in touch with oneself); body language; honest self-exploration and awareness workshops Training in decision making
Reduction of normal tension, anxiety, conflict	Alcohol, barbiturates, OTC sedatives, tranquilizers, cannabis	
Emotional relaxation	Alcohol, tranquilizers, cannabis	
Mood alteration	Stimulants, alcohol, cannabis	
Psychological or emotional insight	Psychedelics, cannabis	
Avoidance of decision making	Any	
Privacy, aloneness	Alcohol, narcotics	
Rebellion; assertion of independence or defiance of authority	Any, especially illicit or forbidden substances	
Intensification of personal courage	Stimulants, alcohol	
Increase in self-esteem	Any, especially alcohol, stimulants, and cannabis	
	INTERPERSONAL	
Peer recognition and acceptance	Any	Creation of alternate peer groups; involvement in positive group activities (e.g., 4-H, college, church clubs, etc.) Individual and group counseling on interpersonal problems
Less inhibited, more relaxed relations with others	Any, especially alcohol and cannabis	
Solution of interpersonal problems	Psychedelics, cannabis	

Source: Adapted from Allan Y. Cohen, pp. 14–27.

WHEN THERE IS A NEED OR DESIRE FOR:	DRUGS MOST PROBABLY ABUSED	ALTERNATIVES THAT CAN BE SUBSTITUTED
	INTERPERSONAL	
Escape, release from family problems	Any	Competently run sensitivity and encounter groups dealing with group process
Escape from feelings of loneliness, alienation	Any	Workshops aimed at developing caring, personal responsibility, confidence, trust, and respect for others
Belonging to a group	Any	Social confidence training; assertiveness training; family life and parent education; premarital counseling
		Temporary alternate families, foster homes, "big brothers or sisters" when needed
		Other activities aimed at developing better interpersonal relations
	MENTAL OR INTELLECTUAL	
Reduction of boredom	Any	Games and activities that improve intellectual functioning: puzzles, chess, etc.
Curiosity	Any	Training in problem solving, decision making, memory, concentration and attention, and mind-control techniques such as positive thinking, autosuggestion
Better learning, problem-solving ability	Stimulants, sometimes psychedelics	Intellectual excitement through discussion, reading, organizations, guest speaker lectures
Knowing oneself and one's learning processes better	Psychedelics, cannabis	Use of physical fitness and good health habits to reduce fatigue
Relief of fatigue, increased ability to study	Stimulants	
	CREATIVE OR AESTHETIC	
More creativity	Cannabis, stimulants, psychedelics	Nongraded instruction or experience, both as participant and observers, in desired artistic activities: art, music, drama, etc.
More enjoyment of artistic productions	Cannabis, alcohol, psychedelics	Creative hobbies of all kinds: sewing, cooking, photography, writing, etc.
Creation of subjective states of fantasy or imagination	Psychedelics, cannabis	Communication experience: public speaking, radio clubs, etc.
		Creative games
		Development of community centers for creative arts

TABLE 18.1 *(Continued)*

WHEN THERE IS A NEED OR DESIRE FOR:	DRUGS MOST PROBABLY ABUSED	ALTERNATIVES THAT CAN BE SUBSTITUTED
	EXPERIMENTAL	
Pure fun, pleasure, recreation	Any	Activities that change one's perceptions and consciousness: experiments in sensory deprivation, sleeplessness, fasting (within health parameters), guided daydreams and fantasy (mind tripping), hypnosis (expertly induced), biofeedback
Highs, intoxication, change in awareness for its own sake	Any	
Distortion of senses and perceptions	Psychedelics, cannabis, sometimes stimulants or barbiturates	
Personal involvement to counteract apathy	Any, except tranquilizers	Self-generated play experience
	STYLISTIC	
Need for identification with hero figures; of youth with adults, of adults with youth; of each with peers	Any	Chance to know others, including hero figures, deep and meaningful involvement in nonchemical alternatives
Automatic chemical reliance; the use of a substance to correct any perceived problems	Any	Involvement in antidrug or alternative programs
Desire for immediacy of achievement; impatience and intolerance with delay of gratification	Any; tranquilizers, volatile chemicals, sometimes OTC drugs	Exposure to the philosophy of enjoying the *process* of attainment, not just the *product*; example of parental and other adult abstinence and wise use of drugs
	SOCIAL OR POLITICAL	
Identification with antiestablishment forces	Cannabis, psychedelics, sometimes any illicit drug	Any positive activity that makes the person part of the political-social system: political campaigning; lobbying; running for office; volunteer services to poor, church, synagogue, youth, schools, etc.; work with drug abusers; environmental protection activities; ACTION
Rebellion against disliked laws	Cannabis, other illicit drugs	
Overcoming discouragement or desperation with social-political future	Any	
Causing a change in public consciousness; disruption of system	Psychedelics	Citizen "potency" training in how to deal effectively with the powers that be
		Development of responsible roles for youth and others in community organization and governance

WHEN THERE IS A NEED OR DESIRE FOR:	DRUGS MOST PROBABLY ABUSED	ALTERNATIVES THAT CAN BE SUBSTITUTED
	PHILOSOPHICAL	
Purpose and meaning in life	Cannabis, psychedelics, others	Seminars, courses, workshops on values, morals, systems of belief; reading philosophical literature; values clarification
A belief structure	Cannabis, psychedelics, stimulants	
Personal identity	Psychedelics, cannabis, others	
Development of lifestyle	Any, especially cannabis, psychedelics	Exposure to individuals committed to varieties of personal philosopies
Overcoming frustration from lack of meaningful vocation and work	Any	Maximization of ethnic, racial, and minority roles
	SPIRITUAL OR MYSTICAL	
Intense spiritual experiences, mystical states, communication with God	Psychedelics, cannabis	More exposure to various systems of belief, techniques of applied spirituality; study of spiritual literature
Overcoming frustration with organized religion	Psychedelics, cannabis	Meditation, yoga (especially nonphysical), prayer, contemplation; spiritual song and dance
Enrichment of unorthodox spiritual methodology—yoga, etc.	Psychedelics, cannabis	New approaches to traditional religions
	MISCELLANEOUS	
Risk taking, danger	Any, especially the more dangerous ones	Exhilarating risk-taking activities: scuba diving, sky diving, skiing, surfing, etc.
Adventure, exploration	Any	Exploration of new physical environments and places: flying, wilderness camping, travel, etc.; outward bound survival training
"Vacuum phenomenon," or "What else is there to do?"	Any	
Economic profit	Any illicit substance	
Combination of motives, needs, aspirations	Any	
Reaction to extreme mental or physical discomfort, as in withdrawal, pain, confusion	Any	Involvement in new projects (business, recreation, community, academic) that involve risk and new frontiers Competence and self-reliance training in areas important to vocational and occupational goals, family, and household operations and management, child care, nutrition, etc.

> cating that they wouldn't dream of blunting their perception chemically before walking into a new situation. Afterwards, maybe—to celebrate—but not before. (*b*, p. 151)

Indeed, teaching children at an early age to find "intoxication in life" is an important drug preventative. Allan Y. Cohen, director of the Institute for Drug Abuse Education of the JFK University, sees childhood as the first in a three-stage program for introducing alternatives:

- *The first stage: prevention* Something should be done before an individual has begun the drug-abuse cycle. A natural "immunity" to serious drug dependency can be built by helping young people to develop coping skills, personal values, and appreciation for life (see Chapter 2).
- *The second stage: early intervention* If casual experimenters who have yet to become heavily involved or psychologically committed to a drug-abuse lifestyle are exposed to meaningful alternatives, they can be guided away from escalation of drug use and prepared for a more chemical-free existence.
- *The third stage: rehabilitation* When drug use has severely limited the individual's options and resulted in powerful physical or psychological dependency, alternative programs must be stronger and especially sensitive to the physical-psychosocial needs of severely dependent individuals. Success is more difficult to achieve at this stage.

Finding Alternatives

As can be seen in Table 18.1, we may look for alternative roads to high in many directions: within ourselves and in relationships with friends; in relationships with family or community; in our own culture or others. We can become concerned with the ultimate uses to which we put our time, lives, and natural resources, and with how these uses will affect the quality of life now and in the future. We can learn to stretch ourselves, to widen our experience, to become turned on to many things, including ourselves.

Alternatives should not be presented to the drug user or potential user either as reward or punishment. Anyone can devise alternatives, users as well as nonusers, but unless they are realistic and meaningful, and acceptable and attractive to the people they are meant to help, they will not work.

Offering alternatives is not substituting a game of checkers or basketball for a fix of heroin. To be helpful, alternatives must truly give meaning to life and the skills to cope with that life. They must be beneficial alternatives, not damaging ones. Drag racing a car on the highway, or irresponsible sex, or watching TV every waking hour cannot be considered sound alternatives to drug abuse. Like drug abuse, these alternatives are no help to the individual in solving the basic problems of life.

What Kinds of Alternatives?

Some communities, schools, clinics, groups, and individuals have begun to provide alternatives.[1] In New York City, thousands turned out for nondrug highs at a multimedia happening at a usually somber office building. Dancers performed in the windows, lobby, and plaza of the skyscraper; flutists played in the fountains; and windowwashers on scaffolding painted a stripe down the entire 40-story facade of the building. In Blandings, Utah, Navajo teenagers found meaning as they preserved the oral traditions of their people by describing them in booklets and on animated film. In the lower Naugatuck Valley of Connecticut, a "community" of some 300 young people originated an exciting conglomerate of fulfilling activities: operating a radio station, a copper-leather boutique,

[1] Ideas from Messolonghites.

I play it cool and dig all jive,
that's the reason I stay alive,
My motto is, I live to learn
to dig and be dug in return.
Langston Hughes, p. 11

and a job corps; providing short-term housing for runaways, legal aid referral, and counseling; participating in photography, drama, music, and writing workshops, in encounter and sensitivity programs, and in church-based coffee houses; and much more.

Individuals who want to begin finding non-drug highs must loosen inhibitions, release pent-up energies, see with eyes that have never seen before, listen with ears that have been deaf, learn who they are and what their needs and desires are.

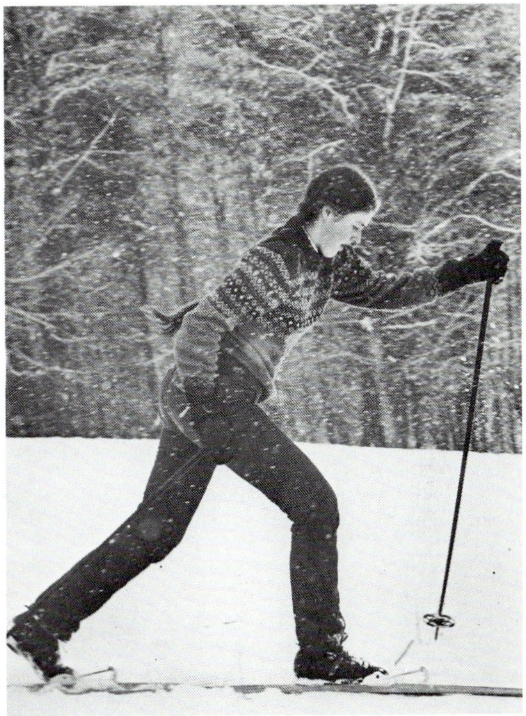

Peter Miller/Photo Researchers, Inc.

Alternative roads to "high": cross-country skiing is one of many satisfying physical activities that can serve as an alternative to substance abuse.

LOOKING BACK

REVIEWING CONCEPTS IN CHAPTER 18

- A major problem many persons face is what to do when a friend or loved one has a drug problem.
- A person who has a panic reaction (bad trip) to a drug needs reassurance and help in keeping in touch with reality.
- A person who is unconscious, convulsive, or vomiting uncontrollably, who has extremely high or low body temperature, or who is incoherent or violent (from drug use or any other cause) needs immediate medical help.
- Additional drugs of any kind should never be given to a person having a bad reaction to a drug. To aid the treating physician, efforts should be made to find the drug that caused the reaction.
- Withdrawal can vary from very mild to severe enough to cause death, depending upon the drug, the individual, and the degree of dependence.
- Drug "cures" can rarely be forced; the individual involved must want to give up the habit.
- Drug abuse is an illness that requires treatment, not punishment and scorn.

- Helping a person get off drugs is only the beginning; rehabilitation that leads to or reestablishes self-confidence and self-respect, and help in finding alternatives to drug abuse are a necessary part of the treatment.
- A wide variety of treatment services are available to the drug-dependent person today; which treatment is best depends upon the individual, the drug, and other factors.
- Some persons support the British-style concept of government control of distribution of all types of drugs to addicts, but the concept is very controversial.
- As with other health problems, prevention is the best treatment of drug abuse. To this end, a change in viewpoint is needed, both among individuals and in society at large about how to get highs in life without chemical assistance. Many people today are seeking and finding alternative roads to high.

V

V

LOVE AND THE HUMAN LIFE CYCLE

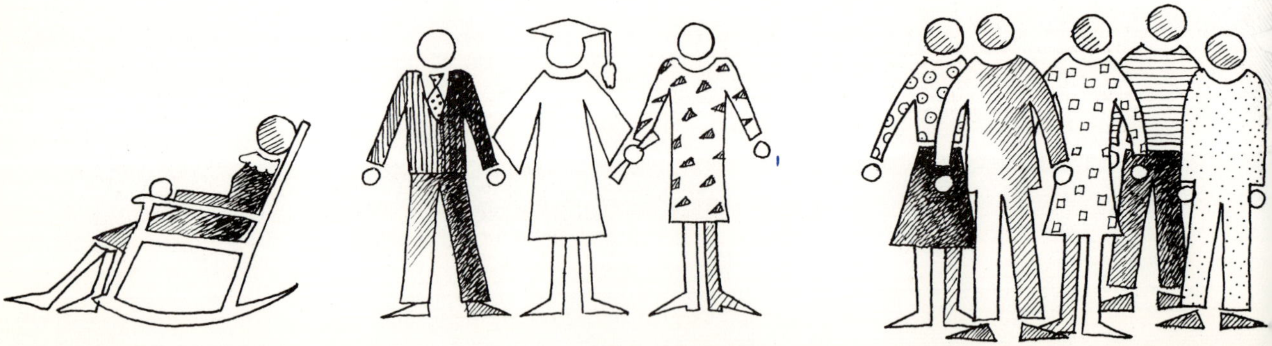

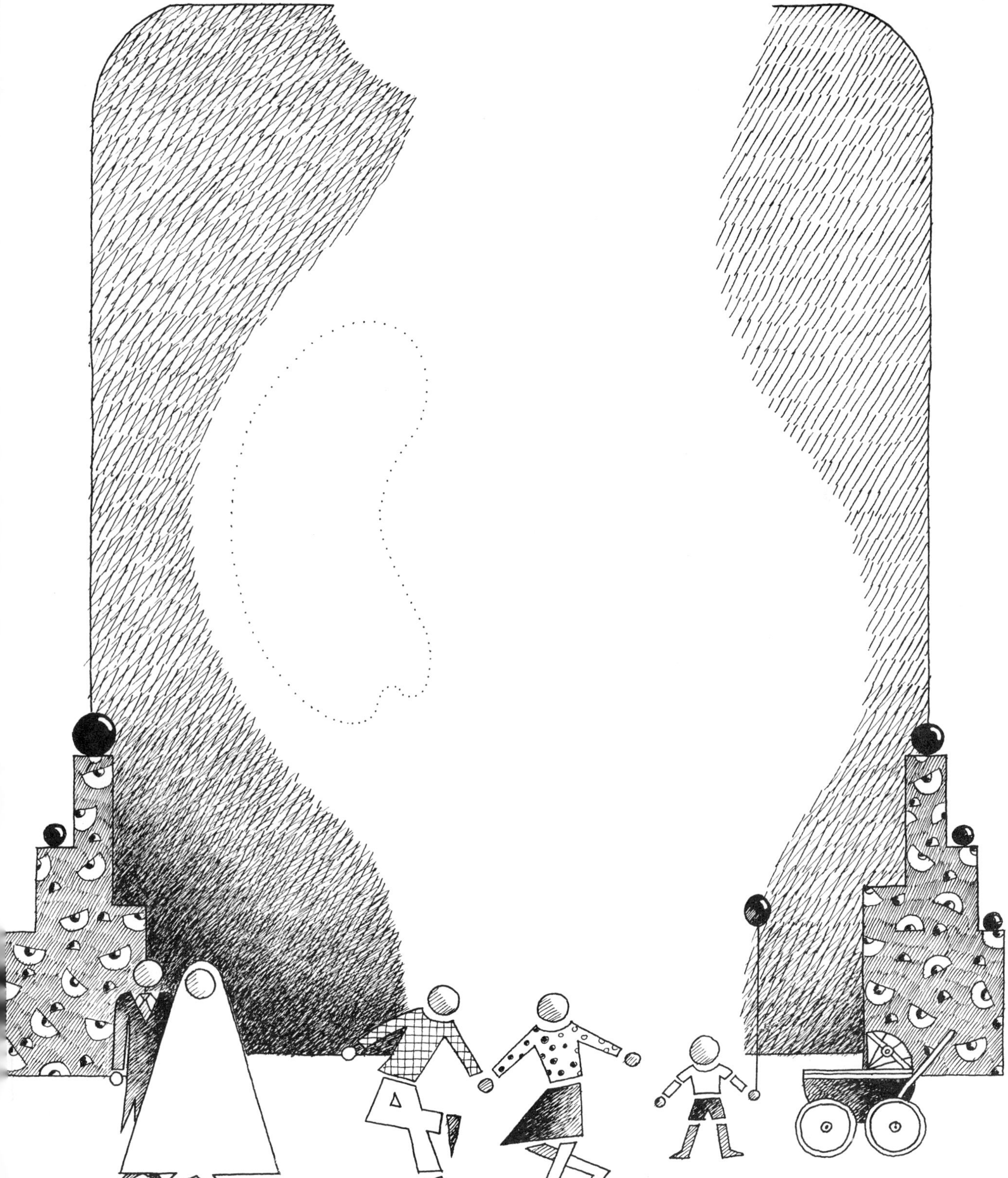

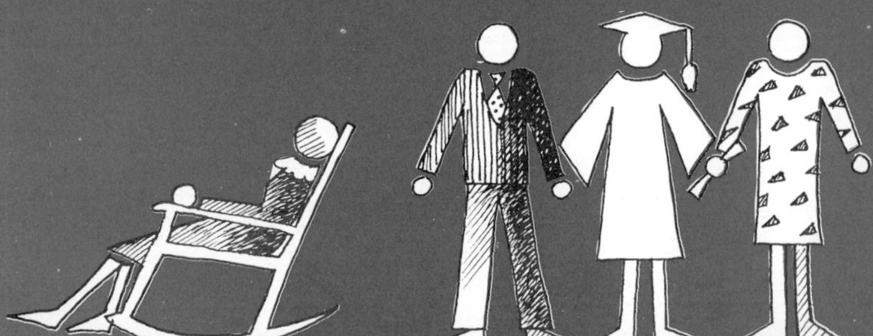

19 MALE AND FEMALE: HUMAN SEXUALITY

WHAT'S AHEAD IN CHAPTER 19 What is sexuality? What factors are believed to influence the differences between the sexes? What are the controlling substances in the reproductive system? What are the myths about menstruation and how do they influence a woman's reaction to her monthly periods? How can discomfort during menstruation be reduced? What are the problems that affect the male/the female reproductive organs? When do they signal the need to see a physician? How is a good sexual relationship built? Is perfecting one's technique all that is necessary? What factors influence sex drive? Is there a "best" level everyone should strive for? What is orgasm? How important is it to the enjoyment of sexual relations? Should intercourse meet a set standard of pleasure for everyone, everytime? What are the causes of inadequate sexual response? How can individuals find help in overcoming such difficulties?

- A toddler snuggles against his mother's comforting bosom after scraping his knee in a fall.
- A white-haired couple fondly clasps hands at their fiftieth wedding anniversary party.
- A couple of 10-year-old boys tease a pair of female classmates.
- Two lovers entwine in a tender embrace after intercourse.
- A teenage girl falls "in love" with her history teacher.
- A father watches with awe and pride as his wife is delivered of their first child.

Sometimes we think of sexuality as relating only to the genital organs and intercourse. But, in fact, it embraces all the subtle and not-so-subtle relationships and differences that exist between male and female as well as some relationships that exist between male and male and female and female.

In an age of liberation movements and battles for equal rights, we often tend to gloss over the differences between males and females, but the differences are very real indeed. However, they in no way indicate the superiority of one or the other sex. For example, there are differences between the "average" male and the "average" female in size, bone structure, muscle development, voice, health, and longevity (women live longer, are generally healthier). The differences are not absolute. There are often wider differences between individuals in each gender than there are between average males and females. The difference between the tallest woman and the shortest is much greater than the difference between the average woman and the average man.

There also appear to be some differences in temperament, personality traits, and intellectual interests. How many of these male-female differences are biologically determined by genetics or hormones and how many are determined by societal conditioning (little girls are "sugar and spice and everything nice," sensitive, and nurturing, while little boys are "snips and snails and puppy dogs' tails," aggressive, and assertive) is a hotly contested issue today.

But there is no debate over the existence, and importance, of the basic biological differences between the sexes. Without them, there would be no future generations to carry on any debates at all.

BIOLOGICAL DIFFERENTIATION

The Reproductive Systems

During the first five weeks following conception, males and females appear to develop identically, though in each embryo there is hereditary material that will dictate whether it will be a boy or a girl. At about the sixth week for males, and as late as the twelfth week for females, the sex glands, or *gonads* (testes and ovaries), begin to develop. During the third fetal month, the testes begin to secret the hormones that program male development of internal and external sex organs and masculinization of the brain. Without reprogramming by male hormones, the fetus will develop as a female, for it appears that all human fetuses are originally programmed that way. Because *re*programming is necessary for the development of the male, more things tend to go wrong in the sexual development of boys than of girls.

Since male and female reproductive systems share a common beginning, it is hardly surprising that the two, though outwardly very different, are similar (see Figure 19.1). Their functions are complementary. The male reproductive system (Figure 19.2) is involved in producing the sperm and propelling it safely to its rendezvous with the ovum or egg in the female's fallopian tubes. The female reproductive system (Figure 19.3) is geared toward producing the ovum, guiding it to its meeting with a sperm, and then nourishing and protecting it as it grows and develops during nine months of pregnancy. Controlling all this activity are the sex hormones.

The Controlling Sex Hormones

Sex hormones, chemical substances produced by the gonads and the pituitary gland, dictate the development of genitalia before birth; of the secondary sexual characteristics at puberty (facial hair in males, breasts in females, pubic and underarm hair, changes in voice and body shape); and of sexual behavior. Each sex has a small amount of the other's hormones, which are probably produced in the adrenals and to some extent in the ovaries and testes. High levels of male hormones (androgens) in a woman can lead to growth of facial hair and other masculine characteristics; high levels of female hormones (estrogen) in a man can lead to development of breast tissue and feminine traits.

Hormones also control the reproductive

Erika Stone/Peter Arnold

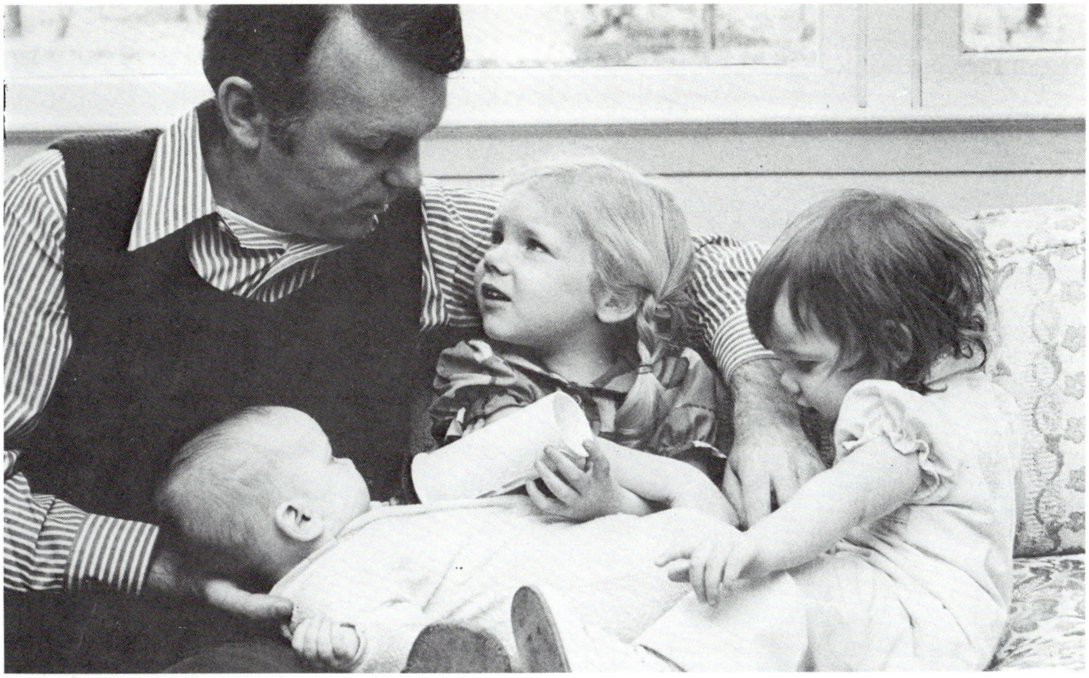

In the past decade, differences between male and female roles in United States society have narrowed.

Freda Leinwand/Monkmeyer

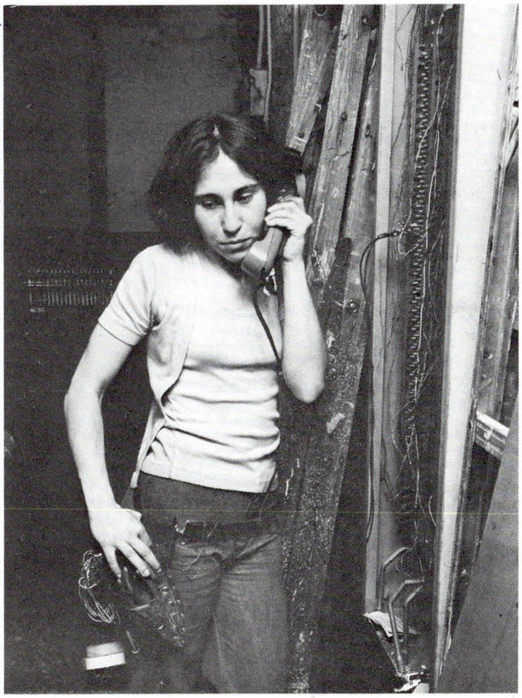

functions that begin at puberty: *spermatogenesis* in males, the production of millions of sperm that may be ejaculated in *nocturnal emissions* (erotic dreams ending in orgasm), or as the climax of masturbation, or intercourse; and the *menstrual cycle* in females, the ongoing cycle of production each month of an egg (ovulation), preparation for its fertilization and implantation in the uterus, and then, if fertilization does not take place, a sloughing off of the unutilized materials in the uterine wall (menstruation; see Figure 19.5).

Like other hormones (see Chapter 9), the sex hormones operate on a complex feedback system, with the hypothalamus and the pituitary gland playing master roles. The pituitary, stimulated by LH- and FSH-releasing factors from the hypothalamus, produces LH

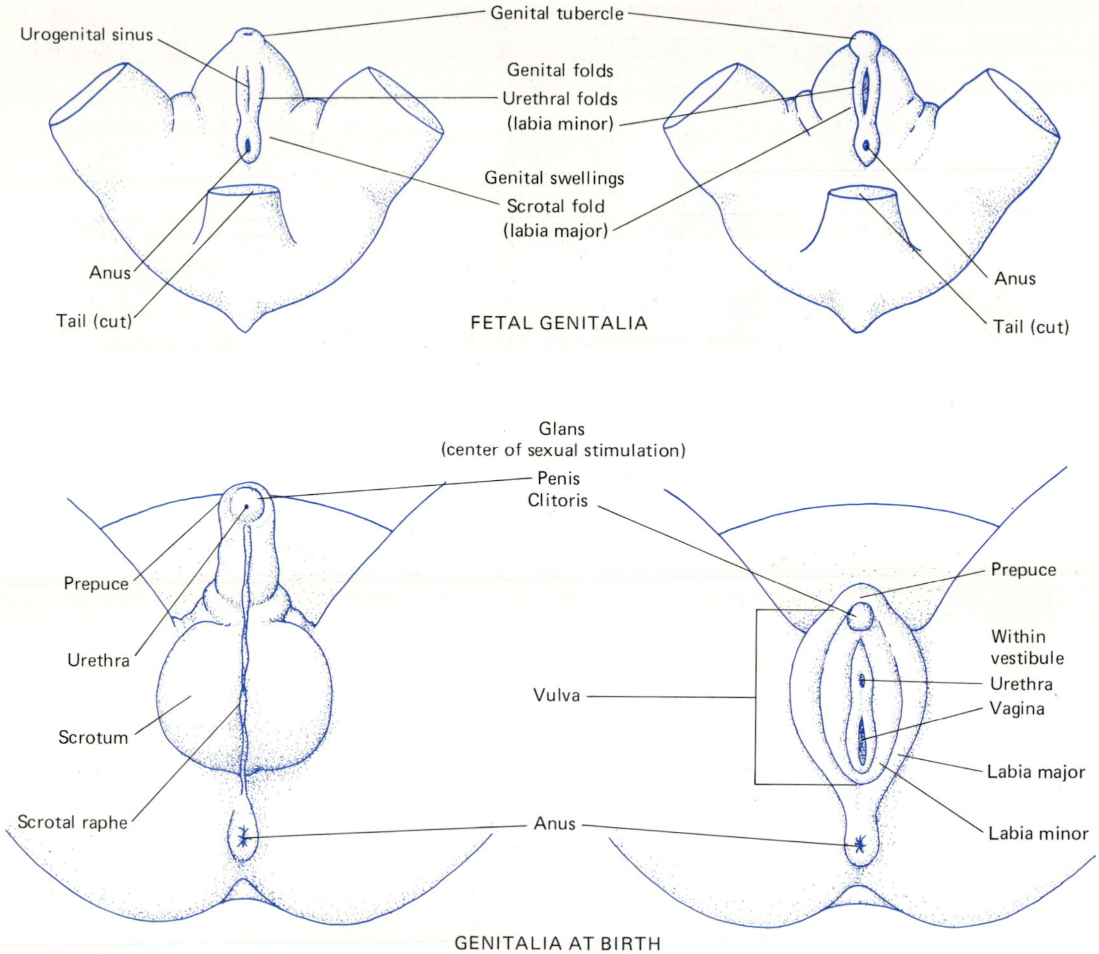

FIGURE 19.1 A comparison of male and female genitalia. Male and female genitalia start out identically in the fetus. Even at birth, and into maturity, there are many similarities. [*Adapted from Tobin and Ng.*]

(luteinizing hormone) and FSH (follicle-stimulating hormone). These in turn stimulate the gonads to produce their hormones (androgens, including testosterone in the male, and estrogens and progesterone in the female) and the gametes (sperm and ova).

Although sperm production continues uninterrupted from puberty to old age, ovulation rarely begins when menstruation does and is often irregular at first. Early periods, too, may be erratic. Once ovulation becomes regular, the ovaries continue to produce an egg a

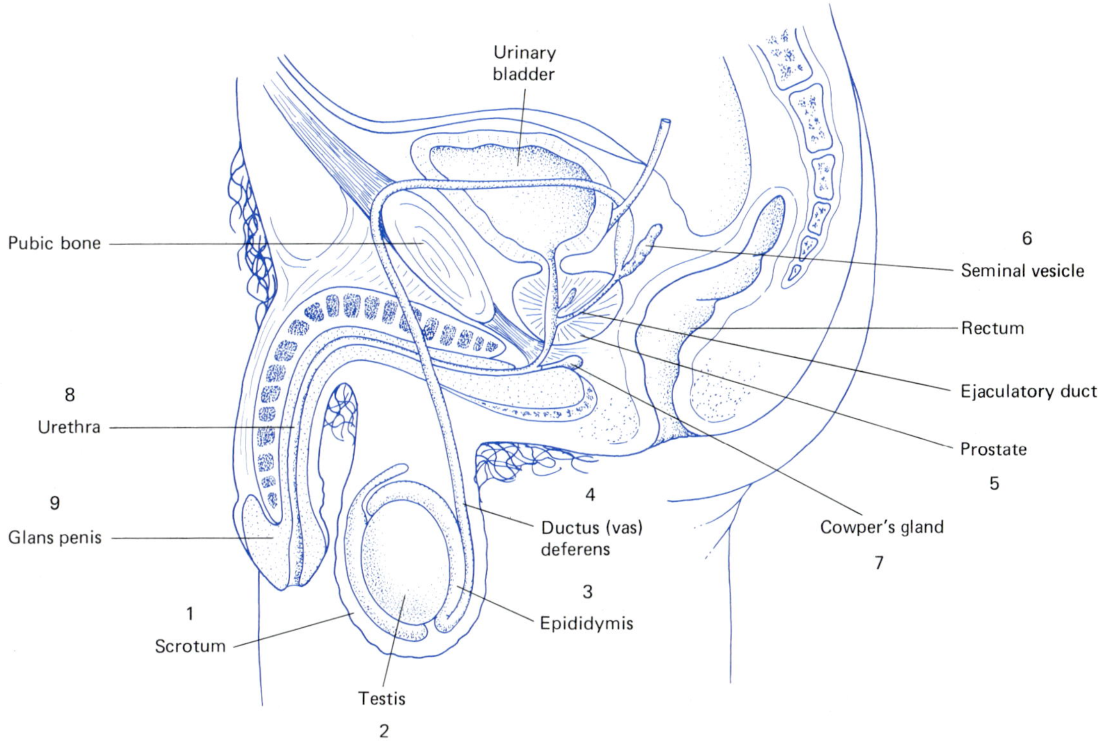

FIGURE 19.2 Male reproductive system.

1 *Scrotum* Pouch that stores and protects testes, keeping them at 2 or 3°F below body temperature (needed for sperm production) by drawing close to the body in cold weather, lowering in hot weather.

2 *Testes (testicles)* The male gonads, which produce sperm and male hormones in 800 narrow tubules, from puberty to old age.

3 *Epididymis* Tightly coiled 18- to 20-foot tube attached to each testis; stores mature sperm for 30 to 60 days.

4 *Ductus (vas) deferens* Tubes that carry mature sperm to the ejaculatory ducts, and also store sperm between ejaculations. Cutting or tying causes sterility.

5 *Prostate* Produces some of the semen that carries sperm; prostate muscles help eject semen.

6 *Seminal vesicle* Produces some of the semen that carries sperm.

7 *Cowper's gland* Secretes a lubricating liquid to prepare urethra for semen, lubricate tip of penis prior to coitus. Secretion contains some sperm.

8 *Urethra* Thin tube running through penis that carries both sperm and urine (from bladder), but not at the same time.

9 *Penis* External male sex organ that deposits semen in vagina during intercourse. [*Adapted from McCary, p. 62.*]

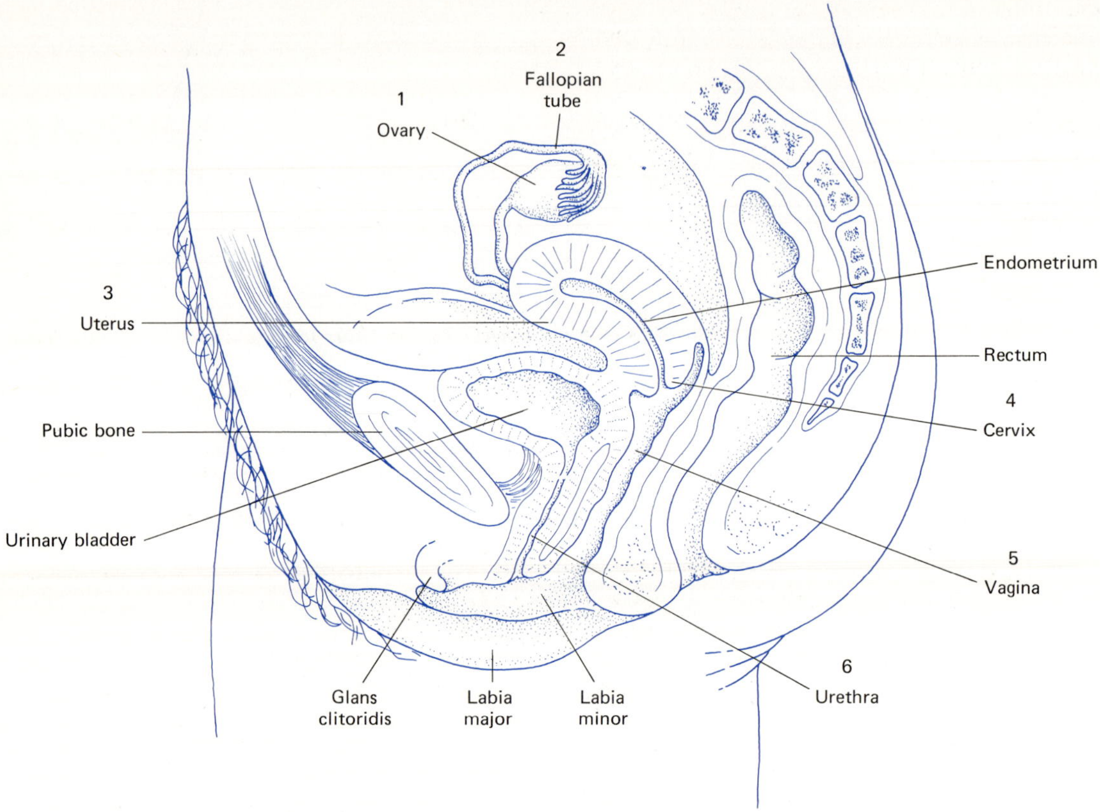

FIGURE 19.3 Female reproductive system.

1 *Ovaries* The female gonads, $^4/_5$ to 1 inch long. Produce ova in unripe follicles nestling in their fibrous framework; secrete hormones that regulate menstruation. Removal of both ovaries terminates possibility of childbearing and produces "surgical" menopause.

2 *Fallopian tubes* Narrow tubes between ovaries and uterus. Waving of tiny fringes (fimbria) at ovary ends creates a current that encourages the newly expelled ovum into tube, where it is moved along by hairlike cilia. If sperm penetrates ovum in tube, conception takes place. If both tubes are blocked or damaged, cut or tied, or scarred by VD, normal pregnancy cannot take place.

3 *Uterus or womb* A fertilized ovum implants in the lining (endometrium) of this muscular organ and grows into a fetus. Remarkable elastic quality allows uterus to stretch to hold full-term baby; muscular contractions expel infant at birth. Removal of uterus ends childbearing but not sexuality.

4 *Cervix* Narrow neck or opening of uterus. Expands considerably during childbirth; has no nerve endings, and so no pain is felt during stretching or treatment.

5 *Vagina* Four-inch canal from vulvar opening to cervix, ordinarily collapsed but can expand to allow for birth of child or to accept penis during month (in rare cases, there may be two eggs released together, which can, if fertilized, result in nonidentical twins) until menopause, usually between 45 and 55. At this time, production of the hormone estrogen drops, and menstrual flow diminishes and finally stops entirely. (Menopause is further discussed in Chapter 24.)

HEALTH PROBLEMS OF THE REPRODUCTIVE SYSTEMS

The Male

There are no specialists to deal with health problems that are specific to males, though urologists (urinary system specialists) do handle some of them. It has been suggested that a new medical specialty, possibly called andrology (*andro* = male), is needed. Meanwhile, the male with questions about his reproductive organs must turn to a family physician, internist, or urologist, who may or may not be well trained to handle them. Most common concerns include:

Penis size Normal penises vary considerably in size, from about 2 to 10 inches in the relaxed state. During erection, however, the smaller penis enlarges more than the longer one, so that most are very similar in size when erect. Penis size has little or nothing to do with the pleasure of either the male or his partner during intercourse, because the flexible vagina adjusts to virtually any size. If the penis fails to develop at puberty (a condition called *microphallus*), however, hormone therapy may be necessary.

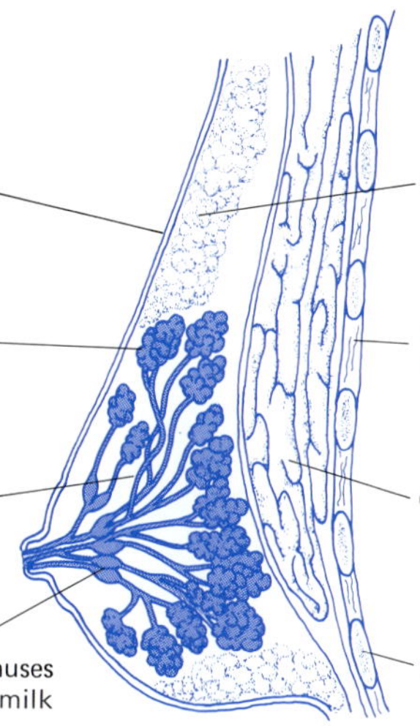

FIGURE 19.4 Mammary gland (breast). Breasts are formed prenatally in both males and females. At puberty, female hormones stimulate further growth of breasts.

Breasts serve both erotic and nurturing functions. Normal breasts vary greatly in size and shape; size is dependent upon amount of fat and connective tissue, and upon heredity. Breast size, shape, and color may change during sexual excitement and menstrual cycle, and even more during pregnancy and nursing. One breast, usually the left, may be larger. Exercise *cannot* change breast size, but can develop muscles under the breast, giving the appearance of firmness and larger size. Going braless can cause ligaments to break down and breasts to sag if they are average or large; weight loss can also result in sagging. Little bumps and dark spots on the nipple are normal. Hairs can be removed safely with tweezers, ingrown hairs with hot soaks.

intercourse. Moist mucous membrane lining is sensitive; glands secrete lubricating fluids on sexual stimulation.

6 *Urethra* Tube for emptying urine.

7 *Hymen* Ring of tissue (not shown in drawing) that may narrow entrance to vagina, rarely completely blocking it. May stretch or tear during strenuous exercise, masturbation, medical examination, tampon use, or first intercourse. A tough, thick hymen may hinder intercourse and should be removed by doctor. [*Adapted from McCary, p. 79.*]

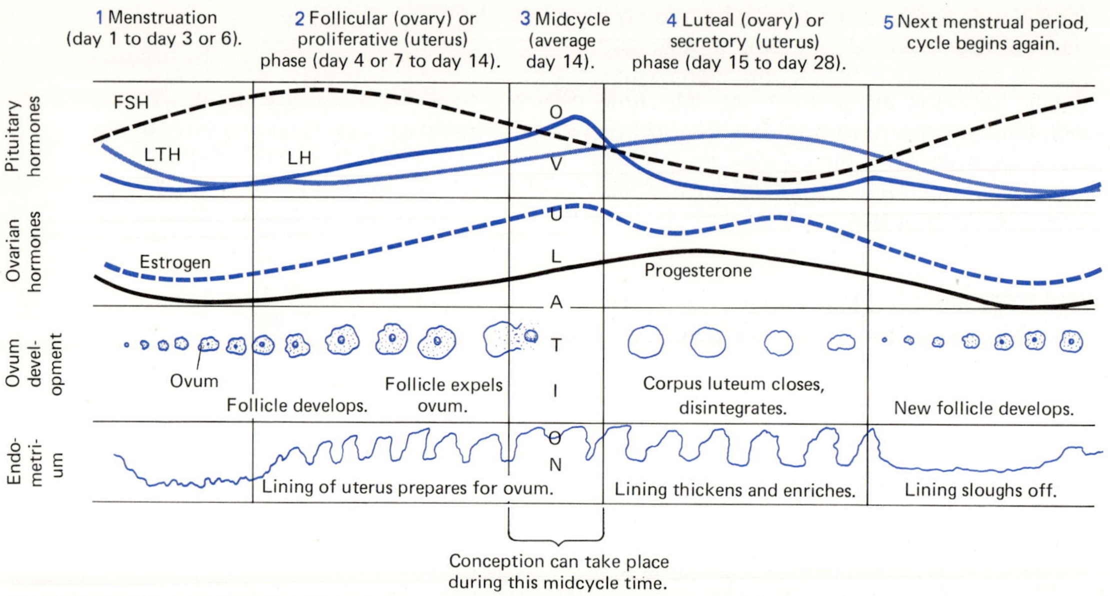

FIGURE 19.5 The menstrual cycle.
1 During and following menstruation, FSH levels rise, prompting an immature egg follicle in one ovary to grow and begin to mature.
2 As the follicle matures, it secretes large amounts of estrogen, which causes the endometrium to thicken in preparation for the fertilized egg and signals the pituitary to stop production of FSH and increase LH. When LH and estrogen levels peak, the mature follicle bursts and propels the ovum toward the fallopian tube, the process of ovulation.
3 On the average, ovulation occurs on day 14 of the menstrual cycle, but it can vary from day 9 to day 18 and even beyond in rare cases.
4 The empty follicle, prompted by LH, closes and becomes a corpus luteum. LH and LTH stimulate the corpus luteum to produce progesterone and estrogen, which encourage buildup of the endometrium. If conception does not occur, high progesterone levels suppress LH and LTH, causing the corpus luteum to degenerate and ending progesterone production. This, in turn, leads to the next stage.
5 There is a new sloughing off of the endometrium, resulting in a new menstrual period and the beginning of a new cycle.

With few exceptions, this 300-year-old statement still stands:

> The Vagina is made . . . that it can accomodate itself to any penis, so that it will give way to a long one, meet a short one, widen to a thick one, constringe to a small: so that every man mite well enough lie with any Woman, and every Woman with every Man. . . .
>
> *The Anatomy of Human Bodies Epitomised*, 1682

Menstruation: Facts, Not Fallacies

The first menstrual period, the *menarche*, usually occurs in the United States between ages 10 and $16^1/_2$, with the average just over 12 years. A century ago, it was about 16. The reasons for earlier maturation are uncertain, but both improved diet and social conditions have been suggested. Young girls may await the event with dread or with happy anticipation, depending upon how they have been prepared. Knowing the facts of menstruation can remove the mystery and fear:

- Cycle lengths vary; 28 days is typical, but cycles can be longer or shorter by several days.
- Duration of flow varies; a 3- to 6-day period is typical, but longer or shorter duration can be normal.
- Exercise is not only permissible during menstruation, but often helpful in decreasing discomfort.
- Sexual relations, though taboo in some cultures, are not harmful during the period.
- Bloating caused by water retention is common, and cutting down on salt just prior to the period can minimize that difficulty.
- Virgins *can* use tampons, an internal form of protection, if the hymen is sufficiently open or elastic.
- About half of all women suffer some premenstrual discomfort, pain, depression.
- Bleeding between periods is not normal (though some women experience slight staining during ovulation about halfway between periods) and should be investigated by a physician.
- Some menstruating or premenstrual women experience increased levels of anxiety or tension; women commit more crimes, have more automobile accidents, do worse on exams during the menstrual period (Dalton; Neu and Dimassio; Tiger). However, many female athletes have won events during their periods. Some menstrual and premenstrual tension may be "learned."

Undescended testicles In the fetus, the testes develop in the abdominal cavity, dropping into the scrotum just before birth. In about 1 to 7 percent of males, one or both testes fail to drop. Most will descend by the end of the first year. For those that do not, surgery or hormonal treatment may be necessary to prevent sterility and the higher rates of cancer of the penis that occur in men with undescended testicles.

Gynecomastia Enlargement of the breasts can occur in males. Most frequently, it is simply a tender nubbin of tissue under the nipple, but in the obese it can be quite disfiguring. The condition usually disappears without treatment within 6 to 36 months. It may be associated with estrogen treatment or possibly with heavy use of marijuana, or it may be of unknown origin. Rarely, swelling is great enough to cause extreme embarrassment and distress. In such cases, plastic surgery readily remedies the condition.

The Female

Women who have health problems related to their reproductive systems can turn for help to a family physician, an internist, or a specialist in women's problems, the obstetrician-gynecologist. Though some women have promoted the concept of women's self-care because of dissatisfaction with care provided by male physicians, most have rejected the

WHEN TO SEEK HELP
For "Male" Problems

- Premarital or birth control counseling
- Discharge or bleeding from the penis
- Sores, blisters, pain in genital area
- Itching in genital area (jock itch)
- Painful intercourse or impotence
- Lump or irregularity in penis or scrotum
- Burning on urination; difficult urination
- Undescended testicles or testicle

idea of taking care out of professional hands. They have, instead, often opted to discuss the sometimes demeaning attitudes of physicians with them, hoping to effect a change. The most common "female" problems are:

Vaginitis This inflammation of the vagina is usually signaled by vaginal soreness, itching, burning, and/or discharge. It can be caused by an infectious organism, by strong chemicals (such as those in a douche), by an irritating foreign object, or by an antibiotic or other drug that upsets the chemical balance of the vaginal canal. The condition is so common that nearly every woman experiences it at least once in a lifetime. The most common causes of infection are *Trichomonas vaginalis* (a parasite) and *Monilia* or *Candida* (yeasty fungi). Though symptoms are less noticeable in the male, men can both "catch" and transmit these infections via sexual contact. This has led some observers to label them "ping-pong" infections (see STDs, Chapter 8).

WHEN TO SEEK HELP
For "Female" Problems

- Premarital and birth control counseling
- Prepregnancy examination
- Amenorrhea (absence of menstruation)
- Any staining or bleeding between periods
- Heavy yellowish or smelly vaginal discharge
- Painful menstruation or painful intercourse
- Lump or other irregularity in a breast
- Sores, itching, pain in genital area
- Burning or difficult urination

Dysmenorrhea Painful menstruation or menstrual cramps, called dysmenorrhea (*dys* = painful + *men* = month + *rrhea* = flow), can be caused by a physical abnormality of the reproductive organs. But psychological causes (tense feelings about feminity, sexuality, and menstruation itself) are more common, especially in young women.

Amenorrhea An absence of menstruation, called *amenorrhea* (*a* = without), can result simply from fatigue, climate change, tension, or excessive weight gain or loss, or it could signal pregnancy or serious illness. It is frequently related to heavy physical training, as in sports or dance.

Cystitis Symptoms of bladder infection, very common in women, include a burning sensation on urination, frequent urination, and sharp pain in the lower abdomen that may be severe during intercourse. Causes include infection, especially in women who have lowered body resistance, psychological stress and fatigue, and pressure on the bladder from frequent intercourse. Treatment consists of increased fluids (not coffee, tea, or alcohol), careful personal hygiene, warm baths or heating pad, medication if needed, and in some cases, psychotherapy. If intercourse is the cause, emptying the bladder before and after, and using lubricating jelly if needed, may be helpful.

BUILDING A GOOD SEXUAL RELATIONSHIP

The sexual relationship means different things to different people. For some, it is strictly for procreation; for others, it is recrea-

SELF-CARE

Avoiding Genital Area Infection and Irritation

- Wear cotton underwear, and change it daily; avoid wearing tight under or outer pants; don't wear panty hose under slacks; skip panties or pajama bottoms at night.
- Wash or bathe daily; avoid perfumed soaps, sprays, and powders; don't use other people's washcloths, towels, or underwear.
- Wash genital area before and after intercourse, and make sure your partner does the same.
- Women, wipe anus from front to back.
- Eat yogurt when taking antibiotics to help restore bacterial balance.
- Don't sit around in a wet swim suit.
- Use a lubricating gel (not Vaseline) if needed during intercourse.
- Women, douche only on medical advice; keep the equipment clean.
- Men, clean under the foreskin if you are uncircumcised.

tion. For still others, it is the consummation of a deeply felt love. It is as old as humankind, and for a loving couple, it is ever new.

The development of a good sexual relationship does not begin under the sheets with foreplay. It is built day in and day out by the courtesy, understanding, trust, patience, and good humor that go into a loving union, and by touching, kissing, and caressing at times when intercourse is not the object.

Factors that Affect Sexual Motivation

- *Genotype* A tendency toward high, low, or medium arousability may be inherited.
- *Hormone levels* Low levels of male hormones appear to reduce arousal in both men and women.
- *Stimulation of the nervous system* Stimulation through the five senses (sight, hearing, touch, smell, and occasionally, taste) causes arousal.
- *Prior sexual and social experience* Pleasurable prior experiences make for easier arousal; unpleasant experiences make arousal more difficult in the future.
- *Time since last orgasm* Recovery time varies from individual to individual and influences arousability.
- *Environment* Food and drink (too much or too little), drugs, disease, time of year or month, temperature, social conditions, atmosphere, and so on can all influence desire.
- *Cultural influences* Religious laws, for example, can be restraining; pornographic films can be encouraging, though restrictive laws stimulate some people.
- *Stress* Worry, fear, anger, frustration, pain, discomfort, and distraction can all affect sexual drive.
- *Age* Sex drive is reported highest in males between 18–20, in females around 40; it often declines with age because of illness, lowered hormone levels, reduction in sensory response of the skin, poorer circulation to genital areas, infrequent opportunity, societal pressures, and expectation.

Source: Adapted from Goldstein, p. 97.

Charles Gatewood

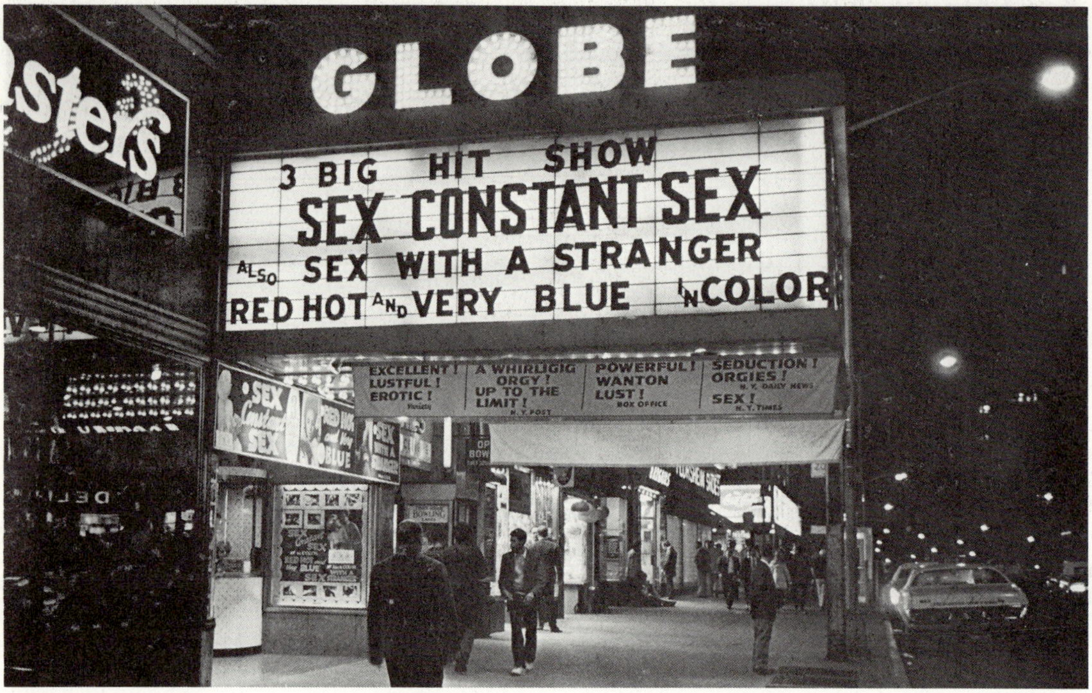

Differences between males and females in the degree of sexual arousal on visual stimulation have been attributed by some to learning, by others to inherent drives.

Sexual Motivation

What is considered "normal" sexual motivation or sex drive varies from person to person, from time to time. The sex drive differs from other human drives in that we can survive indefinitely without its being fulfilled. It is unlike the reaction to hunger or thirst in that the body's tissues do not become starved by abstinence (Beach and Jordan). Celibacy sometimes hurts, but no one ever died from it.

Many things influence the ability to be sexually aroused. Psychological readiness is particularly vital. Without it, the male cannot have an erection and take part in intercourse; the female may passively submit, but does not truly participate and cannot reach orgasm. Worry about making his partner pregnant may make a man suddenly impotent. Fear that "the children will hear us" may prevent a woman from achieving orgasm. A couple who ordinarily have a robust sex life may have absolutely no interest in sex during exam-time stress.

Sexual motivation and what stimulates it differs in men and women, but it is uncertain how much of that difference is attributable to nature and how much to nurture. Some authorities believe that sex motivation is a learned appetite, while others contend that basic drives are inherent and only the trend they take is learned.

Precoital Stimulation

A variety of early experiences condition the individual to view certain stimuli as sexually arousing. A particular song or words of endearment, an erotic picture, an enticing scent or style of dress, can all contribute to readi-

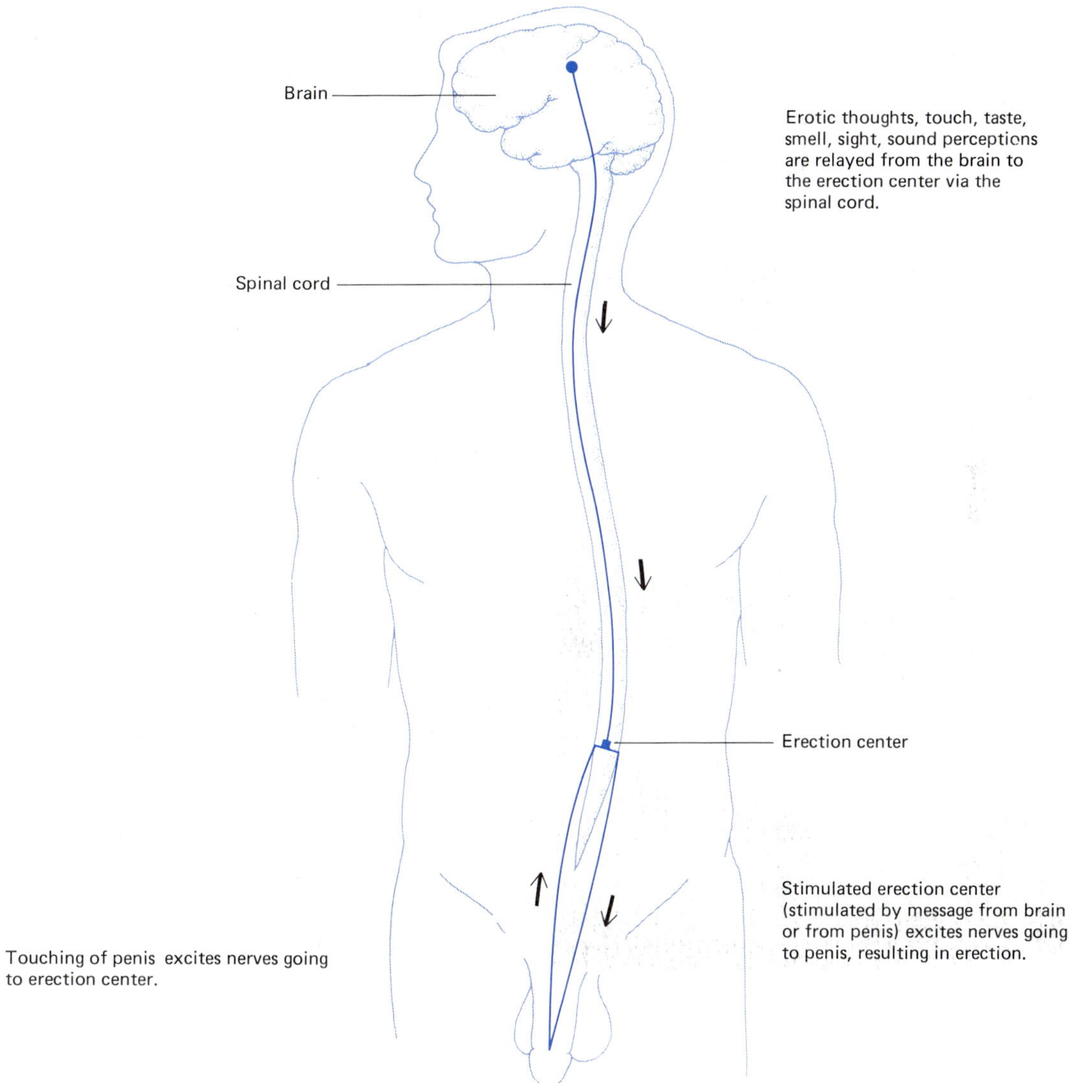

FIGURE 19.6 How erection may be stimulated either by a message from the brain or by direct stimulation of the penis. The penis can be stimulated to erection by visual, psychological, or physical stimulation and is under control of the higher brain centers. Erection is an involuntary reflex and cannot be willed; trying too hard can sometimes make erection impossible. Erection occurs when the three cylindrical sections of erectile tissue in the penis become engorged with blood and fill out the loose skin of the organ. Ejaculation begins with many contractions all along the route from the epididymis through the vasa deferentia. The seminal vesicles and the prostate also contract, ejecting semen into the urethra to combine with sperm. Sphincter muscles surrounding the opening of the bladder close tightly to prevent urine and semen from mixing. After ejaculation (orgasm), the excess blood drains out of the penis back into the circulatory system, and the penis becomes limp. [*Adapted from Goldstein, p. 25.*]

ness for the actual sex act—coitus or intercourse.

The use of the senses, especially touch, for sexual arousal is known as petting or, if it leads to coitus, as foreplay. Stroking of the body's *erogenous* zones, areas of the skin with many sense receptors, is a major way of causing sexual arousal. Other than the genitals, the areas reported most often to be erotic are the breasts in women, the thighs in men. Individuals can learn through trial and error just which areas are most sensitive for them.

The most common approaches to foreplay include general hugging and caressing, ordinary kissing, tongue kissing, manual and/or oral stimulation of the female breasts and genitalia, manual stimulation of the male genitalia, oral stimulation of the male genitalia (*fellatio*), the female genitalia (*cunnilingus*), or the anal area (*anilingus*). Also important to sexual arousal are a relaxed and receptive mood; verbal endearments; variety in setting, techniques, and position; lack of distractions; good communication; mutual trust, patience, and absence of exploitation; and the desire of each partner to give as well as receive pleasure.

Petting not leading to intercourse is often engaged in during the dating and courtship periods. Many authorities believe such sexual experimentation is a crucial prelude to satisfying sexual intercourse later. Some persons move on to coitus with a loved partner before marriage; others continue to use petting, often to orgasm, until marriage.

Coitus

The culmination of the sexual act—*coitus* from the Latin "a coming together," *intercourse* from the Latin for the act of "running between," or *copulation* from the Latin "coupling or joining"—is the insertion of the penis into the vagina. In humans, it is an act that, contrary to popular belief, does not "come naturally." The facts of life are passed on from one generation to the next in ways that vary from society to society. Many persons find they continue to learn about sex and to improve their lovemaking techniques as long as they are sexually active. Others settle into a pattern of sexual activity early and stick with it from then on.

The positions in intercourse are almost infinite. The most common throughout the world appear to be those in which male and female are face to face (Ford and Beach), probably because stimulation of the mons veneris and the clitoris are most pronounced this way. Kissing, fondling, whispered endearments, and ecstatic sighs continued during coitus increase stimulation. Experimenting with different positions, locales, and times can add variety and renewed stimulation to a relationship that is becoming routine. Some couples utilize "play acting" for the same purpose.

The First Sexual Experience

Mark Twain once said that Niagara Falls was the second biggest disappointment to honeymooners. One reason the first sexual experience, whether before or after marriage, is so often a fiasco is lack of experience. Making love, like any other skill, takes practice. Another reason is social conditioning: the combination of repressive ideas about sex (many children are still raised with them) and the Hollywood image in which men are always virile and experienced and women cuddly, willing, and able often imposes a great burden, particularly on men.

Developing skill in lovemaking requires mutual respect, patience, kindness. Each partner must communicate to the other what feels good, much as we do when someone scratches our back: "A little to the right, a little higher; ummm, that feels wonderful!" We get out of lovemaking what we put into it.

Good preparation can help make the first experience more successful. That includes a

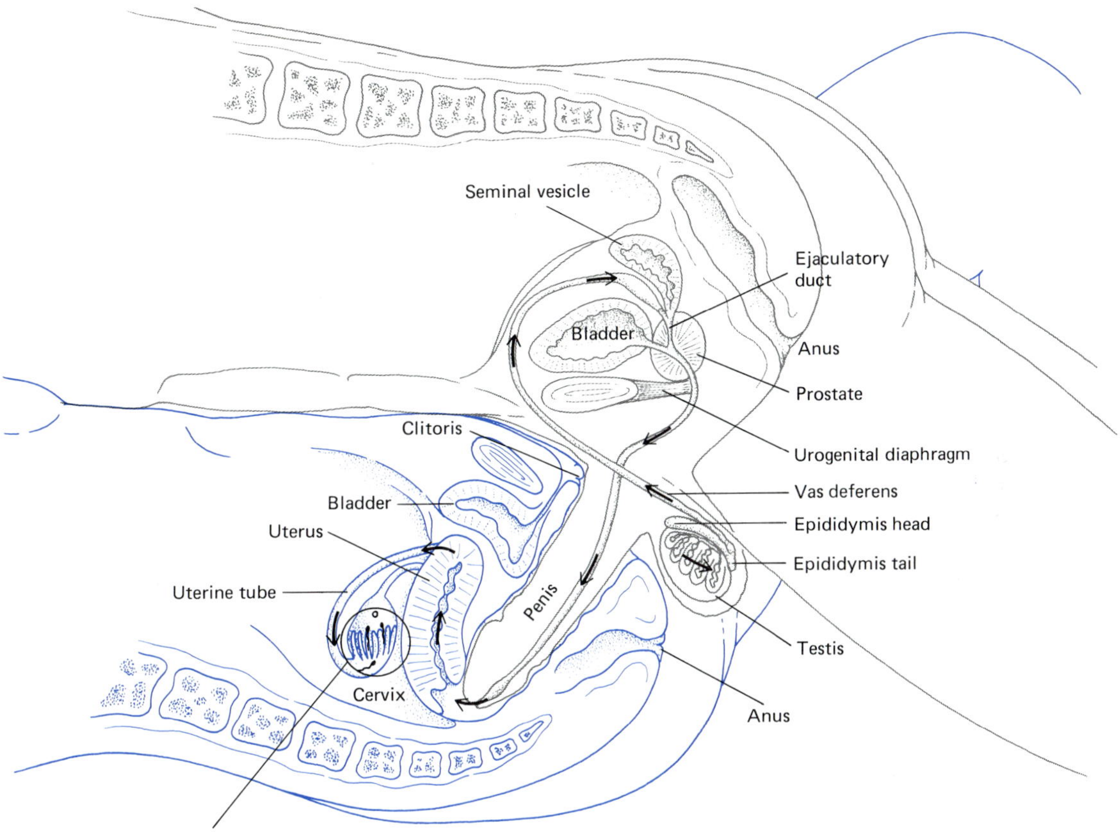

FIGURE 19.7 The human couple in coitus (woman's right thigh omitted to reveal inner structures). Path of sperm from testis to site of fertilization can be seen. [*Adapted from Elson, p. 604.*]

thorough medical examination for both partners so that any condition (such as a tough hymen in the female) that could interfere with intercourse can be taken care of in advance. The physician can also test for venereal disease and can advise the couple on appropriate birth control measures. Some scientific readings on sexuality and sex techniques may be helpful, too. For persons who have serious concerns about their sexuality or are fearful of engaging in coitus, counseling is advisable.

Understanding Orgasm

If arousal reaches a climax, there is orgasm: the pleasurable, relief-giving, seizurelike moment of supreme physical and emotional gratification. William Masters and Virginia Johnson, who have carried out extensive laboratory studies on hundreds of men and women engaged in sexual activities, describe orgasm as being very similar for both males and females, except that in the male there is almost always ejaculation. Orgasm affects the

Vaginal stimulation is like a warm bath of pleasure; my whole body responds to it. In clitoral stimulation my whole body is rigid with the expectation of continuing pleasure. Vaginal is like a hum, but clitoral is a high pitched note. From clitoral, my body demands to be satisfied; from vaginal my body is content if it's not. (Quoted in Fischer, p. 219)

entire body: Breathing quickens, pulse and heart rate increase, muscles tense, genital organs become engorged with blood. In 3 to 10 seconds, it is all over, and the body quickly returns to its prearousal state, though breathing, heart rate, and blood pressure may race for several minutes.

Though 95 percent of women are capable of attaining orgasm at some time in their lives, only 70 percent in the Kinsey study were able to attain it during their first year of marriage (*b*), in part due to good-girls-don't-enjoy-sex conditioning. Of course, most eventually discover that good girls do. The kind of orgasm women experience has been a subject of considerable contention. Freud believed women could experience two types of orgasm, vaginal and clitoral, but deemed vaginal to be the more mature response. He labeled women who could not achieve vaginal orgasm as "vaginally frigid." Masters and Johnson, however, concluded that there is only clitoral orgasm, that during intercourse it is the stimulation of the clitoris, not the vagina, that triggers orgasm.

Other studies, including one by Dr. Seymour Fischer, have tended to dispute their findings and support Freud's theory of two types of orgasm, though not the superiority of vaginal experience. Most of the 300 women Fischer interviewed reported that clitoral orgasm produced a higher charge, though vaginal orgasm could be more emotionally satisfying. Two-thirds declared that if they had to choose between the two, their choice would be clitoral.

There has been much debate about whether or not women can have multiple orgasms. Some authorities believe that there may be several clitoral peaks reached before orgasm, which are mistaken for orgasm itself—and thus the impression of multiple orgasm (Vincent). Masters and Johnson claim not only that serial orgasms are genuine, but that most women can experience them. Such debate has not always led to more satisfying sexual relations. Instead, for many couples, it has led to concern about the adequacy of sexual response. Many women do not experience multiple orgasms, and some experience none at all. Is this a serious problem?

Not according to Dr. Philip Sarrel and Lorna Sarrel, spouses and co-therapists in sex counseling at Yale University, who comment:

> Our preoccupation with female orgasm amounts to a mass hang-up . . . there is no reason why a woman must experience orgasm. It is not necessary for health (although some few women can develop a chronic aching in the pelvic area from continuous sexual excitation without orgasmic release), nor is it necessary for conception. The only reason for having an orgasm is that it feels wonderful, but so does kissing and having your breasts kissed, and touching his penis and seeing his pleasure in you. A woman must let her body respond; it can't be forced or willed to respond. In fact, the more conscious she is of a goal, the more focus she puts on performance, mechanics, the more anxious wondering she does, the least [sic] likely she is to have an orgasm. . . . (*a*, p. 181)

Dr. Fischer's study seems to substantiate the belief that the absence of orgasm has no negative effects except in people who worry about missing it. Low orgasmic women in his study were no more irritable, tense, or anxious than high orgasmic women.

Simultaneous orgasm, in which both partners reach climax at the same time, is often touted in sex books. But physiologically, simultaneous orgasm is difficult to achieve because the rhythm of the male and female orgasm generally differ. Most couples find separate orgasms very satisfying, as each enjoys the climax of the other.

INADEQUATE SEXUAL RESPONSE

The Female

Frigidity, characterized by a lack of sexual desire and an inability to respond adequately to the sexual experience, may be psychological or physical. Psychological problems may stem from repressive attitudes learned in childhood, from an upsetting or unsatisfactory earlier experience, from an upbringing that valued careful control of emotions, or from the inability to communicate with or fully trust one's partner. Satisfying sexual intercourse requires the ability to abandon controls and give oneself fully. Physical problems, not common in young women, include: *dyspareunia* (painful intercourse), caused by vaginitis, by inadequate lubrication (lubricating gel will help), or (after menopause) by thinning vaginal membranes; *vaginismus*, an involuntary tightening of the vaginal outlet so that the penis cannot penetrate (psychological counseling may help).

The Male

Impotence Masters and Johnson describe two types of impotence in males: *primary*, in which the man has never had an erection or never been able to maintain an erection long enough to have intercourse; and *secondary*, in which he has had erection, either through masturbation or intercourse, but has since lost the ability to maintain it. Again, causes may be psychological or physical. Deep-seated primary impotence may originate in early childhood when the boy was taught that sex was dirty or that his penis was an evil object, or as the result of an upsetting sexual observation of or encounter with his mother. Secondary impotence can occur following a very unpleasant sexual experience—especially a first one—or can result from general depression or other emotional problems. More recently it has been reported in young men who feel pressured to "perform" by their female partners.

Opinions on Sexual Experimentation

Yesterday's perversion is today's deviation and tomorrow's variation. (Lief, psychiatrist, director, Center for the Study of Sex Education in Medicine, University of Pennsylvania, p. 3)

The problem of the deviate is that he doesn't know how to love on a mature plane. He knows only the masturbatory pleasure of his own physical sensations. Since this is unrequiting, he finds it necessary to embroider the act, searching vainly for the satisfaction that is always just beyond reach. . . . Only when one is mature enough to enjoy empathic love—to share his partner's pleasure and to value it as being equally or more important than his own—does he know true intercourse. . . . People who know the real thing don't need these peculiar substitutes. (Bates, *a*, Michigan internist, p. 152)

So long as [people] are not exploiting or violating the rights of others . . . any way is the "right way" sexually. (Harper and Stokes, p. 78)

Any kind of sex, from the kinkiest to the straightest, can be an extension of a disordered personality or a way of relieving tension or perfectly normal. (Alex Comfort, author of *Joy of Sex, b*)

Bob Levin/Black Star

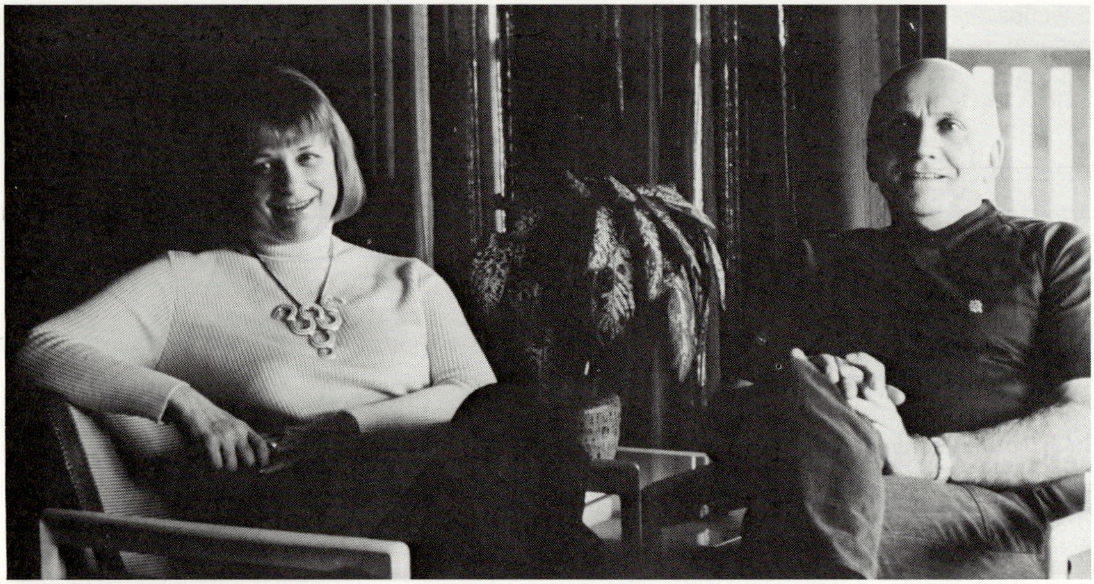

The research of Virginia Masters and William Johnson into human sexuality has led to the development of sex therapy techniques for treatment of inadequate sexual response that have been of help to thousands.

Physical causes of impotence include acute illness, chronic diseases such as diabetes or hypothyroidism, and use of alcohol or other drugs. Masturbation cannot cause impotence, but worrying about it might. An occasional episode of impotence is normal, and is experienced by almost every man at one time or another. If neither partner becomes anxious about the incident, it will probably not recur, but if it is treated as a matter of great moment, it could grow into a chronic problem. Before this happens, the couple should see a physician.

Premature ejaculation An occasional expulsion of semen before coitus actually begins, or immediately upon insertion into the vagina, is normal, particularly if there has been a long break between sexual experiences or if the period of foreplay was overextended. Handling the penis of an inexperienced male may also cause ejaculation, but this can usually be prevented by avoiding direct stimulation and donning a condom immediately upon erection. Consistent failure to withhold ejaculation until intercourse, however, is a serious problem and, like impotence, can compound itself. Failure leads to failure. However, this is one of the easiest of male dysfunctions to cure. Help is also available for the male who cannot ejaculate in the vagina, a condition called *ejaculatory incompetence*.

Other male concerns *Dyspareunia* (painful intercourse) can also be a male problem. It may be caused by an inflammation or infection of the penis (sometimes due to poor hygiene or contact with an infected partner) or by scars in the urethra from an old gonorrheal infection. *Phimosis*, an uncomfortable condition caused by a tight, restrictive foreskin, can be corrected by circumcision.

You have one principal sex organ; it's between your ears.

When Help Is Needed

A physician who feels competent to discuss or counsel on sexual matters may be helpful. One who does not feel able to deal with the problem may refer patients to sex or marriage counselors, to psychologists or psychiatrists, or to a physician with training in sexual counseling. If at all possible, both partners should seek counseling together. Sex is a problem two people share; treating just one of them is often unsuccessful.

Some 3500 to 5000 sex treatment clinics in the United States now offer various types of sex therapy. The best known and most imitated approach is Masters and Johnson's "sensate focus," which reconditions sexual behavior through a gradual exploration of the sex partners' bodies accompanied by constant communication of the feeling of pleasuring one another. During early sessions, no intercourse is permitted, even if an impotent husband should have an erection. After each session, separate and joint interviews are held with therapists and new instructions given. From love play, the couple moves to touching genitals. Performance fears are minimized because the focus is not on performance but on enjoying one another. Not until the last stage is intercourse permitted, when both are ready. Results: Masters and Johnson report a 74.5 percent success rate (*b*).

Of course, perfecting technique can only be useful when love is already on the premises; it will not improve the sexual relationship in a weak marriage with a serious communication problem. Nor is it necessary for everyone. Some couples with solid marriages and just ordinary sex lives are perfectly happy that way. Others may be anxious to do better. That is as it should be. Sex patterns need no more be uniform than any other elements of lifestyles. Liberation as applied to sex means that each couple is free to develop its own style of relating and loving.

HEALTH CONSUMER TIP

What You Should Know about Sex Therapy Clinics

Poor therapy can be harmful, and so careful shopping is a must. Fees in sex treatment clinics range upwards of $40 per hour and may involve as much as $1500 to $2000 for a two-week course with follow-up. Although many centers claim to follow the Masters and Johnson technique, Dr. Johnson at one point noted that possibly only 50 clinics out of thousands meet all the standards for good treatment.

Ask your physician, a school health officer, Planned Parenthood, or the gynecology or psychiatry department of the nearest medical school to suggest a clinic or private therapist. Clinics affiliated with a university teaching hospital can be expected to be of good quality.

To evaluate a therapist, check credentials, as for a psychotherapist (page 50), and look for training in both psychotherapy and sex therapy from a hospital or its affiliate or from a reputable clinic. Avoid therapists (or clinics) that promise instant results, ask for full payment in advance, or make sexual advances.

Nothing good is going to happen in bed between a husband and wife unless good things have been happening between them before they go into bed. There is no way for a good sexual technique to remedy a poor emotional relationship. For a man and a woman to be delighted with each other in bed, both must want to be in that bed—with each other. (Masters and Johnson, *c*, pp. 107–108)

LOOKING BACK

REVIEWING CONCEPTS IN CHAPTER 19

- Sexuality encompasses all the subtle and not so subtle differences and relationships between male and female, as well as some relationships between male and male and between female and female. It is not limited to the genitals.
- Differences between males and females are dependent upon genetics, hormones, and environment. There is disagreement about the relative importance of each of these factors.
- Reproductive organs in males and females share a common origin. Their activity and development are controlled by the sex hormones.
- The many myths about menstruation cause both confusion and fear. Menstruation, however, is a normal process that should normally in no way disable a woman.
- Building a good sexual relationship requires patience, practice, and trust, as well as good communications. Sexual and emotional relationships are interrelated, each affecting the other.
- Sex drive is not static; it varies from person to person and time to time. There are no optimum levels. Unlike such drives as hunger and thirst, the fulfillment of the sex drive is not necessary for individual survival. It can be influenced by many factors, both physical and emotional.
- Orgasm, the climax of sexual stimulation, almost always occurs in men engaged in sexual intercourse, but some women find it difficult to achieve. 95 percent of women are capable of reaching orgasm at some time in their lives. However, orgasm is not essential to every good sexual relationship.
- Inadequate sexual response can have a physical cause, but it is more often traceable to psychological hang-ups from childhood or from earlier and unsatisfactory sexual encounters. Therapy can often help.
- Sex therapy administered by poorly trained, unqualified persons can be more harmful than helpful. Help should be sought from qualified professionals only.

20

OTHER MODES OF SEXUAL EXPRESSION

WHAT'S AHEAD IN CHAPTER 20 How have attitudes toward modes of sexual experience outside the traditional Judeo-Christian concept of marital sex changed since ancient times? In recent years? What does current medical opinion have to say about masturbation and the effects it might have? How widespread is the practice? What are the factors that might be considered by someone involved in a decision about premarital intercourse? Is sex before marriage always bad? Always good? Are there alternatives for young people who want a satisfying relationship without actual intercourse? What are the various opinions about homosexuality—what it is, what causes it, how or whether it can be treated? Can you recognize the homosexual? Should homosexuals have "equal rights"? How have rape laws often protected the criminal rather than the victim? How is this changing in some places? Are there ways of reducing the likelihood of rape? What are the effects of rape on the husband or boyfriend of the victim?

With the proliferation of porn shops, massage parlors, and X-rated movies, it is easy to believe that ours is the most sex-saturated society in history. Of course, this is not so. The degree and intensity of practices deviating from the traditional concept of "sex within marriage with one partner of the opposite sex" has varied widely over the centuries.

Ancient ritual orgies, Roman and Greek sex manuals for heterosexual and homosexual activity, even Victorian pornography easily rivaled and often surpassed modern sexual practice.

Among the forms of sexual expression that fall outside the traditional Judeo-Christian boundaries are masturbation, sex before marriage, homosexuality, and rape, an antisocial sexual practice. Because these practices are common enough to touch on the lives of nearly everyone, it is important to explore and understand them.

MASTURBATION

Masturbation, the self-stimulation of the genitalia or other parts of the body for sexual pleasure, is the most common form of sexual expression other than heterosexual intercourse. Yet it is still looked upon by many as a harmful aberration. When children play with their toes, parents are delighted and make a game of it. When children take pleasure in playing with genitals, parental reaction is often quite different, ranging from distraction among more enlightened parents to the cry, "No! Naughty!" coupled with a sharp slap on the hand. Though all parents teach the proper names for parts of the body (eyes, ears, nose, toes, and so on) to young children, many often concoct such nonwords as "whatsis" and "pee-pee" for the genitalia. The pre-Freudian concept that children are sexually innocent has been exploded, but its fragments are yet to be tidied up.

Children toying with their genitals are not truly masturbating. But the guilt they learn to associate with the pleasure of this early self-stimulation can carry over into fear and guilt about masturbation and sometimes into attitudes about other forms of sexuality. Today's pediatric authorities suggest parents ignore a child's genital play unless it begins to interfere with other activities, in which case it may be a symptom of an underlying physical or emotional problem.

Masturbation itself, in spite of all the thrice-told tales about its inducing madness and causing everything from pimples to cancer, is, by scientific standards, perfectly normal and harmless. Doctrines of some religious faiths, however, view it as morally wrong. Guilt over the practice can lead to psychological problems.

Masturbation is so common that between 85 and 96 percent of males and between 50 and 80 percent of females in Kinsey's survey indicated they had masturbated. The practice is most frequent after puberty and before regular patterns of sexual intercourse are established. Frequency among teenage boys averages about 2.5 times a week and then tapers off. For women, frequency varies from as rarely as once or twice a year to 10 to 20 times a week and generally increases until about age 45 (Kinsey et al., *a, b*). Sexual fantasies often accompany masturbation.

Adults may use masturbation to supplement sexual intercourse or to replace it during illness, late pregnancy, separation from their mates, and often mutually, when contraception is not available or a couple feel unready to become involved in the possible consequences of intercourse.

SEXUAL RELATIONS BEFORE MARRIAGE

For a time during the 1960s, there was some doubt that the sexual behavior of young people was any different from that a generation earlier. But by the 1970s, it became clear that there had been a significant shift, particularly in females. While Kinsey in 1953 found 3 percent of women had coital experience by age 15, Robert Sorensen found in 1973 that 30 percent had. Both Kinsey and Sorensen found a tendency toward having a single partner for whom there was a feeling of love and away from sexual adventurism or promiscuity. But a 1977 report found 50 percent of experienced teenage girls had had more than one partner (Kantner and Zelnik, *b*).

TABLE 20.1 Sexual behavior of American adolescents*

	TOTAL	BOYS	GIRLS	13–15	16–19	WHITE	NONWHITE
Virgins, all	48%	41%	55%	63%	36%	55%	49%
Virgins, no beginning sexual activity	22	20	25	39	9	25	23
Virgins, with petting experience	17	14	19	12	21	20	9
Nonvirgins, all	52	59	45	37	64	45	51
Nonvirgins having sexual relations with only one partner at time of interview	21	15	28	9	31	19	14
Nonvirgin "adventurers" moving from one partner to another	15	24	6	10	18	11	18
Nonvirgins, inactive, who have not had intercourse for more than 1 year	12	13	10	15	10	11	14

*This represents a nationwide cross section of adolescents. Sexual behavior in any particular area of the country may vary considerably.
Source: Sorensen, p. 122.

Possibly at the root of the changes were women's feelings about themselves and about sexuality; the new openness about sex in our society leading to a single standard of sexual behavior for both males and females; increased opportunity because of more young people being unchaperoned, having access to automobiles, empty homes, and open college dormitories; and better and more available forms of birth control.

Making a Decision

While the question rarely arose for their parent's generation, today's young people find the question of whether or not to engage in sexual activity comes up early and often. That many young people make no conscious decision, but simply progress into intercourse in a relationship, can be deduced from Sorensen's finding that fully 55 percent took no birth control precautions at all the "first time." However, many young men and women prefer to make a conscious when-where-and-with-whom decision. They do not want it made for them by social pressure, marijuana, alcohol, or the passionate impulse of the moment. Sex education pioneer Dr. Mary Calderone believes the decisions should not be made outside the fabric of the rest of their lives: "Sex is not just a series of genital acts. It plays an integral part in all our relationships, not just in bed. It is the key to our being" (*b*).

Reasons for sex before marriage In making a decision, it is valuable to know why one wants to engage in coitus. Among the most common positive reasons are love, the need for intimacy or a meaningful relationship, the development of one's sexuality, or a trial run for marriage. But some people use or are used by sex. Sex is a way to satisfy curiosity; to enjoy new experiences or gain popularity and approval; to escape from life's pressures or loneliness; to punish parents, spouse, or former sweetheart; to defy society, to attain status, maturity, "adulthood"; to win a boyfriend or girlfriend, a spouse, a career, or other benefits (Gadpaille, *b*; Sorensen). Some young women have sought to use sex as a wedge into the man's world by taking a traditionally male, nonromantic, no-strings-

Laima Druskis/Editorial Photocolor Archives

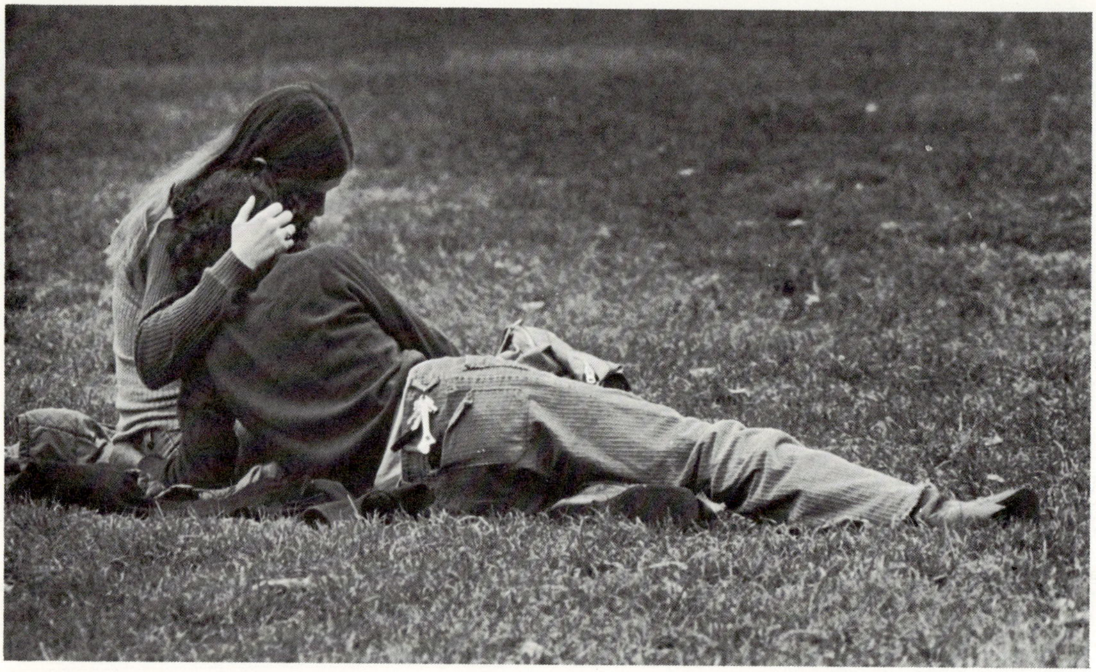

Finding one's place in the spectrum of sexual value systems is an important step in making a decision about premarital sex.

attached view of sex. But for many women who grew up with the old values of love, commitment, marriage, and motherhood fastened to sex, this role has been difficult, and sexual liberation has not brought the hoped-for self-esteem and identity (Bardwick).

Sexual value systems Next it is important to explore the spectrum of sexual value systems and find one's place in it. Ira Reiss has described four viewpoints in this spectrum:

1 *Abstinence before marriage* Sexual intercourse for both males and females should be reserved for marriage, often the choice of those with strong beliefs in religion or in the concept of family and fidelity.

2 *The double standard* Premarital sex is fine for males, but female virginity is prized, a view often held by those with traditional concepts of male/female roles.

3 *Permissiveness with affection* Coitus between unmarrieds is acceptable where deep mutual affection and a stable relationship are shared, an increasingly popular standard.

4 *Permissiveness without affection* Intercourse between mutually consenting unmarrieds, with emphasis on physical attraction and desire rather than love, is permissible, a less widely observed standard.

Some authorities (Sorensen, Gadpaille, *b*) have suggested that our society has eliminated another option: noncoital sex including

Everybody must develop their own standards of sexual morality. Hopefully it will include a sense of responsibility, adventure and respect. (Calderone, *b*, p. 39)

Several friends and myself went down to see this girl with the expressed purpose of losing our virginity. It was worth $25 to have the act behind me. (Male student at Ivy League school, quoted in Packard, p. 196)

Once you've had sex, you know, you're really like trying to justify it in your own mind. I mean, so you change your views really drastically. (A 17-year-old female, quoted in Sorensen, p. 187)

There's a feeling you can be reborn, if just by being sexually intimate with a person. With the kids I talk to, intimacy is much more crucial than sexual performance. They want to see in themselves the capacity to be close, trusting and giving, and to be able to receive these things back. (Tom Cottle, Boston psychotherapist, quoted in Woodward, p. 118)

"If you really love me, you'll sleep with me."
"If you really love *me*, you'll stop pressuring me."

petting to orgasm. Intercourse is generally considered to be the only valid expression of sexual love. Of course, it is not the only way. And the option of noncoital sex is often a more suitable choice for the young sexual beginner and an essential step in the development of sexuality, self-understanding, and understanding of one's partner. Yet many young people skip this stage and go right to intercourse.

The consequences The effects of premarital intercourse are also to be considered when making a decision:

- *The physical consequences* These effects, particularly pregnancy and venereal disease, are perhaps the most obvious. The hazards from each can be reduced (though not totally eliminated) by a couple's planning in advance which birth control method will be used, what course of action will be taken should a pregnancy occur, and by each taking tests for VD as part of a preintercourse medical examination. (See Chapter 22 for birth control information; Chapter 8 for VD.) More recently, another physical hazard has been observed: Women who begin to engage in sexual activities in early adolescence and have several partners have a higher risk of cancer of the cervix, possibly because of herpes virus infections.
- *The psychological consequences* These are difficult to assess, and observers have evaluated the effects differently (see the sidebar on premature sexual relations). "No one knows," suggests Dr. Calderone "what effect sex, precociously experienced, will have on the immature mind. Sex experienced before confidentiality, empathy and trust have been established can hinder and may destroy the possibility of a solid permanent relationship" (*a*, p. 4).

  There is no conclusive evidence that premarital intercourse is either always beneficial to the development of personality, mental health, and sexuality, or that it is always harmful to them. It is most likely to be harmful when it is misused (as a coping method, as a way to cover up problems) or when an individual has deep feelings of guilt.
- *Effects on future marital happiness* Again, information is sketchy and not definitive, but there appears to be a slight edge for those who marry as virgins or who have not had a variety of sexual partners before marriage.
- *Effects on others* A commonly heard philosophy today is "anything goes as long as no one gets hurt." In deciding about premarital intercourse, those who hold that view may wish to consider the effect it may have on others: Is it possible that a future husband or wife may feel some resentment

Opinions on Premarital Sexual Relations

Premarital intercourse may draw the couple closer together in deeper unity and sharing; or through conflict in initial and continuing motivation, it may create distrust, suspicion, and disrespect. . . . (Rev. Perry LeFevre, dean, Chicago Theological Seminary, pp. 22–27)

I feel it (sex with my boy friend) is right at this point . . . it brings a special tenderness. (A 17-year-old girl, quoted in Lake, p. 111.)

When a person's earliest experience with sex is associated . . . with apprehension, guilt and disappointment, later lasting relationships are consciously handicapped . . . (and) sexual response is less than it should be. (Beverly Mead, psychiatrist, *a*, p. 22)

. . . Sex is not, normally, in the least wrong when it is carried on between consenting adults for their cooperative enjoyment. And even when it is foolishly performed—when, for instance, it is continually done with an unsatisfactory partner, or is allowed to encroach too seriously on other enjoyable and necessary aspects of life—it is still only a mistake, an inefficiency, and hardly a heinous, sinful crime. . . . The real "loss of reputation" that [a woman] is likely to feel if she engages in premarital affairs is the definitional one she sets up in her own head. In other words, the same old guilt. . . . (Ellis, pp. 51–52)

What of the currently spreading pattern of "intercourse with affection" but without commitments? This will result in serious, long-range adverse effects. Planned dissociation of sex and love commitment generates both a public climate of opinion and an individual state of mind that will deprive marital intercourse of its personally perceived and socially acknowledged significance as an exclusive expression of mutually shared conjugal companionship. (Father Thomas, Georgetown University, *d*, p. 27)

I have been convinced by the young that the new relationships are a noble experiment that should be allowed to run its course. . . . The pendulum should be allowed to swing. It will swing back (at least part way). It's much more in keeping with human nature to make sex a private thing and to have some elements of exclusivity. (Blaine, M.D., former chief psychiatrist, Harvard Health Service, *b*, p. 38)

Among primitive peoples, as with lower animals, sexual mating begins with physiological readiness. As mankind advanced, a delay in sexual activity was necessary to give intellect a chance to develop before it was swamped by the sex drive. Successful civilizations have depended upon this delay. (Paul Popenoe, Sc.D., president and founder, American Institute of Family Relations, *b*, p. 118)

about an earlier relationship? What about the unborn child that might accidentally be conceived? What if such a pregnancy should force the partners into a premature marriage? What will be the effect on each partner if the relationship breaks up on a one-sided or otherwise unpleasant note? How does a roommate feel about being put out on weekend nights? Or how do parents feel about what may seem an abandonment of their values and mores? Will there be an effect on society, on the concept of marriage, family, and fidelity?

The Right to Abstain

One result of the current openness about sex is the pressure that some young people feel

I had several sexual experiences when I was a freshman. I was lonely, and bewildered and needed to be wanted. I didn't enjoy sex. The next morning I usually hated myself. That was nearly 2 years ago. I haven't had intercourse since and I feel like a virgin. That one messed-up year isn't going to ruin my life. Now I'm waiting until I meet the man I want to marry. (Female student, Eastern school, personal interview, 1977)

My parents have a very strict code. . . . I've been taught to think for myself. I lead a happy, satisfying life without sex. I can handle a deep relationship that does not include going to bed. . . . (Woman student, quoted in Woodward, p. 125)

I really liked this girl when I was a junior in high school. She wanted to have sex, so finally we did. It was awful. I was really shook up. I decided then and there that I was going to wait until I was older and until I was sure that I had the right girl, one I wanted to marry. And that's what I'm doing. (Male student, Midwestern college junior, personal interview, 1975)

I'm into women's lib, and I'm learning to be my own person. That includes the right to say no! (College freshman in Lake, p. 158)

to conform, a pressure that is the flip side of the pressure a generation or two ago "to remain a virgin." Some have engaged in intercourse just to shake off the onus of virginity. Others find it better to lie than to admit to virginity.

Millions of young men and women, however, find virginity no disgrace. Eighteen percent of boys and 23 percent of girls in Sorensen's study rejected the idea of premarital sex out of hand, and 41 percent of males and 55 percent of females among these 13- to 19-year-olds were still virgins. By the time they reach the altar, their numbers will have dwindled to 10 to 15 percent of men and 30 percent of women. In addition, there are young men and women who, having sampled sex early and found it wanting (often because of traumatic or unpleasant experiences), have adopted a "secondary virginity," abstaining from coitus until a later, perhaps better, time. Sorensen found 10 percent of boys and 13 percent of girls in his sample had been inactive for a year or more after having previously experienced coitus. Many persons recognize that sexual energies can be expended in many ways: through art, religion, music, athletics, as well as through sexual activity.

HOMOSEXUALITY: VARIATION IN SEXUAL CHOICE

Homosexuality has emerged from the closet and this has led to greater understanding of homosexual men and women in the community. But we are a long way from understanding homosexuality (*homo* = same). It is an excellent example of a subject in which opinions of eminent authorities differ completely, partly because of the lack of well-controlled studies, partly because of the emotionalism attached to it.

What Is Homosexuality?

To begin with, authorities do not agree on what homosexuality means or who is a homosexual. Some consider the homosexual one who engages in physical contact with a person of the same sex which both recognize as being sexual in nature and which ordinarily results in sexual arousal. Others consider a person who is erotically aroused by another of the same sex to be homosexual even if he or she does not follow up with actual sexual behavior. Still others see as homosexual the shared understanding of sexual preferences

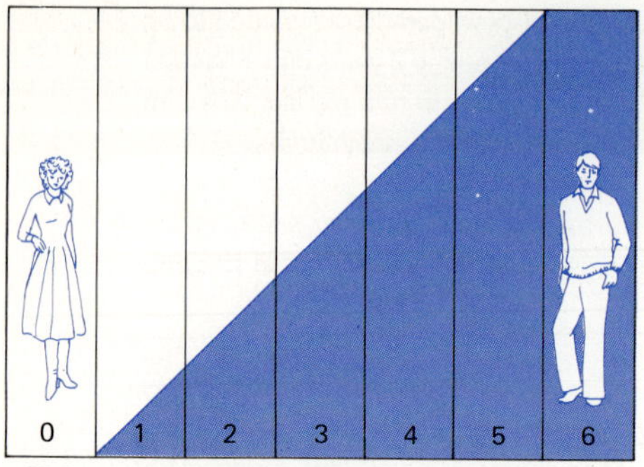

80.6 5.6 2.6 1.3 1.8 1.9 2.3

Percentage males in each category (3.9% no sexual contact)

FIGURE 20.1 Kinsey's heterosexual-homosexual rating scale. Based on both psychological reactions and actual experience of white college males, age 20, ratings are as follows:

0 Exclusively heterosexual, with no homosexual arousal or contacts.

1 Predominantly heterosexual; only incidental homosexual arousal or contact, which may result from curiosity, may be forced, or may occur under influence of alcohol or drugs.

2 Predominantly heterosexual, but more than incidentally homosexual.

3 Equally heterosexual and homosexual; bisexual. No strong preference.

4 Predominantly homosexual, but more than incidentally heterosexual.

5 Predominantly homosexual, but incidentally heterosexual.

6 Exclusively homosexual, in both response and activity.

[*From Kinsey et al., a, pp. 638–643.*]

for members of one's own sex and participation in the gay subculture.

Kinsey suggested that most people are neither wholly heterosexual nor wholly homosexual, but rather fall along a wide spectrum (see Figure 20.1). He found, too, that approximately 60 percent of men and about 33 percent of women in his surveys had experienced at least one homosexual contact by age 15 (Kinsey et al., *a, b*). More recently, Sorensen found the figures for his 13- to 19-year-olds to be only 11 percent for boys and 6 percent for girls, possibly as a result of the opportunity for greater heterosexual activity. The percentage of active homosexual adults in the United States has been estimated at anywhere from 2 to 6 percent for males and about half that for females.

The typical adolescent homosexual experience begins between ages 10 and 15, when sex hormones begin to flow (Fink). A boy may be sexually attracted to his mother. The feeling frightens him. He and a best friend engage in homosexual play, which seems safer than his yearnings for his mother. For 90 percent of such youngsters, homosexual activity is abandoned when opportunities for acceptable heterosexual activity become available. If this transfer to the opposite gender is not made, however, a permanent pattern of homosexuality may be set.

Homosexual behavior may surface, too, in the absence of heterosexual outlets for sexual urges, as in prisons, military camps, or single-sex boarding schools. This is not considered true homosexual behavior by those who believe homosexuality implies the inability to function heterosexually. In the same category is the behavior of the occasional feminist who sleeps with other women to prove her sisterhood or of experimenters who try homosexual relations as a lark, on a dare, or out of curiosity or spite. According to Dr. Charles Socarides (*a*), a psychiatrist active in treatment and study of homosexuals, it is important to differentiate between "obligatory" homosexuals (who can't help themselves) and nonobligatory or episodic homosexuals who engage in homosexual activities out of choice.

The confusion over what homosexuality is or is not has created concern among young people who have engaged in sexual activities with friends of the same sex during adolescence, who have difficulty relating to peers of the opposite sex, or who have a deep friendship with someone of the same sex. They wonder, "Am I homosexual?" Most often they are not. A preference for a homosexual or heterosexual lifestyle usually becomes confirmed sometime between 17 and 21, although some discover latent homosexual leanings in their twenties and thirties (Robert Gould).

What Are Homosexuals Like?

Contrary to the stereotypes of effeminate male with high-pitched voice and boyish female with a "butch" haircut, the majority of homosexuals cannot be distinguished by their appearance. They come from all walks of life and every socioeconomic group, and apart from sexual orientation, they differ little from the general population in lifestyle, religious and cultural mores, political attitudes, and mental health.

Though in some persons, homosexuality is a reflection of a disturbed personality (Robert Gould), many homosexuals appear perfectly normal and show no more neuroses, psychoses, or bizarre behavior unrelated to their homosexuality than heterosexuals. Is their sexual orientation alone reason enough to consider them victims of a psychiatric condition?

Answers of leading authorities vary. Their positions run the gamut from "homosexuality is a mental illness" to "homosexuality is simply a sexual variant, much as heterosexuality is." The condition has been called "an alternative lifestyle," a "disorder," a "dysfunction," a "loss of function," "normal," "abnormal," and none of the above.

The leadership of the American Psychiatric Association (APA), in a move to free homosexuals from the stigma which has led to discrimination in housing, jobs, and public accommodations—and which, many therapists believe, has also brought unnecessary psychological suffering—voted in 1974 to remove "homosexuality per se" from the list of psychiatric disorders. Instead it should be considered, they said, as a "sexual orientation disturbance," and that only when the individuals are "either disturbed by, in conflict with, or wish to change their sexual orientation." A hotly contested and criticized referendum of the APA membership upheld this position, but, as can be seen in the sidebar on homosexuality, this did not settle the matter.

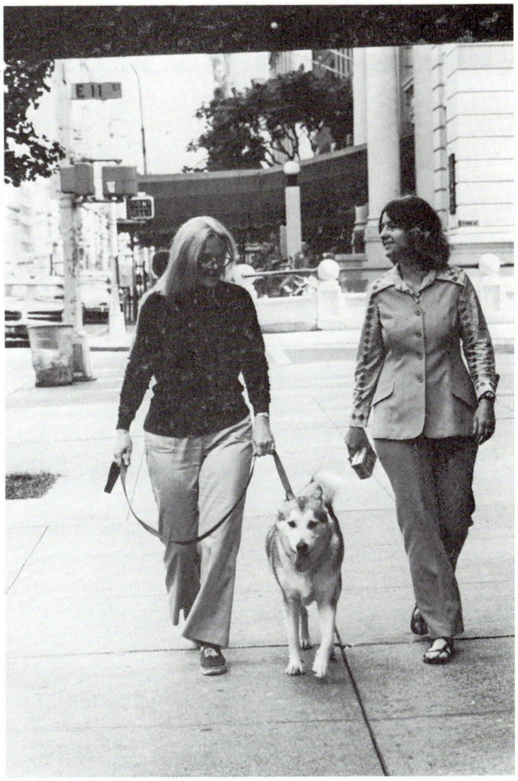

Chie Nishio/Nancy Palmer

Contrary to stereotypes, homosexuals, apart from their sexual orientation, differ little from the general population in lifestyle, religious and cultural mores, political attitudes, or mental health.

Sexual Behavior of Homosexuals

Many people have an image of homosexual relationships as brief encounters in gay bars, men's rooms, and parks. These do occur, especially for secret homosexuals who cannot risk being involved in a long-term affair.

Opinions on Homosexuality (Illness or normal sexual variation?)

We're not saying that it is normal; we're not saying it is abnormal . . . [they] are not really psychiatric terms. . . . I have to say that it is easier for me to say how it should not be characterized than how it should be. I don't regard homosexual behavior as optimal as heterosexual behavior. I would agree with Freud that something happens in the development of the sexual instinct that leads one to be incapable of or not interested in heterosexual functioning. I am loathe, however, to apply the word "disorder" because of its many implications. (Spitzer, p. 5)

A homosexual adult is a person whose heterosexual function is crippled much like the walking function of a person with two paralyzed legs. Can we call this normal? . . . For some to suggest that we can take the most severely injured homosexual—the one who is unable or unwilling to change—and call him normal and then take the least injured—the one who . . . wishes to revert to a male/female relationship—and decide he has a sexual orientation disorder, to me seems wild. (I. Bieber, *b*, p. 5)

. . . in ancient Greece it [homosexuality] was institutionally approved and practiced in the very highest circles . . . . Much of the "disease" that homosexuals suffer from in our culture is not because of their homosexuality at all, but is a consequence of the prejudice and discrimination that they encounter in a hostile society. . . . (Marmor, pp. 10, 15)

[Homosexuality] is *not* a normally equivalent sexual alternative. . . . [It] is a manifestation of disordered psychosexual development. (Gadpaille, *a*, p. 25)

The person who is sick and in need of therapy is not the homosexual fired from a job but the employer firing him . . . not the homosexual who gets beaten up, but the thugs who go out to "roll queers"; not the homosexual who gets entrapped or enticed into a solicitation, but the policeman volunteering for such a duty . . . not those homosexuals who seek their sex in semipublic places, but the society that provides them with no other social resources and . . . has forced them to accept the only outlets available to them and then blames them for the damage it has wrought. (Kameny, President of Mattachine Society, p. 26)

Sexual behavior in lower animals is heterosexual. Such behavior is instinctual and insures the existence of the animal kingdom. Man is an animal. . . . [In addition] just as a man may kick his dog when he doesn't dare kick his boss, so too a man (or woman) may discharge his sexual drive onto a person of the same sex when he is afraid to do so with the opposite sex. (Voth, pp. 15–16)

Between 10 and 20 percent of homosexuals report that they have often picked up sexual partners in public terminals, and a larger proportion in public or semipublic places. But many homosexuals form permanent or semipermanent relationships that are in many ways similar to heterosexual ones, involving love, sharing, and caring as well as sexual contact.

The Possible Causes of Homosexuality

As with almost everything else about homosexuality, there is little agreement about cause. Many influences are suspected, and they probably overlap and interact. They include the following.

Heredity and hormones Jon K. Meyer, Di-

Freud described several elements in male homosexuality: (1) a narcissistic search for a love object symbolizing one's self and focused on the male genitalia; (2) an unconscious attraction to mother which is, of course, forbidden and which is converted to an avoidance and fear of all women; and (3) an associated unconscious castration anxiety and fear of punishment by males. He developed a similar definition for female homosexuality with, however, a difference in the nature of the castration anxiety.

rector of the Sexual Behaviors Consultation Unit at Johns Hopkins University, declares: "There is absolutely no good evidence that genetic constitution, fetal hormone environment, or adult hormonal imbalance contribute in any way to eventual gender role or sexual object choice" (p. 37). But others urge more study. They point to: (1) twin studies showing that when one identical twin has homosexual tendencies, the other does, too, while nonidentical twins, with their differing hereditary makeup, demonstrate no such correlation (Kallman); (2) several recent studies that have found hormonal differences in homosexuals when compared to heterosexuals, though it is uncertain whether the hormones are cause or effect; (3) rat studies that indicate prenatal hormone imbalance may cause a mixup in the sexual orientation of the brain, something as yet undemonstrated in humans.

Environment Strong evidence points to early family influences as a cause of homosexuality. Some researchers, however, believe an innate tendency is necessary for environmental influences to be effective. Male homosexuality has been shown in some studies to be traceable to a close-binding, overprotective mother who babied and favored the child, made him dependent on her, used him as an ally against the father, preferred him to her husband, and was both puritanical and seductive (I. Bieber et al.). Fathers in these studies appeared to be either weak and ineffectual, spending little time with their sons, or actively inhuman. These studies, however, have been criticized because of the limited population they examined.

Studies of female homosexuals are even less reliable, and thus little is known about the family that rears the lesbian. It is suspected that fathers probably exert powerful influences on the sexual object choice of their daughters by being puritanical while masking sexual interest in them. Daughters often fear their fathers (Gadpaille, *b*). One study found that homosexual girls could not find qualities in either parent to which they could trustingly relate (Kremer).

Of course, many heterosexuals come from families such as those described above, and many homosexuals from other types of families. Thus some other factors may also be at work in the development of homosexuality.

The impact of peers at certain stages in a youngster's life may be one of these. A boy who is less rough-and-tumble than other boys, or a girl who likes sports and hates to dress up may be challenged by friends as "a queer," "a fag," or a "lezzy." An uncertain youngster may then decide, "Maybe they're right." Though, of course, they're usually wrong.

It has also been suggested that lack of success or fear of failure in a heterosexual encounter can also push a borderline adolescent over the brink. Whether or not a seduction by an older homosexual can do likewise is controversial.

Can and Should the Homosexual be Treated?

Adult homosexuals may desire two kinds of help: They may wish to revert to heterosexual behavior, or they may wish to learn to live happy homosexual lives. The latter is much more likely than the former. A variety of treatment approaches—psychotherapy, behavior modification, aversion therapy, and

Sex was just never mentioned in our house, but I got the strong message that it was something dirty you did with girls. Nobody ever said anything about boys. . . . (A male homosexual in psychotherapy, quoted in Hatterer, p. 34)

others—have been tried with varying degrees of impact on sexual orientation or behavior. Most important is a therapist experienced in working with homosexuals and understanding their situation (Socarides et al.). The likelihood of changing sexual object choice is increased when the individual is under 35, strongly wishes change, respects his father, has attempted heterosexual intercourse, and has dreams with heterosexual content (I. Bieber et al.).

Some authorities, such as Dr. John Money, believe that obligatory homosexuality is not reversible through treatment. The late homosexual physician Howard J. Brown maintained that though some who engage in both homosexual and heterosexual behavior might shift their object preference, this shift did not result from therapy. Psychiatrist Warren Gadpaille (*a*), who has successfully treated many young homosexuals and potential homosexuals, argues therapy can help. Socarides believes not only that treatment is possible but also that saying homosexuals are "normal" denies them the right to help: "True, it is difficult to know one is ill, but it is far worse to keep experiencing symptoms and yet be told by supposedly qualified people that: 'You're all right. . . . Relax and enjoy it.'" (*b*, p. 123).

Today many homosexuals are pressing for civil rights legislation that will prohibit discrimination in jobs and housing.

Howard Petrick/Nancy Palmer

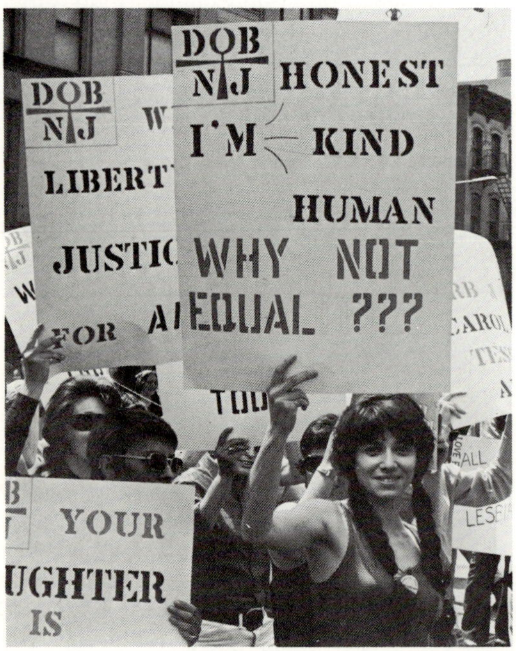

Gay Liberation and Society

Using the preferred term "gay," hundreds—attorneys, teachers, doctors, writers, athletes, public officials, and so on—have come out of the closet to announce their sexual orientation to the world. They have organized homophile groups, public meetings, civil rights demonstrations, gay bars. The majority of homosexuals, however, are still under cover—fearful of losing jobs, friends, community status. Some still fear the threat of blackmail.

A chief goal of the Gay Lib movement is public acceptance of homosexuality as an alternative lifestyle. A national campaign to pass civil rights legislation to protect the rights of gay people to jobs, housing, and public accommodations has met with mixed success. In some cities, bills have been passed; in others, they have met stiff opposition from conservative elements. Gay civil rights groups have been more uniformly successful on college campuses. According to the National Gay Student Center, there were some 250 officially recognized homosexual student groups at schools across the country in 1974.

OTHER VARIATIONS IN SEXUAL BEHAVIOR

Bisexuality "More and more students are calling themselves bisexuals," says John B. Sturrock, director of a major college mental health center. "To be AC-DC, to swing both ways, has become almost a vogue thing. I think bisexuality can indicate some psychosexual confusion. When life is generally confused, bewildered and uncertain, then this surely must show up in sex [as well as in] politics and economics" (Klemesrud, p. 38).

Many other reasons have been suggested for the apparent upsurge in bisexual behavior, including the many liberation movements advocating indifference to gender and freer attitudes toward sexuality. Some experts see bisexuality as a "normal and healthy" lifestyle that has been inhibited only by social brainwashing and cultural taboos. Others believe it is "contrary to nature, which over the millenia went to a great deal of trouble to differentiate sex organs and properly align them for reproductive acts."

Transvestism The tranvestite (*trans* = cross + *vestite* = dress) feels a compulsion to dress up in the clothing of the opposite sex. The condition, which probably affects less than 1 percent of the population (D. G. Brown), may stem from childhood trauma, often the rejection of the child's sex by parents. Most transvestites are men; most are not homosexual. They usually fulfill a sexual need by wearing frilly women's underclothing beneath their male outerwear. A rare few masquerade completely in clothing of the opposite sex.

Transsexualism In the transsexual, there is a total incompatibility, a gender identity inversion, between the individual's genetic sex and the self-perceived gender. This happens most often in males; though they have completely normal male genitalia and reproductive systems, they feel emotionally and psychologically like women. The urge is so strong that many are willing to undergo hormone treatment and surgery to have their genitals removed and refashioned into female genitalia. They are not homosexual. They desire, and often find, heterosexual relationships with "straight" men.

Pedophilia Adults with pedophilia (*pedo* = child + *philia* = love) usually derive erotic pleasure from relationships with children, often young relatives or children of friends. These "child molesters" are probably much more common than generally supposed; they compose 30 percent of all sex offenders.

Sadism and masochism These deep-seated complementary disturbances involve a need to connect sex with torture and pain of partner (*sadism*, after the Marquis de Sade, who practiced and wrote about it) or of self (*masochism*, after Austrian novelist von Sacher-Masoch, who wrote of and experienced it).

Bestiality Kinsey et al. (*a*) found 17 percent of boys who grew up on farms had reached orgasm through relations with animals. Some believe this outlet for sexual gratification is no different from masturbation, unless it becomes a replacement for and refuge from heterosexual relations.

Fetishism Fetishists, mostly male, derive sexual excitement directly from an inanimate object (an article of clothing, for example) that substitutes for the real, but "dangerous," love object. Masturbation is often involved.

Exhibitionism Thirty-five percent of arrests for sexual violations are for men who expose their genitals in public. These exhibitionists usually crave attention and have deep-seated psychological problems.

Voyeurism and scoptophilia The reverse of exhibitionist, these individuals draw erotic pleasure from compulsively viewing sexual acts or genitalia (scoptophilia) or nudes (voyeurism). When the need is not compulsive and their "peeping Tom" activities simply substitute for unattainable coitus, the condition is referred to as *pseudovoyeurism*.

RAPE: WHEN SEXUALITY GOES AWRY

When sexual impulses get out of hand, when hostility, anger, and frustration seek release through asocial sexual outlets, rape—*the penetration or partial penetration by a male of a female, not his wife, without her valid consent, by compulsion, through violence, threats, stealth, or deceit*—may be the result. On rare occasions, the victim may be a child or an adolescent boy, but in most cases it is a female between the ages of 18 and 25 (Harper and Stokes).

Intercourse need not be forced to be considered rape. Sexual relations with a female minor (how young depends on the state) is considered "statutory rape," even if she consents or initiates the contact. The rationale? She is too young to understand the nature of her consent. In a few states, an adult woman who seduces a boy legally a minor can also be charged with statutory rape. Forced intercourse within marriage is not *legally* considered rape.

The rapist has been shown by studies to be most often in his mid-twenties, from a low-income family, culturally deprived, mentally retarded, or of low-normal intelligence (Gebhard et al.; Rubin). He is likely to come from a broken or unstable home where he received little supervision, often has an alcoholic father, is generally emotionally immature, and frequently is physically unattractive. There is some evidence that some chronic sex offenders may suffer from brain dysfunction.

Many rapes are committed by the "boy (or man) next door." An informal survey by Andrea Medea and Kathleen Thompson for their book *Against Rape* found that 57 percent of women respondents were raped by men they knew, sometimes relatives or friends. A study in a college setting found that often, when sexual intimacy reached the brink of intercourse and the female refused to go further, the male became forceful. In most cases, they were deterred by the female's "screaming, fighting, crying, and pleading." Fewer than 1 percent of the women reported the assaults (Kanin).

Rape as a Crime

Rape is a violent crime and one of the most rapidly increasing offenses in the United States. Its incidence is spiraling even in formerly immune suburbs and rural areas. According to the FBI, a reported rape takes place every 10 minutes. But so many go unreported that the true figure may be as high as one a minute. Most occur at night in the victim's car or apartment, in shopping center parking lots, elevators, dark alleys and hallways, or wooded areas (Harper and Stokes).

In the past, rape was a crime in which the accused received more protection than the victim, and convictions were rare. Many states required a corroborating witness. Since most rapes are conducted without an audience, crying rape was considerably easier than proving it. The victim's past sexual history could be brought into evidence, but the accused rapist's past activities, including previous rape charges, could not, unless he took the stand himself. The basic philosophy appeared to be that men needed protection from false rape charges and that the woman who is raped is "looking for it." The courtroom scene was such an ordeal and so fruitless that few women pressed charges.

But recent pressures from women's groups, civil libertarians, and law enforcement officials have persuaded legislators it is time for a change. In some states, a woman's previous history is no longer relevant, and the

AP Wirephoto

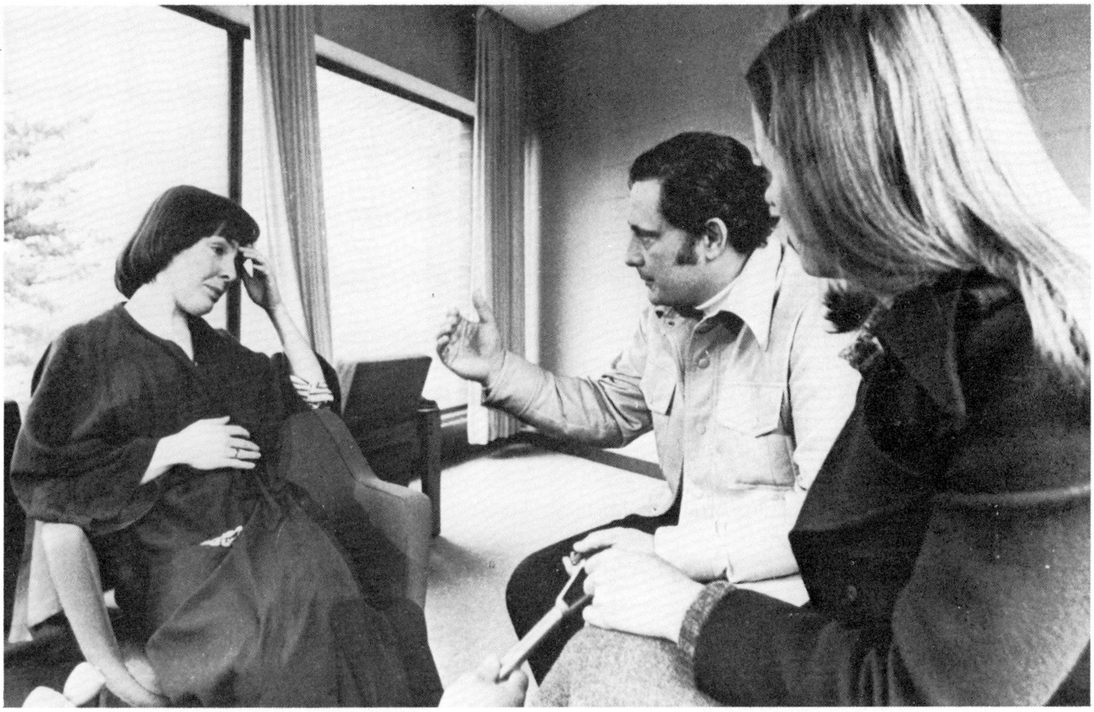

The acting out of a rape report with a professional model is part of a special police training program at Brandeis University. Programs such as this, designed to increase police sensitivities and improve rape investigations, are being established throughout the country.

need for a corroborating witness has been eliminated.

Reporting a Rape

For many women in the past, reporting a rape to the police was "like being raped again." Treatment was often brutal and insensitive. This, too, has begun to turn around. Many communities have set up rape squads staffed by policewomen or specially trained policemen. In others, rape centers offer 24-hour telephone counseling and someone to accompany the victim to the police station.

It is recommended that a woman who has been raped report the attack to the first person she sees, unless that person is an unknown male. She, or the other person, should notify the police or the local rape center immediately. She should not shower or change clothes until after an examination by her private physician or at a hospital to medically establish the fact of rape, determine the extent of injury, if any, test for VD, and determine the possibility of pregnancy. If pregnancy seems possible, she may be given a "morning-after" pill (see Chapter 22).

Rape from the Male Point of View

A TV film once depicted a rape in which the victim was a man. But the differing nature of

How to Avoid Rape

A special note for women and girls Rape is not 100 percent preventable, but the National Rape Center suggests steps a woman can take to reduce the chance of being victimized:

1 Always lock car doors, whether you are in the car or not. Before getting into an empty car, check the floor of the rear seat in case someone is lying in wait. Keep the windows rolled up most of the way and doors locked when driving alone. Be alert at red lights and crossings. Don't walk alone through dark or deserted parking lots or public garages.

2 Always lock the door of your apartment or room, whether you are in or out; don't leave it unlocked even "for a moment." Never open the door to an unexpected stranger or chance acquaintance. Have a chain put on the door, and keep it secured while you check who is there. Reject unexpected deliveries, unless the delivery person has proper identification. Windows accessible from ground level or a fire-escape should be kept locked, and even barred in some neighborhoods. Keep drapes or shades drawn at night. Women living alone can deter potential rapists by using initials instead of first names in telephone books and on mailboxes.

When you go out, leave outside and inside lights on. Have your key ready before you get to the door. Don't enter your apartment or room if a door or window appears to have been forced or left open. Never let a strange man in to use the telephone; instead, make the call for him.

3 Avoid walking on deserted streets, in dark parks, in other isolated places, or through groups of men you don't know. Don't arrange to meet someone on a street corner. Don't board an empty subway car (particularly the first or last) or catnap on a bus or train. Don't hitchhike.

4 Don't dress or walk in a seductive way when alone. Wear shoes and clothing that you can run in if necessary, not 2-inch platforms or tight pants or skirts. Walking alone, especially when you are "high," upset, or distracted, makes you doubly vulnerable. Check behind you occasionally. Look "put together"; look as if you know where you are going.

5 If someone suspicious seems to be following you, don't hurry home to your empty room or apartment. Stop at a store or at the student center instead, and get a reliable escort; or telephone the police or campus security. If someone seems to be loitering in your apartment house or dormitory lobby, head for the nearest crowded spot—a coffee shop, store, student center. If you are approached when walking alone, make a good loud disturbance. A police whistle is a good way to get help or scare off an assailant; police in some cities distribute whistles free. If someone in an automobile behaves suspiciously, run in the opposite direction, again making a racket. But try to keep your cool. If a stranger gets on an elevator with you, step off. Use an excuse such as "I forgot my mail" if it makes you more comfortable.

6 Weapons are controversial; a dangerous one can be used against you. Mace is classed as a dangerous weapon. But a juice-filled plastic lemon or a spray deodorant aimed at close range at the eyes can temporarily stun the attacker, giving you a chance to run. Use a sharp hat pin or throw handbag, books, packages at him. You can also kick (a knee in the groin can be very discouraging), scratch, or bite. All this is intended to give you a chance to make tracks fast, not to start a fight. You can't win one unless you are a judo or karate expert. *If the attacker displays a gun, knife, or other weapon, fighting back could be a fatal mistake.*

7 If someone you know becomes overly aggressive sexually, be assertive. Don't be embarrassed to say, "I'm leaving now" or "Please go," when you suspect someone you know has less than honorable intentions.

A note for men Men can help protect women friends and loved ones from attack by walking or driving them home at night and being sure they are safely inside before leaving.

sexuality in males and females makes it unlikely that such rapes will ever become epidemic. While women can be forced to submit to intercourse without arousal, men cannot be forced to have an erection. Moreover, men are generally larger, stronger, and better equipped to resist attack.

But rape does affect men, primarily when a woman or child they love is rape's victim. The first reaction is one of shock and often fury. But sometimes that fury turns, against the man's own will, on the victim. He fights, but sometimes cannot overcome, the suppressed, unverbalized feeling that she could have resisted. Maybe she enjoyed it or led the rapist on. His own insecurity may figure in: "Maybe someone else is better." An unreasoning jealousy may be another factor. As a result of such feelings, many relationships break up after a rape.

If a man whose wife, daughter, or girlfriend has been sexually attacked has difficulty coping with his feelings, he should see a sensitive counselor—a clergyman, a physician, or the specially trained counselors at some of the new rape centers.

Rape also has an impact on a man falsely charged with rape. On rare occasions, an unstable woman may charge a man with rape when no coitus, or when consenting coitus, has taken place. New laws may give men less protection in such cases, but steps can be taken to avoid false charges. Men can avoid forcing a girl to submit, even if they have had relations with her previously, and can be wary about exploiting a woman sexually; she could cry rape to get revenge. Responsible sexual attitudes and behavior are probably a man's best guarantee against the damaging charge of rape.

Recovering from Rape

For many women, rape is the most traumatic experience of their lives. (Burgess and Holstrom). Those with strong, loving support from family and friends recover most quickly; those attacked suddenly, especially in their own homes, and those with psychological or emotional problems often tend to recover slowly.

LOOKING BACK

REVIEWING CONCEPTS IN CHAPTER 20

- Attitudes toward modes of sexual expression that differ from the traditional concept of "sex within marriage with one partner of the opposite sex" have varied over the centuries. The "sexual revolution" is nothing new.
- Today, scientists believe that masturbation is a normal aspect of sexual behavior for many people. It is not known to cause any negative aftereffects, other than those of misplaced guilt.
- Attitudes about and toward sex before marriage are changing and have led to a change in behavior, but the promiscuous sexual adventurer is still in the minority. Most unmarried young adults prefer love relationships to casual affairs.
- The effects of premarital intercourse on young persons vary depending upon the individual's background, beliefs, hopes for the future, maturity, etc. It is impossible to generalize that it will be "good" or "bad" for all.
- A sexually intimate relationship that stops short of intercourse can be satisfying

and meaningful for some young people. Abstention before marriage can also be considered a reasonable sexual lifestyle.

- Concern about their maleness or femaleness is common among young people, and so is some homosexual experience in early adolescence. But most persons grow up to live heterosexual lives.
- Homosexuals do not fit stereotype molds; they usually look and act like other people.
- Because of lack of sound scientific information, there is much disagreement about homosexuality—its causes, its "cures," and whether it is a disorder, a dysfunction, a personality defect, or an alternative lifestyle.
- The gay civil rights movement is attempting to end discrimination in housing, jobs, and public accommodations.
- Rape laws that formerly protected the male from false charges of rape are now changing to offer more protection to the victim.
- New police rape sections, often staffed by women, now make it easier for women to report rapes. Still, the experience of reporting can often be as traumatic as the rape itself.
- Not all rapes can be prevented, but women can take precautions that will reduce the likelihood of such an event.
- Husbands and boyfriends of rape victims, as well as the victims themselves, often need help in sorting out their feelings about the rape.

21 COURTSHIP AND MARRIAGE: CHANGING INSTITUTIONS

WHAT'S AHEAD IN CHAPTER 21 How have attitudes toward marriage been changing? What factors might be considered in selecting a mate for life? How can one distinguish between love and infatuation? What areas is it often suggested a couple planning marriage agree about in advance? What elements are found in happy marriages? How can the honeymoon be used to improve the chances of marital success? How can the major adjustment problems of the first year be minimized? What are the risks and benefits of a campus marriage? How can these risks be reduced? How can negotiation and renegotiation improve a relationship? What is the best course when a marriage is having serious trouble? What are the alternatives to marriage? Why are more persons opting for these than in previous generations?

Much as the 1960s were labeled by some as the era of the death of God, so the seventies were heralded as the decade of the death of marriage. Sociologist David Cooper wrote a book called *Death of the Family*. Futurist-author Alvin Toffler confidently prophesied that traditional marriage was on its way out. Divorce rates climbed dramatically, free and unfettered relationships developed as acceptable alternatives to marriage, the musty images of the Old Maid and the Lonely Bachelor were replaced by the Swinging Singles. Radical feminists called for female independence and applauded women who rejected "stifling" marriages.

Yet, in spite of the doomsayers, marriage,

John Launois/Black Star

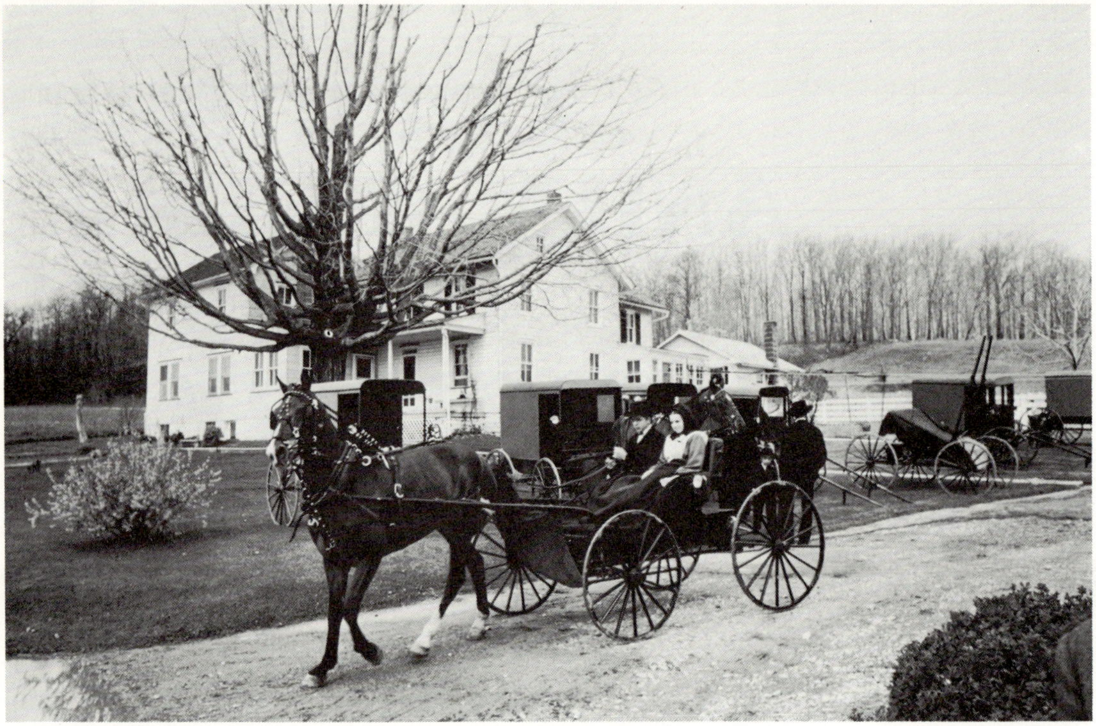

While prescribed courtship rituals still exist in some areas, as among the Amish, most young Americans set their own courtship patterns.

like God, has remained popular. In fact, more people were marrying in 1975 than ever before, and surveys showed a vast majority of young adults desirous of marrying at some time. Despite divorce rates, most married people appeared pleased with their lot. A series of interviews with more than 2000 Americans found 58 percent of married couples were completely satisfied with their relationships and only 3 percent were more dissatisfied than satisfied (Campbell et al.).

COURTSHIP

Courtship, the period of time leading up to marriage, is not unique to humans. Many animal and bird species enjoy elaborate courtship rituals. Prescribed rituals still exist in some contemporary societies, but in the United States such rituals have been replaced by casual patterns set by the couples themselves. Even the concept of formal engagement is no longer considered an obligatory prelude to marriage.

Studies of college couples have shown that nearly half wait a year or longer before becoming engaged or reaching an "understanding" (see Table 21.1, part *a*). Not all engagements end in marriage; however, informal understandings are more likely than formal engagements to break up (part *b*). The most common reason given for the broken engagement is the lack of readiness of one or the other partner (part *c*). Taking time to get to know one another before marriage apparently leads to better marital adjustment (part *d*).

However the courtship period is organized, it clearly plays a crucial role in the later success of marriages. It is a dress rehearsal for a performance that may run for a lifetime—a familiarizing, getting comfortable period in which to make sure the casting is right before the curtain goes up. It is not a time to pretend, to cover up differences in lifestyle, values, desires for children, religious practices, and so on, but a time to be oneself. Some of the things courting couples consider are discussed below.

TABLE 21.1 Engagements and college students

a AVERAGE LENGTH OF TIME ELAPSED IN 546 COURTSHIPS BETWEEN FIRST DATE AND ENGAGEMENT

	NUMBER	PERCENT		NUMBER	PERCENT
1-2 weeks	11	2	5-8 months	105	19
3-4 weeks	15	3	9-11 months	39	7
1-2 months	50	9	1-2 years	142	26
3-4 months	70	13	More than 3 years	114	21

b PROPORTION OF ENGAGEMENTS THAT BREAK UP

Break up: one-third to one-half
  72% informal engagements
  28% formal engagements
Marry: one-half to two-thirds

c REASONS FOR BREAKING ENGAGEMENTS GIVEN BY 810 STUDENTS

CAUSE OF BREAKUP	MEN	WOMEN	CAUSE OF BREAKUP	MEN	WOMEN
Parents	11%	12%	Contrast in background	11%	14%
Mutual loss of interest	8	8	Incompatibility	10	15
Partner lost interest	13	10	I was not ready	18	25
I lost interest	18	22	Partner was not ready	7	18
Separation	19	19			

d DURATION OF ENGAGEMENT AND MARITAL ADJUSTMENT

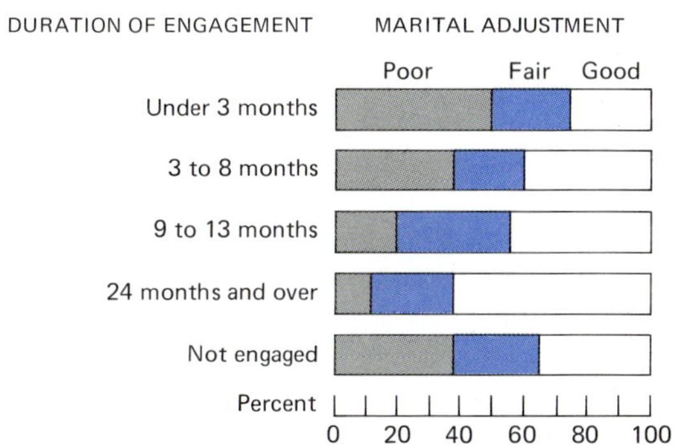

Source: a to *c* Landis and Landis, pp. 187, 191, 192; *d* Landis and Landis, p. 201, from Burgess and Cottrell.

Keep your eyes wide open before marriage, half shut afterwards.
Ben Franklin, *Poor Richard's Almanac* (1738)

Is It Love?

Bells ring. Chills run up and down your spine. You mope endlessly when you're apart. It must be love. Either that or mono. More likely mono.

Psychiatrist Harry Stack Sullivan suggests a more practical definition of love: "When the satisfaction or the security of another person becomes as significant to one as one's own satisfaction or security, then a state of love exists."

Mature love, rarely seen in young, inexperienced persons, is not instant, "at-first-sight" fireworks, but requires time to grow and grows richer with time. It is expressed in many ways, involving the whole person and not only the body. It is more fulfilling than frustrating, even when things go wrong. Though its central theme is "we," instead of narrowing one's life, mature love broadens it. A sound, loving relationship gives strength, brings out the best in both partners, is relatively jealousy-free. Mature love differs from infatuation, or being "in love," which is more likely to be self-centered and based on a physical attraction (Gadpaille, *b*). The ability to love, in contrast to the ability to lust, is learned from the moment of birth onward.

In an infatuation relationship, the loved person is idealized, and there is stubborn resistance to granting importance to faults or to recognizing major incompatibilities that could lead to serious future problems. Infatuation-love is really blind, but many persons marry while still under its spell.

What Is the Potential Mate Really Like?

It is important to understand that "marriage is not a reform school" (J. Thomas, *a*). The diamond-in-the-rough does not suddenly become polished; personalities do not change magically and radically once the wedding ceremony is performed. Marriage will not provide solutions for such problems as drinking, drug abuse, or the inability to hold a job. Nor will conflicting views on the desirability of having children or a two-career family melt away after marriage vows are taken.

Approaching the choice of a mate rationally may seem coldly calculating—more like choosing a car than a spouse. But consider, which is the more important decision? Here are some points worth exploring.

Background Husbands and wives who share common racial, religious, ethnic, educational, and socioeconomic backgrounds and experiences bring similar expectations about marriage and male-female roles to the relationship, and are more likely to hold the same values and desire the same lifestyles than are those from differing backgrounds; thus they may find less conflict to resolve. Their marriages are less likely to end in divorce.

Goals Understanding and accepting one another's goals for life, as well as for marriage and family, valuing the same things (whether skiing or politics, travel or religious observance) will increase the odds for marital success.

Personality How does the potential mate treat his or her family? (Once married, you will be family, too.) How does he or she treat the waitress, the service station attendant, salespeople, friends? Does he or she disparage members of other racial or religious groups? Make mountains out of anthills? Is he or she honest? Cheating in school, lying on income tax, or other types of dishonesty may forecast what marriage will be like. Is the prospective partner always right? Is someone else always to blame? Such persons may be incapable of admitting mistakes or saying "I'm sorry" (a difficult trait to live with). Does he or she have a sense of humor (a difficult trait to live without)? Does he or she have an explosive temper, drink too much, abuse drugs, or use a car as a weapon, gunning it to illegal speeds, cursing other drivers, jumping lights? These are all possible signs of deep-seated problems.

Preparation for Marriage

A recent newspaper article reported that 450 hours of training are required for a license to work in a massage parlor in one state. No training at all is required for a marriage license in any of the 50. California does insist on premarital counseling before persons under 18 are permitted to wed. The Roman Catholic Church requires premarital counseling. But though sex education has worked its way into most school systems, only a handful of high schools and colleges have instituted courses in marriage and the family.

Marriage counselor Clark Vincent blames our laxness on the misguided impression:

> . . . that a successful marriage "just naturally happens" unless the participants are stubborn, evil, or pathologically ill. . . . The myth of naturalism obscures the fact that marriage is the most complex relationship any two people will ever enter into—a relationship for which they usually receive less preparation than for driving a car. . . . We would hardly blame the "engineer" whose bridge collapsed in a society that provided no training for engineers; but we do blame, and even shame, those who terminate a marriage for which they received no preparation. Building successful marriages should be as important to a society as building durable bridges or highways—and indeed it is. Unfortunately, however, society fails to recognize that the former occurs no more naturally than the latter. (pp. 258–259)

Vincent asserts that the United States, proud of its continuing education programs in everything from social dancing to Swahili, has neglected not only preparation for but ongoing education in marriage survival techniques. Until education for marriage becomes

Marriage Agreements

Cooking: Breakfasts during the week are divided equally; husband does all weekend breakfasts (including shopping for them and dishes). Wife does all dinners except Sunday nights. . . . Whoever invites guests does shopping, cooking, and dishes. . . .

Laundry: . . . Wife does home laundry. Husband does dry-cleaning delivery and pick-up. Wife strips beds, husband remakes them.

Children:

1 Mornings: . . . Every other week each parent does all.

2 Transportation: . . . Parts occurring between 3 and 6 PM fall to wife. She must be compensated for extra work from husband. . . . Husband does all weekend transportation and pick-ups after 6.

When this excerpt from the marriage agreement of feminist author Alix Cates Shulman and her husband was published, it raised a flurry of enthusiastic and antagonistic responses. Most couples, however, seem to prefer subtler covenants with less the stamp of a Chrysler–United Auto Workers bargaining session.

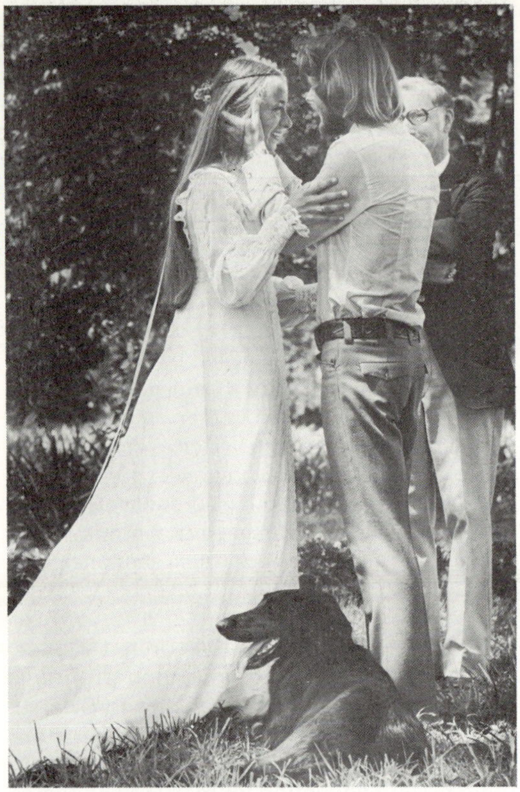
Bruce Roberts/Photo Researchers

Many young couples today incorporate their marital goals into their wedding rites, composing their own vows.

commonplace, interested persons will have to educate themselves. They can take marriage courses when available, read books on marriage and male/female relations, profit from experiences and suggestions of married acquaintances, and seek premarital counseling from a skilled and sensitive clergyman, physician, or professional counselor.

NEGOTIATING THE GOALS OF THE MARRIAGE RELATIONSHIP

What is wanted and needed from marriage differs from person to person. Before the wedding day, a couple should discuss their wants and needs. Their joint goals can later become part of their marriage vows, a formal contract, or an informal agreement. Postponing discussion of sensitive issues simply ignites a time bomb with a long fuse. Some of the decisions that couples can work out in advance include:

- How will decisions be made?
- How much togetherness will there be, in work, play, vacations?
- How, and by whom, will the family be supported? If there will be two incomes, how will the monies be allocated? How will they be banked?
- How will household chores be handled?
- Will there be children? How will their care be shared?
- If there are now, or someday may be, two careers, how will priorities be set? Whose career will come first?
- Will there be a dominant personality in the home? Or will there be a split dominance, each taking charge of certain areas?

The best-laid plans, of course, can go astray. Couples need to be ready to renegotiate if change (in individuals, goals, circumstances within and outside the family) comes, as it so often does. An already married couple, coming upon change, can sit down with a similar list and renegotiate.

MAKING MARRIAGE WORK

Though the externals of every marriage differ, there are internal elements that are basic to almost every successful union: genuine interest in one another; conscious effort to help one another realize potential and grow in confidence; spontaneous expression of emotion and affection; shared backgrounds, understanding, and commitment; mutual admiration and respect.

Sociologist George Shanker points out that many marriages fall short of these goals because they carry into the home the virus of competitiveness that infects the larger society. Each puts the other down to bolster his or her own ego. Such intrafamily competition demolishes the supportive environment that a family should offer: a haven from pressures, a place to relax and to be oneself without feeling threatened or defensive. In place of competition, a happy marriage employs compromise, negotiation, and mutual support. An interdependence develops between the partners that many authorities find essential to a good relationship (Gadpaille, *b*).

The First Year

The most difficult period of adjustment in a marriage is generally accepted to be the first year. Couples who have used their courtship wisely will have made a good start on getting to know one another. But even those who have lived together will have much to learn after the wedding ceremony. Commitment puts a new face on an old relationship.

A timeworn vaudeville sketch depicts the dismay and disappointment of a newlywed as his wife disrobes in their nuptial chamber, removing her wig, padded bra, false eyelashes, and finally unscrewing a wooden leg. The "natural look" and uninhibited courtships make such deceptions unlikely today. But in subtler ways, the mask does begin to slip after the marriage, and the real person underneath is revealed. By the end of the first year, one study found, a majority of couples became aware of unexpected differences in such areas as religion, in-law relations, attitudes toward time, social lifestyle, recreation, ways of showing affection, communications, finances, and sex (Landis and Landis).

Dr. Tom McGinnis in *Your First Year of Marriage* suggests that individuals who are prepared to find their mates and marriages a little less than perfect, who accept and accommodate themselves to each other's minor foibles (leaving the cap off the toothpaste or dishes in the sink, occasional lack of tact, a

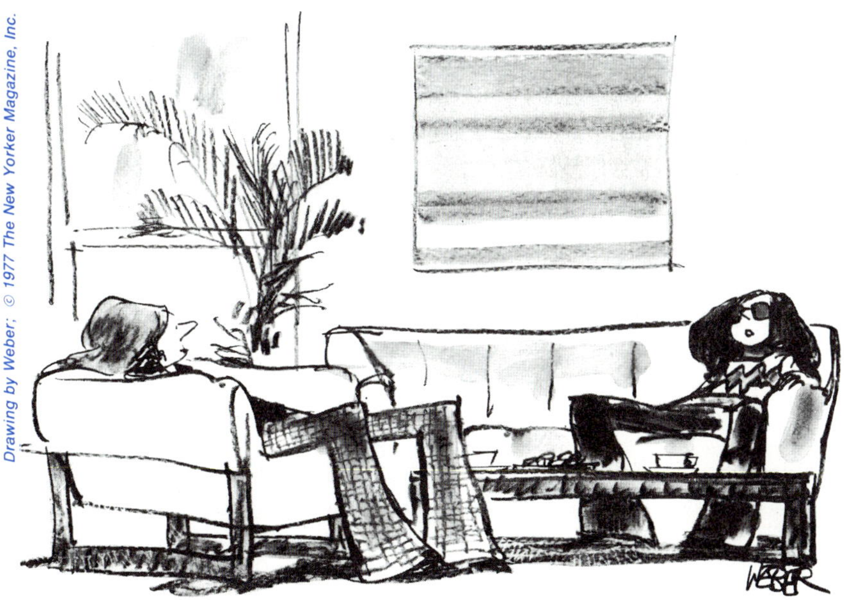

"They have this arrangement. He earns the money and she takes care of the house."

The good marriage is somewhat like a trapeze act. To begin with, it requires a certain aptitude, a basic wish to work with one other person in some death defying venture. Then it takes a good lot of practice before the real soaring begins. Success requires each partner to be independent, to be strong in a critical way, to be responsible for the unit. Through trust and timing and a certain tension, each can help the other reach new heights. Or just enjoy the flying. (Streshinsky, p. 169)

tendency to be late frequently) are well on their way to mutual understanding and long-term marriage survival. Let us look at the major challenges to young marrieds.

The honeymoon Honeymoons are not purely excursions into sensuality. They provide a necessary opportunity for a couple to adjust to one another without distraction from in-laws, friends, jobs, school. The honeymoon should be viewed as a marriage workshop, with plenty of anxiety, disappointments, and mistakes, as well as some pleasant surprises.

In-laws Parents on both sides (most often the mother-in-law) are often a cause of early marital friction, particularly if the young couple lived at home or were totally dependent upon parents for support up until the wedding. Young couples can set the stage for good in-law relationships early, even during the courtship period, by agreeing to let parents know that, though they love and respect them and are interested in their counsel, marriage decisions will be made jointly by husband and wife and no one else. They might remind parents that many pages before the Bible spoke of honoring father and mother, it said, "Therefore shall a man leave his father and mother, and shall cleave unto his wife, and they shall be one flesh" (Genesis 2:24).

Open communications Ideally, openness begins to develop during courtship. Each partner learns to understand and express his or her feelings and thoughts and to listen to and understand the feelings and thoughts of the spouse. Helpful pointers about good communication include: (1) Be sure you know what your mate is really saying. Don't jump to conclusions; if you're not sure, ask. (2) Be sure your mate knows what you are saying; be specific, clarify. (3) Watch for significant body language (a frown, a clenched fist, a tapping foot) which may indicate true feelings even better than words.

Disagreements If a couple never quarrel, either they do not care enough to disagree or they are bottling up their feelings, in which case the bottle is sure to explode ultimately. *Intimate Enemy* co-authors Dr. George R. Bach and Peter Wyden suggest that constructive quarreling is necessary for a healthy marriage and that smothering differences or arguing in a hurtful way can lead to real or "emotional" divorce.

Learning how to handle disagreements intelligently is an important marriage skill that can be learned in the first year or the fortieth. Dr. McGinnis offers some guidelines:

- The couple can try to determine what the underlying disagreement is, rather than debate surface issues. The battle over who should do the dishes may simply be a symptom of the husband's ignoring his wife because he has been heavily involved in a business crisis.
- If there is strong disagreement about a decision, husband and wife can explore some of the following questions: How does the decision relate to their basic marriage goals? Who is more concerned with the decision? Who must live most closely with it? How do friends and relatives solve such a problem? Is it worth doing something daring if both cannot agree?

As the mechanism for decision making becomes familiar, disagreements become less difficult to handle, especially if two senses are exercised: humor and perspective.

The Campus Marriage

Despite the trend toward remaining single longer, many young men and women marry while still in college. Although divorce rates are highest for marriages where the partners are under 21 (U.S. Department of Commerce), a campus marriage offers many advantages to an emotionally mature young couple. They may find that, once married, they can concentrate more effectively on schoolwork, are less frustrated and tense, and have a home that offers a welcome sanctuary from the pressure cooker of campus competition. But there are many pitfalls, each of which should be honestly examined before the wedding.

The reason for the marriage A young marriage may be built on quicksand if it took place because of: feelings of inadequacy and lack of self-esteem; a desire to become part of the adult world and counteract the adult-status frustration of college; a need to escape parental restrictions; parents who prefer the couple to marry rather than "live together"; or a pregnancy that neither partner wants to abort.

Money problems If both partners are to continue in school, financial difficulties may be severe. Often parents will continue support, but the money may come with strings attached. When parents do not provide support, education and future plans may have to be shelved or altered in order for the couple to survive. If either or both is forced to sacrifice educational or career dreams, resentment can mount, explode, and subsequently destroy the union. Explosions may also occur because of inexperience in handling bills and debts that may quickly collect.

Scheduling A couple juggling school, marriage, and work schedules may find they have less time to spend together than before marriage. Housekeeping chores may prove unexpectedly time-consuming, and a fair sharing and scheduling of responsibilities needs to be worked out and adhered to.

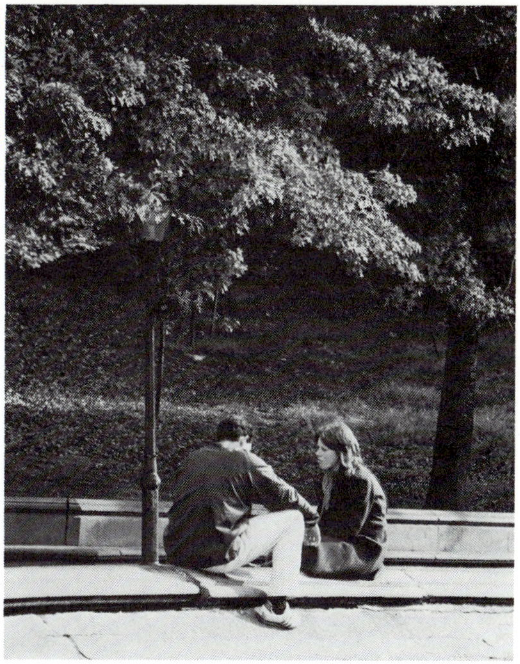
Erika Stone/Peter Arnold

Good communication is an important element in successful marriage.

Help for the Troubled Marriage

Few marriages fail when both partners are sincerely willing to work at them. Without that effort, few marriages succeed. If a marriage runs into trouble, couples can often learn a system of negotiating or bargaining that can help them. Here is how one such system, developed by Dr. Philip Croce, works. First, both partners must be willing to accept a set of four ground rules on faith:

1 If there is a problem that produces friction, the partners share the responsibility equally.

WHERE TO GET HELP
To Save a Troubled Marriage

Not everyone who hangs out a shingle offering marriage counseling is a qualified professional. In many states there is no licensing required. A qualified counselor will have years of specialized training; a degree in counseling, psychology, social work, or psychiatry from a recognized institution; and probably membership in one of the professional organizations listed below. Counseling need not be prohibitively expensive; many community mental health centers make it available for minimal or no cost at all.

For the name of a qualified counselor, write or call any of the following professional organizations:

National
- American Association of Marriage and Family Counselors, 225 Yale Avenue, Claremont, CA 91711
- American Psychological Association, 1200 17th Street, N.W., Washington, DC 20036
- National Association of Social Workers, 2 Park Avenue, New York, NY 10016
- American Association of Pastoral Counselors, 201 East 19th Street, New York, NY 10003
- American Psychiatric Association, 1700 18th Street, N.W., Washington, DC 20009
- American Academy of Psychotherapists, Directory Editor, 1101 Third Street, S.W., Washington, DC 20001

Community
- Family Service Association of America, 44 East 23rd Street, New York, NY 10010
- National Association for Mental Health, 10 Columbus Circle, New York, NY 10019
- Psychiatric Outpatient Clinics Of America, 504 Wolf's Head Building, Oil City, PA 16301

Religious
- National Council of Churches of Christ in the U.S.A., Department of Family Life, 475 Riverside Drive, New York, NY 10027
- National Catholic Welfare Conference, Family Life Bureau, 1312 Massachusetts Avenue, N.W., Washington, DC 20005
- Jewish Family Service Agency, 33 West 60th Street, New York, NY 10023

2 They are in love with one another, even if they feel numb, angry, jealous, or depressed, and even if they temporarily doubt that love.
3 The perfect partner does not exist, and so they must discard the "grass-is-always-greener" fantasies.
4 They will both have to change equally or there will be overt or covert resentment.

The bargaining itself is easy and interesting, though, of course, it will not work for everyone. The couple examine the problems that have been causing friction. They may see different causes, but at this point the causes are not important. Each jots down a list of all the things he or she thinks the other can do to ease the friction. Now the bargaining begins: "If you do this, I'll do that." The next step is to live up to the bargains. Each can be reminded by the other of failure to keep the bargain. By mutual agreement, this is not "nagging." As time goes by, new lists are drawn up and

Improving a Good Marriage: Marriage Encounter

The word "encounter" conjures up a picture of nude touching sessions, of shouting and screaming matches, or of group confessionals. Such sessions for married couples have been almost uniformly condemned by professional marriage counselors. Widely respected, however, is Marriage Encounter, Inc., founded by a Spanish priest in the 1950s. It has spread worldwide and now has units for Jewish and Protestant couples as well as for Catholics. Groups meet for encounter weekends, with the basic goal of learning and renewing communication skills. Though the *teaching* is done in a group, the *communication* is done by the couples in the privacy of their own rooms. Members warn that encounter is not for unhappy or shaky marriages but rather a way of improving and enriching good ones and enlivening dull ones.

bargained. Later lists are more likely to get to basic problems and causes than earlier ones. Reaching the desired result may take months, even a year or more. Setbacks may occur. But if both really try, marital problems can sometimes be ironed out in this way.

When self-help fails, a couple should seek outside counseling, preferably together, before their differences become irreconcilable. They may turn first to a trusted cleric or family doctor. Many are trained counselors and can handle marital conflicts themselves; others can offer a sympathetic ear and recommend a professional counselor.

WHEN MARRIAGE FAILS

Even skillful counseling cannot keep some marriages together. A couple may reach a point in their relationship where they find there is nothing left. Though to outsiders and friends they may look perfectly content, their ability to meet change and growth in one another's lives has broken down. All attempts to revive the relationship fail, sometimes because the attempts are weak, inadequate, or without professional guidance. The only solution appears to be divorce.

It is a solution to which more and more Americans are turning. A woman born between 1935 and 1939, it is estimated, has a 1 in 4 chance of divorce before she is 50. In 1890, there were 18 marriages for every divorce; in 1973 there were just over 2 marriages for each divorce. The ratio continues to narrow. Sociologist Harold T. Christensen believes there is a separation or desertion for each divorce, which means that the chances that a couple who marry today will stay together are about 50-50. Their chances are somewhat better if they have a college education, have a higher than average income, and are white.

Contributory Factors to Marital Breakup

In no two divorces are the problems and causes exactly the same. But the overall divorce picture is affected by some common situations or attitudes both within the marriage and outside it:

1 Unfulfilled (often unrealistic) expectations for romance, success, excitement, whatever
2 Neighbors or friends who are divorcing, influencing a couple to assess its own relationship critically
3 Stress on self-fulfillment and assertiveness where the concept of "I" becomes more important than "we"
4 A wife who is convinced that the only way she can prove herself as a person is to get out from under the domination of her husband and become self-supporting

Thoughts on Divorce

During my marriage I had blamed most of my problems on our relationship. After I was single again, I was surprised to find myself . . . still subject to mood swings, anxiety and frustration—only this time I had no one to blame but myself. (Green, p. 51)

I suppose if I had it to do all over again I would have stayed married to Ike St. John. He was a good husband and in the long run I think I would have been happier. I think people get divorced too easily. (St. John, p. 12A)

. . . the divorced man is likely to be alone much of the time, and the absence of any family life can also leave a keen ache. . . . Suddenly, too, he has to handle new and irksome tasks, like attending to his laundry, meals and housekeeping, and this upsets him further. . . . It is the unendingness of alimony payments that drives men crazy. It turns a man's mind to fantasies of murder and escape. (Epstein, p. 29)

I needed to get married for security and identity, and Jim needed a child-wife to make him feel like a hero. My woman's group pressured us not to tolerate that kind of screwed-up marital situation. People would put you down and make you feel guilty for allowing yourself to be "oppressed." You were supposed to split and find yourself—to become a new woman. (Streshinsky, p. 212)

5 Disagreement about the structure and support of the family, particularly the woman's role
6 Breakdown of the extended family (several generations living and interacting together), removing the support of close relatives and pushing the couple into a totally self-sufficient unit that becomes stifling
7 A longer lifespan, leading couples whose children are grown to suddenly find they have another 20 or 30 years together and not much left in common
8 A greater acceptance of divorce and eased divorce laws

Sometimes divorce is not desired, but becomes inevitable. Perhaps a blow-up occurs. One angry partner calls an attorney as a bluff. From that point on, the couple find themselves in a fight to the finish, particularly where divorce proceedings are of the adversary type, pitting one spouse against the other. The introduction in many states of a no-fault divorce (in which neither party need be charged with adultery, cruelty, or other grounds for divorce) may help ease the situation, allowing couples to reconsider their relationships in a calmer atmosphere.

Children and Divorce

Children are often the unintended victims of divorce. Parents become so involved in attacking one another that they ignore the effects of their belligerence on the young. Even when the divorce is over, parents may continue to use the children as pawns in an emotional battle. And children learn to use their parents in the same way. As difficult as divorce is for children, living in an intact home in which "emotional divorce" has taken place, where bickering and backbiting or simply chilling silences replace love and affection, may be even worse (Despert).

Divorce Takes Effort

Divorce is not just emotionally and financially draining; it is hard work as well. An intelligent divorce, particularly where children are involved, takes a great deal of planning, energy, goodwill, and cooperation. It has been suggested that if couples would put equivalent effort and goodwill into trying to save their marriages, the divorce rate would certainly drop.

ALTERNATIVES TO MARRIAGE

Living Together

Psychiatrist Nathan Ackerman once said that marriage is a symbol of readiness to cope with commitment and responsibility. "Marriage," he said, "is yes or no, not maybe."

Today a growing number (some 250,000 listed in the census of 1974) of couples are opting for "maybe." The phenomenon of living together blossomed so swiftly that sociologists were not ready with a name for the relationship. Among those suggested: unlawful union, unmarried living together (ULT) or living together unmarried (LTU), consensual union (CU), and unmalia (unmarried liaisons).

There are many reasons for such relationships. Some say that living together allows more emotional and personal freedom than marriage and that the lack of reliance on "a piece of paper" makes for a more honest relationship. Others, who point to the 35 percent divorce rate, see it as an easier union to break. For still others, it is a trial marriage, a chance to test a relationship. And finally, for some, living together is just a good experience—no pretensions, no nonsense, no strings attached.

Couples living together often agree to structure their relationship loosely, with freedom, including sexual freedom, for each. Yet most remain faithful, and ironically, when the permitted freedom is acted upon, guilt and a sense of betrayal are often felt. Couples living together try hard to avoid traditional roles, but often the males fall into the typical "husband" role, and the females into classic

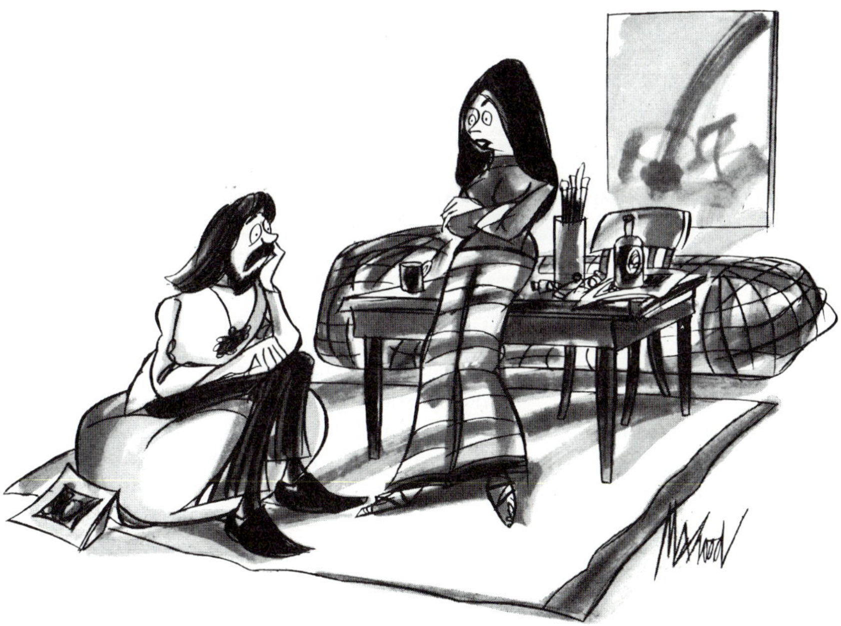

"I thought people had to be married for the magic to go out."

To Tell or Not to Tell

If you suspect your parents won't budge an inch in their moral stand, if you feel that they'll be deeply hurt, that there will be unwanted changes in your relationship with them, or even that they'd really be happier not knowing the truth, your candor would be pointless—even a big mistake. It's wise to examine your own motives, too—sometimes people use "truth" as a weapon against others. But if you really believe your family will come to accept your living arrangement, there are advantages to confiding in them. Keeping up a pretense both lends romantic unreality to your situation and comes between you and your parents, tainting what could be an open, loving relationship.

There are good and bad ways to tell them, if that's what you decide to do. It's not wise to meet them at the airport with the introduction, "This is my roommate, Jeff." Breaking it to them by letter is safest, according to Stanford University counselor James Fadiman. Then, by the time you see each other, some of the initial shock will have worn off.

If you can anticipate what your parents' objections might be, it will be easier to deal with them. They may see your living together as a personal affront, a rejection and thus a judgment of the way they've been living—namely, married—for years. (Sarrel and Sarrel, *b*)

"wife" roles (Mainardi; Whitehurst; Clatworthy).

Because the freedom to walk out is always there, each partner lives with the unsettling threat of imminent loss of mate. The burden of living with this lack of commitment is one of the major problems that unmarried couples, who make up 20 percent of the case load of some marriage counselors, bring to counseling sessions.

Many young couples, nevertheless, feel strongly that living together is a good experience. Some who have married after such a relationship point out how it helped their marriage:

> It helps to know how someone will react in all kinds of silly situations that you don't come across in dating—like how angry they get because dinner is cold or what they are like before their morning coffee. How do they deal with being frustrated or depressed? Do they express what they are feeling or keep everything inside? Living together, you find out.

In spite of such testimonials, there is no evidence that the marriages of those who have lived together before the ceremony are more successful than the unions of those who have not. For most couples, the relationship changes drastically once the marriage commitment has been made. In addition, many well-suited couples living together break up permanently over small disagreements that they would probably have made an effort to resolve had they been tied to one another by a "piece of paper."

Few unmarried relationships endure as is. Those that develop into matches where caring about the other replaces caring about self move on to marriage. The others rarely survive the first year's renewal of the lease.

Staying Single

It has been reported that some 40 million single Americans, nearly half aged 19 to 29, nearly 60 percent female, spend some $205 billion a year in the single-minded pursuit of happiness (*U.S. News and World Report*). To the outsider, their lives appear all flashy sports cars, skiing at Aspen, sunbathing in the Aegean, and perpetual romance. In reality, the picture is not so rosy.

The incomes of single people employed full time are lower than those of married people,

Richard Wood/Taurus Photos

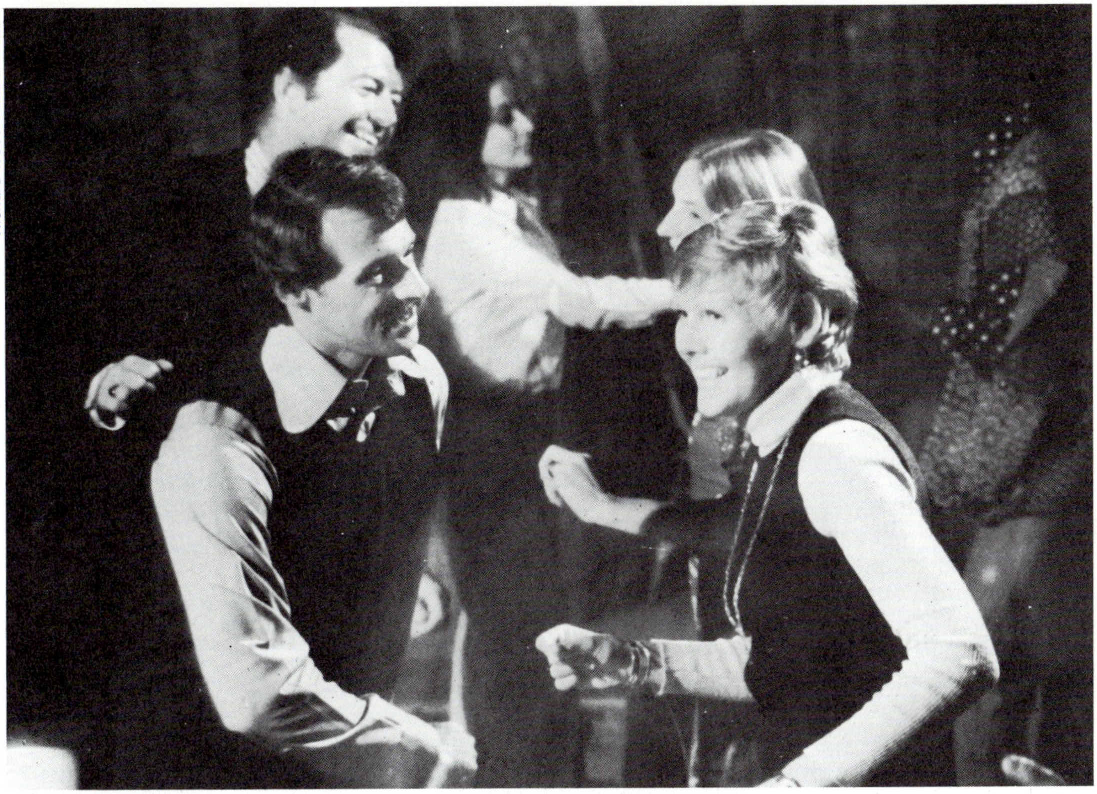

The old stereotypes of bachelor and spinster are rapidly disappearing as increasing numbers of Americans choose a single lifestyle.

although the gap is narrowing. Single people are less likely to hold professional, managerial, or administrative jobs, though their level of education is a shade higher than that of married people. They tend to die earlier, particularly the male. Females living alone are especially vulnerable to violence in some areas.

There are many reasons behind a decision to remain single, not just for a few extra years of independence, fun, and experimentation, but for life:

1 *The population explosion* Many people feel less need to have children.
2 *The sexual revolution* Availability of intercourse outside of marriage eliminates sex as a reason for marriage.
3 *Women's liberation* Women nowadays are better trained, more able to be self-supporting.
4 *The acceptance of single parenthood and abortion as alternatives to the shotgun wedding.*
5 *The new emphasis on individual freedom and fulfillment.*
6 *The high cost of rearing children, both emotionally and financially.*
7 *Increased male self-sufficiency around the house.*

In deciding between marriage and the single life, individuals consider the benefits of marriage: a full-time companion, in times of joy and of sorrow; a regular sex partner; someone to grow with; the fulfillment of children to nurture and give one "immortality"; someone to count on when health fails or things get rough; and especially as the years wear on, a friend to ward off loneliness. They weigh these factors against the benefits of the second: freedom; independence; less economic hassle; more chance for travel and excitement; no children to tie one down or to worry about; more variety in friends of both sexes; more variety in sexual opportunity.

Other Alternatives

Some other alternatives to traditional marriage are only just emerging, such as the homosexual marriage. Others are apparently dipping in popularity. The number of young people going to live on communes is down since 1972. Wife swapping and the swinging married life seem to be losing favor. Group marriages, in which three or more partners share board and bed and children, appear to be very short-lived. Larry and Joan Constatine report that, of the group marriages they studied, only 44 percent lasted even a year. After five years, no more than 7 percent were still hanging in there.

Future Alternatives

Many observers of the family scene have, in recent years, suggested a revamping of the present marital system. Though proposals vary, they usually include a formalized trial marriage or confirmation period, with no children permitted, that would last a year or two and then be finalized. Other suggestions have included periodic reevaluation—for example, when the children have grown and left home—at which time the couple decide whether to continue the marriage. Couples could have serial marriages, as many now do by following the divorce-remarriage route. None of the authors has suggested how to resolve matters when one partner wants to stay married and the other does not.

H. L. Mencken once said, "For every human problem, there is a solution that is simple, neat and wrong." It remains to be seen whether the newly suggested solutions will be superior to those that have been with us for so many centuries of courtship, marriage, and divorce.

LOOKING BACK

REVIEWING CONCEPTS IN CHAPTER 21

- Some social commentators suggest that marriage as we know it is on the way out and that other forms of the male-female relationship will replace it. So far there is no clear evidence that this is happening.
- Love (when the other's satisfaction and security become as important as one's own) differs from being "in love" (a state of infatuation which is based on a physical attraction and is relatively self-centered).
- Though love is blind, the potential mate needs to be examined with eyes wide open. Many authorities suggest that the absence of preparation for marriage and premarital counseling is one of the reasons for the high failure rate of American marriages.
- Most couples decide before marriage what kind of arrangement they wish to have, how they will share responsibilities and tasks as well as free time.

- In order to offer a haven from the competitive society in which we live, marriage must be free of intrafamily rivalry. Spouses should offer each other mutual support.
- The first year, because of the difficulty of adjustment, is often the most difficult. Good communications, negotiations, and compromise can ease the adjustment.
- Campus marriages can succeed, if they take place for the right reasons and if the couple can remain relatively independent of parents on both sides.
- Counseling help for a troubled marriage is most effective if both partners participate in the sessions; it takes two to cause the problems and two to cure them.
- Many persons today are opting for alternatives to marriage, though few select alternatives permanently. Most persons eventually marry.

22

WAYS AND MEANS: FAMILY PLANNING AND BIRTH CONTROL

WHAT'S AHEAD IN CHAPTER 22 What are the various ways in which humans have tried to prevent a frequent result of intercourse: the birth of offspring? What are the advantages and drawbacks of each method? Which are most effective? Which are *not* effective? Are the same approaches best for everyone? Whose responsibility is birth control? What factors should be considered by a couple making a decision about birth control? How does the irreversibility of sterilization influence those thinking of using it for birth control? What are the various points of view about abortion? What elements might a couple, or a woman alone, consider in thinking about abortion? What are the alternatives for the unmarried pregnant woman? For those who select abortion, when is the best time?

Since ancient times, the human race has attempted to interfere with what often seemed the inevitable outcome of sexual intercourse: the production of offspring. There have been five basic ways in which this has been done: *contraception* (*contra* = against), which prevents the conception that would occur as a result of the meeting of sperm and egg; *contraimplantation*, which prevents a fertilized ovum from implanting itself in the uterus and commencing growth; *sterilization*, which permanently blocks conception; *abortion*, which removes the product of conception; and in some societies, *infanticide* (*cide* = kill), which eliminated born but unwanted children.

Today, the first four approaches are used by both married and unmarried couples who do not want to have children, and are used by married couples to time and space their offspring in the most desirable way: *family planning.*

DECIDING ABOUT BIRTH CONTROL

Those who participate in sexual relations, in or outside marriage, have a decision to make about contraception. Before making it, they should: (1) thoroughly inform themselves about all methods of contraception and about such birth control techniques as sterilization and abortion; (2) learn the benefits and risks of each method; (3) decide whether pregnancy is an acceptable risk; (4) consider personal convenience and preference as well as health needs; (5) apply personal values, including religious ones, to the decision.

Because no birth control method is without hazard (either the method itself, or from the risk of a pregnancy that might result), risks have to be weighed against benefits. There is no one best contraceptive and the choice for each couple may be made for different reasons. More important than the contraceptive chosen are the care and consistency with which it is used. (See Figure 22.1.)

CONTRACEPTION

Formulas for contraceptive potions, employing such ingredients as crocodile dung, honey, and acacia tips, have been found among ancient Egyptian cosmetic recipes. The Bible tells of Onan using what appeared to be "withdrawal" (removal of the penis from the vagina before ejaculation) in order to avoid carrying out his obligation to make his dead brother's wife pregnant. Ancient Chinese men scorned such profligate waste of "seed." They did not ejaculate at all because they believed that recycling the semen to the brain would increase the lifespan. Advice on how to accomplish this remarkable feat? Think of the woman as ugly and hateful; gnash the teeth.

If early birth control methods sound laughable, consider the contemporary experience of a newlywed couple who, on their wedding night, suddenly realized they had forgotten to "take precautions." The husband unceremoniously dumped his wife into the bathtub, then hurried to the nearest all-night pharmacy for a vaginal douche—which is no more effective in preventing conception than the bath or crocodile dung. There are, however, a good many effective contraceptives today, and they are more widely used than ever before in history.

Married couples in the United States are reaching the point of near perfect contraception use. By 1973, 70 percent were believed to be using some form of birth control. Of the remaining 30 percent, many were pregnant, trying to become pregnant, or infertile. The

While family planning and use of effective contraception have grown significantly in this country, the young teenager remains at great risk of unwanted pregnancy.

Erika Stone/Peter Arnold

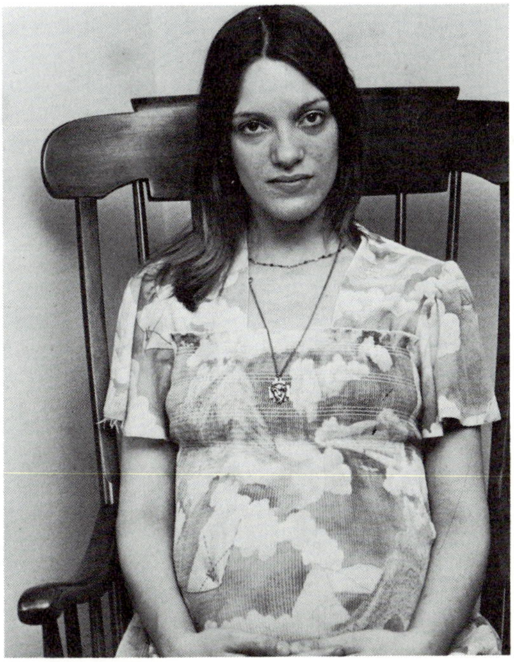

Positions of Major Religious Faiths on Birth Control

Protestant Most Protestant denominations view the purpose of marriage as including not only parenthood but the nourishment of mutual love and companionship of husband and wife as well as service to society. They hold contraception to be morally right when the motivations of the couple are right. Factors to be taken into account include the right of children to be wanted, loved, educated; the health and welfare of the mother; and socioeconomic conditions (National Council of Churches).

Roman Catholic The traditional Catholic position embraces the concept of family planning as a means to responsible parenthood, but holds that this can be achieved only through the rhythm method and only when serious cause—medical, eugenic (potential hereditary disease), economic, or social—is present. Catholic couples having such cause can practice the rhythm method without the permission of their priests (G. Kelly).

Liberal Catholic clergy and laypeople take a more lenient view, seeing other forms of birth control as no different from the rhythm method except that they are more effective. A papal commission appointed by Pope John XXIII concluded:

> The regulation of conception appears necessary for many couples who wish to achieve a responsible, open, and reasonable parenthood in today's circumstances. If they are to observe and cultivate all the essential values of marriage, married people need decent and human means for the regulation of conception. (Guttmacher, p. 133)

Jewish Birth control is sanctioned to some degree by all the major branches of Judaism. Sex in marriage is recognized as having two functions: (1) begetting children, and (2) enriching the relationship between husband and wife. The birth control methods most acceptable are those that interfere least with normal intercourse, such as the Pill and the diaphragm (Feldman). The liberal *Reform* movement has declared that "parents have the right to determine the number and to space the births of their children in accordance with what they believe to be in the best interests of their families" (Central Conference of American Rabbis). The more moderate *Conservative* movement has affirmed the use of contraception on economic as well as health grounds when "the earning capacity of the family makes the postponement of childbearing or the limitation of the number of children socially wise and necessary" (Rabbinical Assembly of America). *Orthodox* rabbis, on the other hand, permit birth control methods used by the woman but only when the physical or mental health of the mother is jeopardized and only on rabbinic approval (Rabbinical Alliance of America).

> Family planning gave us a new life. My husband and me, we got five kids. We was having one every year. Nobody would rent us an apartment with so many. We had to stay in our little three room walk-up in a terrible neighborhood. But the clinic saved us. It's been five years since the last baby. We've been saving money instead of paying doctor bills. Now we're moving out to Long Island . . . to a house of our own. God bless these people for what they did for us. . . .
>
> A woman at a family planning clinic in New York City

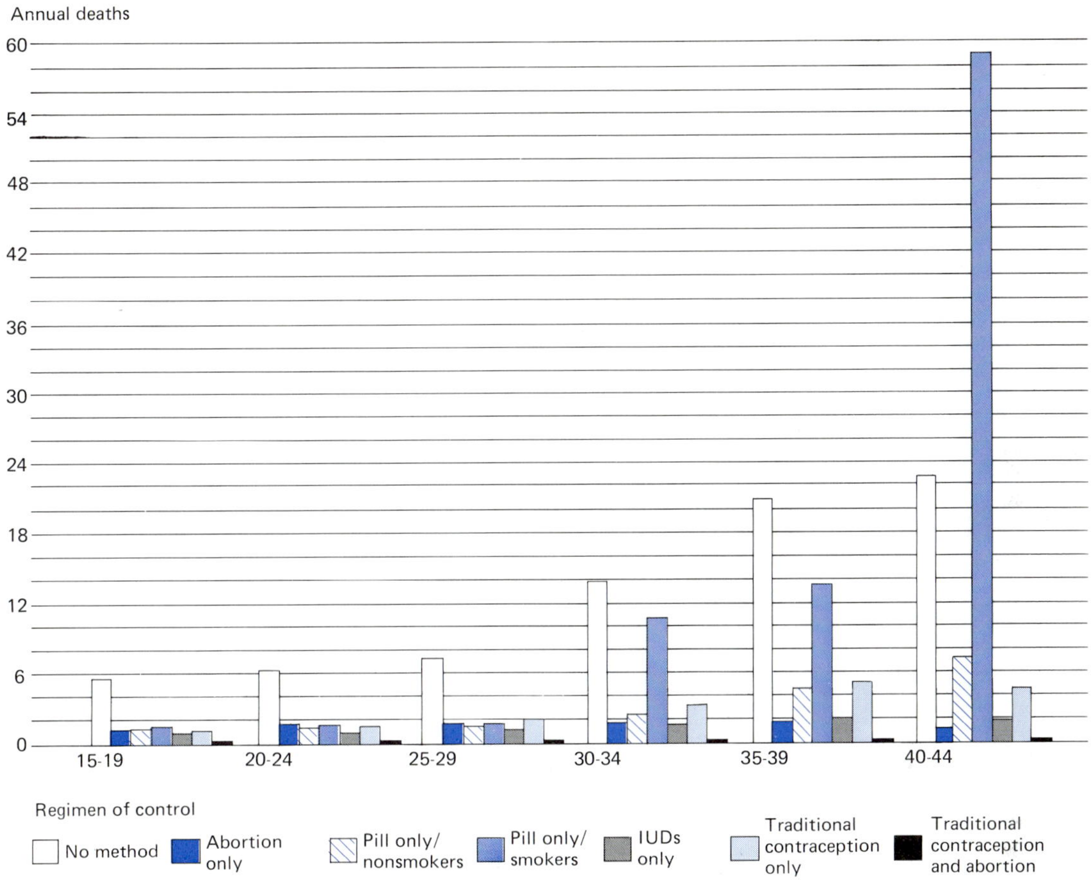

FIGURE 22.1 Annual number of deaths associated with control of fertility and no control per 100,000 nonsterile women, by regimen of control and age of woman. The main risk for traditional forms of birth control—the condom and the diaphragm—is from pregnancy when the methods fail or the individual uses them incorrectly. The risk with the Pill and abortion is from the methods themselves. Riskiest birth control, even more hazardous than pregnancy and childbirth, is the Pill used by women over 40 who smoke. The safest form of fertility control at all ages is the condom or diaphragm backed up by abortion should pregnancy occur. [*After Tietze, b, p. 76.*]

oral contraceptive, the "Pill," is the most widely used method among women married fewer than 10 years. Sterilization is first among couples married longer. The IUD (the intrauterine device) is third. But recent findings about possible dangers of the Pill and the IUD have induced a slight shift toward such "old-fashioned" contraceptive methods as the diaphragm and the condom (Westoff and Jones).

The greatest growth in family planning is evident in low-income couples, previously subject to a weary cycle of recurrent pregnancies. Today the lower-income family has almost attained the level of effective contraception usage experienced by higher-income couples.

One segment of the population, however, the young teenagers, remains at great risk of unwanted pregnancy, out of ignorance or inability or unwillingness to obtain birth control information. Though the percentage of teens using contraceptives is growing (up from 18.4 percent in 1971 to 30 percent in 1976), 25 percent *never* use contraception (Kantner and Zelnik, *c*). First intercourse usually occurs without contraception, often so as not to interfere with the spontaneity and naturalness of the act. Contraception use is higher among older teenagers. Kantner and Zelnik (*b*) found some 80 percent of 19-year-old college students using some form of birth control. Of the estimated 4 million sexually active female teenagers, about 1 million become pregnant each year and an estimated 600,000 live births result (MMWR, *c*).

Nearly half the teenagers in one study who did not use contraception believed they could not become pregnant for reasons like: "I'm too young" or "It's the wrong time of the month" or "I don't do it often enough." One-quarter either did not know what to do or were unwilling to bother. A small percentage refrained from contraception because boyfriends objected, or because they believed birth control to be wrong for religious or other reasons (Kantner and Zelnik, *a*).

The Oral Contraceptive

Some 50 million women around the world use oral contraceptives (OCs)—the Pill. The goal of the Pill (not one pill, but 40 different brands, containing varying ratios of the female hormones estrogen and progesterone) is to prevent the monthly release of an ovum. It accomplishes this by supplying estrogens and/or progesterone, mimicking the hormonal conditions of pregnancy, during which ovulation does not occur. In additon, it causes the cervix to produce a thick mucus which is difficult for sperm to penetrate, and keeps the uterine lining too thin to properly nourish a fertilized ovum should one somehow run the blockade. Controversy about the safety of the Pill has reduced use in the United States.

Benefits Aside from its high contraceptive effectiveness and the fact that it does not interfere with the enjoyment of sex, the Pill has other benefits. It often helps regulate a woman's menstrual cycle, eases acne, slightly increases breast size and reduces incidence of benign breast nodules, eases menstrual discomfort and reduces iron loss by reducing blood loss. As a side benefit, women on the Pill may receive improved medical care because they must return to physician or clinic for regular checkups before receiving refills.

Risks Because 15 to 20 years of regular use by a large population are needed for full evaluation of a drug, the full story on OCs may not be in until the 1980s. What do scientists suspect so far?[1] Young teenagers and women over 40 appear to be at greatest risk. The Pill may stop growth in young women by making them chemically mature artificially; it makes older women, especially those who smoke, much more susceptible to heart and blood vessel damage.

A variety of other problems have been linked to the oral contraceptive, including increased risk of venous thrombosis (blood clots in the vein), elevated blood pressure and serum cholesterol levels, erosion and ulceration of the cervix, noncancerous liver tumors, gallbladder disease, and some types of infection, possibly because the pills interfere with the immune system. About 10 to 30 percent of women on the Pill report mood changes,

[1]Compiled from Royal College of General Practitioners and Kaiser-Permanente reports, the Vessey et al. study, and an interview with Dr. Heinz Berendes.

Randy Matusow

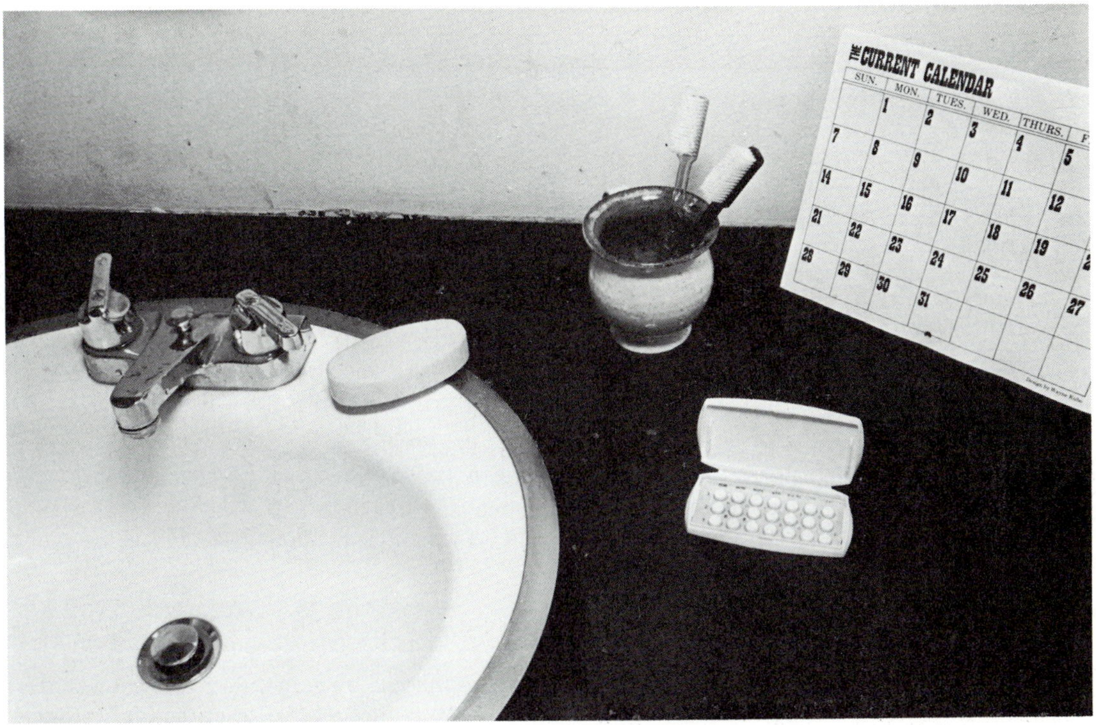

With oral contraceptives, as with other medications, risks must carefully be weighed against benefits before a decision to use them is made.

especially depression. These changes may be related to salt and water retention or to the vitamin B_6 deficiency caused by the Pill. Reports of reduced sexual interest are balanced by other reports from women who claim improved sex drive because they no longer fear pregnancy.

Metabolic changes in Pill takers may lead to earlier risk of diabetes in susceptible women, to epilepsy, migraine headaches, skin disorders, and facial paralysis, but cause and effect have not been proven. Such relatively minor annoyances as varicose veins, hyperpigmentation (darkening) of skin, hair loss, breast tenderness, headache, and absence of menstruation have also been noted. Nausea and vomiting have been experienced by some Pill takers, and it is important to remember that when vomiting takes place right after a pill is swallowed, the medication is lost and the dose must be repeated.

The only oral contraceptives definitely linked to cancer have been taken off the market. But it is too soon to state categorically that a link will not be found with other OCs. Several studies have found a linkage, however, between birth defects and use of the Pill just prior to or during pregnancy. Authorities recommend that women discontinue the Pill three months before they plan to attempt pregnancy, with a temporary switch at that time to another form of contraception. This will give the hormones time to clear from the body before the baby is conceived. There is some indication that Pill users who have not borne children previously may have difficulty conceiving (Vessey et al.).

Why do physicians continue to prescribe

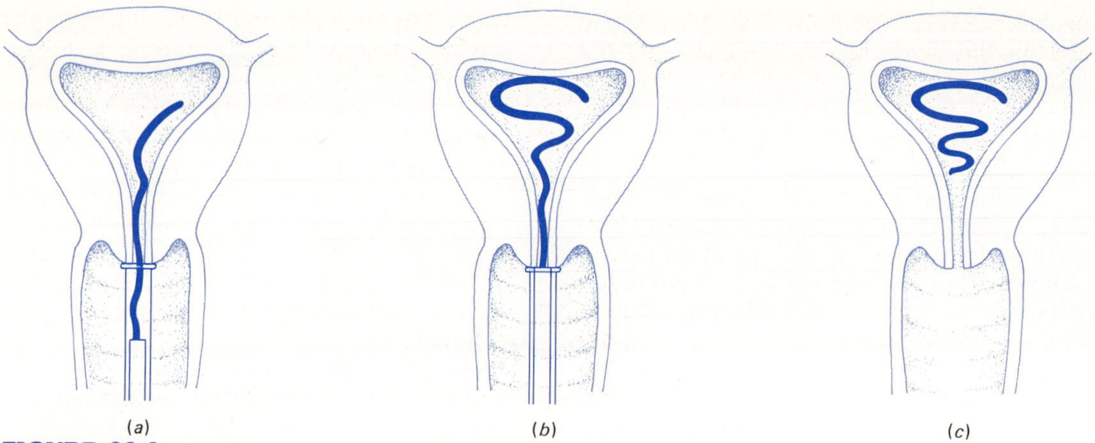

FIGURE 22.2 The IUD is inserted by a physician. Here the Lippes loop is drawn through an insertion tube and inserted through the vagina into the uterus (*a*). As the insertion tube is removed, the loop uncoils in the uterus (*b*). When it is fully in place (*c*), threads extend slightly below the cervix to allow the loop to be removed when necessary.

OCs in the face of the many reported risks? It must be remembered that, for younger women, the risks are still statistically lower than those of pregnancy and childbirth, which are often the alternative to this contraceptive. For women over 40, and those over 30 who smoke, however, the Pill presents a hazard greater than pregnancy.

A woman thinking of using the Pill should expect a thorough medical examination, including an evaluation of her medical history. She should be informed of all the risks and of alternative methods of birth control. In the absence of such a careful procedure, she should turn elsewhere for contraceptive advice. She should also be on the alert for symptoms of serious side effects: severe headaches or abdominal pain, shortness of breath, loss of vision or eye problems, sudden chest, arm, or leg pain.

The Intrauterine Device

In ancient times, camel drivers used to place small olive-sized stones in the uterus of a female camel on long desert treks to avoid impregnation by romantic male camels. Today, the contraceptive of choice for millions of women in the United States is a device called the *intrauterine device* (IUD), which is similarly inserted in the uterus. Scientists are not much more clear on why this prevents pregnancy than the camel drivers were. But current thinking is that the presence of a foreign object inhibits the implantation of the fertilized egg. Thus, the IUD is not, strictly speaking, a contraceptive, but a contraimplantation device.

Benefits IUDs (metal or plastic shaped into spirals, T's, Y's, M's, and other forms) are flexible enough to be inserted into a narrow tube that is slipped through the vagina into the uterus. When the tube is withdrawn, the IUD snaps back into its original shape. Some newer IUDs contain hormones which are released gradually, enhancing the contraceptive effect (these need periodic replacement). The wide variety of designs allows for individualization. Avoidance of pregnancy is about 97 percent assured if the woman experiences no discomfort or problems and the IUD is not expelled. Except for occasional checking to see that the device has not been expelled, the IUD is the contraceptive demanding the least attention. If pregnancy is desired, a physician removes the device.

Risks Possible drawbacks include bleeding, pain, and discomfort in some women; embedding in the uterine wall which can make removal difficult and dangerous; perforation of the uterus, and increased susceptibility to vaginal infection. Sometimes the IUD is spontaneously expelled, and if this should happen without the woman realizing it, risk of pregnancy is naturally high. More serious, however, are FDA-compiled reports of spontaneous abortions, blood poisoning, and scores of deaths when women have become pregnant with the IUD in place. The IUD most responsible for these complications, the Dalkon Shield, has been removed from the market.

IUD packaging now includes written warnings to physician and patient about potential risks. A woman who becomes pregnant while wearing an IUD should have the device removed if she wishes to continue the pregnancy. Though pregnancies have been known to go full term with the IUD in place, risk of a tubal pregnancy, miscarriage, serious infection, or even threat to life is great. Overall medical opinion, however, holds that, under normal circumstances and with careful use, the IUD is a relatively safe and effective method of birth control. The latest refinements have cut down on complications.

The Vaginal Diaphragm

When, near the end of the nineteenth century, a German doctor came up with the idea for a gadget to cover the cervix, or mouth of the uterus, his early diaphragm was not a first. A century earlier, that eminent romantic, Casanova, is said to have devised a similar one from a partially scooped out lemon. Casanova's cap not only kept sperm from entering the uterus, but the citrus had a slight spermicidal (*cide* = kill) effect as well.

Today's diaphragm is soft rubber rimmed with a flexible metal ring, made in a variety of sizes. It must be fitted by a physician or in a family planning clinic, and should be refitted periodically, especially after childbirth, when the cervix has been stretched. As important as the fitting are the how-to-use-it, how-to-check-it instructions. A woman unsure about how to insert the diaphragm is likely to discontinue its use or to position it incorrectly, risking pregnancy. Extremely active intercourse can dislodge the diaphragm. (See Figure 22.3.)

The diaphragm should always be used with a spermicidal jelly or cream, which prevents sperm from moving around the diaphragm and into the uterus. The diaphragm should not be removed nor the gel or cream douched away for six hours following coitus. After each use, the diaphragm should be checked for leaks, washed with soap and water, powdered, and stored carefully. Before having intercourse a second time, the woman must insert another application of spermicide into the vagina without disturbing the diaphragm.

Benefits Correctly used, the diaphragm offers 96 to 98 percent protection against pregnancy. It facilitates intercourse during menstruation, safely blocking flow for up to 12 hours.

Risks There are no serious health risks, but the device may be difficult for a virgin to insert and thus is probably not the best initial contraceptive. Some women spurn the diaphragm, because they see the insertion of a device just prior to intercourse as "too calculating" or disruptive of the romantic mood. This objection can be overcome by routinely inserting the diaphragm before going to bed each night, and being sure to renew the spermicidal gel if several hours pass before intercourse takes place.

The Condom

Casanova, said to pride himself on never getting one of his many lady friends pregnant, was reportedly among the first to use the

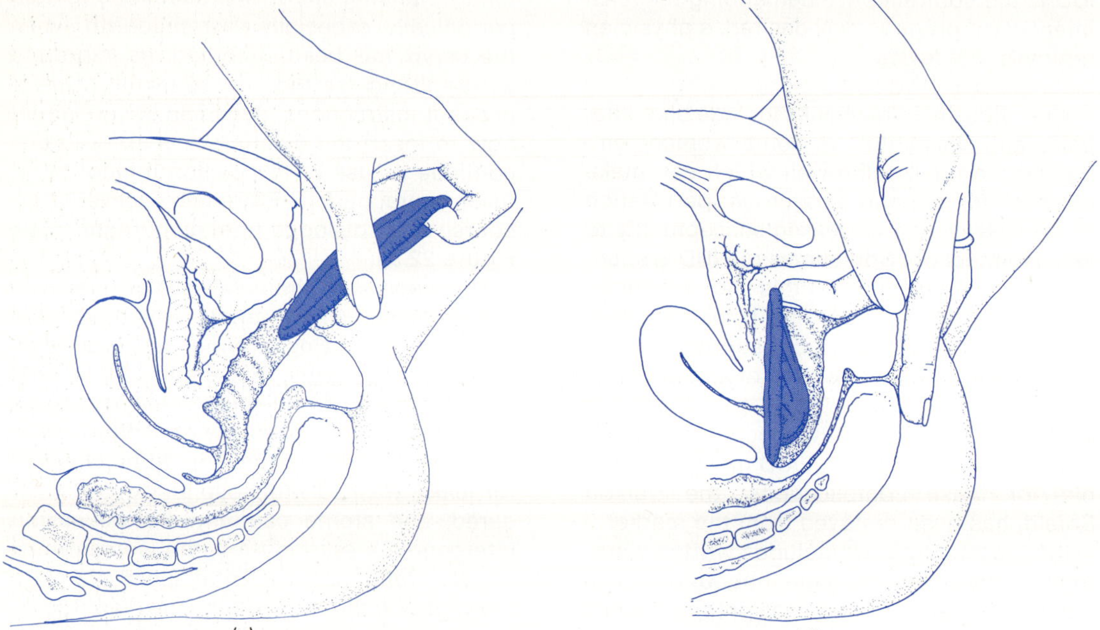

(*a*) (*b*)

FIGURE 22.3 Insertion of the diaphragm. Before use, the diaphragm should be held up to the light to check for pinhole leaks. Then both surfaces should be covered with contraceptive jelly or cream. Compressed as shown above (*a*), the diaphragm can be inserted while the woman is in a squatting position, or in any comfortable position. It should be pushed downward, then tipped to fit behind the pubic bone, until the far end slips into position in the space behind and below the cervix. The woman can check for proper positioning by feeling the cervix through the diaphragm with her fingers (*b*). [*Adapted from* Koromex Diaphragm Patients' Manual Method of Insertion, *Holland-Rantos Co., Inc., April 1973.*]

"sheath" for birth control rather than disease protection. In those days, the condom was made of animal intestine and tied with a ribbon. Today's condom (also called a *rubber, prophylactic,* or *contraceptive*) is usually made of rubber to exacting manufacturing standards and may be sold dry or prelubricated. Natural "skins" made of sheep intestines are available, too, but at a much higher cost for their assertedly superior sensitivity.

Benefits In many ways, the condom is the ideal birth control choice for young, sexually active persons. It is inexpensive and easy to use, requires no prescription, and helps protect against VD. As state laws restricting advertising and display of condoms are struck down, they are becoming more readily available.

Risks The condom causes no harmful side

effects and adds protection against VD, but it is slightly less reliable than the pill or IUD—about 97 percent effective when used properly and teamed with a spermicidal cream or gel. Some couples reject it because they believe it will interfere with sexual pleasure by literally coming between them. Others view the slight decrease in sensitivity as an advantage, allowing the man to withhold orgasm longer. The objection that stopping to put the condom on interrupts the mood of precoital love play can be met by donning the condom as part of shared foreplay.

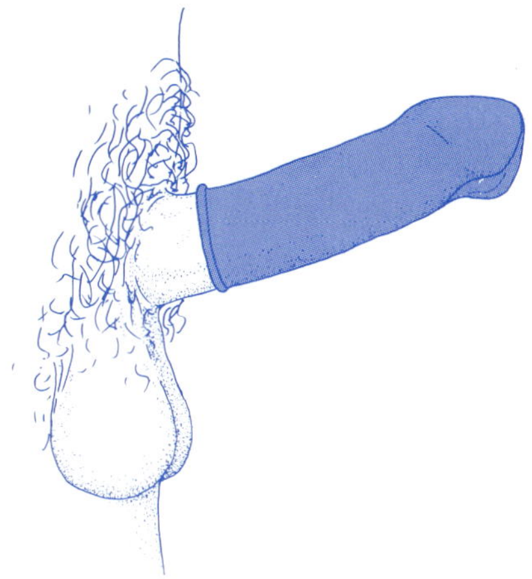

FIGURE 22.4 The condom should be worn so that the tip forms a 1/2-inch reservoir, to prevent splitting under pressure of ejaculation. Some condoms have built-in reservoir tips. To prevent leakage around the edges of the condom, the rubber rim should be gripped firmly as the penis is withdrawn from the vagina following intercourse. Condoms should be kept in their protective foil wrappings until use; old ones, including those in vending machines, may become cracked and dry. Vaseline used as a lubricant can damage the rubber.

Foams, Gels, Creams, and Other Spermicidal Agents

These contraceptive products, not to be confused with lubricating gels and creams often found on the same pharmacy shelves, have a sperm-killing effect. Creams and gels should be used only with condoms or diaphragms. Foam used alone is one of the less reliable contraceptives. Pregnancy rates vary widely from 1.8 to 38.7 pregnancies per 100 women, depending upon the study (Bernstein). Spermicidal agents are most effective when applied no more than half an hour before intercourse. Some doctors recommend doubling suggested doses. These products *should not* be washed or douched away for at least six hours after intercourse and should be reapplied for each intercourse. Spermicidal suppositories, too, are sold, but they are even less reliable. A new suppository-like contraceptive introduced in the United States in 1977, however, after several successful trials in Germany, promises only a 1 percent risk of pregnancy. It melts on insertion in the vagina and forms a protective shield over the mouth of the cervix.

Benefits Spermicidal agents are readily available without prescription.

Risks Though they can cause irritation, spermicidal agents are generally safe. Greatest risk is from pregnancy.

Abstinence

Some persons choose to abstain from intercourse rather than risk pregnancy or contraceptive hazards. This may be abstinence for a night, when no birth control devices are available, or it may be long-term abstinence, when a couple decide to wait for marriage. Such couples may substitute mutual petting and other noncoital forms of lovemaking.

Periodic Abstinence, or the Rhythm Method

The only birth control method sanctioned by the Roman Catholic Church limits inter-

The Rhythm Method

1 *The calendar method* A woman keeps a record of her monthly menstrual cycles for three to six months. She then calculates:

- Day *A* = the number of days in her shortest cycle minus 18
- Day *Z* = the number of days in her longest cycle minus 11

Thus if her longest cycle is 30 days and her shortest 28, she figures:

- Day *A* = 28 − 18 = 10
- Day *Z* = 30 − 11 = 19

Her fertile period (unsafe for intercourse if she does not want to become pregnant) runs from *A* to *Z*, days 10 to 19 of her menstrual cycle, counting the first day of her menstrual period as 1.

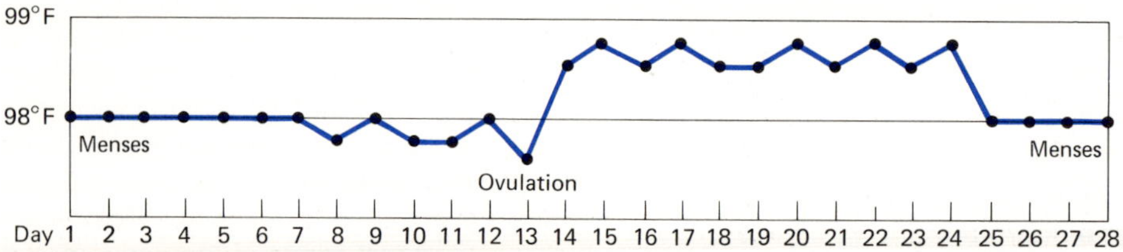

2 *The basal body temperature* The BBT can help to pinpoint more accurately the unsafe period of ovulation. To get the BBT, the woman takes her temperature every morning *immediately* on awakening, before speaking, sitting up, etc. In most women the temperature will drop and then rise abruptly at the time of ovulation as seen above. Three full days after ovulation, intercourse can be resumed.

3 *Other indications of ovulation* Further indications of the release of the ovum may be low abdominal pain (*mittelshmerz*), slight staining in midcycle, a change in the mucus consistency in the vagina. The rhythm method works best when the couple consult a physician or family planning clinic and then follow directions faithfully.

course to "safe" or nonfertile times of the month. It can be fairly effective for women whose monthly periods are absolutely regular, who are meticulous about recordkeeping, and who know how to say no. However, rhythm use is dwindling in the United States.

Rhythm is based on physiology. The single egg released by a woman's ovary each month survives only 12 to 24 hours. Sperm can survive for 48 to 72 hours or more after ejaculation into the female. That leaves about $3\frac{1}{2}$ days during which pregnancy can occur—usually about 14 days before the onset of the next menstrual period. To be fairly certain of avoiding conception, a female with a 28-day cycle must abstain from intercourse for eight days during this fertile time. But for some women, often young ones, whose periods are irregular or widely spaced, the period of abstention can widen to 14 days or more.

The time of ovulation can be more accurately pinpointed by charting basal body temperature (BBT) as shown in the sidebar above. Further confirmation may be found by examining mucus secretions in the vagina which become thick, clear, and lubricating at ovulation, probably to help the sperm's passage. A combination of calendar, temperature, and mucus observation has yielded results in some studies comparable to diaphragm and condom effectiveness. In these studies, couples avoided intercourse from the end of the menstrual cycle until at least three days after ovulation. The method requires good rapport between partners and acceptance of fairly long periods of abstinence. It can be upset by stress, illness, or climate changes which can alter the menstrual cycle.

Withdrawal

This ancient method of withdrawing the penis just before ejaculation, also called *coitus interruptus*, is not effective contraception. Some semen containing sperm often escapes into the vagina before ejaculation. And it is not very satisfying and not easy to interrupt intercourse just before climax. While not recommended, withdrawal can be useful, if risky, when no other birth control is available.

The Morning-After Pill

This after-the-fact medication causes some nausea, but is 100 percent insurance for terminating a possible pregnancy when administered within 72 hours of the suspected conception. However, the FDA has licensed it only for emergencies, such as rapes, because it contains diethylstilbesterol (DES), a form of estrogen, the long-term safety of which is suspect. A woman who has taken the medication and then discovers she was already pregnant from an earlier intercourse should see a physician immediately, because the fetus may be endangered by the drug.

Non-Birth Control: The Douche

Douching, often thought of by the inexperienced as birth control, is virtually useless. It can force sperm further up into the cervix and uterus and, if used too frequently, can lead to vaginal irritation.

Contraceptives on the Horizon

In 1972, the World Health Organization, concerned about burgeoning world populations and the failure of some birth control programs, greatly expanded its search for simple and improved methods of fertility regulation. Presently under study are:

- Pills for the male to reduce sperm count but not libido
- A once-monthly pill for women
- Contraceptive injections, monthly or even annually, for both males and females
- Implantation in the woman's uterus, or under the skin of a man or woman, of time-release hormone capsules
- A ring to fit in the vagina that releases hormones at a regulated rate
- Heat applications to the testes (infrared, microwave, and ultrasound) to provide temporary sterilization
- A vaccine containing antibodies to human chorion growth hormone (HCG) that will turn off HCG and, thus, pregancy, should it occur
- A vaccine containing antibodies that will attach themselves to mature eggs and reject sperm

VOLUNTARY STERILIZATION: PERMANENT BIRTH CONTROL

In our era of concern about overpopulation, it is hardly surprising that voluntary sterilization has become a major form of birth control, used worldwide by 1 in 10 couples of childbearing age (Stokes). In 1970, only 100,000 male sterilizations and far fewer female sterilizations took place, and most of those were for medical reasons. By 1977, about 7 million Americans had been sterilized, and the procedure had become the method of choice for couples married a decade or more, as well as for couples who have had all the children they want.

Watriss-Baldwin/Woodfin Camp

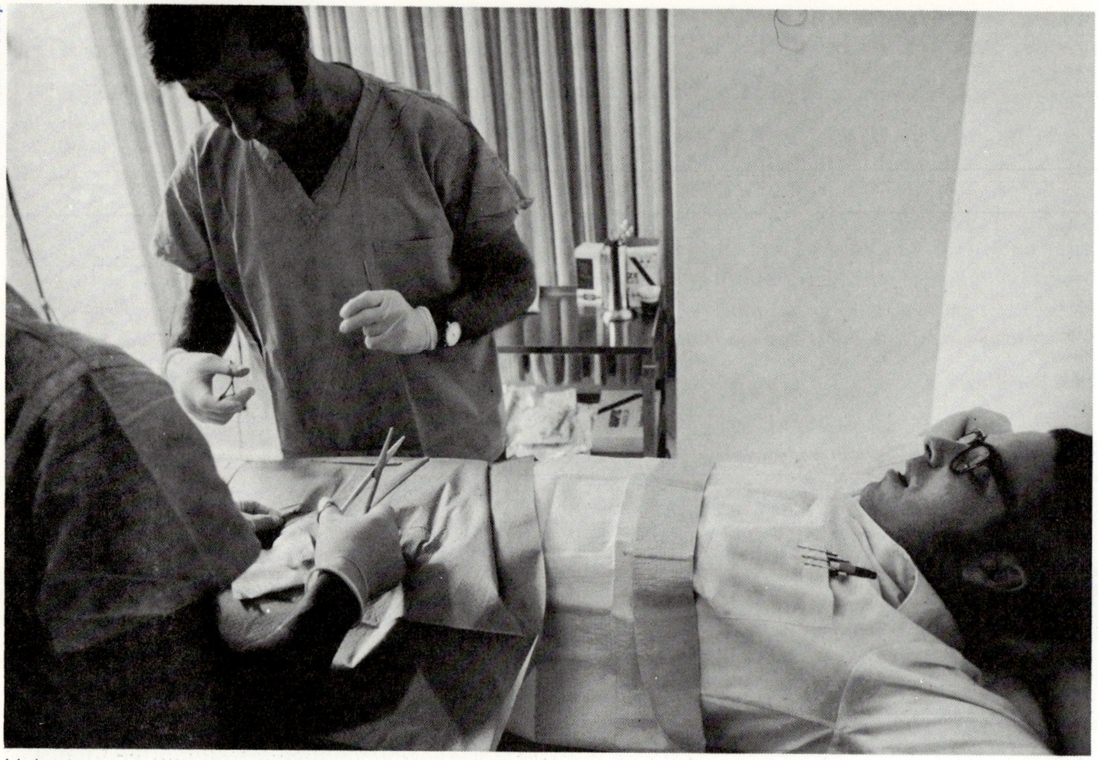

Voluntary sterilization has become a major method of birth control, as increasing numbers of males undergo this simple vasectomy procedure and more females undergo the slightly more complicated tubal ligation.

Types of Sterilization

The goal of sterilization in the male is to prevent the ejaculation of sperm, and in the female to prevent passage of the ovum through the fallopian tubes. A number of approaches are in use or under study.

Male sterilization, vasectomy In the most common method, the surgeon makes a small incision in the scrotum. The vasa deferentia, tubes that transport sperm from testicles to penis, are cut or tied. The surgery takes about 15 to 45 minutes, can be performed under local anesthetic in the physician's office, and is relatively safe and inexpensive. There may be some pain and discomfort and occasional complications, but most men go home after a half hour's rest and resume normal activities. However, they will not be sterile until sperm already in the tubes have been ejaculated—often about 12 ejaculations. Other birth control is needed until two consecutive sperm-free semen samples have been tested.

Female sterilization The woman's fallopian tubes are tied, clipped, cut, or blocked following either incision or puncture of the abdominal wall, or entry through vagina or cervix. The method used will depend on the situa-

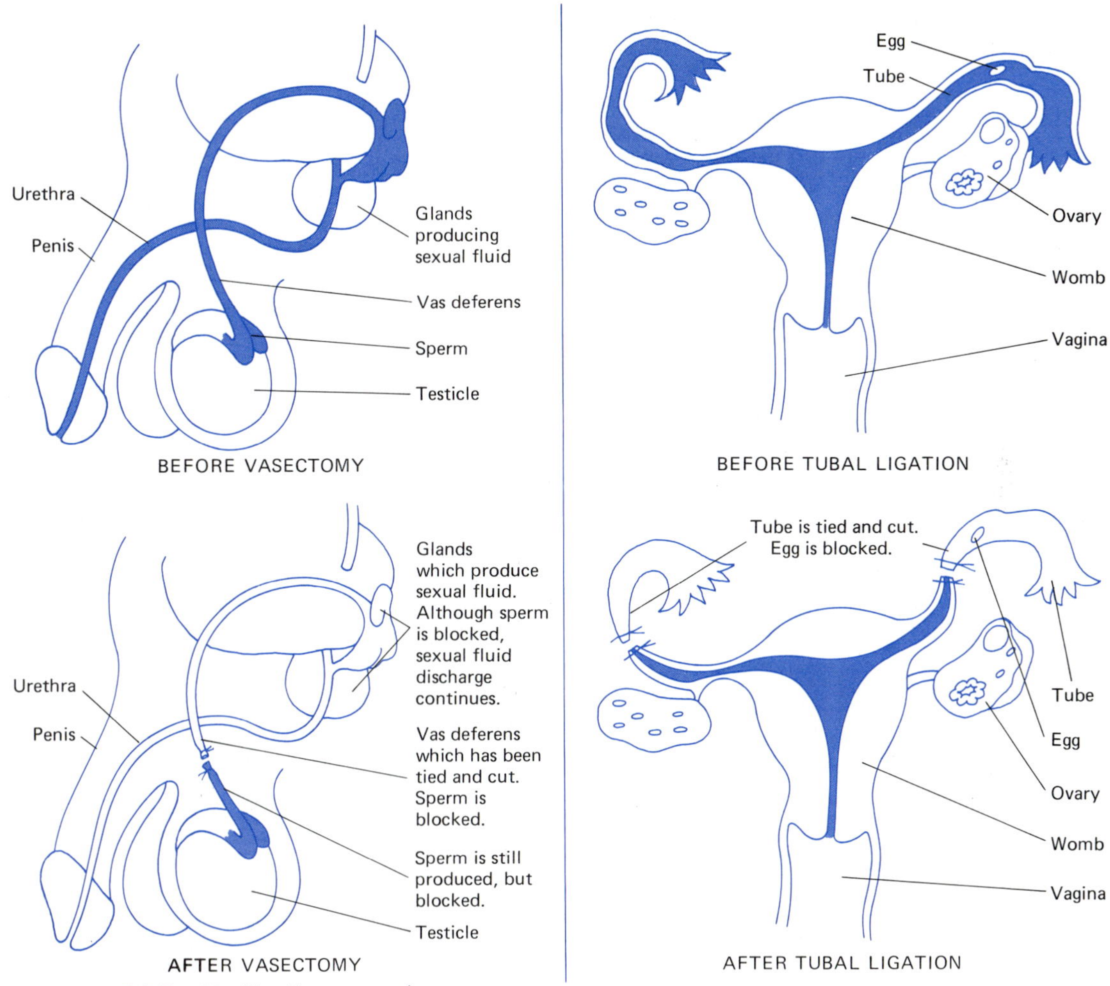

FIGURE 22.5 Sterilization procedures.

tion. In most cases, the major abdominal surgery is avoided and the procedure is performed in the doctor's office or clinic and need be followed by only a few days' rest.

Risks and Benefits

Sterilization is the ultimate in birth control. Once done, it requires no further attention. It does not interfere with intercourse and eliminates the fear of pregnancy which often hampers sexual pleasure. And the risk of pregnancy is nil, except in rare cases of spontaneous rejoining of severed tubes, or when the male has an unsuspected third vas that continues to deliver sperm. However, there are disadvantages to consider before a decision is made to undergo sterilization.

Irreversibility All present sterilization procedures for males or females must be considered permanent. Candidates for sterilization should be certain they will not want children in the future and should consider the possibilty that their life situations might change (divorce and remarriage, or death of a spouse or of a child, for example) and alter their feelings about having more children.

A few vasectomies have been reversed experimentally. But even such successful reconnecting of the tubes does not guarantee fertility. Some 50 to 60 percent of sterilized men show antibodies to their own sperm and these antibodies may continue to destroy sperm even after the vasectomy is reversed. Some men buy future fertility insurance by storing semen in frozen semen banks. But sperm in frozen semen tend to lose their motility (ability to move well) and are frequently ineffective in impregnating a woman (Lader).

Physical risks All surgery carries some risk, but serious complications are not common in sterilization. The long-term physical effects, if any, of vasectomy are unknown. A few studies have hinted at changes in the immune system, beyond the appearance of sperm antibodies, but they have not as yet been substantiated.

Psychological risks Sterilization does not appear to affect masculinity, femininity, or sexual performance, but guilt or fear could cause frigidity or impotence. The major psychological risk is a decision to undergo sterilization that is thoughtlessly arrived at, made for the wrong reason, or not mutually agreed upon by both partners in a marriage. Sterilization will not cure a rocky marriage or a poor sexual relationship, though it does remove the fear of pregnancy. It is birth control—nothing more, nothing less. To be sure patients understand this, many surgeons insist on psychological counseling before sterilization.

ABORTION

Humans who have tried and failed to prevent conception have continually sought ways to end unwanted pregnancies. A toxic poison sometimes succeeds in killing a fetus, but usually kills the mother as well. Efforts at extracting the fetus with an improvised instrument, while offering the possibility of success, carry the risk of a punctured uterus, hemorrhage, and fatal infection. It has often been considered safer—for the mother—to carry the infant to term, deliver it, then leave it somewhere to die, or swaddle it warmly, ring an orphanage bell, and then run.

Today, abortion, made safe by newly developed medical procedures, is believed to be the most widely practiced form of birth control in the world, in spite of strong opposition from many quarters (Lieberman and Peck). In the United States in 1975, 854,853 legal abortions were reported, making abortion the most frequently performed surgery after tonsilectomy. An estimated additional 750,000 women, mostly poor or from rural areas—are believed to have desired abortions they were unable to get.

The average abortion in 1976 was performed on a young, white, unmarried woman in the first 12 weeks of her pregnancy. The death rate was a low 1.0 per 100,000, making it safer than several other forms of birth control and considerably safer than pregnancy (MMWR, *b*).

Modern Techniques

Abortion is the expulsion of the fetus from the womb, ending pregnancy before the fetus can survive on its own. Abortion can be spontaneous, as in a miscarriage. It can be accidental, as in an automobile crash or a fall. Or it can be induced by medical means for therapeutic purposes (to protect a mother's health or because there is something wrong with the fetus) or because the woman does not want to continue the pregnancy for *any* reason (often called *abortion on demand*).

First-trimester abortion Abortions performed during the first three months (trimester) of pregnancy are considered safest. Two basic techniques are used:

- *Dilatation and evacuation (D and E)* For this safest, most popular abortion technique, the vagina is prepared with an antiseptic spray. A device called a speculum is then inserted to hold the vagina open, and the cervix is injected with a local anesthetic. A series of dilators, each larger than the one before, is inserted into the cervix to stretch it to about the diameter of a fountain pen. Next a small motorized "vacuum" is used to suction out the contents of the uterus. The entire process takes 1 to 5 minutes. The doctor double-checks with a curette, a small spoonlike instrument with serrated edges, to be certain no remnants of the pregnancy are left.
- *Dilatation and curettage (D and C)* This once-popular method has largely been replaced by the vacuum technique. The vagina and cervix are prepared and dilated in the same way as in a vacuum curettage. Menstrual-like cramps may be felt at this point by some women. A curette is inserted into the uterus through the dilated cervix, and the implanted embryo is scraped loose and removed, terminating the pregnancy.

Second-trimester abortion About 15 percent of women who wish abortions delay until after the first three months. Their reasons may be financial, psychological (they cannot make up their minds or face the fact of their pregnancies), or physiological (they fail to realize they are pregnant, possibly because they menstruate irregularly). Some women seek late abortions because of a life-threatening physical problem that arises during pregnancy, others when prenatal testing reveals an actual or potential defect in the developing fetus. Second-trimester abortions are generally less safe for the mother and more traumatic emotionally because the fetus is fully formed and "looks like a baby."

Since the fetus and its surrounding materials, amniotic sac and placenta, are too large after the third month to be curetted out, other procedures are used. Most common is "salting out," in which a saline solution is injected into the amniotic fluid to stimulate labor contractions. The woman, usually hospitalized, remains awake so she can report any potentially dangerous symptoms to the physician. Contractions may begin in from 5 to 48 hours and the minilabor may last several hours until the fetus is expelled. Prostaglandins, a group of hormones that regulate many body functions, have also been used to stimulate abortion, but complication rates are higher than for salting out.

Complications

Physical Though normally safe, abortion (like any medical procedure) is not entirely without risk. With the D and E and the D and C, there is a slight risk that the uterus will be punctured, that abnormally heavy bleeding (hemorrhaging) or infection may occur. To avoid the entry of germs into the uterus, postoperative restrictions are placed temporarily on tub baths, tampons, vaginal sprays, and intercourse. Serious complications can result from saline abortion, but may be minimized by prompt competent treatment.

Repeated abortions, particularly if close together, can lead to a stretched out or "incompetent" cervix, later unable to retain a wanted pregnancy to full term. Illegal abortions, performed by untrained persons or by the pregnant woman herself, carry a risk of death estimated at 8 times that of legal abortions (Cates and Rochat).

Psychological Psychological damage is reported to be uncommon, but it does occur. One young woman with a rocky marriage describes what happened when she learned she was pregnant:

> . . . I wasn't upset at all when I went into a local abortion clinic. . . . But as the doctor was aborting the fetus, I felt for the first time that there was life inside me, that I was destroying a baby. I got hysterical—even after I returned home from the clinic, I was uncontrollably upset for weeks. . . . I think of that every year. I had a miscarriage about six years ago, and after the first year I sort of stopped thinking about it. . . . It's a natural problem. But this—the abortion is something I did. It's destroying life. And it's not easy for me to live with that. (Geacintor, p. 7A)

Controversy over Legalization

Less than a decade ago, any discussion of abortion was purely academic. The only legal abortions in the United States were performed to save the mother's life and had to be so certified by a hospital committee. Most women carried unwanted babies to term. A few went abroad for safe legal abortions. Hundreds of thousands turned to sleazy, incompetent, and unscrupulous back-street abortionists or, if they couldn't pay the price, attempted, in desperation, to do the jobs themselves with coat hangers or Clorox. They often paid with their lives.

A few licensed physicians risked jail terms to perform abortions. Dr. W. J. Bryan Henrie, a compassionate Oklahoman whose home town threw a huge party for him when he was released from prison, explained why:

> It took three women to persuade me to perform abortions. Two were butchered by incompetents, and were brought to me in critical condition. The third was a wealthy woman, terrified because she had become pregnant two years after her prominent husband had been sterilized, who came to me for an abortion. I explained the law to her, and turned her down. Next day, she drove her car into a crack-up at 100 miles an hour. That was the last time, until I went to prison, that I ever turned down a request. (*b*)

Groups and individuals concerned with the high death rate from illegal abortions, with the large numbers of unwanted and uncared-for children born each year, and with the right of women to control their own bodies began to lobby in the 1960s for changes in antiabortion laws. By 1970, several states had eased regulations against abortions, and Washington, Hawaii, Alaska, and New York has passed legislation that virtually allowed abortion on demand.

In 1973, all remaining laws restricting a woman's right to an abortion during the first 12 weeks of pregnancy were nullified by the Supreme Court's decision holding that "the right of privacy . . . founded in the 14th Amendment's concept of personal liberty . . . is broad enough to encompass a woman's decision whether or not to terminate her pregnancy." It suggested that during the first three months the state could not restrict abortion on the grounds of the mother's health, since mortality is lower during first-trimester abortions than during normal childbirth. Nor could it restrict on the basis of protecting the child, because the fetus is not yet viable. The decision, said the court, must be left to the pregnant woman and her doctor.

The ruling added that during the second and third trimesters regulations could be laid down to protect the mother's health and the life of the fetus after it becomes viable—about 28 weeks, said the Court, although others have declared it to be as early as 20 weeks.

What are among the results of abortion liberalization? An evaluation noted a dramatic drop in illegal abortions, in the number of births, and in deaths associated with abortion, from 292 per year in 1958–1962 to 44 in 1975. There have been no indications that women in the United States are abandoning other forms of birth control in favor of abortion (Tietze).

Making a Decision

Abortion is a simple procedure, but not so the issues encrusting it. Positions and priorities

Daniel S. Brody/Editorial Photocolor Archives

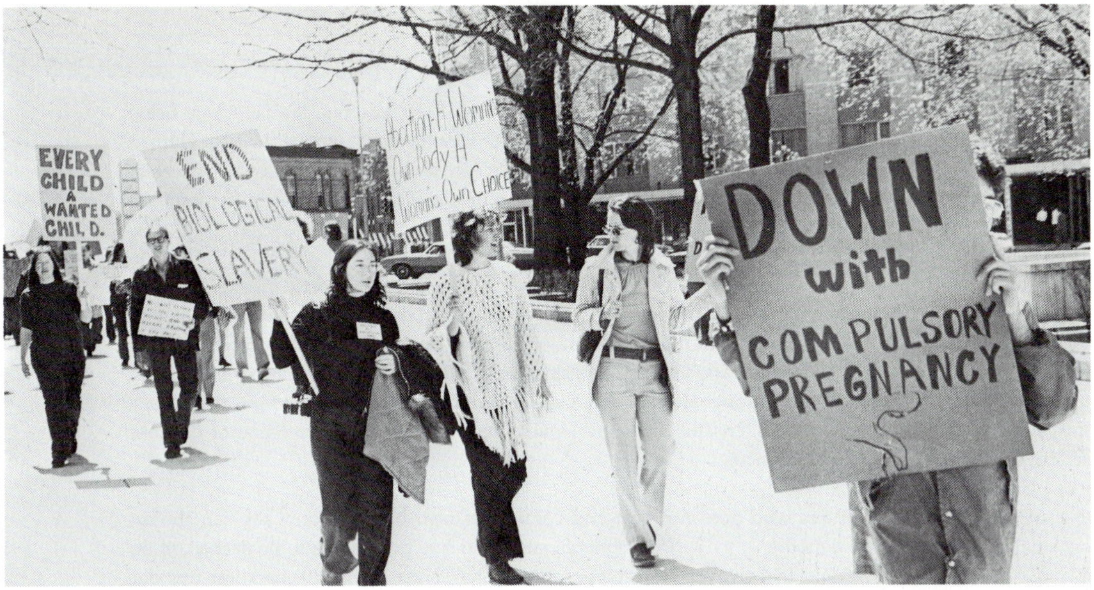
EVERY CHILD A WANTED CHILD
END BIOLOGICAL SLAVERY
DOWN with COMPULSORY PREGNANCY

Paul S. Conklin/Monkmeyer

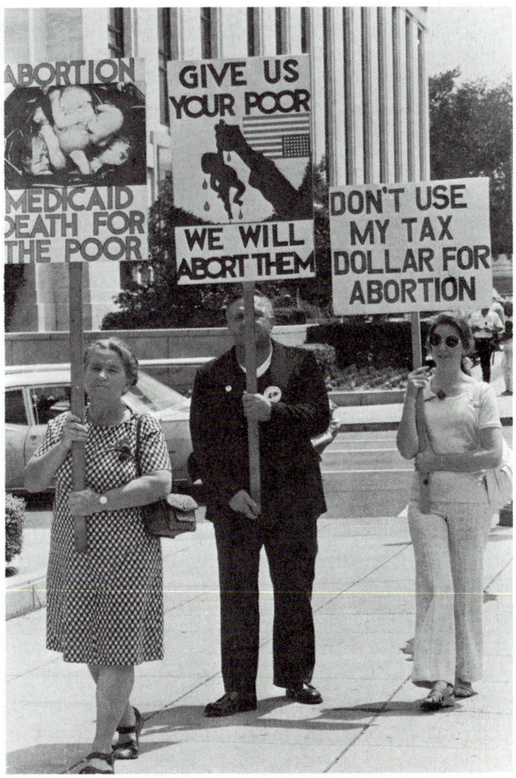
ABORTION
MEDICAID
EATH FOR
THE POOR
GIVE US YOUR POOR
WE WILL ABORT THEM
DON'T USE MY TAX DOLLAR FOR ABORTION

Because of related emotional, religious, and political issues, abortion has become the most controversial form of fertility control in the United States.

of sincere, good, and well-intentioned people vary. Some put the unborn fetus first; some the health and happiness of "born" children; others the future of the mother, the family, or society (see the sidebar). Like other moral issues, abortion is emotionally charged, difficult to legislate to everyone's satisfaction, and very personal. Because a decision should be made very quickly once a determination of pregnancy is made, many women, often with the help of husband or sexual partner, give considerable thought in advance to "what will happen if. . . ."

Here are some of the factors a pregnant woman, married or not, might consider in thinking about one of the most difficult decisions she may ever have to make:

1 *Her own health* Does the physician feel that pregnancy and a new baby would endanger the mother's physical or psychological health?

Opinions on Abortion

Abortion is essentially the last stage in a series of possible birth control measures, the first stage being abstention from sex and the intermediate stages being the use of various contraceptive devices. Human beings are always producing sperm and ova and making decisions about when to terminate their development. All these cells are alive, and all are potential human beings. Thus, in my view, abortion is no more wrong than the practice of celibacy. . . . (Henrie)

. . . We reject the opinion of the U.S. Supreme Court as erroneous, unjust, and immoral . . . the Court has apparently failed to understand the scientific evidence clearly showing that the fetus is an individual human being whose pre-natal development is but the first phase of the long and continuous process of human development that begins at conception and terminates at death. . . . Ultimately (their decision) means that the fetus, that is, the unborn child, belongs to an inferior class of human beings whose God-given rights will no longer be protected under the Constitution of the United States. (National Conference of Catholic Bishops and U.S. Catholic Conference)

No woman can call herself free who does not own and control her own body, or until she can choose whether or not she will be a mother. . . . The first right of every child is to be wanted, to be desired, to be planned with an intensity of love that gives it its title to being. (Margaret Sanger, some 50 years ago, founder of Planned Parenthood)

Far be it from me to weight the decision for or against abortion. . . . And yet as the mother of a child retarded from PKU, I can ask myself. . . . if I had rather she had never been born. . . . Now with full knowledge of anguish and despair, the answer is no, I would not. . . . I would have chosen life. . . . I fear the power of the choice over life and death in human hands. (Buck, Foreword)

I'm in favor of abortion. . . . I've had more than one. They were horrible experiences—demeaning, tawdry, denigrating, and, at the time, criminal. Today, we have three wonderful, wanted children. We're prepared for them economically, emotionally and hope to enrich their lives. (Pogrebin, p. 6A)

Psychic life before birth is far from negligible. . . . The foetus experiences well-being or discomfort. When asleep, it may dream. At term it has behind it sensory and affective past.

Before seeing light and uttering its first cry, IT IS ALREADY SOMEONE! (Rostand, p. 14)

2 *Condition of the fetus* Do prenatal tests or prenatal trauma or illness of the mother indicate that the fetus may be defective in some way?

3 *The present family* Are there already more children in the family than parents can handle, either financially or emotionally?

4 *Beliefs* Is there a strong religious or ethical conviction that abortion is wrong, that it is equivalent to murder, that it would bring shame upon the family?

5 *Agreement* Do both partners fully accept the idea of abortion, without strong pressure from one upon the other or from outside?

6 *Age* Do either or both of the parents feel they are too young or too old to have the child?

7 *Future plans* What will the couple have

Alternatives to Abortion

Single women and girls who become pregnant and find both abortion and forced marriage unacceptable, or who are uncertain about which route to follow, can turn to such organizations as Birthright for help in their decision making. Birthright offers a full range of services from counseling and help in talking with parents (for girls under 18) to free pregnancy tests (some 50 percent of worried young women turn out not to be pregnant), medical aid and legal advice, education, employment and housing assistance, maternity clothing, adoption aid for those who wish it, and baby clothes and furniture for women who decide to raise their babies alone. In 1974 there were over 400 Birthright chapters in the United States and Canada.

to sacrifice (education, career, financial security, freedom, retirement) for the baby? Will they resent these sacrifices?

When the pregnant woman is unmarried, there are several additional questions she might consider:

1 How did she become pregnant? In most cases, pregnancy implies a certain degree of consent. Did she secretly hope to tie her man down? Is she trying to get away from a very difficult family situation? Or to compensate for a recent death in the family? Is she anxious to begin the mother experience—looking for someone to love who, she may naively assume, will make no demands?
2 What is her relationship with the father? Is she prepared to marry him? Does she *want* to marry him?
3 Other than marriage, what are the alternatives to abortion? Would she want to raise the child alone? Or carry through to delivery and then give it up for adoption?

OBTAINING INFORMATION ON BIRTH CONTROL OR FAMILY PLANNING

Seventy percent of all major colleges in the United States offer family planning services or referral. Some church-related schools, of course, do not supply such information on principle. Students in need of advice and unable to obtain it on campus may look to one of Planned Parenthood's 800 clinics around the country which provide counseling and assistance regardless of age or marital status. Or they may turn to a local birth control clinic, a public hospital, or a private obstetrician-gynecologist.

Once a pregnancy has occurred, help or advice is available from Planned Parenthood, Clergy Consultation Service, Birthright, local health departments, and some college health services, as well as from private physicians. Abortion consultation firms charging a fee should be avoided, for they are often exploitive.

LOOKING BACK

REVIEWING CONCEPTS IN CHAPTER 22

- Temporary birth control can be achieved in several ways: abstinence from sexual activity; use of devices (mechanical or chemical) or procedures that prevent the meeting of sperm and egg; use of devices that prevent the implantation of a fertilized egg in the uterine wall; removing a developing embryo early in pregnancy (abortion).
- Permanent birth control can be achieved through sterilization of either the male or the female. These procedures are at present largely irreversible, and thus the decision is for a lifetime.
- Deciding whether or not to use some method of birth control and which to use requires understanding the risks and benefits of each and applying one's own values and religious beliefs to the decision.
- The risk of complications from pregnancy, though small, is greater than the risk of complications from many birth control methods.
- Abortions are safest when performed very early (within the first three months) in pregnancy.
- Though some birth control approaches are used by men and others by women, it is considered best for both partners to share the responsibility for and the decision making about the actual choice.

23

CREATING NEW LIFE: PREGNANCY AND CHILDBIRTH

WHAT'S AHEAD IN CHAPTER 23 What are sound reasons for having children? Where does commitment fit in? How do spacing and timing of children influence health of children and mother? What signs suggest the possibility or probability of pregnancy? What are the sure signs? Why is medical care from early pregnancy important? What are some of the complications of pregnancy and how can some of them be avoided? What are some of the causes of infertility? What modern techniques are used to overcome them? What factors determine what a baby will be like? How much influence do the prospective mother and father have? What is the role of genetic counseling? How can the health of a baby be safeguarded during delivery? What are the relative advantages and disadvantages of breast- and bottle-feeding? How important are mother and father in the early development of the infant? Which factors are crucial to good parenting? How common is parent abuse of children? What are the most important things to remember about the "special" child and his or her needs? What kind of future can be expected for a mentally retarded child born today? What kind of people abuse their children? Can they be helped to end the abuse?

PLANNING A FAMILY

To Be or Not to Be a Parent

Now that question can be asked. In earlier generations, everyone was expected to "be fruitful and multiply." Today, as a result of sophisticated birth control methods, abortion, and perhaps most important, changing social attitudes, there is a genuine choice. It is a choice that is relatively easy for some. But for most people, the decision to have or not to have children is not so easily reached. They must explore their own feelings and values as well as such considerations as those discussed below.

Physical or genetic risks If genetic counseling (discussed later in this chapter) or family history indicates a strong possibility that offspring will bear some serious hereditary disease, a couple might well decide against having children, or in favor of adopting them. If one or both parents are physically or mentally handicapped to the extent that caring for a child might be difficult or impossible, this too might be a reason to forgo parenthood.

Reasons for wanting children Persons who want children for mostly negative reasons (to prove virility or femininity, for security in old age, as a sign of achievement, to mend a marriage, to please parents who want grandchildren, to meet society's expectations, to use as extensions of themselves, to fulfill their dreams) are often poor candidates for parenthood.

Those with positive reasons (to share a happy home with others; to nurture a small and helpless creature and help it grow into a loving, healthy, and independent human being; to satisfy an indefinable urge to have their own children, because they have always liked children) are more likely good parent material.

Willingness to make a commitment "Commitment is the key to happier, healthier babies," according to Dr. T. Allen Merritt, perinatologist (*peri* = about + *natus* = birth + *logy* = study). A committed mother takes good care of herself when she is pregnant, is willing to forgo her two packs of cigarettes and to switch from soda pop to milk for the sake of her baby.

The father, too, must make a commitment—not just during pregnancy, by supporting his wife and sharing in preparations for the baby, but throughout the child's growing years. He, like his wife, may have to forgo a career opportunity in order to best meet the needs of their children.

Adults who suspect that the need to make sacrifices for offspring would make them resentful probably will not make good parents. It all comes down to the familiar line (you may have used it yourself): "I didn't ask to be born." Children do not ask to be given life. It is a parental decision, and once made, it is a parental responsibility.

Competence To drive a car, one must demonstrate competence. It has been suggested that we should also be required to demonstrate the ability to parent well, and even that potential parents should be licensed (McIntire). Of course, in a free society, such licensing is unlikely. Each of us must decide on his or her own competence for parenthood. Society can help by making parenting education readily available.

When to Start a Family

A couple decide they will have children. When should they have them? *Age* is one consideration. Though there have been documented reports of births to women as young as 5 and as old as $57^1/_2$, the healthiest babies are born to mothers in their twenties. Babies born to women under 16 or over 40 are at greatest risk of being premature, stillborn, or having birth defects. *Financial readiness* is another factor. A couple should be financially secure enough to handle the cost of a new baby as

Opinions on Motherhood

. . . My husband and I do not want children. We are tired of the polite slogans, the halfway, too-late measures. . . . Within the 15 to 35 age group, there is a population doubling; and as the children grow, requiring schools and cars and housing, the bulldozers move. And we are sick of being brutalized by bulldozers. Once there were good and valid reasons to have children. Once, it was inevitable . . . human survival depended on human fertility. Once, the attainment of adulthood was marked by a desire to share one's values and delights in life with one's own children.

But these things are no longer true. Today, conception and sterilization can be chosen; there is a world outside the home for women; our survival now rests with our ability to stop smothering the eco-system with our numbers; and parenthood, today, seems to us the very opposite of adulthood.

Many marriages do not survive the stress of parenthood; the birth of children too often means the dissolution of romance; the loss of freedom; the abandonment of ideals to economics.

Writer R. H. Gardner asked a poignant question once, "How many young men's dreams," he wondered, "have been sacrificed to the need for separate bedrooms for the children, an education at the college of their choice?" How many? Would anyone like to count?

A woman's ideals and her involvement with the larger world of the community can suffer, too. With 100 carpools every year, she simply has less time to care about the problems of the inner city. She knows there is a wider world outside, but she must teach the alphabet, direct the play group. The talents and energies of too many of our women are largely lost to the stricture, and the routines of motherhood.

Surely, it is wrong to think that we should all be parents. . . . It would be far wiser to regard parenthood as a specialized occupation—and childlessness as our cultural norm.

Mother's Day is over. (Peck, p. 31)

Motherhood's not dead. It's growing stronger because women who don't really want children aren't having them. . . .

Parenthood doesn't limit horizons, it broadens them. It doesn't stifle idealism, it increases it. (A parent has a reason to make the world better.) Perhaps it does occasionally get in the way of petty ambitions, selfish dreams—but they're not the stuff that idealism is made of.

During more than twenty years of parenting three wonderful children, my husband and I have travelled the world (with them), struggled to improve the community (for them), been stimulated to a changing world with a new focus (by them). Is this loss of freedom? The abandonment of ideals? Dreams are more often sacrificed for fear of trying than because of children; children just serve as a convenient excuse.

And which woman has more time and energy to devote to causes? The career woman working eight hours a day, or the mother with kids safely in school looking for a cause? Check the lists of volunteers in an organization—you'll see who finds the time and takes an interest in the outside world.

And is the mother who is "teaching the alphabet" or "directing a play group," doing less about the problems of the world than the career woman skiing at Aspen or even one who tutors a ghetto child? The future depends on our children, and the woman who has the talent and intelligence to nurture a child, but chooses childlessness, is the one who is squandering her talents and energies. She leaves no one else to carry on the battle for a better world when she is gone.

Mothering can never die as long as women know the joy of a life squirming within them, experience the satisfaction of a sighing suckling baby at the breast, hear a tiny moppet with jam-stained face or a balky teen struggling for independence mutter, "Mom, I love you." It will never die as long as one man and one woman love each other enough to preserve that love through a child. (A mother of three, personal correspondence with the authors) well as the possible loss of income if the mother decides to give up her job. *Emotional readiness* is important, too. A husband-wife relationship needs to grow strong before it is ready to face the challenge of a third party. Potential parents must be mature enough to put the interests of another human being before their own.

On the other hand, older couples who are set in their ways often find it difficult to accept the inconveniences of parenthood, and have less patience and energy for coping with small children. And those who wait until the late thirties to have children will be tied down well into middle age. Still, any couple, at any age, with a strongly shared desire for children can be good parents.

Spacing of Children

A pause between children refreshes parents harassed by too many diapers to change and too many noses to wipe. It also gives each infant, in turn, the individual attention of parents and a better chance for a healthier emotional climate in which to grow. Moreover, intervals of about three years between births assure a healthier mother and baby. And, not unimportant, later college tuition costs will be more spread out.

How Many Children?

It has been reported that a Russian couple had 69 children (16 sets of twins, 7 sets of triplets, and 4 sets of quadruplets). American women today, however, average 2.1 children (U.S. Department of Commerce). Limiting family size has become desirable to many because of the population explosion, because statistically each child born after the third has an increased risk of birth defects, and because large families can be a strain and expense in a society where another child is no longer an extra pair of hands to work the farm, and where children are no longer cheaper by the dozen.

Sex Selection

There is some evidence that parents may soon be able to select the sex of a planned child. One method of planned sex determination relies on the fact that sperm carrying male chromosomes are lighter and faster and have a shorter life than sperm carrying female chromosomes. Several studies have shown that couples who have intercourse two to five days before ovulation are very likely to have girl babies; those who have coitus one day before to two days after ovulation are most likely to have boys (Benendo). Further study is needed to substantiate this evidence. Another approach to sex planning, one that raises many ethical questions, involves determining the sex of a fetus early in pregnancy and aborting if it is not of the desired sex.

Preparing for Conception

Before a decision to have a child is acted upon, both husband and wife should have prepregnancy medical examinations so that any potential problems (such as diabetes in the mother, VD in either, or inadequate diet) can be evaluated and, if necessary, treated. The physician will also advise how long a precautionary waiting period should be allowed between the termination of oral contraception and conception; will remove an IUD if one is in place; and will warn against any unnecessary exposure to medication or other drugs, or to x-rays or other substances hazardous to the unborn.

PREGNANCY

"I have finally done it; I am elated and terrified. For the first time in my life, I feel like a woman. . . . What is happening to my body?" (McBride, p. 22). These words from a woman pregnant for the first time sum up the feelings of the expectant mother, the tug-of-war between joy and fear. They make it clear that "expecting" means more than awaiting a

Culver Pictures

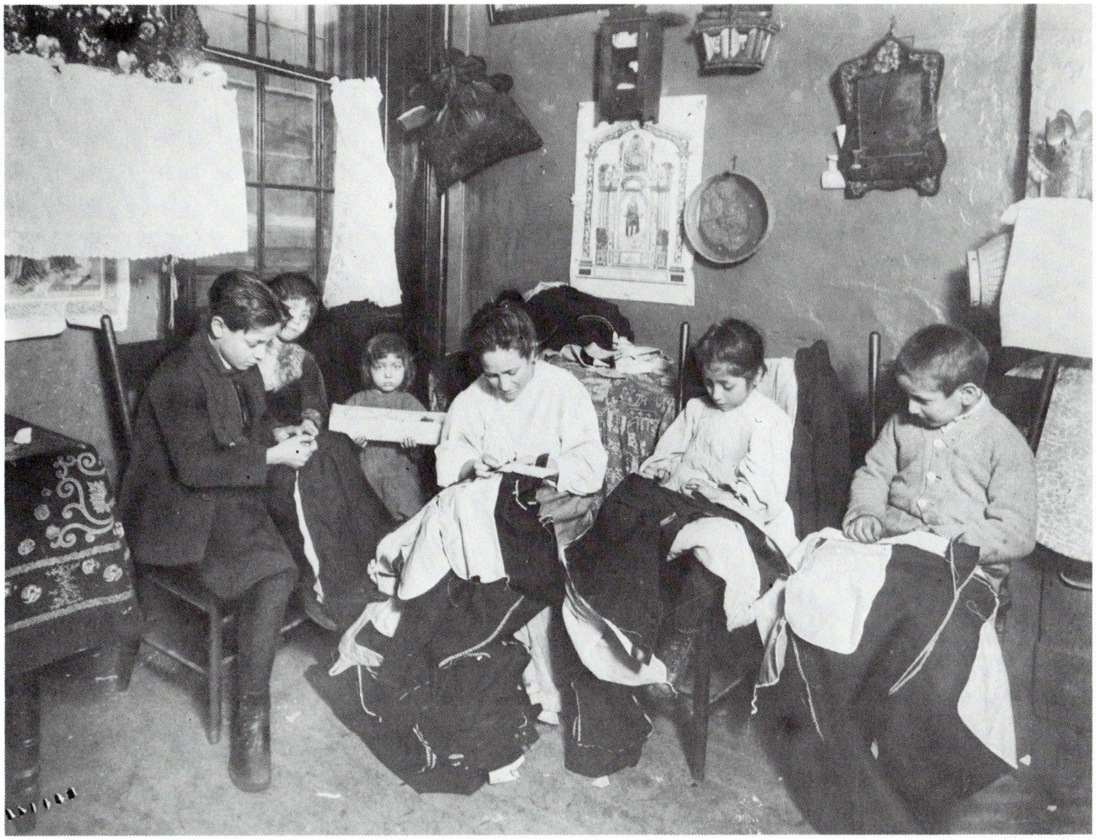

In the past, each additional child meant an extra pair of hands, and children were "cheaper by the dozen." Today, because of the population explosion and the strain and expense of large families, most couples prefer to limit family size.

baby. It also means expectations about the child and how it will change one's life: "What will my baby be like? Will I be all right? Will my baby? Will I be a good mother?" The expectant father feels the same mixed emotions. He is excited by the expectation of fatherhood, frightened by its responsibilities. He feels love for his wife and pride in her, as well as fear that he may lose her to "the baby," and he may be faintly jealous of all the attention she gets. A clear understanding of what is happening physically and psychologically during pregnancy can help ease the anxieties of expectant parents.

Signs of Pregnancy

A missed menstrual period can mean joy for the woman who hopes she's pregnant, misery for the woman who is "scared to death" she is. But because many other factors can delay a period, absence of menstruation is not proof positive of pregnancy. Instead it is *presumptive*; it indicates a possibility of preg-

Hella Hammid/Photo Researchers

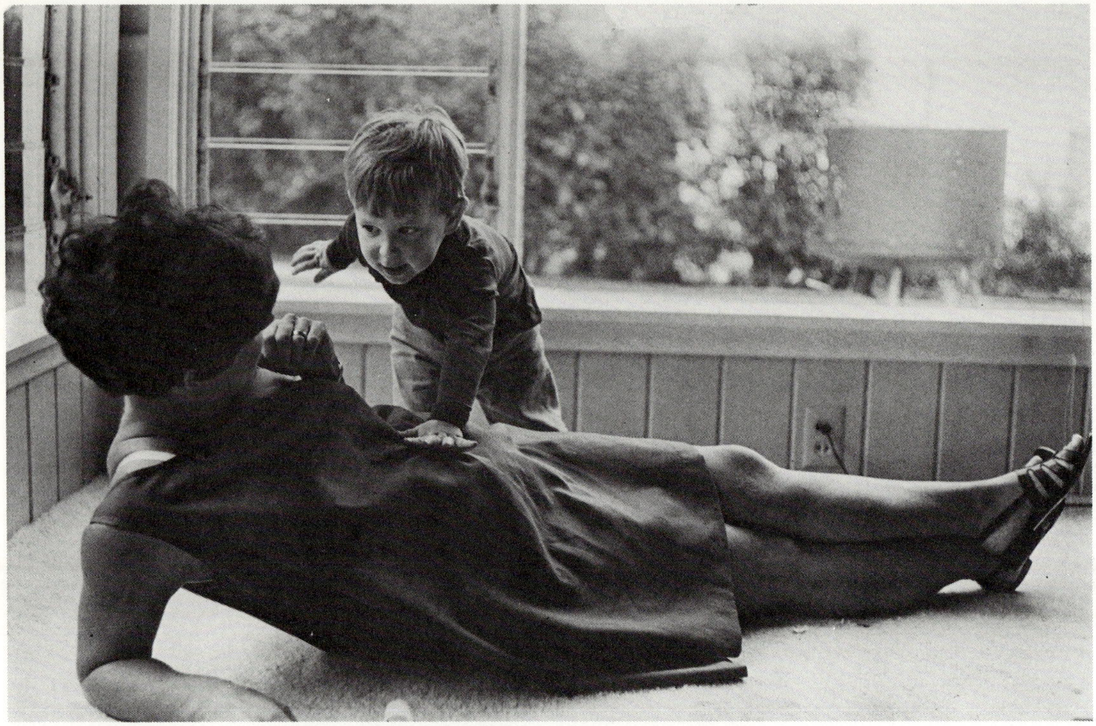

"Expecting" means more than awaiting a baby.

nancy. In Table 23.1, you can see the other signs of pregnancy: *probable* (more definite than presumptive), and *positive* (occurring only when a woman is pregnant).

A pregnancy test[1] at a lab, the doctor's office, or with a do-it-yourself kit can usually confirm pregnancy, though there are occasional false-negative or false-positive results. The physician's examination at the first visit can also confirm pregnancy. A woman who believes she is pregnant should see her doctor as soon as possible after the first missed period. She will receive a thorough examination, tests to rule out VD, anemia, kidney problems, diabetes, heart disease, possible Rh incompatibility, and any other condition that might interfere with a normal, healthy pregnancy.

As pregnancy progresses, some women may feel moody, or may suffer from backaches or varicose veins. But the radiant good health most women enjoy during pregnancy makes it clear that it is not a state of illness. It is a condition to enjoy.

WHEN SOMETHING GOES WRONG

Most pregnant women look and feel "in the pink." And the vast majority of newborns are vigorous and healthy. Occasionally, however, there are complications that endanger both mother and child.

[1]Planned Parenthood, health clinics, and some school health services can refer the possibly pregnant woman for a pregnancy test. She should avoid commercial referral services, whose chief interest is to "steer" women to assembly-line abortion clinics.

TABLE 23.1 Signs of pregnancy

WHEN SIGNS APPEAR	SIGNS A WOMAN NOTICES	SIGNS PHYSICIAN FINDS	OTHER POSSIBLE REASONS
	PRESUMPTIVE (indicating pregnancy is possible)		
Very early	Breast changes: tingly, tender, swollen, color of areola deepens		The Pill, menstruation to some extent
2–7 weeks	Morning sickness (any time of day) in about half of women; becoming less common		Many diseases
Entire pregnancy	Amenorrhea (absence of menstruation)		Travel, fatigue, exams, stress, fear of pregnancy, disease
12–16 weeks and late pregnancy	Frequent urination		Urinary infection, nervousness
First 3 months	Food cravings, stretch marks, dark pigmented line from navel to pubis	Changes in color of vaginal and cervical tissue as blood flow to them increases	
	PROBABLE (indicating pregnancy is probable)		
2–8 weeks		Softening of uterus and cervix	
3 months	Enlarging abdomen	Enlargement of uterus, change in shape of uterus	Tumor
Throughout		Intermittent painless contractions	
14–16 weeks	Fetal movements—"quickening"		Gas; bowel contractions
	POSITIVE		
12–16 weeks		Fetal heartbeat	
16 weeks		Fetal movements felt through abdominal and uterine wall	
16 weeks after missed period		X-ray, ultrasound (can be done earlier)	
2 weeks after missed period		Pregnancy test (test for HCG)	

Miscarriage

About 15 percent of all pregnancies end in miscarriage, or spontaneous abortion. Very early miscarriages may not be noticed at all; they may just appear as slightly delayed menstrual periods. Later miscarriages can be recognized by the passage of fetal or placental material and usually a considerable amount of blood. Following a miscarriage, the physician may perform a D and C to "clean out" the uterus and prevent bleeding.

FIGURE 23.1 Nine months from conception to birth*

CONCEPTION AND FIRST WEEK

The ovum, swept from the ovary into the fallopian tube, is penetrated (fertilized) by a single sperm. It continues toward the uterus, dividing into a ball of cells. At about the end of the first week, it implants itself in the wall of the uterus.

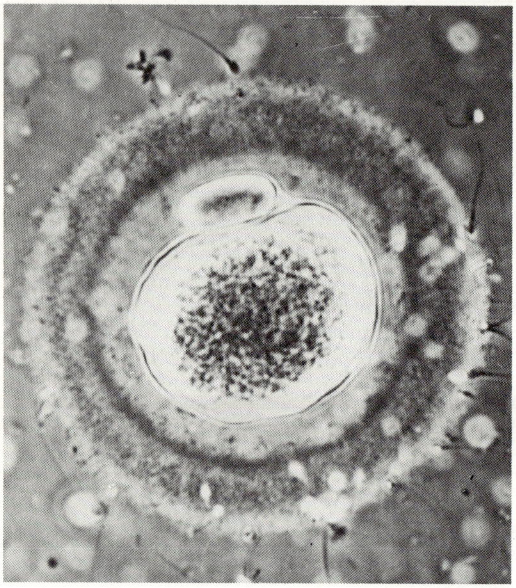

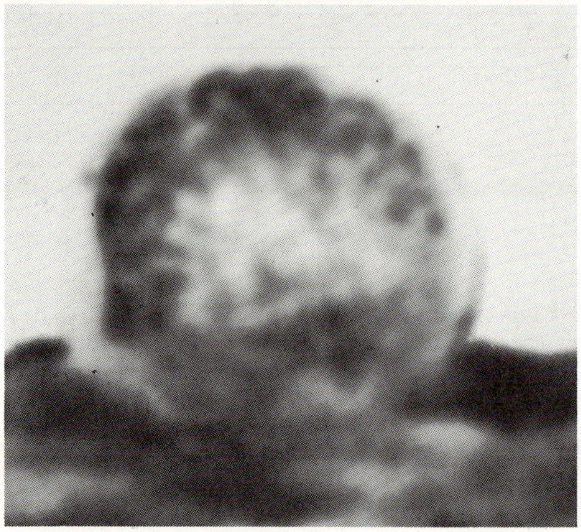

Fertilized ovum implanting on uterine lining one week after fertilization.

Living human ovum at moment of fertilization.

SECOND WEEK

The embryo elongates, and cells begin to differentiate, becoming nerve cells, bone cells, blood cells, etc. A watertight "balloon," or amnion, forms around the embryo and fills gradually with amniotic fluid which will protect and insulate the developing infant. Around it forms the chorion, from which the placenta will develop. The human chorionic gonadotropin hormone (HCG) begins to circulate, probably inhibiting menstruation.

FOURTH WEEK

The placenta, hooked up to the embryo via the umbilical cord (a two-way pipeline which carries nourishment from mother to child and waste products from child to mother), continues growth. The embryo now has three layers of cells. The outer layer will become skin, hair, oil and sweat glands, and the nervous system; the middle layer will become muscles, bones, blood vessels, kidneys, genitals, and connective tissue; and the inner layer will evolve into the digestive tract, lungs, and the urinary tract. The primitive mouth, throat, brain and spinal cord form, and a small U-shaped tube, soon to become a heart, begins to pump blood. Arm and leg buds appear.

*Photos courtesy of Landrum B. Shettles.

FOUR TO EIGHT WEEKS

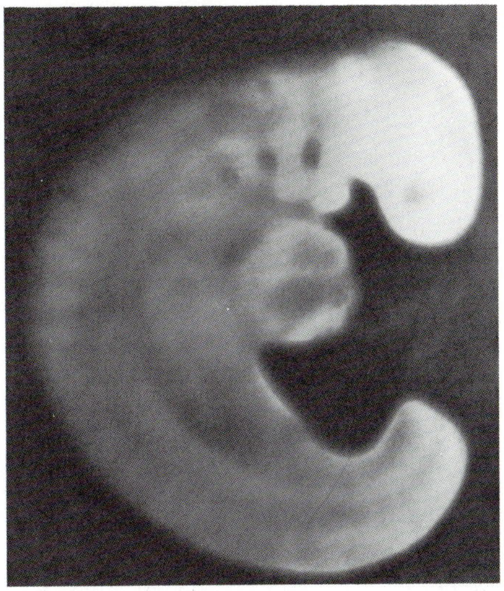

Liver, kidneys, reproductive and digestive tracts, and the spinal cord (the end of which looks like a tail, but is not) are developing. Eye, ear, and nose, and teeth buds and the skeleton become apparent toward the end of the month. Movements of the embryo, just becoming a fetus, are too miniscule to be felt by the mother.

Living human embryo four weeks after fertilization.

EIGHT TO TWELVE WEEKS

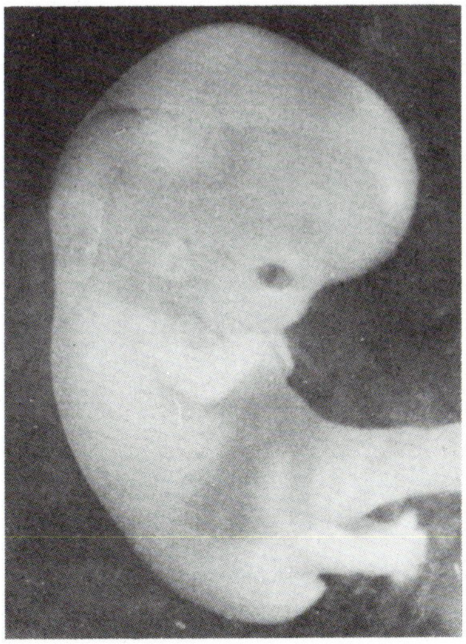

The fetus, a tiny "intranaut," moves around weightlessly in amniotic fluid, attached to the placenta life support system via the umbilical cord. It can swallow, inhale and exhale, make a fist, and do somersaults. Many organs are functioning. Its features have family resemblance.

Living human fetus eight weeks after fertilization.

FIGURE 23.1 *(Continued)*

TWELVE TO SIXTEEN WEEKS 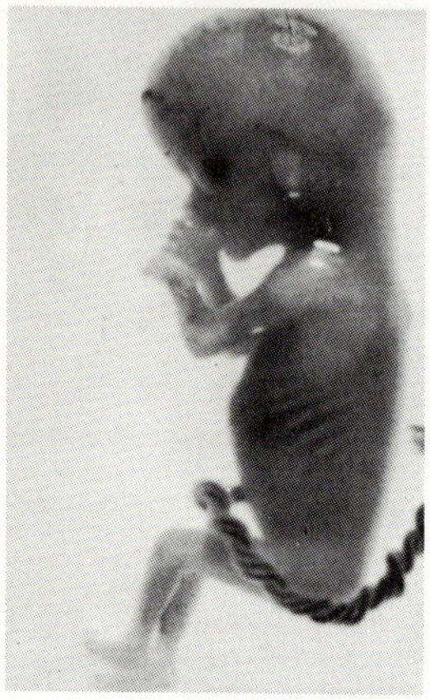	The fetus may suck its thumb. The heartbeat becomes recognizable through a stethoscope. Toward the end of the month, or at the beginning of the next month, kicking movements of the fetus can be felt. Fetus twelve weeks after fertilization.
SIXTEEN TO TWENTY WEEKS	Downy hair begins to grow on scalp, brows, and lashes. All organs continue to develop.
TWENTY TO TWENTY-FOUR WEEKS	Eyes open or close at will. The fetus responds to loud sounds. The body systems are rapidly maturing, but only rarely will a sixth-month baby survive if born prematurely.
LAST TRIMESTER (THREE MONTHS)	Growth and maturing continue. Each day the fetus remains in the uterus, the better its chances of survival at birth.

WHEN TO SEEK HELP

Problems in Pregnancy

A pregnant woman should notify her doctor at once if any of the following signs appear:

- Bleeding from the vagina
- Severe or continuing nausea and vomiting
- Continuing or severe headache
- Swelling or puffiness of the face or hands
- Marked swelling of the feet or ankles
- Blurring of vision or spots before the eyes
- A marked decrease in the amount of urine passed
- Pain or burning on passing urine
- Chills and fever
- Sharp or continuous abdominal pain
- A sudden gush of water from the vagina before the baby is due
- Severe, prolonged pain in the side or small of the back
- No movement of the fetus for more than 6 to 8 hours

Determining the Due Date

The human gestation period, or pregnancy, averages 266 days from conception or 280 days from the first day of the last menstrual period (LMP). The estimated day of confinement (EDC) can be calculated by using Nägele's rule:

$$\text{LMP} + 7 \text{ days} - 3 \text{ months} + 1 \text{ year} = \text{EDC}$$

For example, if Rosanne is pregnant and her last menstrual period began on September 14, she adds 7 days, which brings her to September 21. She then counts back 3 months to June 21. One year from last June 21 is her EDC or due date, but delivery 2 weeks earlier or later is not at all unusual.

Many women blame themselves following a miscarriage, recalling some overexertion or other activity that might have caused it. But the real cause in early pregnancy is much more likely to be an abnormality in the embryo or a faulty implantation in the uterus. In late pregnancy, the cause is more often the mother's ill health or an incompetent cervix, one that is stretched out and will not hold the growing fetus.

Can a threatened miscarriage signaled by bleeding or staining and pain be prevented? Experts differ on this. Some prefer to take no action—on the assumption that if a miscarriage occurs, the fetus is probably defective. Others may prescribe medication and rest. No definitive studies document which course is best. In cases of habitual or repeated miscarriage, there may be a hormone deficiency, a defect in the mother's anatomy, inadequate nutrition, overweight, subnormal sperm from the male, or a psychological problem. Treatment may include diet, vitamins, hormones, and the avoidance of drugs, alcohol, tobacco, and stress.

Rh Incompatibility

About 85 percent of Americans inherit an Rh factor in their blood; they are Rh-positive. The other 15 percent do not; they are Rh-negative. Both groups are equally healthy. But the children of an Rh-negative woman and an Rh-positive man are at risk of erythroblastosis fetalis, a potentially fatal disease characterized by jaundice (yellowness), anemia, and brain damage. The process begins when the woman is exposed to Rh-positive cells during the delivery of a child with Rh-positive blood or via a transfusion of Rh-positive blood. In subsequent pregnancies, these antibodies attack and damage the blood cells of any fetus with Rh-positive blood. Once, this condition killed some 2600 newborns a year. Now it has been almost totally eliminated by prompt diagnosis and treatment. Care can begin while the baby is still in the uterus. If moderate or severe Rh incompatibility is determined through amniocentesis (see Figure 23.7), and the fetus is mature enough, doctors may induce labor immediately or deliver the baby surgically in order to avoid further damage of the infant by its mother's cells. At delivery, a complete exchange transfusion is carried out to replace the infant's Rh-positive blood with Rh-negative blood. If the fetus is not yet sufficiently mature for delivery, the exchange transfusion may be carried out while it is still in the uterus. A more recent treatment approach is to give the Rh-negative mother an injection of a serum (within 72 hours following the birth of each Rh-positive child or aborted fetus) that prevents the development of the harmful antibodies. This serum will not work for a woman who has already developed the antibodies.

Infertility

Like Abraham and Sarah in the Bible, many couples today find it difficult to conceive at all. Biblical aid came in the form of divine intervention. The modern couple, though not necessarily abandoning prayer, are likely to seek help from a family physician, an obstetrician-gynecologist, or a fertility specialist.

Of couples attempting to conceive, about one-third will succeed the first month, 60 percent by the end of three months, and 85 percent of those who conceive at all will do so by the end of the first year (Guttmacher). Conception will be impossible for 1 couple out of 10. Young couples who have been unsuccessful after a year of trying should visit a physician. Couples over 35 should see a doctor after six months without success.

The source of the problem may be easy to pinpoint: chronic or acute disease; infrequent or too frequent intercourse or intercourse at the wrong time of the month (see page 484, sidebar); hot baths or saunas taken by the husband before intercourse (they re-

Other Common Complications of Pregnancy

Tubal pregnancy The embryo develops in a narrow fallopian tube causing pain on one side and vaginal bleeding. If surgery to remove the growing pregnancy is not performed immediately, the tube will burst, preventing any future conception in that tube and causing risk to the mother's life.

Preeclampsia and eclampsia These conditions, occurring late in pregnancy, affect about 5 percent of pregnant women. Symptoms of preeclampsia include: increased blood pressure; swelling of hands, feet, face; water retention; rapid weight gain; headaches; and protein in the urine. Prompt treatment prevents the condition from advancing to the convulsions and coma of eclampsia, which are fatal to about 13 percent of afflicted mothers and half their unborn children.

Abruptio placenta The premature separation of the placenta from the inner wall of the uterus occurs during the last three months of pregnancy in about 2 percent of pregnancies. It can range from a mild separation with no symptoms to a severe separation. The latter results in heavy bleeding and cuts off the infant's oxygen supply, causing its death unless it is delivered immediately—usually surgically by Caesarian section.

Placenta praevia When the fertilized ovum implants itself low in the uterus instead of in the normal position near the top, the placenta grows near the cervix. This can interfere completely with the development of the fetus and cause a spontaneous abortion. If the fetus continues to develop, the placenta may be torn away from the uterus when the painless contractions of late pregnancy begin. Bleeding may result. Bed rest can be helpful, but if bleeding is severe immediate delivery becomes necessary. Even if the fetus is mature enough to survive, lack of oxygen or other complications during the delivery can lead to a variety of birth defects, cerebral palsy, for example.

WHERE TO FIND HELP
Fertility Specialists

Ask your family doctor, obstetrician, or write to the American Society for the Study of Sterility, 920 South 18th Street, Birmingham, AL 35205.

TABLE 23.2 Common fertility problems

FINDING	MALE OR FEMALE	POSSIBLE CAUSE	POSSIBLE REMEDY
Ignorance about intercourse, fertile times, etc.	Both	Poor sex education	Sex counseling, medical guidance.
No ovulation	Female	Malformed or damaged ovaries (often caused by VD); hormone imbalance; depressed thyroid activity	Fertility pill; early treatment of VD; hormone therapy; thyroid hormone.
Fertilization does not take place	Female	Blockage in tubes or somewhere else between ovaries and vagina that prevents passage and meeting of egg and sperm; woman's allergy to husband's sperm; infection causing blockage somewhere along tract	Surgery to clear blockage, remove tumors, etc.; culdoscopy or other method to clear tubes; in the future, possible replacement of tubes; allergy to sperm is difficult to treat; antibiotics for infection; in vitro (test-tube) fertilization in some cases.
Repeated miscarriages	Female	Defective embryo (early miscarriage); damaged or abnormal uterus unable to hold or nurture fetus (sometimes due to multiple abortions)	Better diet, prenatal care, genetic counseling; surgery may help; bed rest and medication may help after third month.
Insufficient numbers of sperm; sperm that don't move properly; abnormally shaped sperm	Male	Hormonal inadequacies; ill health; tension; tight pants; hot baths prior to coitus	Hormone therapy may help; abstinence prior to fertile time may help; treatment of underlying illness; relief of tension (vacation, rest, outdoor exercise, etc.); dietary treatment; caffeine as a stimulant.
Impotence, premature ejaculation	Male	Psychological problems; physical illness	Sex therapy or counseling; treatment of underlying illness.
No sperm production	Male	Blockage or abnormality somewhere between testes and tip of penis; hormonal or physical abnormality	Surgical correction; hormone therapy; artificial insemination using sperm from an unknown donor.

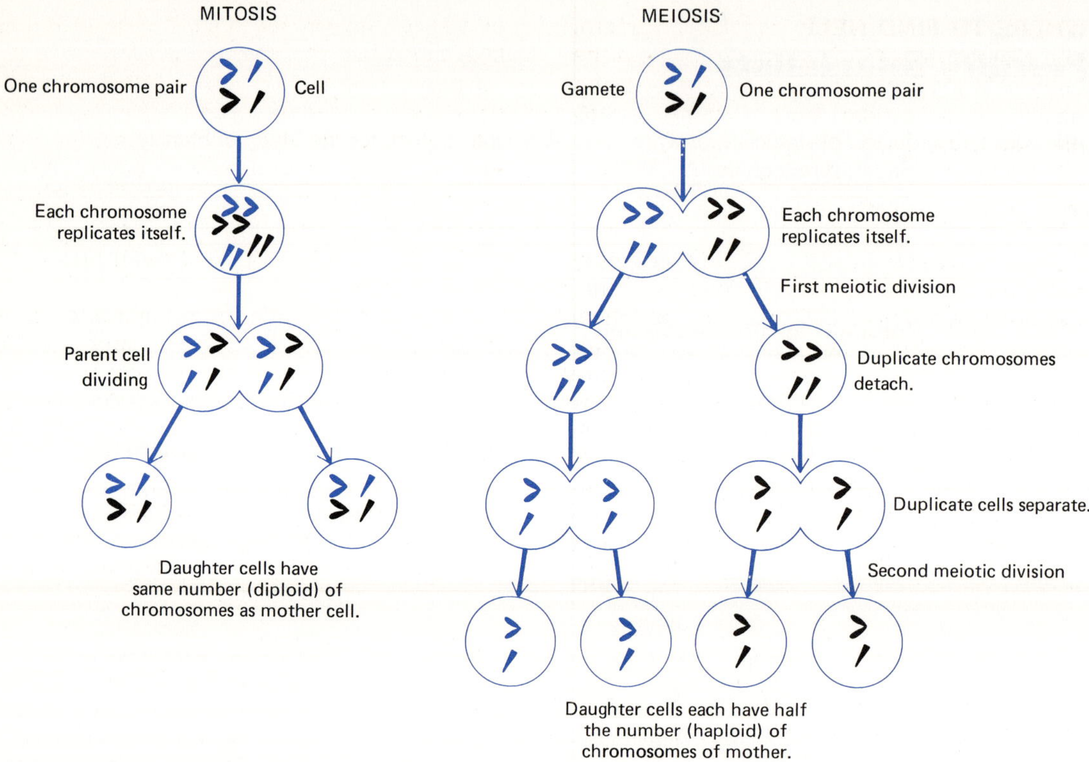

FIGURE 23.2 Mitosis, division of an ordinary cell (with four chromosomes) as compared with meiosis, division of a sex cell, or gamete (with four chromosomes). [*Adapted from Goldstein, p. 13.*]

duce sperm production); occasionally, ignorance about how coitus is performed. Further testing will be necessary to discover fertility problems such as those in Table 23.2.

Very often, all possible physical causes are ruled out and the barrier to conception proves to be psychological. Maybe the couple are trying too hard; they both become tense and upset. The harder they try, the worse the problem becomes. In cases where the wife has not been ovulating or menstruating because of tension, a fertility drug, Clomid, may do the job. But Dr. Wallace L. Herrmann, developer of the drug, warns that it should not be used unless a woman's basic anxieties about sex, marriage, and motherhood have been worked out. A pill can help a woman become pregnant, but it cannot make her happy about a baby that, deep down, she does not really want (Kasindorf).

WHAT THE BABY WILL BE LIKE: GENETIC DETERMINANTS

Will the baby be a girl or a boy? Will it have its father's blue eyes, or its mother's musical talent? Will it grow up to be tall or short? Most important, will it be healthy? The role of heredity is vital. Parents are kept in suspense for nine months, but hereditary characteristics are determined at the moment of conception—the instant the father's sperm penetrates the mother's ovum. And unless the baby is an identical twin, there never was and never will be another human being exactly like him or her.

The Process of Heredity

The gametes or germ cells The baby's story really begins when its parents' own reproductive cells are formed. Take a hypothetical couple, Lisa and Brian. Lisa is 23, but her reproductive cells began developing more than 23 years ago, when she was still in her own mother's uterus. By the end of the fifth prenatal month, she had millions of these cells. Later these *primary oocytes* began to disintegrate and disappear. Only 3000 to 4000 were left by the time Lisa was 7 years old. Of these, 350 to 400 would become mature eggs or ova to be released once a month during Lisa's childbearing years.

Brian's sperm cells were not as clearly developed prenatally as Lisa's. But the material was there for the billions of sperm cells that would be produced in his lifetime. When he reached the age of maturity, the ongoing process of sperm production began, taking about 2½ months from spermatogonia to mature sperm.

Sperm and ova differ from other body cells in that they contain only half as much of the genetic material that dictates what an organism will be like, whether it will be man or mouse, large or small, healthy or sickly. In other human cells, the hereditary material is contained in 22 pairs of autosomal (*auto* = self + *soma* = body) chromosomes that ordain an individual's characteristics and in an additional pair of chromosomes that deter-

FIGURE 23.3 Meiotic division in the human male (spermatogenesis) and the human female (oogenesis). [*Adapted from Goldstein, p. 13.*]

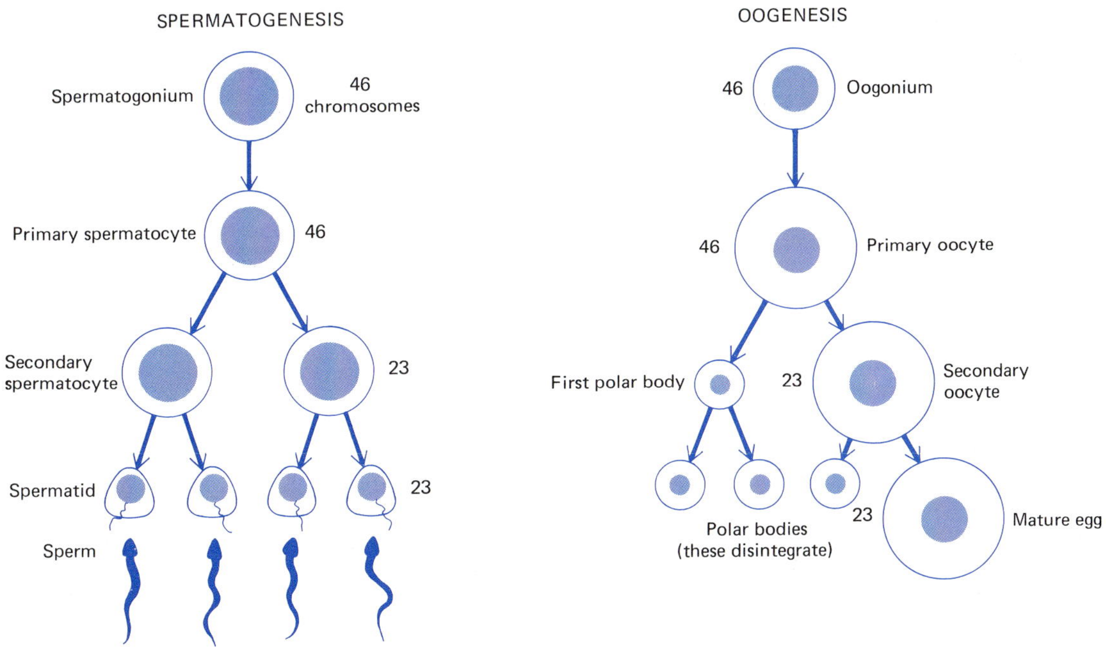

mines sex. These cells contain the *diploid* or full number of chromosomes, half of each of the 23 pairs coming from each parent.

Figure 23.3 shows why sperm and ova have only 23 single chromosomes, the *haploid* or half number. If they had the full 46 chromosomes, the new individual formed when they joined would have double that number. In future generations, chromosomes would multiply at a chaotic rate, and the human cell with 48 chromosomes—and the human being we know—would disappear.

The genetic code Chromosomes (*chromo* = color + *soma* = body), so called because of the way they absorb color from certain dyes, are coded spiral ladders composed of a genetic material called *deoxyribonucleic acid* (DNA). Each segment of this ladder, from 500 to 2000 rungs, is a distinct *gene* carrying explicit directions for a particular trait: curly hair, big feet, aquiline nose. Each of these genes has an opposite number in the corresponding chromosome from the other parent.

The genetic code has been compared to a recipe. Say you are baking a devil's food cake. With all the right ingredients, proper pan, correct oven temperature, you get a perfect, light, moist chocolate cake. Leave out one or more ingredients, put in the wrong ones or the wrong amounts, and the cake is hard or mushy or tasteless, has bumps and lumps, or is not a cake at all.

When the genetic recipe goes wrong, the results are much the same, ranging from minor imperfections to incompatibility with life. If, when Lisa's oocytes were forming, or during the first division of the ovum later to be fertilized by Brian's sperm, a TA rung in a DNA ladder broke off and was replaced by a TG, the resulting child might have a birth defect. If the defect were extremely serious, Lisa might suffer an early miscarriage. Such accidents to genetic material, whether they occur spontaneously or are caused by radiation, illness, drugs, or factors unknown, are called *mutations*. The mutation can be passed on to all future generations descending from surviving offspring, or it can be lost in the process of cell division.

Patterns of Inheritance

There are several patterns, not all fully understood, by which hereditary traits are passed on from parents to children. They include:

Single gene heredity In this hereditary pattern, the individual has *one pair of genes* for a given trait—one of the pair from the mother, the other from the father. Each gene is either *dominant* or *recessive*. An individual who has one dominant gene and one recessive for a given trait is said to be *heterozygous* (*hetero* = different + *zygo* = union) for that trait. The dominant gene is activated for that trait; the recessive gene curls up and does nothing. A person who has two recessive or two dominant genes for a trait is said to be *homozygous* (*homo* = same) for that trait. In this case the *phenotype* (what actually shows in the person) is the same as the *genotype* (the genetic makeup) (see Figure 23.4). Differences in environmental conditions or genetic background may affect whether or not a trait will show up and to what extent.

Sex-linked or X-linked heredity Sex or gender is passed on through the X and Y chromosomes. All normal females have two X chromosomes (XX) and all normal males have an X and a Y chromosome (XY). A mother can only pass on an X chromosome; a father can pass on either an X or a Y, for each sperm contains one or the other. Thus the father determines the sex of the child. (This fact would have come as a surprise to kings who divorced or even beheaded wives who did not bear them sons.) The X chromosomes carry other genetic material as well, and it is now believed that the Y may, too.

Polygenic heredity Many traits (height, intelligence, hair color, for example) are probably controlled by several genes, thus allowing

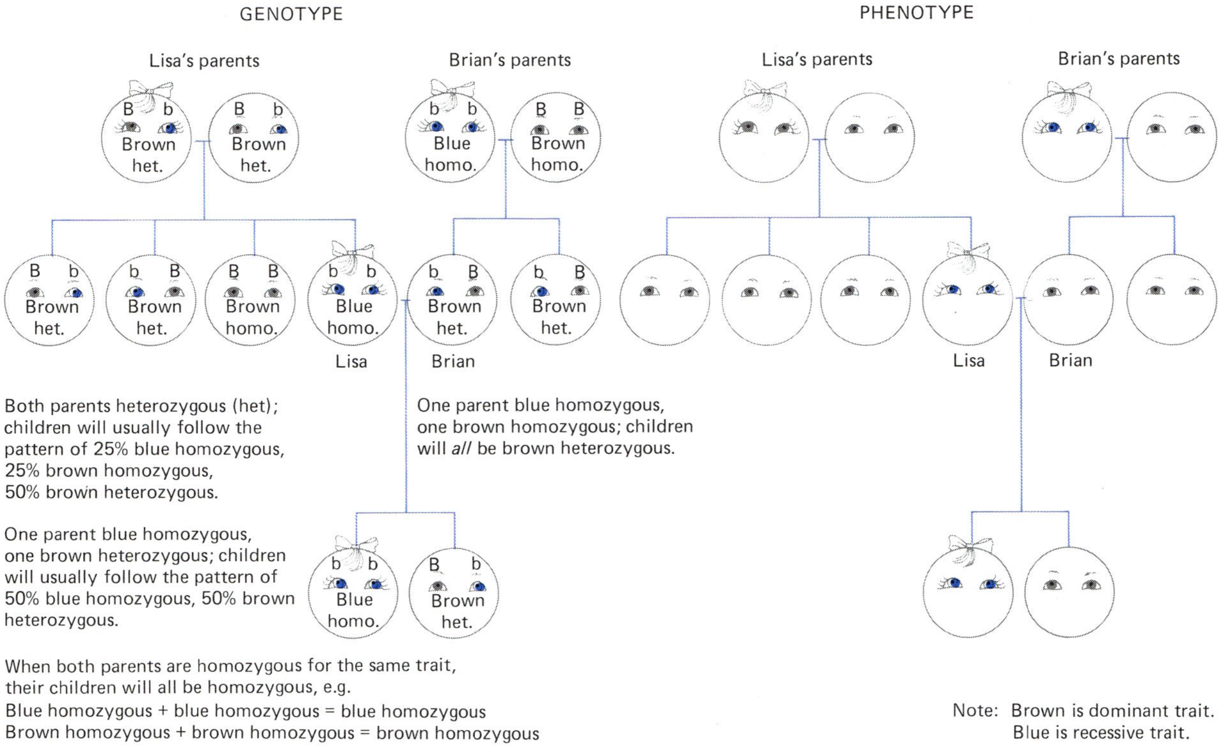

FIGURE 23.4 The genotype (genetic makeup) and phenotype (actual appearance) of the families of Lisa and Brian, with respect to eye color, according to Mendel's law.

March of Dimes

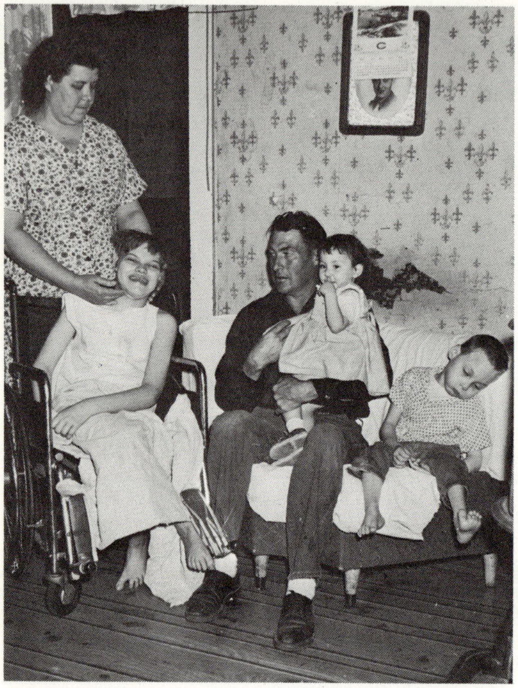

After having had two children with PKU defects, these parents were able to obtain early preventive treatment for their third child, who developed normally.

for wide variations in offspring. Ten children of the same set of parents may, for example, all be of different heights and intelligence, and have different hair color.

Disease Inheritance

About 15 years ago, Ellen Green gave birth to a darling little boy, David. The first couple of months, he thrived. Then, gradually, he stopped lifting his head, stopped smiling, stopped cooing, began having convulsions. By the end of his first year, he was a vegetable. Mercifully, David died during the next year. His parents, anxious for a family, tried again. This time, a lovely little girl was born. Like her brother, Jennifer grew and thrived. Her parents prayed that, unlike her brother, her growth would continue. Fearful of loving and losing again, they tried not to become too wrapped up in this warm and sunny infant. But Jennifer crept into their hearts anyway. And the pain was even greater the second time around, for Jennifer, too, became sick and died. Both children were victims of Tay-Sachs disease, an inherited disorder that primarily strikes children of Jewish persons of East European descent (see Table 23.3).

Some genes carry hereditary material for a disease or defect. The Greens had passed such genes on to their children. All of us carry some deleterious genes for mild or serious disorders, but they rarely show up. When they do show up they cause 80 percent of all birth defects and at least 40 percent of infant mortality. More than 3000 genetically conveyed diseases have been identified, and nearly 12 million Americans are affected by them to some extent. Estimates of individuals born with major or minor defects range from 7 to 14 percent or more of the population (Apgar and Beck).

Many inherited defects or diseases show up at birth (PKU or cystic fibrosis); some show up during infancy (Tay-Sachs); others in the teenage years (Wilson's disease); and still others in adulthood (Huntington's chorea and late-onset diabetes).

Though genetic diseases such as hemophilia were described even in ancient times, they have taken on new significance since they have replaced infectious diseases as the major threat to newborns. Because they take their toll early in life, they destroy more productive years of life than cancer and heart disease.

The four major patterns for inheritance of defects parallel ordinary inheritance: *dominant inheritance*, in which the harmful gene is dominant and can be passed on by only one parent; *recessive inheritance*, in which the harmful gene is recessive and two of them, one from each parent, are necessary for the trait to show; *sex-linked inheritance*, in which the female X chromosome carries the deleterious gene and the male child is the one

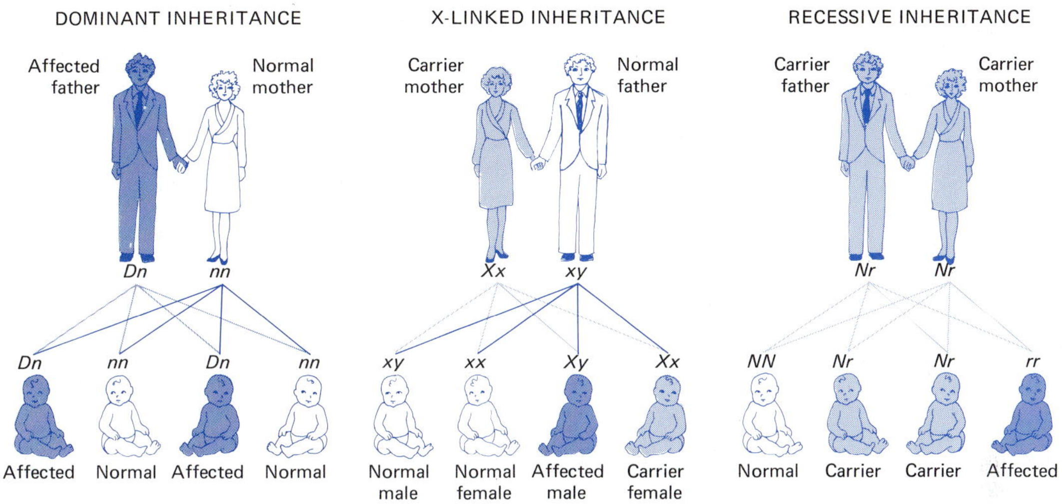

FIGURE 23.5 How laws of disease inheritance work. In *dominant inheritance,* one affected parent has a single faulty gene (*D*) which *dominates* its normal counterpart (*n*). Each child's chances of inheriting either the *D* or the *n* from the affected parent are 50 percent.

In the most common form of *X-linked inheritance,* the female sex chromosome of an unaffected mother carries one faulty gene (*X*) and one normal one (*x*). The father has a normal male X and Y chromosome complement. The odds for each *male* child are:

1 50 percent risk of inheriting the faulty *X* and the disorder
2 50 percent chance of inheriting normal *x* and *y* chromosomes

For each *female* child, the odds are:

1 50 percent risk of inheriting the faulty *X*, to be a carrier like mother
2 50 percent chance of inheriting no faulty gene

In *recessive inheritance, both* parents, usually unaffected, carry a normal gene (*N*) which takes precedence over its faulty recessive counterpart (*r*). The odds for each child are:

1 25 percent risk of inheriting a "double dose" of *r* genes which may cause a serious birth defect
2 25 percent chance of inheriting two *N*'s, thus being unaffected
3 50 percent chance of being a carrier with *Nr* [*Adapted from U.S. DHEW, aa, p. 17.*]

affected (see Figure 23.5); and *polygenic or multifactorial inheritance*, in which the interaction of several genes, with or without the influence of environmental factors, is responsible for the defect or disease. Disorders can also be inherited through abnormalities in the chromosomes themselves.

There are some 3000 known inherited diseases. Some are so rare they have not even been named; others (such as sickle-cell anemia, cystic fibrosis, and hemophilia) are fairly common. About two-thirds are believed to be *inborn errors of metabolism*, chemical mistakes caused by genes that carry incorrect

TABLE 23.3 Major inherited diseases

HOW TRANSMITTED	EXAMPLES	DIAGNOSIS	CHARACTERIZED BY	INCIDENCE	PREVENTION†	TREATMENT	OUTLOOK
Single gene recessive (Both parents must pass on recessive gene carrying disorder.) Odds: 1 in 4 if both parents carry gene	Cystic fibrosis (shortage of pancreatic enzyme)	Saltiness of perspiration	Heavy mucus secretions block digestive and respiratory function; fertility problem in adults	2 to 5% carry gene; 1 out of 1000 babies born with it (whites); 2000/yr	Early treatment prevents severe symptoms	Special diet and enzyme preparation	Without treatment few live to adulthood; with, 50% survive.
	Phenylketonuria (PKU) (abnormal buildup of phenalaline)	Test of blood from heel of newborn	Severe brain damage; retardation, hyperactivity, destructiveness; fair coloring	1 out of 10,000; 310/yr	Treatment by first or second week; carrier identification	Special diet	Untreated, 90% are institutionalized.
	Sickle-cell anemia‡ (hemoglobin abnormality, sickling and clumping of red blood cells)	Blood test; can also screen for carriers	Excruciating pain when cells clump and block blood vessels; anemia (see text)	Mostly in blacks: 1 out of 400 has disease; 1 out of 10 carries; 1200/yr	None except avoiding childbirth by carriers	Folic acid for pregnant victims; avoidance of stress, fatigue, and cold; transfusions	50% die before age 20; few live past 40.
	Tay-Sachs (excessive glycolipid storage in brain and nervous system)	Blood test; PN*	Deterioration of brain and central nervous system	Almost exclusively Ashkenazi Jews; 1 out of 30 is a carrier; 30/yr	None except avoiding childbirth by carriers, or genetic counseling and prenatal diagnosis	None	Death by third year of life.
Single gene dominant (One parent, affected by the disorder, passes it on to offspring.) Odds: 1 in 2 if one parent carries gene	Osteogenesis Imperfecta	Examination	Brittle bones; bluish "whites" of eyes; deafness (one or more symptoms)	Rare	Diagnosis of disease in adults before childbearing so they can avoid childbearing	Avoidance of injury; no cure	Varies depending on symptoms and severity.
	Marfan's syndrome (spider fingers)	Presence of symptoms	Long arms, legs, fingers, feet; absence of fat under skin; abnormalities of eyes, heart, blood vessels	Rare		Symptomatic	Depends on degree of involvement of heart, blood vessels, etc.
	Huntington's chorea	Presence of symptoms	Loss of motor control; personality changes in mid-thirties	Late appearing		None	Total deterioration 5 to 15 yrs after onset; death.

X-linked or sex-linked (Almost always in males who inherit an X chromosome with defective gene; females must inherit 2 such genes to be affected; female with one gene is carrier.)	Hemophilia (bleeder's disease)	Blood test; PN*	Varies from mild to severe bleeding from even very mild injury (uncontrollable)		Genetic counseling and prenatal diagnosis	Blood transfusions; clotting factor from normal blood	Early death without treatment, near normal life with it.
	Color deficiency	Vision test for color	Mild to severe difficulty in recognizing colors		None	None needed	Should be no problems.
	Duchenne form of muscular dystrophy	Presence of symptoms	Weakness and deterioration of muscles in early childhood	Late appearing	Detection of female carriers	None	Death by preteen years.
Polygenic (These do not follow a neat pattern of inheritance; risk of recurrence in family with one affected child about 5%; probably many genes involved.)	Club foot	Examination	Misshapen foot	9300/yr	Genetic counseling	Surgery, training, splinting	
	Some diabetes; possibly tendencies toward heart disease, cancer, allergy, atherosclerosis, hypertension, schizophrenia and other mental disorders		These diseases are treated at length elsewhere in this book; see Index.				
Chromosome abnormalities (Since there are many genes in each chromosome, even slight damage can cause serious defect; only about 4% inherited; remainder due to chromosome damage.)	Gross disfigurement of newborn; miscarriage		Almost any kind of defect, depending on which chromosome is damaged		Genetic counseling in some cases	None	Usually fatal except when X or Y chromosome is affected or in trisomy 21 (Down); early education improves outlook for Down.
	Down syndrome (Mongolism)	Karyotype PN*	Retardation, thick tongue, slanty eyes, flat face, etc.	1 out of 1500 if mother is under 30; 1 out of 100 if over 40; 1 out of 40 if age 45; 5100/yr	Genetic counseling	Early special education	

*Prenatal diagnosis possible.
†Good prenatal care and genetic counseling when necessary.
‡Incomplete recessive.

United Press International

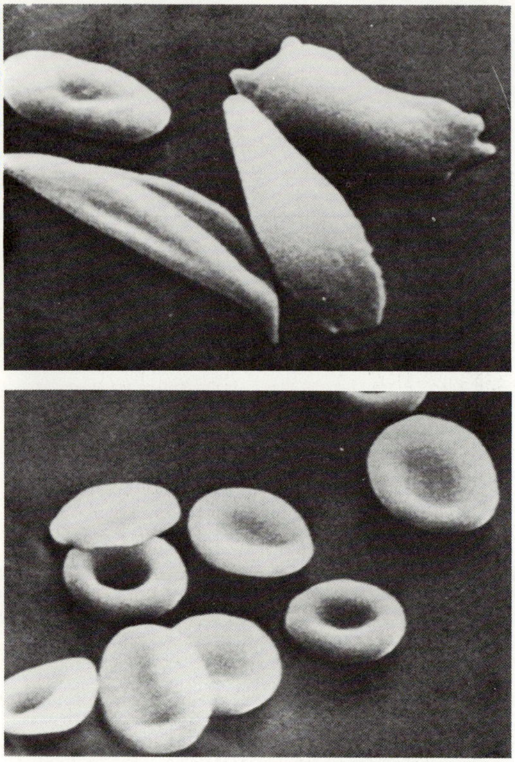

The top photo shows the distorted red blood cells characteristic of sickle-cell disease; the bottom shows normal cells.

blueprints for a needed body enzyme. The most common inherited disorders can be seen in Table 23.3. Two, sickle-cell anemia and Down syndrome, have such an impact that they deserve special attention.

Sickle-cell anemia Life plays strange tricks. What is now the most prevalent and destructive genetic disorder among American blacks evolved as a survival mechanism in Africa. Apparently, individuals carrying one or more sickle-cell genes were protected from deadly malaria attacks. Many with normal genes died of malaria, while those with two sickle-cell genes died of sickle-cell disease. Most likely to survive were those with sickle-cell trait (one normal and one sickle-cell gene) because they were both protected from malaria and free from serious sickle-cell disease. But here in the United States, where malaria is no threat, these survivors are carriers of sickle-cell disease, and if they marry other carriers, they can pass the disease on to their children. They may also occasionally show some symptoms of the disease themselves.

Sickle-cell anemia is the result of a genetic misprint, a misplaced amino acid in the oxygen-carrying hemoglobin molecules of the red blood cells. This leads to a chain of events in which the shape of the hemoglobin molecules becomes distorted, in turn distorting the red blood cell from its normal disc shape to one resembling the familiar farm implement. Sickled cells hook up to one another in such a way that they can block a blood vessel, cutting off blood flow and thus oxygen.

The choking off of oxygen causes further distortion of the hemoglobin, and the cycle continues. The result is excruciating pain, swelling of joints, and eventual damage to organs denied blood. Episodes of sickling can be set off by lack of oxygen from stress, exercise, high altitude. They become less frequent with age, down from 8 to 10 per year in childhood to fewer than 1 per year by age 40. That is small comfort, however, since few sickle-cell victims live to celebrate their fortieth birthdays.

Carriers can be identified by blood tests, but there is nothing that can be done to prevent the disease in some of the offspring of a union between carriers. The suggestion that such unions avoid having children has been widely rejected, since 10 percent of the black population are carriers. Instead it is recommended that research into treatments, such as folic acid for pregnant sickle-cell patients and oxygen to end a sickle-cell crisis, be intensified.

Down syndrome Sometimes called mongolism because of the oriental appearance of its victims, this most common of the chromo-

Nancy Hays/Monkmeyer

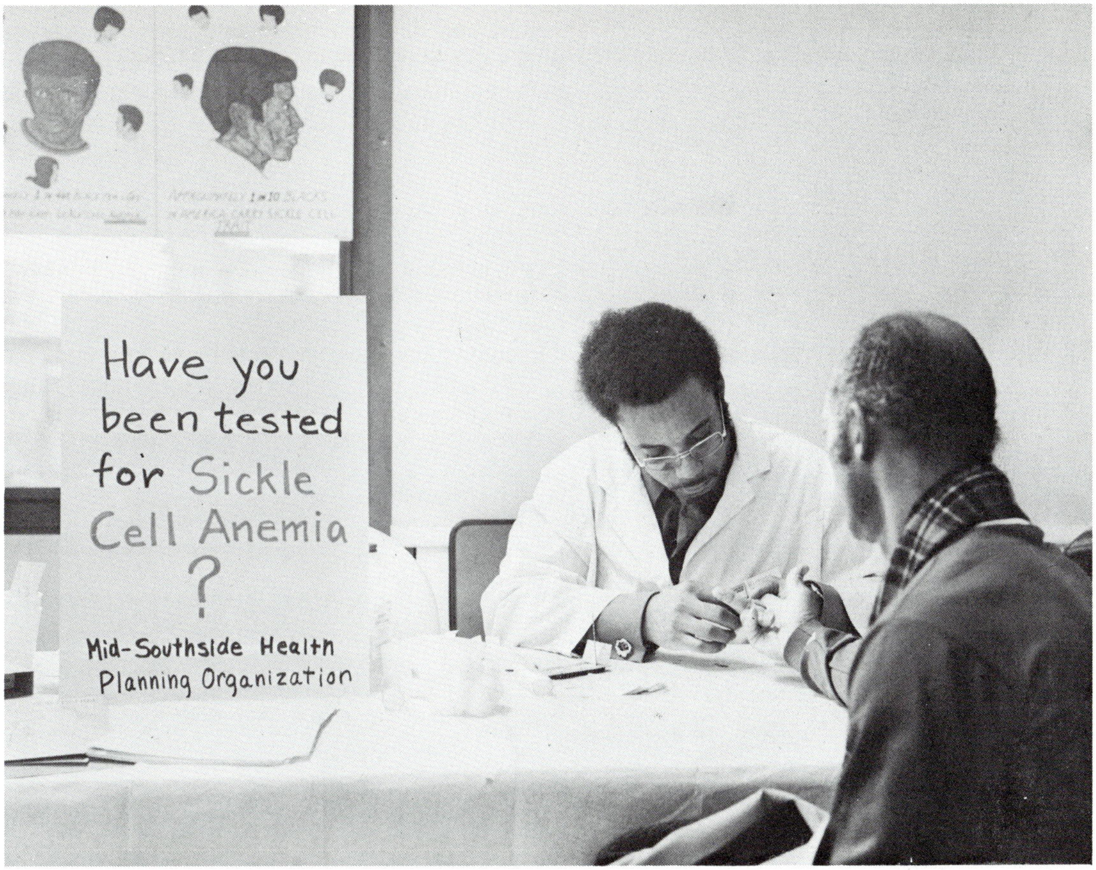
Have you
been tested
for Sickle
Cell Anemia
?
Mid-Southside Health
Planning Organization

The test for sickle-cell anemia is a simple procedure.

somal disorders affects 1 in 700 infants born each year. The cause in each individual case can be determined by doing a karyotype (microscopic examination of actual chromosomes) of skin or blood cells, as shown in Figure 23.6. The disorder results from a surplus of genetic material, usually an extra chromosome 21, a condition called *trisomy 21*. In 95 percent of cases, the excess material results from a flaw in just that one fertilized ovum and is not hereditary. Older mothers, particularly over 40, bear 95 percent of Down babies, possibly because older chromosomes tend not to separate completely during meiosis. If a young woman should bear a child with this defect, chances that any of her future children will be affected are very low.

In another 4 percent of Down syndrome cases, the excess of chromosome material is caused by a *translocation* (a piece of one chromosome, usually chromosome 21, breaks off and attaches itself to another) passed from one parent, most often the mother, to a child who also receives a normal chromosome 21 from the other parent. When one such child is born into a family, genetic counseling is advised before further pregnancies are attempted.

The excess genetic material apparently scrambles the blueprints in the normal chro-

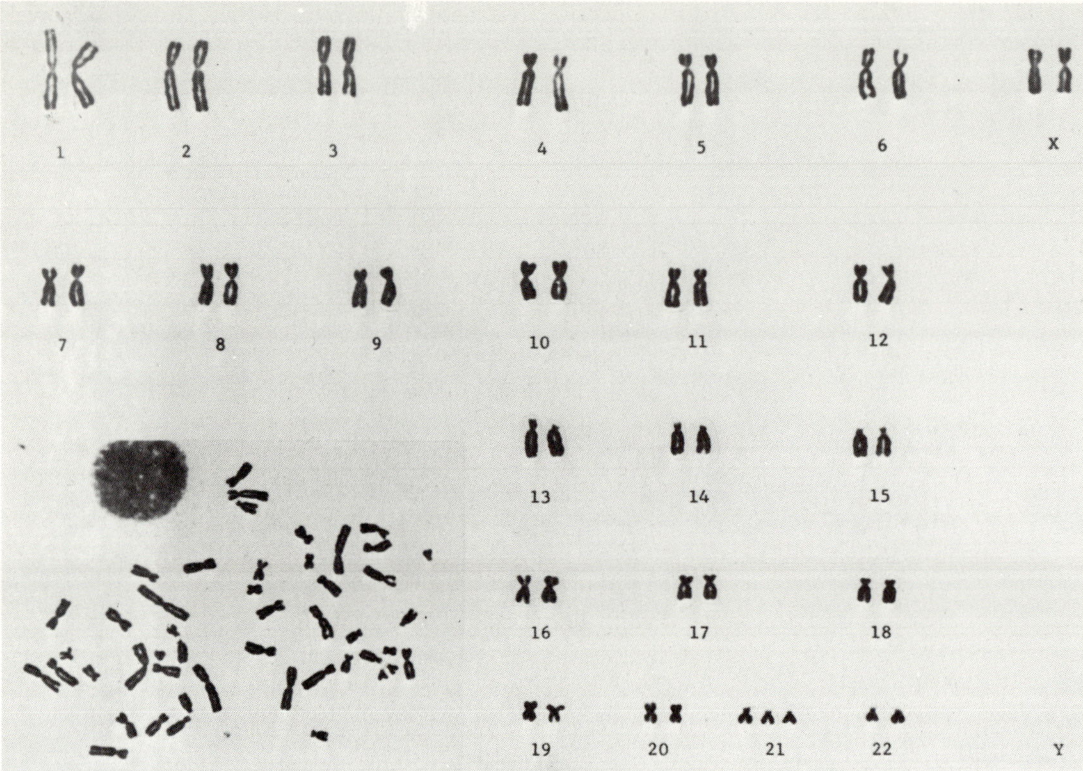

FIGURE 23.6 The chromosomal pattern or *karyotype* of a human female with Down syndrome. Note the two X chromosomes and the extra number 21 chromosome. [*National Foundation March of Dimes.*]

mosome 21 to such an extent that as many as 65 known defects can occur. Mental retardation is the most persistent symptom and Down syndrome is responsible for more retardation than any other single disorder. As better medical care prolongs the lives of Down victims, their numbers increase.

Genetic Counseling

The Greens, the couple described earlier, vowed, after losing two children to Tay-Sachs, that they would never have another child. It was a vow they were happy to break several years later when they heard about genetic counseling. Brand new in the 1960s, genetic counseling is now a rapidly growing field. The most recent compilation of genetic services, both counseling and related labs, lists 903 entries in 58 countries, 398 of them in the United States. The genetic counselor, a sort of heredity bookmaker, is trained to give couples and individuals the "odds" on their having children with birth defects and to help them make decisions on whether or not to have children.

In the case of the Greens, the genetic counselor told them that they were both carriers of Tay-Sachs and that any child born to them had a 1 in 4 chance of acquiring defective genes from both parents and having Tay-Sachs. But odds, including a toss of the coin, can only be counted on in large numbers. Four consecutive tosses may turn up four "heads" or four "tails." A couple carrying Tay-Sachs may have four affected or four normal children in a row.

A 1 in 4 risk was one the Greens would not have been willing to take. But the counselor offered them better odds. He explained that if Mrs. Green became pregnant, he could detect by the 13th or 14th week whether or not the child was going to be normal. If it was not, she would have the option of a therapeutic abortion and could, if she wished, try again. The Greens agreed.

When Mrs. Green was 14 weeks pregnant, the doctor anesthetized her abdomen and, using a long hollow needle in a procedure called amniocentesis (see Figure 23.7) drew some amniotic fluid from her uterus. Examination of cells shed by the fetus showed no signs of Tay-Sachs. The fetus was normal.

Today, some 60 diseases can be detected by amniocentesis. The slight risk attached to the procedure can be minimized by carefully locating the fetus and placenta with ultrasound. Risks are far outweighed by the benefits of being able to evaluate the condition, or chromosomal count, of the fetus before birth.

Prenatal defects are exposed by several other remarkable diagnostic techniques: (1) *Ultrasound* examines the outline of the fetus for abnormalities, much as surface sonar picks up the underwater outline of a submarine. (2) *Amniography* injects a dye into the amniotic fluid, outlining the shape of the fetus on x-ray photos. (3) *Fetoscopy* uses an

Victims of Down syndrome, the most common chromosomal disorder, benefit greatly from early training and loving care.

Bruce Roberts/Photo Researchers

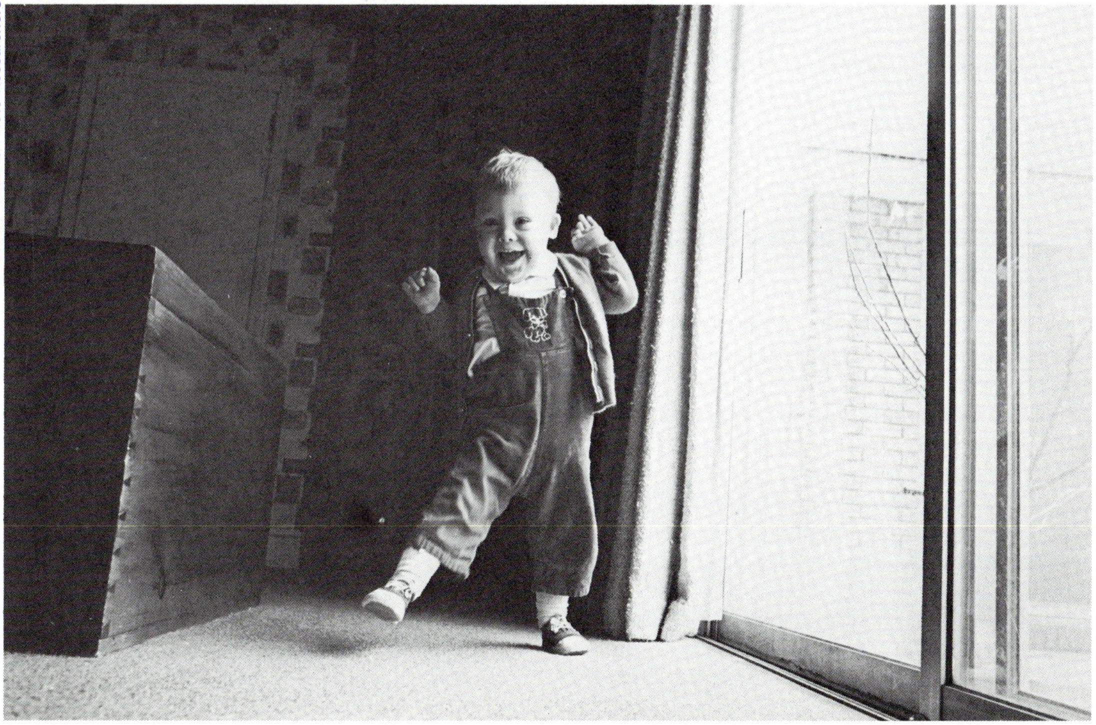

exotic miniature periscope and camera with a fiberoptic bundle of lights (see Chapter 25) to actually view the fetus in the uterus. (4) *Chorionic biopsy* scrapes a bit of tissue from the scalp of the fetus through the opening of the cervix for examination. All this early warning information helps parents make decisions about the future of the fetus and, in some cases, allows a physician to "make house calls in the womb," diagnosing and treating a disorder prenatally.

Not everyone needs a genetic counselor. Happily, most couples can expect to have normal children. But to sidestep tragedy, it is wise for the following individuals or couples to seek guidance:

- Parents who have already borne one child with a birth defect.
- Couples who know of heredity defects on any branch of the family tree.
- Closely related couples (e.g., cousins) who wish to marry, or are married and wish to have children. (When inherited diseases or defects exist in a family, the risk of their emerging is always higher when parents are related—1 in 8 for first cousins.)
- Women over 40, with a much increased risk of having a Down syndrome child.

WHAT THE BABY WILL BE LIKE: ENVIRONMENTAL DETERMINANTS

The other answer to what baby will be like is environment. The belief that a child could be "marked" by something that happened to its mother (be born with an apple-red birthmark because the mother was struck by a falling apple, for example) was discredited more than a generation ago. But today, scientists recognize that what happens to the mother during pregnancy, and to both parents before conception, can have a strong effect on the child. Parents who recognize this can make decisions that will greatly reduce the risk of birth defects and increase chances of a healthy baby.

Mutagens and Teratogens

An estimated 20 percent of birth defects, including 95 percent of cerebral palsy cases, are believed to be environmentally caused (U.S. DHEW, *aa*). Some environmental factors cause changes or mutations in the germ cells of the parents before conception. These factors are called *mutagens* (*mutata* = change + *gen* = cause). Their effects are *genetic*. Other factors can damage the embryo or fetus after conception. These are called *teratogens* (*terato* = monster). The defects caused are called *congenital*. Changes caused by teratogens are not, however, always negative. Mutations can improve an organism as well as harm it. Some of the most common mutagens and teratogens in the environment are discussed below.

Radiation One of the earlier recognized causes of birth defects is radiation—from x-rays, from natural radiation, from atomic explosion, or from defective microwave ovens. The degree of damage is related to the amount and duration of exposure.

Drugs Hundreds of German infants born with shortened or missing arms, legs, or ears after their mothers had taken the drug thalidomide as a sleeping pill alerted scientists to the fact that drugs and other substances could cross the placenta and cause birth defects. It is now known that a wide variety of pharmaceuticals, including hormones, diuretics, antiepileptic medications, barbiturates, tranquilizers, antibiotics, and very large doses of some vitamins, as well as such drugs as alcohol, methadone, heroin, caffeine, and tobacco can cause damage to the fetus. Heavy use of alcohol,[2] even occasional binge

[2]It is strongly recommended that pregnant women take *no more* than 2 alcoholic drinks daily.

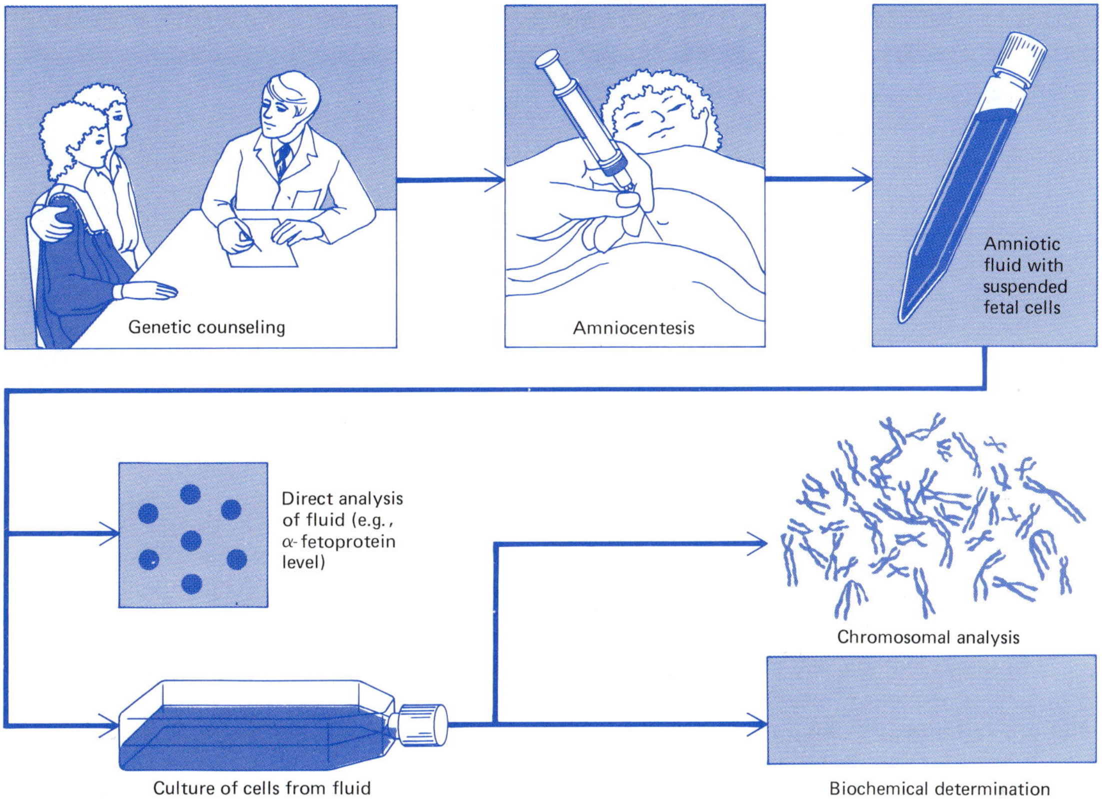

FIGURE 23.7 Amniocentesis, testing the condition of the unborn child. [*Adapted from Karp et al., p. 7.*]

drinking, is so dangerous that it has been suggested that alcoholic women should give serious consideration to early termination of pregnancy. Children of women who average 6 ounces or more of alcohol a day are at very high risk of dying at or just after birth, of being mentally deficient, or having other abnormal features (K. Jones et al.). These symptoms are lumped under the name fetal alcohol syndrome. Children of women addicted to alcohol, heroin, methadone, or other drugs may also undergo withdrawal at birth, sometimes with fatal results. The effects on the fetus of other nonmedical drugs, such as marijuana, LSD, etc., are as yet unknown, but some authorities believe they may pose a threat.

Tobacco, often not thought of as a drug, also presents a hazard to the unborn, especially if the mother smokes after the fourth month of pregnancy. Babies of smoking mothers are more likely to have a low birth weight (under 5.8 pounds or 2500 grams), a serious risk, since LBW babies account for 70 percent of all newborn deaths, and are more likely to have birth defects, to die around birth, to be somewhat behind children of nonsmokers in size and intellectual ability. A

Relationship Between Time of Exposure to Environmental Hazards and Type of Fetal Damage

The time of exposure to a drug or other environmental hazard strongly influences its effect on the fetus. For example, in mothers who took thalidomide the following defects occurred:

AGE OF FETUS AT EXPOSURE	EFFECT
35 days	No ears
39–40 days	Deformed arms
41–44 days	Deformed legs
Over 52 days	No effect

German study further implicated smoking fathers, finding that their children have a 50 percent greater chance of dying around birth, and a 162 percent greater risk of a life-threatening deformity (Mau and Netter, *a*; N. R. Butler et al.). Heavy coffee use by the mother has also been related to prematurity and low birth weight (Mau and Netter, *b*).

Infection The rubella (German measles) virus, as well as several other infections that strike the mother, can cause damage in the fetus, as can be seen in Table 23.4. The fetus is most susceptible during the first three months.

Industrial pollution Technological advanc-

SELF-CARE

Having a Healthy Baby

Parental decision making both before and during pregnancy can increase the chances of a healthy baby. Babies are healthiest when:

- The mother is between 20 and 35 and the father is under 45.
- Both parents are well nourished prenatally and the mother consumes a diet high in nutrients and adequate in calories during pregnancy (she should gain about 20 to 25 pounds).
- Parents have prenatal checkups and genetic counseling if needed.
- The mother receives excellent medical care during pregnancy and delivery.
- Pregnancies are spaced at least two years, nine months apart; families are limited to two or three children.
- Both parents avoid exposure to x-ray or chemicals known to cause mutation prior to pregnancy. The mother should avoid exposure to medication (even aspirin) except on medical advice; to tobacco, alcohol, and other drugs; to x-ray (except when urgent); to pollutants and other known teratogens; to lack of oxygen; and to infectious diseases (taking preventive measures when possible; see Table 23.4) during pregnancy.

TABLE 23.4 Effects on fetus of disease organisms

DISEASE	MONTHS OF RISK	MOST COMMON EFFECTS	PREVENTION/TREATMENT	HOW TRANSMITTED
Gonorrhea*	9	Conjunctivitis of newborn, blindness; serious general infection	Testing/treatment of mother before delivery; drops of silver nitrate in eyes of all newborns	Infant infected during passage through infected vaginal canal
Herpes simplex II	9	Serious infection; can be fatal	Possibly Caesarian section to avoid passage of fetus through vaginal canal	Probably during passage through infected vaginal canal; possibly crosses placenta
Rubella	1–3	Cardiac defects, cataracts, deafness	Immunization of mother before pregnancy	Crosses placenta
Toxoplasmosis*	4–5	Underdeveloped brain, blindness, etc. at birth or later in life	Pregnant women should avoid handling cat litter, eating raw meat	Crosses placenta
Syphilis	5–9	Bone, tooth deformities; progressive nervous system damage; stillbirth; brain damage later in life	Testing and treating mother before fifth month	Crosses placenta after fifth month

*May be no noticeable symptoms in mother.

es designed to make life easier have brought with them dangers for children yet unborn. A long list of chemicals (insecticides, mercury vapors, weed killers, aerosol fluorocarbons, cleaning fluids, vinyl chloride, and plastic by-products) has been linked to birth defects. The inhalation of anesthesia leaking from equipment in hospital operating rooms appears to cause an increase in birth defects in children parented by operating room personnel.

Oxygen deprivation Oxygen shortage due to such factors as injury or illness in the mother that cuts off or reduces oxygen supply, an oxygen-thin atmosphere such as that at high altitudes, or general anesthesia given during surgical or dental care, can lead to low birth weight, prematurity, and sometimes, brain damage.

Dietary deficiency "You are what you eat," a popular radio nutritionist used to say. He might have added, "Your baby is what you eat." Parents, particularly mothers, who were well nourished from childhood through adulthood have a better chance of having healthy children than the malnourished.

During pregnancy, mother and baby are in competition for the nutrients the mother consumes. Very often, the baby is the loser. Yet proper nutrition prenatally may be more important than at any other time in life (Calloway). Both human and animal studies have shown that deficiencies at this time of protein, vitamins, iron, calcium, trace minerals such as copper and manganese, iodine, or calories can lead to low birth weight and/or prematurity, birth defects, mental and physical retardation, and typical deficiency diseases (see basic diet, Table 5.6) (Brody, *a*).

Psychological Environment

Wanted babies of happy, secure women have the best chance of being born healthy, because mothers who are happy about their pregnancies take better care of themselves. Nervous mothers, unwed mothers, and anxious mothers with erratic lifestyles are more likely to have nervous, fussy babies who cry a lot. Rat studies show a clear relationship between prenatal stress and offspring behavior (Joffe). With humans, it is more difficult to find a precise relationship between the mother's mental health and the condition of the fetus, because of the many variables that cannot be controlled, but many scientists believe a relationship does exist. Studies are under way to find out more.

Difficulties During Childbirth

Even at the last moments before birth, the fetus is subject to environmental hazards, among them: a lengthy or difficult labor or delivery, poor use of forceps, too much anesthesia, too much or too little oxygen administered either to mother or newborn.

CHILDBIRTH

Many couples spend hours deciding on a name for the baby, but there are other decisions to be considered. Some will be limited by availability, others by medical necessity. But most expectant parents today find many open options.

What Kind of Childbirth?

The decision about the kind of delivery will be made by the physician in consultation with the expectant parents. Childbirth education can help parents contribute intelligently to this decision. Today, about half of hospitals and many private physicans and clinics in the United States offer such education. Many classes are based on the system introduced in the United States by Ferdinand Lamaze. In Lamaze courses, the physical and emotional changes of pregnancy are explained, and breathing techniques and exercises to be done before and during labor are taught. The father, or a friend or relative, is trained to act as "coach" during practice and actual labor. Group discussions are an outlet for fears and anxieties and offer the kind of support that used to be available from the nearly vanished extended family.

Preparation for childbirth does not mean that a woman commits herself to labor and delivery without medication, but preparation will probably reduce the amount of medication needed. Even for the couple uninterested in "natural" (or "prepared" or "cooperative") childbirth, training can ease the fears and some of the discomforts of pregnancy and childbirth, through knowledge and understanding.

If anesthesia is needed or desired, physician and expectant mother can discuss the options: tranquilizers or analgesics (pain relievers) during labor, local anesthesia such as novacaine which may be needed for the episiotomy (an incision made, if necessary, to temporarily enlarge the vaginal opening), regional nerve blocks to reduce sensation in the lower part of the body, or general anesthesia that puts the mother to sleep. This last is given infrequently today in normal childbirth because of the ill effects it can have on

My husband's a stoic. He never shows his emotions. But when our second child was born, he was in the delivery room. . . . "It's a boy," he said, his voice catching a bit. I took my eyes off the exciting birth scene to look at my husband. Tears were running down his cheeks. I'll never forget that moment as long as I live.

Susan Kilduff, mother, nurse, and Lamaze instructor

Erika Stone/Peter Arnold

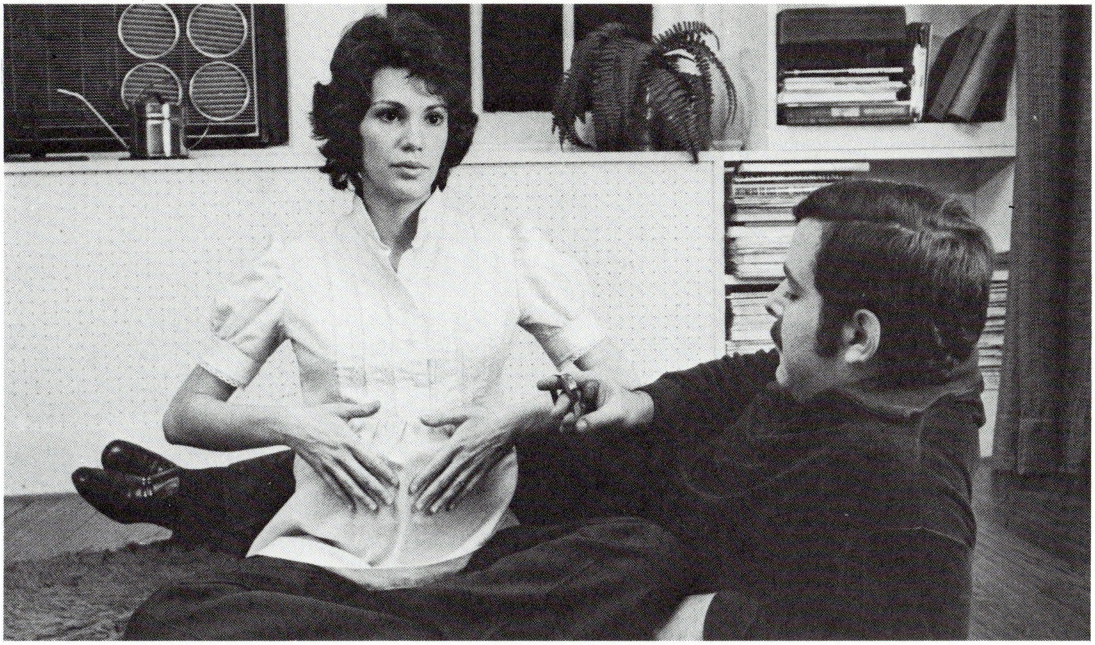

Childbirth preparation, such as the Lamaze technique shown here, can ease the fears and some of the discomforts of pregnancy and childbirth.

Abigail Heyman/Magnum

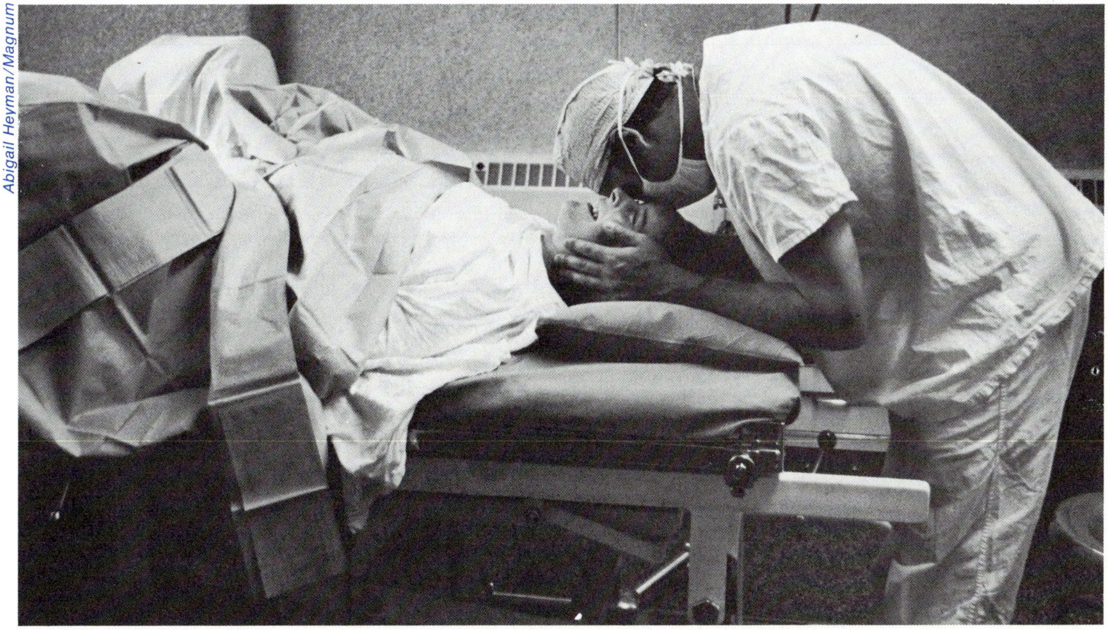

The father is trained to act as "coach" during practice and actual labor.

Childbirth Without Violence

"Hell is not at the end of life . . . it is here. At the beginning. . . . This is birth. This is the torture, the Calvary." So believes French obstetrician Frederick Leboyer who has developed techniques to replace the baby's "inferno" with an environment of peace and tranquility. To accomplish this, he substitutes dim lights, Indian music, fondling, and warm baths in the delivery room for the snug uterine surroundings. He believes the trauma of the ordinary delivery can permanently scar a child's psyche, and a joyful reassuring delivery can have a long-term positive effect.

The Leboyer method, however, has been widely criticized by the medical profession as being antiscientific and without benefit. Leboyer defends his position by claiming to adhere rigidly to all scientific procedures for the health and safety of mother and child. But he avoids many procedures used by others "as a matter of course" (upending and spanking the newborn, for example), using them only when indicated. As much as his colleagues swear at him, mothers whom he has delivered swear by him.

Parents interested in information on Leboyer's methods can read his book *Birth Without Violence.* For prevailing medical opinion, they can turn to their obstetricians.

both mother and child. Since all anesthetics and analgesics cross the placenta, quickly reaching the fetus, the risks of their use should be weighed against the benefits. When needed, they are administered at the very last moment before delivery, so exposure of fetus is minimal. If the baby is too large for the mother's pelvis, or there are other problems, a Caesarian section, in which the baby is removed by surgery through the mother's abdomen, may be necessary. However, Caesarian section, as well as induction of labor through the use of hormones, should be undertaken only when medically indicated and not for convenience.

Who Will Deliver the Baby?

In a one-doctor town, this question may not arise. But most expectant couples have the option of seeking out someone whose philosophy of childbirth comes reasonably close to their own. Some will feel an obstetrician is needed; others would rather have their own family doctor do the job. Board-certified family physicians receive special training in obstetrics and many do deliveries. Some general practitioners have been doing them for years without special training.

A choice only recently available is the nurse-midwife, an RN with special training in obstetrics, who works with low-risk patients expected to have uncomplicated pregnancies and deliveries.[3] Should signs of complications arise, the nurse-midwife calls in the physician under whose supervision she works. Nurse-midwives can give the expectant mother and her family more time and attention than a doctor, and they have received high praise from both patients and physicians.

Where Will the Baby be Delivered?

Many will go to the only hospital in town, or to the one where their chosen physician has delivery privileges. Others, especially those with high-risk pregnancies, will opt for a major medical center. A few will want to have their babies at home because they view hospital care as costly and impersonal. Most,

[3]Lay midwives, of course, have been delivering babies since time immemorial.

however, will not want to risk delivery away from the sophisticated backup equipment of a hospital. Yet they would like a homelike, "natural" setting for childbirth, which is, after all, not a disease. Many hospitals have responded to this desire by making maternity departments more homey—allowing fathers, and sometimes even siblings and friends, to participate in labor and even delivery, and permitting babies to room in with their mothers at least part of the time. Independent "birth centers" have also sprung up to fill this need.

Labor and Delivery

The birth process may take less than 1 hour or drag on for 24 hours or more. When there is concern about the safety of the fetus, its vital signs can be monitored throughout labor and delivery. Such monitoring greatly reduces risk of childbirth injury. Childbirth is usually divided into three stages.

Stage I This longest stage, ranging from 1 to 8 hours in most women, starts with the onset of contractions, with a "show" (slight bleeding from the vagina), or with a leakage of amniotic fluid as the membranes (the amnion) rupture in preparation for delivery. As contractions become stronger, longer, and closer together, the cervix dilates (opens) so the baby can squeeze through during delivery.

Stage II The cervix is dilated. If the baby is positioned head first, if the mother's pelvis is large enough to accommodate the infant, and if there are no complications, the birth will now proceed normally. The woman who is alert and trained can be an active participant by "bearing down" and adding some 40 pounds of effort to the work of the contractions. If necessary, the attending physician will make an incision, the episiotomy, to enlarge the vaginal opening, and will suture (stitch) it up following delivery. The umbilical cord connecting infant to placenta is clamped or tied and cut, leaving the baby on its own, independent of the mother.

If, however, the baby is in a breech position—feet or buttocks first, for example, or there are other problems preventing normal birth, the physician may have to use forceps to help the baby through the vaginal canal, or may have to remove the infant surgically through the mother's abdomen in surgery called a *Caesarian section* (so called because Julius Caesar was reputedly born this way).

Stage III The final stage of labor, delivery of the placenta (sometimes called the *afterbirth*), is more than just an afterthought. If the placenta is not normally delivered within 15 to 20 minutes after birth, the physician or midwife will remove it by hand to prevent hemorrhage.

THE NEWBORN

By the time the newborn—a wrinkled, toothpick-armed little creature with a head misshapen from the tight transit through the birth canal—is nestled in a nursery bassinet, his or her condition has been thoroughly assessed by the medical staff. Obvious physical defects, if any, have been noted, weight checked. Respiration, color, muscle tone, reflexes, and heart rate were checked at 1 and 5 minutes after birth against the Apgar scale. Most infants check out perfectly.

Problems of the Newborn

No time in life is more hazardous than the 24 hours before and after birth. The odds of survival have been improved by neonatal (*neo* = new + *natal* = born) intensive care units set up in medical centers around the nation to care for high-risk infants who are often rushed to them by ambulance or helicopter in special incubators. The babies most often in need of pediatric intensive care are those with the following problems.

Ed Lettau/Photo Researchers

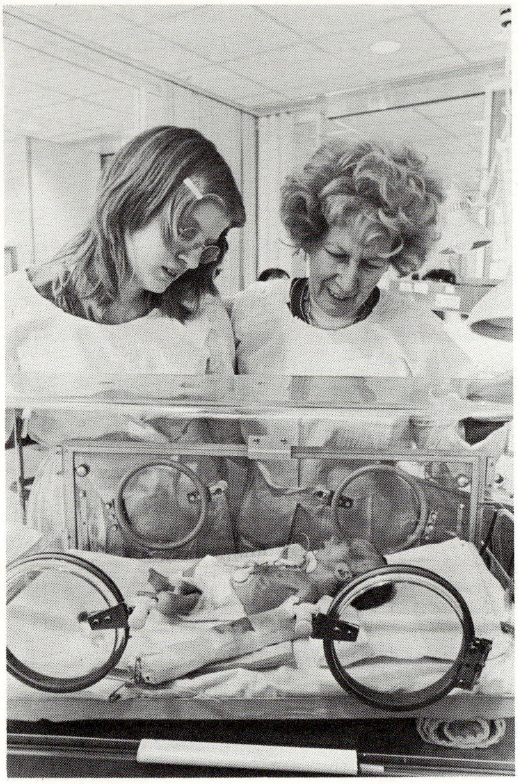

Infants born at low weight for their gestational age are at high risk, whether they are premature or full term.

Low birth weight Infants born at a low birth weight for their gestational age (counted from the first day of the mother's last menstrual period) are at high risk, whether they are premature or full term. LBW babies are prone to respiratory difficulties and have a higher mortality rate, more illness, and more vision, hearing, and mental deficiencies than normal-weight babies.

Respiratory distress syndrome President and Mrs. John F. Kennedy's firstborn son, Patrick Bouvier, died just a few days after birth from RDS, also called *hyaline membrane disease*. Today, though treatment has become more sophisticated, more than 25 percent of newborn deaths, about 11,000 a year, are caused by RDS.

Causes of RDS are not precisely understood, but indications are that its victims' lungs are not fully mature at birth, resulting in severe breathing difficulties. Treatments, sometimes successful, include (1) supplying oxygen to the newborn until its own body system can take over and (2) giving steroids before birth when premature labor is threatened.

Congenital heart and other internal defects. Nearly 1 baby in 100 is born with a malformation of the heart or of a major blood vessel near the heart. Thousands more are born with defects of other internal organs, many so minor they go unnoticed, others so critical that without immediate surgery, the infant cannot survive the first days of life.

In the past, nothing could be done for the more seriously malformed infants. But the remarkable development of minisurgery—delicate techniques utilizing magnifying lenses and miniature surgical instruments—has allowed pediatric surgeons to operate on infant body structures barely visible to the naked eye and to save thousands of newborns.

Early Parental Decisions

Breast- or bottle-feeding? In 1867, Oliver Wendell Holmes the Elder said: "A pair of substantial mammary glands has the advantage over the two hemispheres of the most learned professor's brain in the art of compounding a nutritious fluid for infants." Medical opinion today supports his contention. Breast-fed babies are less likely to suffer from a variety of ailments, including allergies, diarrhea, constipation, colic, diaper rash, and skin eruptions.

Possibly because of the antibodies and other immunological elements received from the colostrum (secreted from the breast during the first few days after birth), they are less

Sudden Infant Death Syndrome

The mysterious death of seemingly normal infants has puzzled humankind for thousands of years. The earliest written account of such a death is believed to be the biblical one described in the book of Kings. In the famous story, a woman whose child had died in the night "because she overlay it" is charged with stealing another woman's baby to replace it. King Solomon, of course, in his great wisdom, was able to identify the rightful mother of the live child. But what Solomon did not know and scholars now believe is that the child died from sudden infant death syndrome (SIDS). The theory that many infants smother because they sleep with their mothers or others is no longer accepted because thousands of babies—10,000 a year in the United States—die similarly while sleeping alone in their cribs.

Theories about what causes SIDS abound and many avenues of research are being followed in an attempt to solve this puzzle. No severe infection is evident in autopsies of SIDS victims, nor is there evidence of choking on food or smothering in bedclothes. One possible explanation is that certain babies, particularly following mild colds, are prone to periods of apnea, or lapses in breathing. These usually last a few seconds, but it may be that, in SIDS cases, they are for some unknown reason extended.

susceptible to many kinds of infections from colds to bronchitis and pneumonia, and probably to enterocolitis, a hazard to premature infants (Santulli et al.). Evidence indicates they may also have healthier teeth and lower cholesterol levels later in childhood than bottle-fed babies (Eiger and Olds). There are, in addition, psychological benefits from the close mother-child contact afforded by breast-feeding (Montagu, *b*).

There are benefits for the mother, too. Nursing helps reduce the uterus to its prepregnancy size more quickly and to control bleeding. Nursing mothers are less likely to become pregnant (though nursing is far from reliable contraception) and are more interested in a rapid return to intercourse than nonnursing mothers. The reasons are unclear, but many studies have shown a correlation between lack of breast-feeding and high breast cancer rates (Hubbard). Mothers also derive psychological benefits; many consider it one of the most rewarding experiences of their lives. And finally, breast-feeding is immediately available to a hungry infant and thus easier for both parents: no formula, no shopping, no bottle heating at 4 A.M.

A recently discovered drawback to breast-feeding is the presence of hazardous chemicals in the milk of mothers who have eaten foods contaminated with such substances as PCBs. It is possible that a diet with no fresh-water fish and low in animal and dairy fats may avoid the problem.

Bottle-feeding, too, can be rewarding and satisfying to both parents and child. Bottle-fed infants thrive physically and if bottle-feeding is accompanied by cuddling, crooning, and affection, the psychological benefits can be maintained. The temptation to leave the baby in the crib with a bottle propped should be avoided.

Though breast-feeding dipped to an all-time low in the 1950s and 1960s, it made a comeback in the seventies, rising from a 30 percent average for 1950 to 1972 to 38 percent in 1975 (*Pediatric News*). Even working mothers have managed to breast-feed, some returning home for noon feedings.

Circumcision The male penis has a natural foreskin covering the glans. Among many peoples, including Jews and Moslems, removal of this foreskin is part of a religious or

WHERE TO FIND HELP

Information on breast-feeding can be obtained from La Leche League International, 9616 Minneapolis Avenue, Franklin Park, IL 60131, or your local La Leche League.

cultural rite dating back into antiquity. Today, the removal of the newborn's foreskin, a process called *circumcision*, has become routine in most hospitals in the United States. Some opposition has developed because, theoretically, the foreskin could have some important but unknown function and because the minor surgery entails some slight risk. Many physicians believe the risk to be reduced by the eighth day, when blood clotting is better developed.

There are tangible benefits in circumcision. Smegma (a sticky secretion of the glands of the foreskin), urine, and other contaminants and irritants can collect under a tight foreskin, irritate the glans penis, and cause infection. Careful cleaning can help avoid this. Then, too, a higher rate of penile cancer has been noted in uncircumcised men. And circumcision eliminates phimosis, in which a tight foreskin causes pain and possible impotence.

PARENTING

A mother's[4] relationship with her baby from birth on has a significant influence on its physical, intellectual, emotional, and social development. Numerous animal and human studies have shown that deprivation of one-to-one care by the mother or a mother substitute leads to abnormal physical, mental, and emotional development and, in extreme cases, even death (Yarrow). Children who do not form an attachment to their mothers later show signs of being unable to form deep attachments (Sheridan).

The father, too, plays an important part in the life of the infant and child (Pedersen and Robson). Not surprisingly, while the mother has been seen as the basic humanizer in the family, the father has been the parent associated with commitment to order (society and family rules), survival skills, and cooperation with the outside world (L. Benson). Studies show that children raised in the physical or emotional absence of a father suffer from a variety of damaging effects (Pedersen et al.; Hetherington, *a, b*; Andry).

As more women find roles outside the home, father will probably become even more important—not as the undisputed master of all the family he was a couple of generations ago, nor as the harried, pressured, too-busy person he often is today, but as an "authoritative father who has a firm hand, quick eye, sensitive ear, open mind and generous heart" (L. Fuchs).

Parenting Styles

There is no best way to rear a child. Each child is different, so is each parent, and circumstances continually change. All parents want to have healthy, happy, successful children, but often their good intentions go astray. It is important that parents realize that they cannot be perfect, that they will make mistakes, that it is less important that they be fairly strict, fairly permissive, or in between than that they be basically consistent and loving. It is also important to be a parent rather than a friend—the roles are different

[4]Little research is available on whether or not the attachment can be split, making it a mother-child/father-child arrangement. Some young couples today, anxious to share parenting, have elected to try to do this. The results are not yet in, though many authorities applaud the attempt.

Erika Stone/Peter Arnold

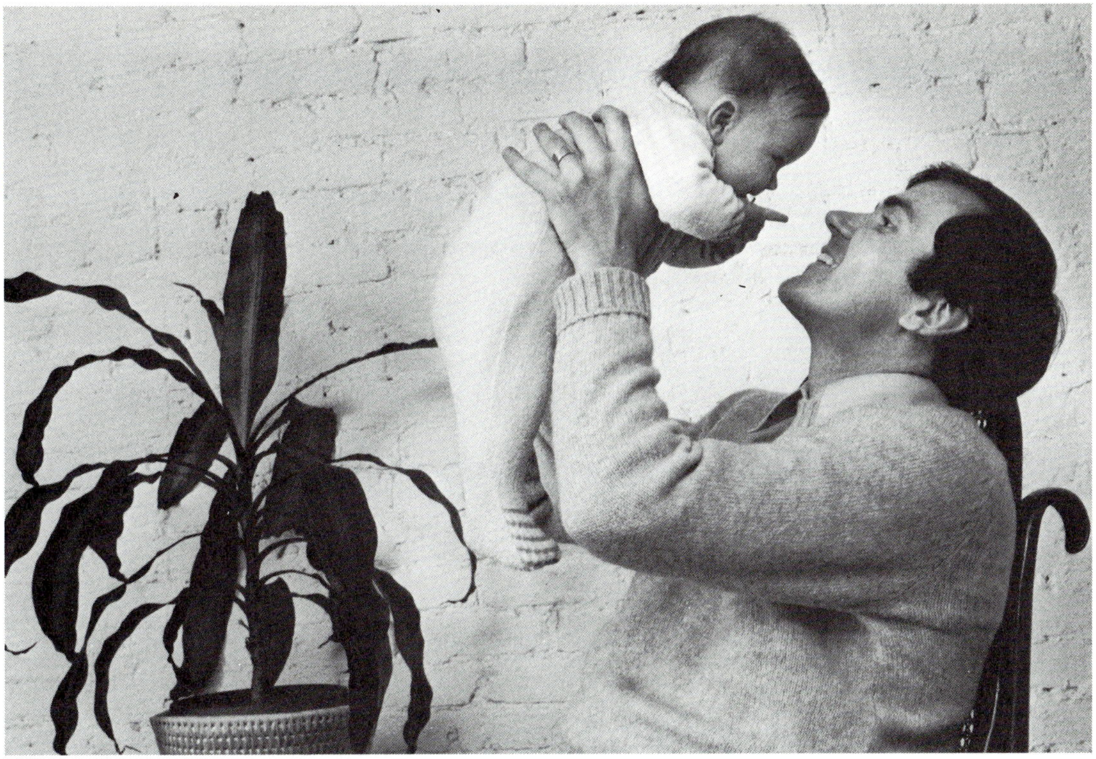

The importance of the father in the family is receiving increasing recognition.

and not interchangeable until the children are grown. Basic parenting principles aimed at rearing children with self-esteem include:

- Teaching decision making and coping skills early
- Combining firmness with flexibility within clearly defined limits
- Listening, really listening, to what the children have to say
- Having positive expectations, for children generally turn out to be what parents and others around them expect them to be
- Respecting and accepting children for what they are rather than for what parents would like them to be
- Supporting the child, giving help in handling fears and problems at the right time and in the right quantity (not too much, not too soon, not too little, not too late)
- Having and communicating values (wishy-washy parents leave children confused)
- Letting go gradually by giving freedom in small doses as children get older

In addition, good parents enjoy parenting. When parenting becomes a burden, the load falls heaviest on the children. Women who are unhappy as full-time mothers may benefit themselves and their families by pursuing interests outside the home. Many parents do not enjoy parenting because they have limit-

WHERE TO GET HELP

For Information on Prevention of Child Abuse

- Parents Anonymous.
- National Center for Prevention and Treatment of Child Abuse and Neglect, University of Colorado Medical Center, Denver, CO 80210.
- Local department of health or child welfare, or any local group formed to help parents and children. Many cities and states have special hot lines set up to serve parents seeking help and to receive reports of child abuse. See your telephone directory.

ed time to give to their children and this time is usually devoted to nuts and bolts parenting. Unless they can make more time for pleasant activities, both they and their children suffer.

Child Abuse

It is difficult to understand a father who hurls an infant across the room or a mother who pours a kettle of boiling water on a crying child. But every year an estimated 1 million children, mostly under age 4, are thus injured by parents or other adults (Besharov). The estimated 700 deaths annually from child abuse make it among the most serious threats to children in the United States and a major "epidemic."

Child abusers are not evil, not even usually psychotic, but they are unable to control the impulse to hurt their young. Often they are part of a cycle of child abuse; 30 to 60 percent were abused by *their* parents (Lauer et al.). Some are alcoholics or drug abusers; others are simply unable to tolerate a baby's crying. Some misdirect anger (which they feel against a parent, spouse, boss, the world) onto the helpless child. A high proportion conceived their child out of wedlock, and they usually are young and have financial problems. They come from all racial groups and all income brackets. Interestingly, very few had pets as children (Lenoski; Lauer et al.).

Most parents who hurt their children can be helped, and often the youngsters can continue to live with the abusing parents while the entire family is in treatment. A variety of programs have opened up in recent years to deal with the problems of the battered child, including residential programs and a variation of Alcoholics Anonymous called Parents Anonymous. Members are encouraged to call one another when they have successfully coped with a crisis, or when they feel one coming on. They are urged to hit chairs, walls, pillows, anything but the children, and to avoid disciplining when they are angry. They also undergo therapy.

The Exceptional Child

Each child is special or exceptional, each is important as an individual, each embodies traits that give him or her the potential to stand out in some way. It may be musical talent or a smile that lights up a room. It may be the ability to slug a baseball a country mile or to understand another's problems. It may be creativity in the kitchen or the laboratory, the ability to work magic with tools or with numbers. A nurturing environment at home and in school helps each human being live up to this potential.

Some children are exceptional because of mental or physical handicaps that require special attention if they are to reach their potential. Like all children, they need good parenting and plenty of love. But they require an extra measure of understanding and patience from parents and others, as well as the expertise of professionals who are learning more every day about bringing exceptional children like these into the mainstream (see Chapter 12 for more on the handicapped). Some of the most common disorders that interfere with normal development are discussed below.

TABLE 23.5 Levels of impairment in retardation*

IQ	RETARDATION	CAPABILITIES
52–68	Mild	Self-supporting with some supervision
36–51	Moderate	Some earning power; needs supervision and protection
20–35	Severe	Unable to learn to read and write but can learn some useful tasks
19 and below	Profound	Total care required

*Intelligence quotient (IQ) obtained on Stanford-Binet and Cattel Scales. The dividing lines are not hard and fast. *Source: Manual on Terminology and Classification in Mental Retardation,* p. 18.

Mental retardation Three out of every 100 Americans suffer from some degree of impaired or incomplete mental development (see Table 23.5). Some have physical defects, some are perfect physically. Some are mentally disturbed, most are not. They can be born into rich homes or poor, and into families with high or low levels of intelligence and education. *Causes*: Genetic, environmental, or unknown. *Prevention*: Testing children for PKU and other disorders at birth and treating those who are affected; preventing lead poisoning of young children, particularly common amidst peeling paint of inner city slums; preventing and swiftly treating such infections as meningitis; reducing smoking and drug addiction among mothers; giving better prenatal care and using fewer drugs during delivery; preventing such viral infections as German measles (rubella) that can be harmful to the fetus; treating for Rh incompatibility and thyroid deficiency; reducing malnutrition and child abuse. *Treatment*: Early identification and training can raise IQs, teach some to read and write, train many to do simple chores around the house and take care of themselves, and prepare those with mild or moderate retardation to be partially or totally self-supporting. The retarded are best cared for in their own homes whenever possible. Next best are small group homes, halfway houses, and foster homes. Large faceless institutions are least acceptable. The goal is not the currently impossible one of making the retarded child or adult "normal," but helping the person to build a life appropriate to his or her abilities.

Minimal brain dysfunction Some 5–20 percent of American children are believed to have MBD. They may be overactive, destructive, or aggressive; have difficulty completing work, or learning to read or write; have impaired motor skills or distortions in the way they see things. Most are of normal or above-normal intelligence. *Causes*: Uncertain; may be genetic or environmental. Age usually improves the condition and many MBD children catch up scholastically by the time they are young adults (Hechtman). *Treatment*: May be controlled through the use of stimulant drugs that paradoxically calm, enabling MBD children to function better in school and out; long-term effects of drugs are unknown. The theory that many of these youngsters are sensitive to food additives and improve on an all-natural sugarless diet is still under study.

Autism There are 2–4.5 autistic children, mostly boys, in every 10,000. They live in a world of their own, do not coo or smile as infants, do not like to be held or cuddled, continue to be unresponsive to people as they grow older, do not use language to communicate. Some are retarded, but not all. *Cause*: Once assumed to be unloving parents, now unknown. Possibly a central nervous system disturbance or chemical imbalance garbles messages the child receives through the eyes and ears, giving a distorted view of reality, with the result that things don't make sense. *Treatment*: Difficult, but possible in some cases, especially if treatment begins by age $2^1/_2$. Behavior modification, traditional psychotherapy, residential therapy, and special stimulation have all been used with some success.

LOOKING BACK

REVIEWING CONCEPTS IN CHAPTER 23

- Today, to have or not to have children is a matter of choice. Many factors go into the decision, but ultimately, both parents must be willing to make a full commitment to the child they wish to bring into the world or to adopt.
- Timing and spacing can influence the health of the prospective child.
- Pregnancy is a time of both joy and uneasiness for expectant parents.
- Many signs of pregnancy can have other causes. Thus, the only way to be certain of pregnancy is to have a medical examination and, if it is early in the pregnancy, a pregnancy test.
- Medical care throughout pregnancy is necessary.
- Miscarriage, or spontaneous abortion, often occurs early in pregnancy when there is something wrong with the developing embryo. Later miscarriage may occur because of an illness or health problem in the mother.
- Many infertility problems can be overcome today in both males and females, and persons experiencing such problems should see a physician.
- What a newborn baby will be like will depend on many factors, including heredity (from both parents), health and age of parents, the environment prenatally (including the air the mother breaths, the food she eats, drugs she takes, diseases she contracts).
- Prenatal examination of the fetus can often determine whether or not the developing infant is normal, and in a few cases, needed treatment can begin even before birth.
- Many approaches to childbirth are available. The choice will depend upon individual preference, hospital regulations, the physician's preference, the condition of mother and child. In general, the less heavily drugged the mother, the better the baby's chances.
- Childbirth preparation classes, no matter what the choice of childbirth procedures, make both parents more comfortable and self-assured, and often make childbirth easier.
- Infants born today, where good medical care and emergency equipment are available, and whose parents are healthy and not exposed to many environmental hazards have a better chance of growing up healthy than infants in any previous

generation. However, the 24 hours around birth remain the most dangerous in the human lifespan.

- Breast milk is the most nutritious and natural food for infants, but infants can also thrive on bottle-feeding, as long as they are cuddled during feeding.
- Both parents can be intimately involved in rearing today's infants, and the role of each parent is vital to healthy development in the child.
- Good parenting comes in many styles, but generally, it is fairly consistent; it is geared to the individual child, the family situation, and the parents' personalities; and above all, it is loving. A good parent-child relationship is one that both parents and children enjoy.
- All children are special; some are very bright, some musically talented, some fine athletes, others good mechanically. Some are special because they are retarded or have learning disabilities. Whatever the specialness, teaching and rearing should be geared to the individual's needs.
- Mentally retarded persons are *not* usually mentally ill. Many can be trained, some can even be educated to read and write, and some can become self-supporting or partially so. Early detection and treatment are crucial. Prevention is even better.
- Minimal brain dysfunction, the group of disorders labeled *learning disabilities*, may or may not be associated with aggressive and overactive behavior. Special help in school can aid youngsters who have these problems to overcome their learning difficulties. The difficulties lessen and often disappear with age.
- Child abuse is a major threat to children in the United States today. Parent-abusers usually cannot control themselves, but with help they can often learn to do so.

24

ROUNDING OUT THE LIFE CYCLE: MIDDLE AND OLD AGE

WHAT'S AHEAD IN CHAPTER 24 What does "old" mean? How does the term differ from "aging"? Why does the problem of the elderly suddenly loom so large? What kind of period is middle age? What factors combine to make it difficult? What lifestyles are common for older Americans? What are the signs of aging—physical, emotional, intellectual, and social? What theories have been put forth to explain aging? Can the aging process be halted? What are the major problems facing older Americans? Are these problems the result of age or of societal conditions? Why do so many people have trouble relating to the elderly? What attitudes are important in dealing successfully with older friends and family? How can the community improve services to the elderly? How can older citizens help themselves? How can you help assure a comfortable, successful, happy old age for yourself?

When you are 4 years old, your 10-year-old brother is "old." When you are 14, any teacher who is over 30 is "old." When you are 24, anyone hitting 40 is over the hill. Bernard Baruch took the position, "I will never be an old man. To me, old age is always fifteen years older than I am." And Charles Judson Herrick said, "You don't grow old; when you cease to grow, you are old."

"Old" is a state of mind, not a specified period of life. Gerontologist and author Alex Comfort suggests that it is a political term used to put out to pasture a group of people who differ from others only in that they have been on earth longer.

Though "old" is a vague term, "aging" is less so. Aging is a biological process, not very well understood, in which the human mecha-

One summer, I picked up Saturday movie money by renting my grandfather to my friends. For a dime, they could watch him whittle a chain and a whistle from one piece of birchwood and, as a bonus, he would sometimes talk as he whittled. During those lazy hot afternoons he told stories of Indians and blizzards, and how barbed wire ruined the wilderness; he made us hear wolves howl and feel the ground shake as the buffalo stampeded. Week after week, Granddad gave my friends and me the gift of his past. He made the way our elders had lived intelligible and real. It was much more entertaining and exciting than the movies I saw with the money I collected. (Curtin, p. 12)

nism is constantly involved from birth until death. Science may eventually slow the rate of aging, but that achievement is probably a long way off. In the meantime, whether you are 18, 38, or 68, you are aging, both biologically and sociologically. How you will fare as you move along the continuum will depend to a great extent upon two factors: (1) how society views aging and the role of those who are past certain chronological stages and (2) how you view aging and what preparations you have made for dealing not just with your biological aging but with the sociological changes you will almost inevitably face: forced retirement[1] with reduced income, loss of personhood, loss of active role in the community, loss of loved ones. Sixty-five is far too late to make these preparations. Just as one can improve the chances of good physical health and long years by practicing preventive health measures, so one can, by planning ahead, assure a more fruitful, invigorating, and happy role in the social scheme in later years.

Two factors have made a major difference in the lot of older Americans:

1 The growing segregation of life-cycle stages because of the disintegration of the extended family, the planned proliferation of homes and retirement villages for the elderly, and the unplanned stagnation of ghettos for the elderly in decaying neighborhoods.
2 The lengthening of the life cycle. In 1900, the average white newborn could expect to live to about 50 and the nonwhite infant only to the early thirties. The cycle then ran from birth to childhood, to a brief (almost nonexistent) adolescence, to adulthood, and for the hardy few, to what we now call *middle age* and they called *old age*. Few lived into their seventh or eighth decades. Today the average child born can expect to live into the sixties or seventies, the middle-aged are relatively young, and nearly 25 million Americans are over 65. The proportion of elderly is expected to continue to rise as the birth rate falls and better medical care and preventive techniques further prolong the lifespan.

[1]Legislation may end forced retirement.

As the population of older citizens grows, it becomes more important for both individuals and the community to explore the needs and problems of this group in order to make intelligent and compassionate decisions about steps to help them and, eventually, ourselves.

THE MIDDLE YEARS

The years between 40 and 60 have been likened to adolescence as a time of painful change and adjustment. In the mid-forties, a woman begins to experience the symptoms of menopause, to feel inexplicably edgy or depressed. She fears loss of her womanhood. She is apprehensive about what will happen when her children leave home. She may be attempting to enter or reenter the job market, and she feels unsure and unprepared.

A man in his middle years may be going through a period of fear and discouragement: "Where am I?" "There's so much I haven't achieved and never will." He may be locked

If you want to be a dear old lady at seventy, you should start early, say about seventeen.
Maude Royden (1876–1956)

The proper study of geriatrics begins with pediatrics.
Journal of Pediatrics

We fear old age, which we are never sure of being able to reach.
Jean de LaBruyere (1645–1696), *Characters,* Chapter VI

into a job he dislikes or afraid of being fired from one he enjoys. He may be concerned about his loss of control of his future, as well as about loss of power, youth and vigor, sexuality, manhood. Unlike women his age, who expect to experience "change of life," he is unprepared for these feelings.

Middle-aged parents share much in common with their often college-aged children, particularly change and uncertainty. Collegians may be pained by fancied inadequacies of their newly matured bodies, or distraught over acne or stringy hair. Their middle-aged parents are distressed that the bodies they have known are changing: Hair is thinning and graying. Middles are migrating. Teeth are being bridged. While the young worry that they may be sexually inadequate, parents fear losing what they have.

Both groups are intent upon establishing identities in their changing life roles, on being "somebody." For the young, this may include speaking or dressing in a certain way or belonging to the "in" group. For parents, it may be living in a status neighborhood, driving a status car, or belonging to a status social crowd.

Emotional and Social Challenges

Pressure is the key word.

- *Financial pressure* Middle-aged adults may be paying or saving for college for their children, helping to support aged parents, and trying to squirrel away a little for the rapidly approaching retirement years.
- *Community pressure* This age group pays the largest share of taxes in the United States, and is expected to take leadership roles in the community (school board, community chest, Scouts, etc.) and participate in decision making.
- *Family pressure* The middle-aged are a generation caught in the middle. On one side are their own parents, often in need of both financial and emotional support and sometimes in need of physical care. On the other side are their children, learning to exercise independence, preferring the counsel of their peers to that of their parents, rejecting family values and sometimes even family contact.

Middle-aged parents watch their maturing children making what they consider mistakes and either remain silent for fear of losing their children's love or carp and criticize in an attempt to hang on to their fading authority. They may be resentful of the young "who do their own thing" but send the bills home to Mom and Pop. Having reared families in an era when the "experts" rather than common sense or parental instinct ran the family, they have little confidence in themselves as parents. Every misstep, or imagined misstep, of their offspring is, they are sure, another sign of their own failure.

Physical Manifestations

In women, middle age is clearly marked by menopause (the cessation of menstruation) and the change-of-life symptoms of climacteric (*klimakter* = rung of the ladder) which may come before, during, or after the menopause. The major physiological occurrence is the reduction of the production of female

Erika Stone/Peter Arnold

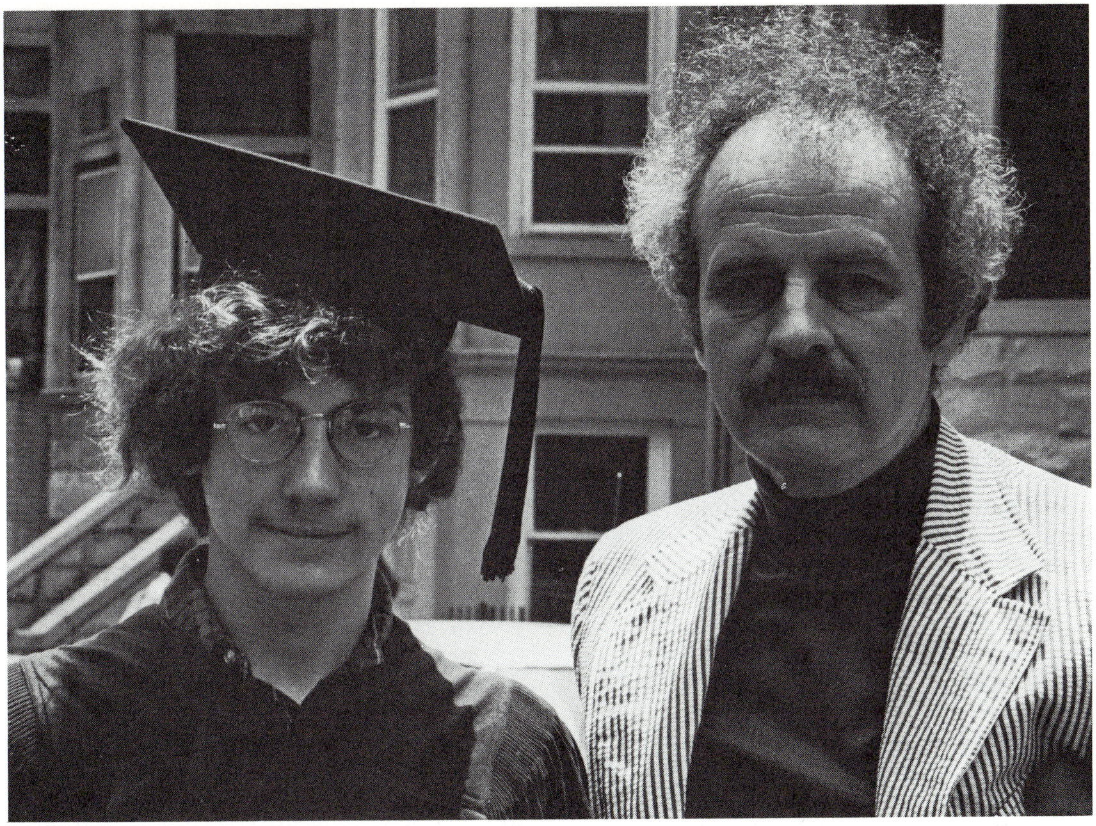

Despite the generation gap, young college students and their parents share similar problems and concerns about changing life roles.

hormones. As a result, the reproductive organs shrink and the linings of the vagina and its secretions thin, sometimes making intercourse uncomfortable without a lubricating cream. The woman at this time may become more susceptible to a variety of illnesses, including cardiovascular and gallbladder diseases and osteoporosis (a weakening of the bones). She may experience hot sweats and flushes and erratic moodiness. Her hormone deficiency may be treated by her physician with a compensating administration of hormones, but the safety of this approach is not fully assured.

In men, the climacteric is much less apparent. According to endocrinologist Herbert S: Kupperman, about 20 percent of men note symptoms between 48 and 58 and another 30 to 35 percent between ages 58 and 68. The major manifestation is a drop in production of male hormones, which may interfere with potency. A variety of other symptoms may appear: physical (urinary difficulties, sweating, flushes, itching, liver spots, headaches, dizziness) and psychological (irritability, fatigue, insomnia, depression, forgetfulness, behavior changes) (Ruebsaat and Hull). Although both males and females often fear that these changes signal the end of a fulfilling sexual relationship, this need not be the case. Sexual activity can, and for many does, continue far into old age.

OLD AGE—A GOOD AGE[2]

- John and Margot Brown are in their mid-sixties. They have just moved to a retirement community. Still vigorous in mind and body, they insist upon independence from their children. Thanks to excellent retirement benefits and social security, they can have the independence they want. Though disengaged from business activities, they are in no way disengaged from life. They have become involved in community activities in their new home, and they enjoy swimming, bicycling, fishing, and an occasional game of doubles tennis. Their social calendar is so crowded, they practically never have an evening to "just sit and watch TV."
- Lena Drake is a widow in her mid-seventies. Though she was independent for many years, she is beginning to slow down. As a result of several mild strokes, she now needs help with her everyday needs. She doesn't want to burden her children, but she is staying temporarily with her son and his wife. Since she strenuously objects to any talk of moving to a home for the aged, the family is perplexed about what to do with a lady they love dearly, but who is becoming increasingly difficult. They are frustrated by her behavior, but feel guilty about their anger.
- Anna and Katherine Stark are elderly sisters, both widows, who live together in a rundown inner-city apartment. Anna's son died a few years ago, leaving her alone except for Katherine. Katherine's children live far from her and she hears from them only at holidays and Mother's Day. The sisters live on small social security widows' benefits and government food stamps, but this does not cover their needs. They get a nutritious hot meal only when they can get to the senior citizens' center a dozen blocks away. The rest of the time, they subsist on tea, canned soups, and soda crackers. They keep a cat as a pet and to kill mice that frequent their apartment. To feed the cat, they rummage through the trash cans in front of a local elementary school after lunch and collect half-empty milk containers and half-eaten sandwiches. Sometimes they find some slices of bologna or egg salad sandwiches they can eat themselves.

[2]This is the title of a book on aging by Alex Comfort.

The elderly persons described above are representative of the wide variety of elderly living in the United States in the 1970s. The majority, 72.7 per cent of the men and 42.5 of the women, live with their spouses independently. Another 14.7 percent of men and 36.2 percent of women maintain their own homes, mostly alone. A smaller percentage, 7 percent of men and 15 percent of women, live with relatives. Fewer than 5 percent live in institutions. The median income for heads of families over 65 was just half the median income for all families in 1970.

Indications of Aging

Aging is determined by genetics and by environmental factors. Lifespan varies from species to species: the elephant averages 50 years; the turtle may reach 150; the modern American human, about 65 to 72 years. What are the indications that the body is aging? What causes aging?

Physical indications The process of aging is not well understood, but it appears that time does wear down the human organism. This "wearing out" occurs at different rates for different parts of the body. With age, hearing, vision, taste, and smell all become less acute. Heart, respiratory, endocrine, and immune systems deteriorate. Skeletal structure loses calcium and turns fragile. The brain

[There is] more danger of the individual rusting out than wearing out.
Sir Humphry Davy Rolleston (1862–1944)

We don't drowse because we're old; we're old because we have gotten to the point of having so few relevant stimuli that we become inattentive, actionless and drowsy.
Alan Gregg (1890–1957)

decreases in size, while the prostate increases. Muscles weaken, and fat increases. About 1 out of 6 aging persons suffers from chronic brain syndrome, often called *senility*, the cause of which is unknown but is attributed by some to atherosclerosis, by others to heredity, metabolic dysfunction, or even a viral source. Senility is at first characterized by loss of memory for recent events, later by progressive memory loss and other personality and intellectual changes. Although that sounds discouraging, overall the health of elderly persons who use available medical services is good. Silver hair does bring some silver linings: The elderly are less susceptible to acute illnesses such as colds and appear to be less buffeted by over- or undernutrition (Ostfeld and Gibson).

Some physical deterioration may be due to cultural conditioning that says older people are ready for the rocking chair. Those who maintain physical activity usually maintain their vigor—the ability to work, to play, to enjoy sexuality. In the Soviet Republic of Abkasia, where retirement is unknown, both men and women continue to work well into their nineties, though at a slower pace, and many live past 100 (Benet).

Emotional indications Depression is the most common psychological symptom seen in the aging. It is often mistaken for senility (Hollister). It can be related to lack of activity, to an absence of friends, to a loss of loved ones, to grinding poverty that contrasts painfully with better days, or simply to the realization that days are numbered and disabilities the only constant companions. Sometimes the psychiatric symptoms are caused by side effects of drugs given for various ailments (Moss, *a*).

Intellectual indications Recent studies have shown that, although reactions are slowed, intellectual capacity is undiminished in most healthy elderly persons until shortly before death (L. Jarvik). There does tend to be a decrease, however, when high blood pressure or other chronic illnesses are present.

Social indications The elderly ordinarily disengage themselves from society gradually, and society withdraws in kind. The steps of this disengagement have been described as: (1) Aging people come to a recognition of their own mortality. (2) They reset priorities, realizing that some dreams will never be achieved. (3) Losses begin to outrun the ability to find replacements; friends die, businesses close, children move away, to be replaced only by memories. (4) New rewards in life (often rewards that have less status in our society) are set. (5) Finally, the aging seek and find freedom from obligations. These steps make the final disengagement—death—easier (Cumming). Not everyone disengages, however. Alex Comfort suggests that the "age-proof people will have none of it and that at any age you can opt out of what you have been doing, often because it is seen to be not worthwhile."

Theories of Aging

No one knows why some people are old in middle age, others still young in old age, nor why, even if we conquer cancer and heart disease, the lifespan is likely to stretch only to

90 years and people will still die of "old age." Many theories have been put forth to explain the aging process. Among them:

1 *The genetic theory* The aging of an individual either (*a*) is preprogrammed in his or her genetic material, or (*b*) occurs at random with the passage of time when a breakdown of genetic material causes the manufacture of error-producing proteins that disturb body function.
2 *The autoimmune theory* With age, the body begins to reject itself and attacks its own cells.
3 *The free radical theory* Free radicals (substances released by polyunsaturated fats) act with cell membranes and certain enzymes to produce oxidation which disrupts cell activity, causing damage to chromosomes and other cell parts.
4 *The RNA tumor virus theory* A virus is transmitted vertically from parent to child, or horizontally from person to person, entering cells and causing them to age.
5 *The wear-and-tear theory* Body parts and systems, like those of any machine, simply wear out after long use.
6 *The waste product theory* Body wastes build up over the years and eventually interfere with cell function.

Research to determine the causes of aging is taking many directions. Among them: the study of human and animal cells and tissues in the laboratory; of persons with rare, early-aging diseases; of the placenta, the shortest-lived human organ; of long-lived humans, their lifestyles and environmental conditions.

Counteracting Aging

These studies have not yet yielded the secret of eternal youth, but they have provided some interesting information. Heredity is an important longevity factor. So is sex: Women (except in areas of poor childbirth care) live longer than men, possibly because of hormonal and metabolic differences, possibly because of differing lifestyles (this may change as women adopt what had previously been male roles). Neither sex nor heredity is controllable, but they may eventually give us clues that will lead to ways of extending the lives of all.

Though the aging process remains as yet undecoded, many factors are known to affect the lifespan directly. People who live longer have usually followed (though not always knowingly) the kinds of preventive measures discussed throughout this book: (1) avoidance of smoking; (2) diet high in necessary nutrients, low in salt, fats (especially animal fats), and refined carbohydrates (especially sugar); (3) little or no exposure to toxic chemicals in air, water, food, or on the job; (4) adequate exercise that continues through middle and into old age; (5) control of high blood pressure or other chronic conditions; (6) lack of continual stress. In addition, those who live well into their eighties and nineties, or even past 100, are most often married, have parented many children, and have continued being active physically, mentally, occupationally, and often sexually.

A variety of approaches to slowing the aging process are under study; these include: antioxidants such as vitamin E and BHT, various hormones and drugs; reduction in food intake (this has extended the lifespan of rats); manipulation of calcium metabolism, which may affect such disorders of aging as osteoporosis, cataracts, and skin wrinkling.

PROBLEMS OF THE ELDERLY

Extending life without improving its quality can only bring misery, as the goddess Aurora discovered when she persuaded Zeus to grant her husband, Tithonus, immortality. Unfortunately, she neglected to petition for eternal youth as well, and as Tithonus grew increasingly infirm, he prayed for death. Indeed, some elderly people, too, pray for death. Pneumonia, which before antibiotics often ended the lives of elderly people who were weakened and sickly, was referred to as "the old man's friend."

Only since the 1960s has the question of improving the quality of life for the elderly been seriously addressed. The later years today have the potential for richness and vitality. But achieving that potential will require sustained efforts by local communities and the federal government, as well as thoughtful preparation by individuals. Major attention will necessarily be focused on these areas of concern:

Retirement

When the elderly were few in number, most continued to work as long as vigor permitted—women usually at household tasks, men at their jobs—though sometimes at a slowed pace. It was not until our society was faced with large numbers of older people, and jobs for younger people became scarce, that the concept of retirement developed.

Must an individual's active working life end at a specific age, 65, for example? Though 4 out of 5 respondents in a *Nation's Business* poll said no, the answer from America's business community appears to be yes. While the number of elderly has rapidly increased, their percentage in the labor force has just as rapidly decreased. Many who manage to hang on to their positions find themselves overlooked for promotions, salary increases, and training opportunities because of the notion that older workers cannot be effective on the job. In fact, older workers, properly placed, function effectively and have greater stability, fewer accidents, and less time lost from work than younger workers. Forced retirement deprives society of their experience, expertise, and wisdom.

Certainly, many retire voluntarily and make highly successful adjustments. But being arbitrarily put "out to pasture," combined with losses of spouses, friends, physical strength, gives the elderly a feeling of uselessness and often gives rise to deep bouts of depression

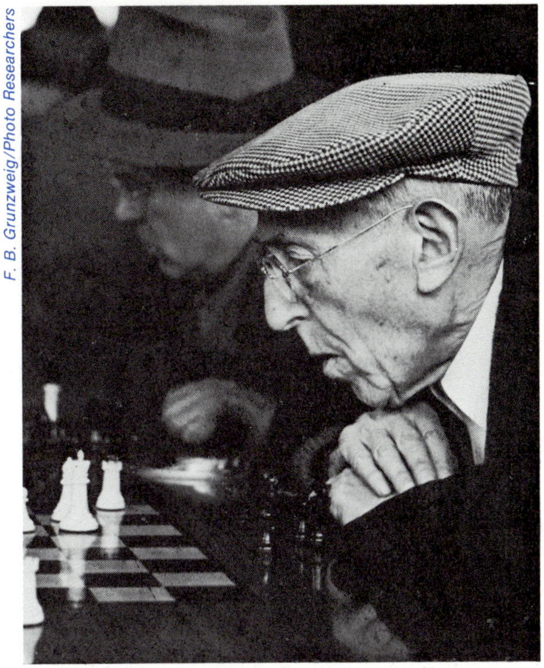

F. B. Grunzweig/Photo Researchers

Contrary to common belief, intellectual capacity is undiminished in most healthy elderly persons.

and even physical illness. As the American Medical Association has pointed out: ". . . a direct relationship exists between forced idleness and poor health . . . chronic complaints develop more frequently when a person is inactive and without basic interests" (in Ossofsky, p. 4).

It has been suggested that retirement be gradual for those who wish to and are capable of continuing at work, with a small reduction in hours and pay each year. It has also been suggested that all work weeks be reduced to 30 hours, so that a much larger work force, including those over 65 who wish to work, can be accommodated.

Finances

In spite of social security and other retirement benefits, 15.7 percent of the elderly lived below the poverty line in 1974. Millions of others above that arbitrary boundary suffered severe financial hardship. Many are forced to abandon the simplest pleasures—an occasional movie, bowling, a trip to visit a friend. Some, too proud to seek welfare or other assistance, live on tea and biscuits.

Health

Medicare is intended to relieve the multiple medical problems of the elderly and has, on the whole, done a good job of it. However, it does not pay all costs, and the percentage left for the senior citizen to handle out of pocket continues to rise.

Sex

"I'm not a dirty old man, I'm a sexy senior citizen" reads a California bumper sticker. There is little doubt that sexual functioning, like other bodily performance, slows with age. The 70-year-old couple may walk rather than jog; their sexual relations will be less frequent and less vigorous than earlier but no less satisfying. Society, however, seems to have concluded that the elderly are "too old for that stuff."

There is no scientific foundation for this attitude. Given the opportunity, those who have been sexually active in their younger years continue to be active in later years. A Duke University study found that 15 percent of men and women actually become *more* sexually active and interested with advancing age. Older women appear less interested in sex and less sexually active than older men for many reasons:

- Many women believe, incorrectly, that their sex lives ended with menopause.
- Many women are widowed and because they reject nonmarital sex, have no potential partner.
- There is a shortage of older men in relation to women; men die earlier, many marry or have relations with younger women.
- Many women were brought up to believe they should not enjoy sex and are therefore not reluctant to abandon it.
- Many women are anxious about their aging bodies and appearance and hesitate to expose themselves in an intimate situation.

In addition, many older people, both males and females, are deprived of the opportunity for a sexual relationship because of lack of privacy, either in a relative's home or in a nursing home. This is true of both married and single senior citizens. Some authorities have urged nursing homes to set aside privacy rooms for aging couples who wish to be alone—to hold hands, to watch TV together, or to be intimate. Even when coitus is not the object, the opportunity to touch, caress, and feel bodily warmth and love can be very comforting (Lobsenz).

RELATING TO OLDER RELATIVES AND FRIENDS

Many younger people find it extremely difficult to deal with the elderly. One reason is the compartmentalization of age groups in our society. Another is the fact that they see in the elderly a picture of themselves in the future—lonely, helpless, waiting to die. Often they prefer to turn their backs on the forecast. Sometimes the difficulty is related to a lifetime of submerged resentment against parents or authority. The resentment is expressed in cutting remarks, in belittling, in treating the elderly like children, in claiming that sex, liquor, late hours, and other forms of fun are not "good" for older people. Another cause of difficulty in dealing with the aged is the recognition that the object of assistance will die eventually no matter what help is given.

Feelings of hostility, fear, and frustration about relations with the elderly are not abnormal. Once recognized, they can usually be overcome. There are some individuals, however, who cannot successfully suppress such feelings. Unless they undergo therapy, their

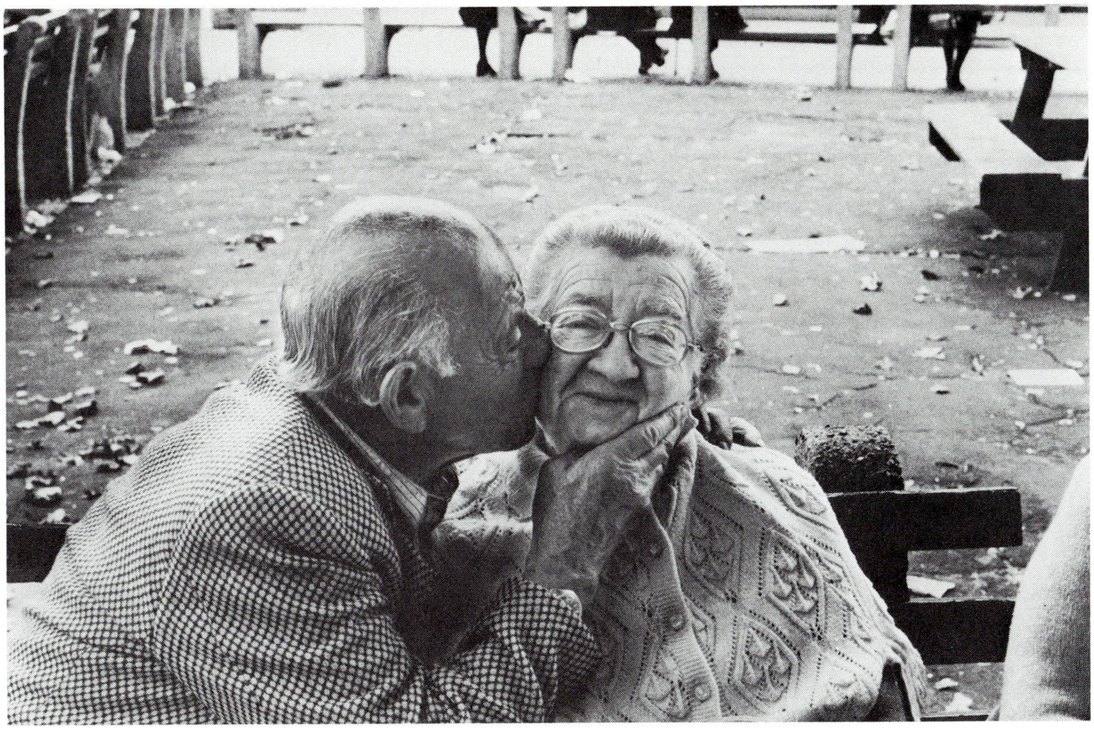

Given the opportunity, most men and women who have been sexually active in their younger years continue to be active in later years.

visits with older relatives and friends should be kept short and sweet.

For those determined to help an older relative, a friend, or even a stranger, Dr. David D. Stonecypher, Jr., gerontologist, suggests some positive approaches. His advice addresses the fact that, though we talk a lot today about death with dignity, we often make life with dignity difficult or impossible for those well along in years. He urges:

1 *Don't dominate.* Older people fear losing control and do not want or need to be treated as children. They should remain in charge of decisions concerning their own lives.

2 *Don't obligate.* Don't do so much for the older person that he or she feels obligated. This increases dependency and breeds resentment on both sides.

3 *Encourage independence.* Sometimes discouraged elderly people view themselves

On Being a Nonperson

How do you think it feels to sit in a restaurant with your son and have a waitress ask him: "How does your father like his eggs?"

as society does—as helpless—and so allow themselves to become dependent.

4 *Don't pass on personal fears or feelings about old age or death.* Older people have enough trouble dealing with their own feelings.

5 *Give the elderly a chance for satisfactions and successes.* Most older people are still quite competent, if a little slow. Encourage them to work if they wish, to do chores, to be useful to themselves and others.

6 *Be honest.* Most older people are experienced enough to know when someone is humoring them rather than telling them the truth. Lying to them weakens their self-esteem, increases their isolation, and destroys trust. Of course, kindness, tact, and discretion *are* needed on many delicate issues.

What the older person needs most is a friend, an ally, a source of protection. This does not take a lot of time, just availability—a visit, a telephone call when needed. How can a little friendship go such a long way? Dr. Stonecypher explains:

> How would a young adult feel if he looked on himself as a dying, abandoned, hopeless person? He would be terribly discouraged, terribly depressed. In so many ways, the old person has found the doors closed to him. He knows better than to seek employment. Yet without involvement in the community, he finds little to say that interests anyone. The world politely but firmly disengages from him. Unspoken but implied in the manner of those who deal with him is the belief that he is a spent creature. . . .
>
> . . . What would be the impact of someone who came along who treated him as a normal member of the community and seemed to enjoy his company? The older person would begin to reassess himself—to see the possibility that he could be interesting and effective. As he learned his opinions were respected (and, Heaven knows, he's lived long enough that his views ought to have some merit), confidence and self-esteem would begin to return.
>
> If the friendship progressed to the point where each member felt he could call on the other for advice and aid, the older person might have all he needed to soothe the frantic feeling of being unable to cope with the world . . . to give [him] a stabilizing sense of support.
>
> Sterile visiting, mere well-wishing, and back-slapping encouragement, of course, are not support. (pp. 124, 125)

COMMUNITY EFFORTS TO AID THE ELDERLY

On every level, from federal government to local community, modest beginnings are being made in the mammoth task of easing the difficulties associated with aging. What is needed?

- *Information and referral services* Many older people and their families do not know where to turn for help, and in most cities there is no central agency that can give them the information they need.
- *Home health services* Visiting nurses, physicians' assistants, and trained health aids are available for older people who cannot easily get to a clinic, hospital, or doctor's office or who need the occasional attention of a health professional in their lonely lives.
- *Nutrition services* Meals-on-wheels delivering food to the homes of the aged, hot meals served at schools or senior citizen centers, food stamps, and supermarket discounts may be helpful to those who get inadequate nutrition because they cannot afford better or because they are too ill, too disinterested, or too confused to prepare good meals.
- *Transportation services* Dial-a-bus, volunteer drivers, and reduced fares are available in many areas for the millions of elderly who cannot use ordinary public transportation because it is too expensive, too far away, or not designed for persons with the infirmities of old age.

Ann Chwatsky/Editorial Photocolor Archives

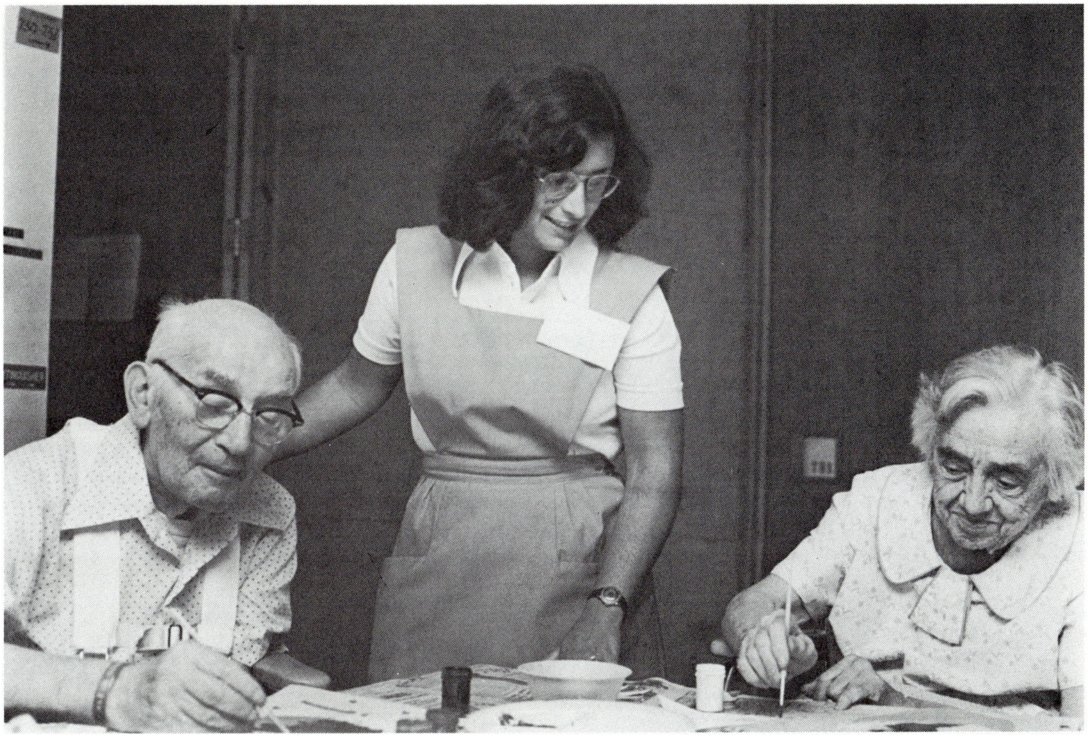

In many communities, college students are directly involved in helping to improve the quality of life for the elderly.

- *Communication services* Television, radio, books, newspapers, and magazines can help to reduce isolation and provide entertainment. Telephones also reduce isolation and provide a way to signal for help in times of emergency. However, 6 million older citizens cannot afford them.
- *Legal services* At low or no cost, there are legal services to help the many older people who are victims of "ageism," are easy prey to con games and other frauds, or are taken advantage of by unscrupulous landlords, business people, greedy relatives.
- *Housing* Appropriate housing for the aged, that is safe, comfortable, clean, and accessible to shopping, transportation, recreation, and medical care, is still relatively rare.

In many communities, college students are directly involved in helping to improve the quality of life for the elderly: visiting shut-ins, driving those who can get around, doing shopping, preparing meals, and most important, giving companionship and support.

SELF-HELP

As much as older citizens need to be helped, they also need to help themselves and others. Senior citizen involvement in community projects—such as RSVP (Retired Seniors Volunteer Program), VISTA (Volunteers in Service to America), SCORE (Service Corps of Retired Executives), and the Peace Corps—gives them a sense of usefulness and

Susan McKinney/Editorial Photocolor Archives

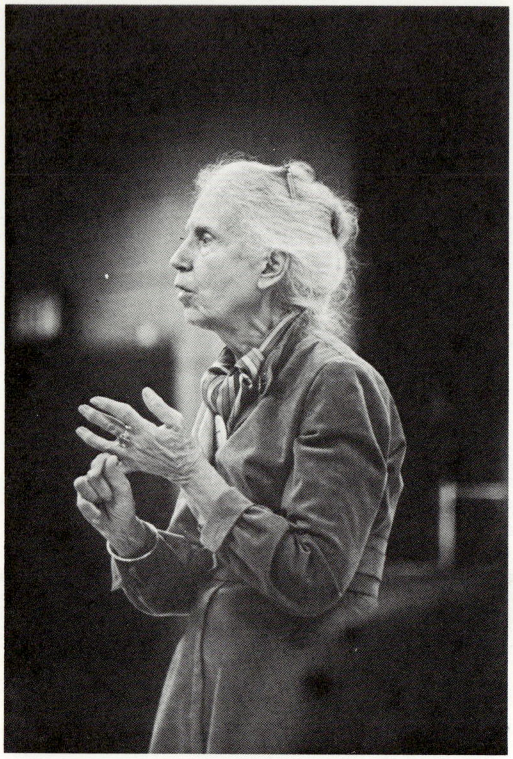

also makes a real contribution to society. Involvement in organizations of older activists, such as the Gray Panthers, that lobby for laws and services to benefit senior citizens gives them the feeling that they still have power—which they do.

The most important aspect of self-help for the elderly begins in youth. Each young man and woman must begin planning for old age—financially, socially, intellectually, vocationally, and avocationally—long before that arbitrary cutoff age of 65.

Maggie Kuhn, founder and head of the Gray Panther movement, urges her fellow senior citizens to organize and work toward needed legislation favorable to the elderly.

LOOKING BACK

REVIEWING CONCEPTS IN CHAPTER 24

- Who is "old" depends upon one's point of view.
- Aging is a biological process involving human beings from birth until death.
- How successfully individuals handle aging depends upon their own attitudes and the attitudes of those around them.
- The increase in the lifespan since the beginning of the century and the growing segregation of the elderly have created a new minority group in our society: senior citizens. It is important that both individuals and the community explore the needs and problems of older Americans.
- Middle age, the years between 40 and 60, has been likened to adolescence as a time of great change and painful adjustment. The problems of the middle-aged may be physical (climacteric or menopause), financial (pressure of college children, parents who need help), social (they are expected to be community leaders), and familial (they are entering a new and unfamiliar stage as children grow and leave home).

- No single stereotype comfortably fits all older Americans. Many live comfortably in retirement. Others continue working productively. Some live below the poverty level. But most, according to studies, appear happy.
- The physical indications of aging include the wearing out of various body parts and chronic brain syndrome. Most elderly people continue to be mentally alert. Depression may often be due to loss, loneliness, or medications. The social lifestyle of some older persons is characterized by a disengagement from life, but many remain very much involved.
- Many theories have been put forth to explain the aging process, but none has yet proved entirely satisfactory or accurate.
- There are no known ways of deterring aging. There are, however, many ways to extend lifespan and its quality.
- Among the problems of the elderly (most of which originate in societal attitudes) are forced retirement, insufficient finances, inadequate medical care, and an unnecessarily early cessation of sexual relations.
- The aging need to be treated with respect worthy of their station in life. They should not be babied, dominated, lied to, or made to feel obligated or dependent. They deserve opportunities for success and satisfaction.
- The community can help the elderly by improving services in many areas.
- The elderly can help themselves by remaining active and insisting upon their earned rights. The most important aspect of self-help for the elderly begins in youth, with planning for old age.

VI
HEALTH AND THE COMMUNITY

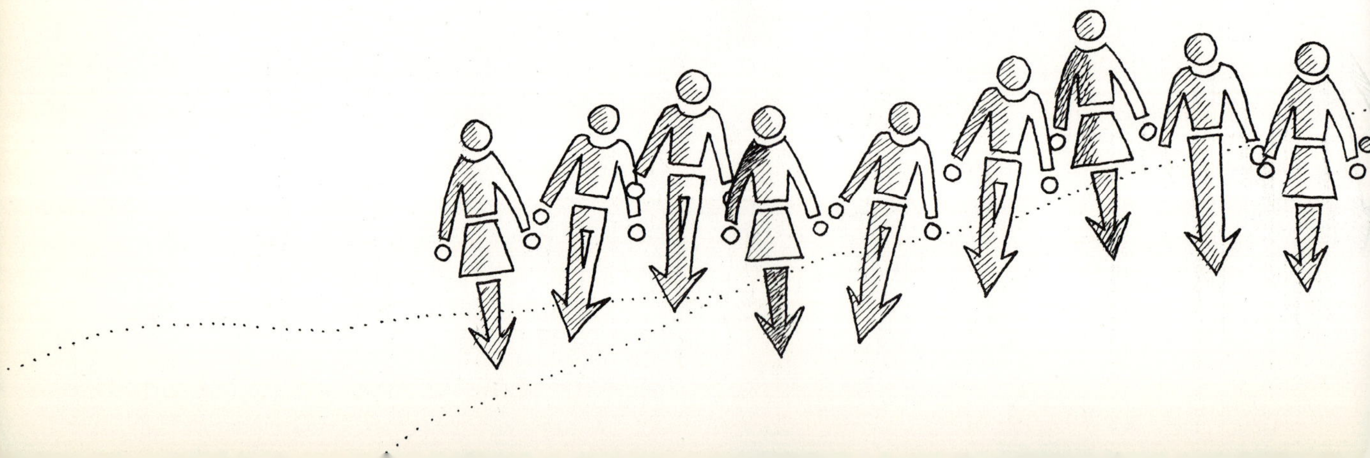

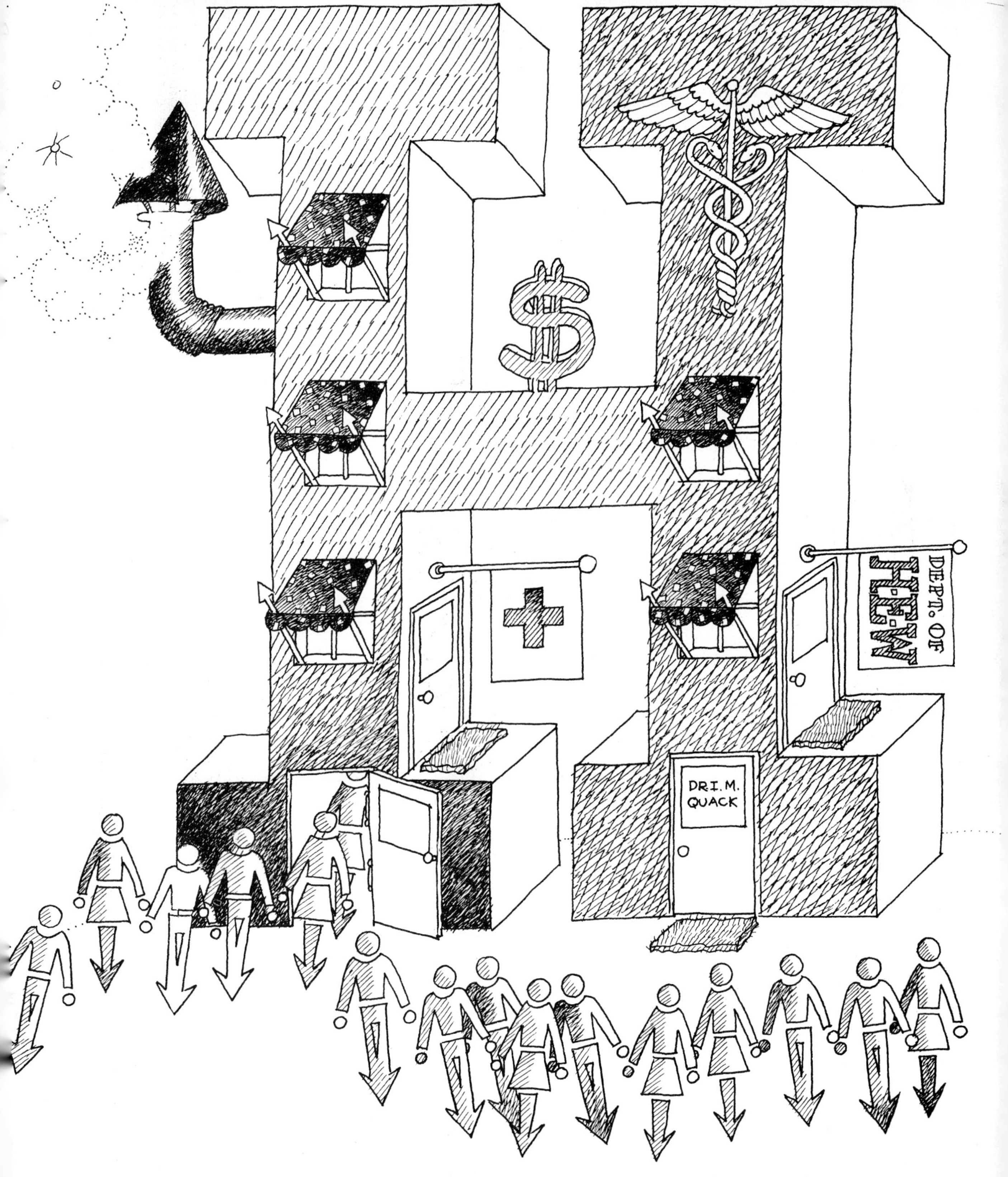
DEPT. OF H·E·W
DR. I. M. QUACK

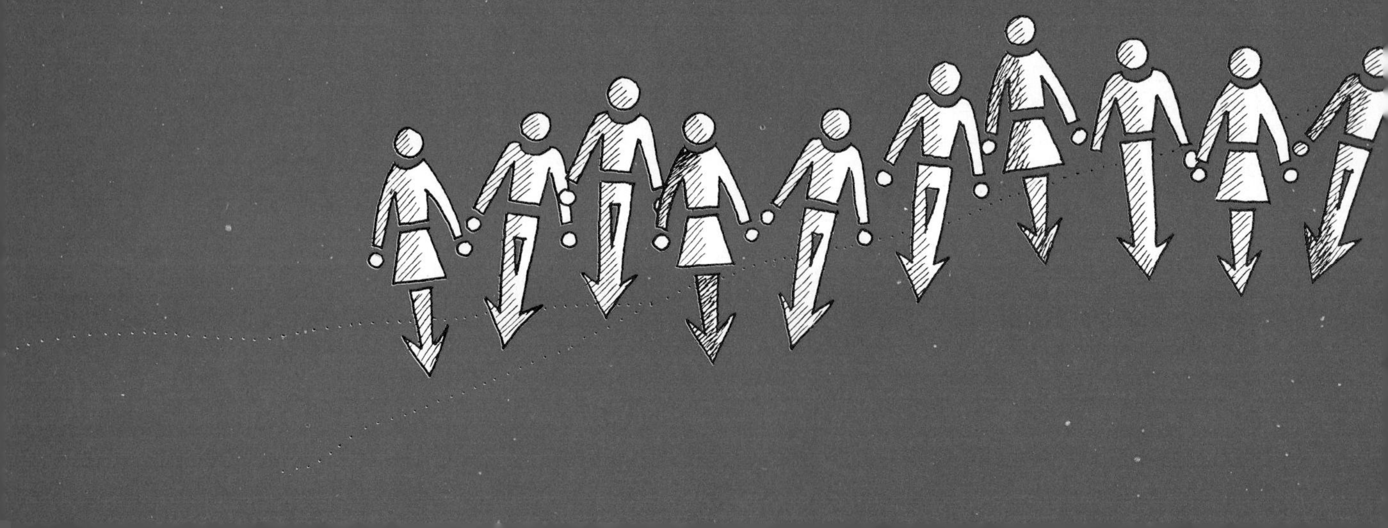

25
THE BUSINESS OF HEALTH

WHAT'S AHEAD IN CHAPTER 25 How, in effect, does a nation choose the level of health of its population? How is the health care establishment in the United States structured? What sectors of the community participate in developing health care policy? What role can the consumer play? In what ways is health care delivered in the United States? What rights are consumers of hospital services demanding? Why have health care costs been rising rapidly? Can the rise be slowed? How is health care for Americans paid for? What factors must be considered in a decision about national health insurance? What contributes to inadequate health care? How can health care be improved? What has been the impact of the proliferation of malpractice suits against physicians, hospitals, etc.? How might this crisis be eased? What are some of the ethical issues that face the medical community and the rest of us? What are the dangers of quackery? What is its allure? How can the quack be recognized? How should the various methods of unconventional care be approached by the intelligent health consumer?

"The right to the preservation of health is inalienable," declared Congressman William Lyman of Massachusetts in 1796. Nearly two centuries later, good intentions notwithstanding, that "inalienable right" is still not assured to all Americans. Health economist Victor Fuchs (*a*) believes that no country is as healthy as it could be; no country does as much for the sick as it is technically capable of doing. It's a matter of priorities and values.

Many of the 50,000 who die annually on the highways could, for example, be saved if known technology could be applied to road and auto design. But the cost would be tremendous. We have not chosen to pay that cost. Likewise we have not made kidney machines available to all those who need them.

Each country, in effect, chooses its own death rate. Some may insist that health is more important than anything else, that if we can squander vast sums on cosmetics, cigarettes, alcoholic beverages, pet foods, and color telephones, then certainly we can afford to spend more money on health. But Fuchs suggests that this is a misleading argument. For there are other worthwhile goals that go unfulfilled because of financial limitations—justice and education, for example. Says Fuchs, "If we are honest with ourselves, there can be little doubt that other goals often take precedence over health. If better health is our goal, we can achieve it, but only at some cost." Thus, community decision making and valuing directly affect the quality and quantity of health care available in the United States today.

The second major influence on health care is the often helter-skelter pattern of its growth and organization. As areas of knowledge developed—in research, disease prevention, delivery of care, public health services, health education—responsibilities were assumed by those who stood ready to receive them, with a sturdy but loosely organized nonsystem of care the result. While some believe such an unfettered design to be appropriate in a society like ours where individual enterprise and innovation are valued, others argue that such a system cannot deliver the best health care at the least cost.

THE HEALTH CARE ESTABLISHMENT

Major roles in health care have been accepted by federal, state, and local governments, the medical profession, and a private sector that includes nonprofit, profit-making and, more recently, consumer groups.

The Role of Government

The piecemeal involvement of the federal government in health through new, and sometimes conflicting or overlapping, layers of legislation has become so widespread that nearly every major government department now regulates, investigates, or educates in some health area. The leading role, however, is played by the Department of Health, Education and Welfare and its subsidiaries (see Figure 25.1).

Local and state health responsibilities are equally diffuse and, at times, contradictory. Feeding of children from poverty homes may fall to the Education Department, while nutritional needs of the elderly are met by the Welfare Department. Because of this fragmentation, someone with a health-related problem often does not know where to turn. Figure 25.2 suggests a procedure that would make entering the health care system at the right point easier.

The Private Sector

The private sector plays its important part in American health care through both voluntary nonprofit agencies and commercial enterprises.

The voluntary agencies The list of voluntary agencies is long. Nonprofit organizations to provide care to the ill and indigent include voluntary hospitals, medical schools, nursing homes, and such uniquely American groups as the National Foundation to Prevent Birth Defects, the American Cancer Society, and the American Heart Association. They fund health research and education, and advise and assist disease victims and their families.

Industry and business United States industry does more than supply health products and services. The producers of pharmaceuti-

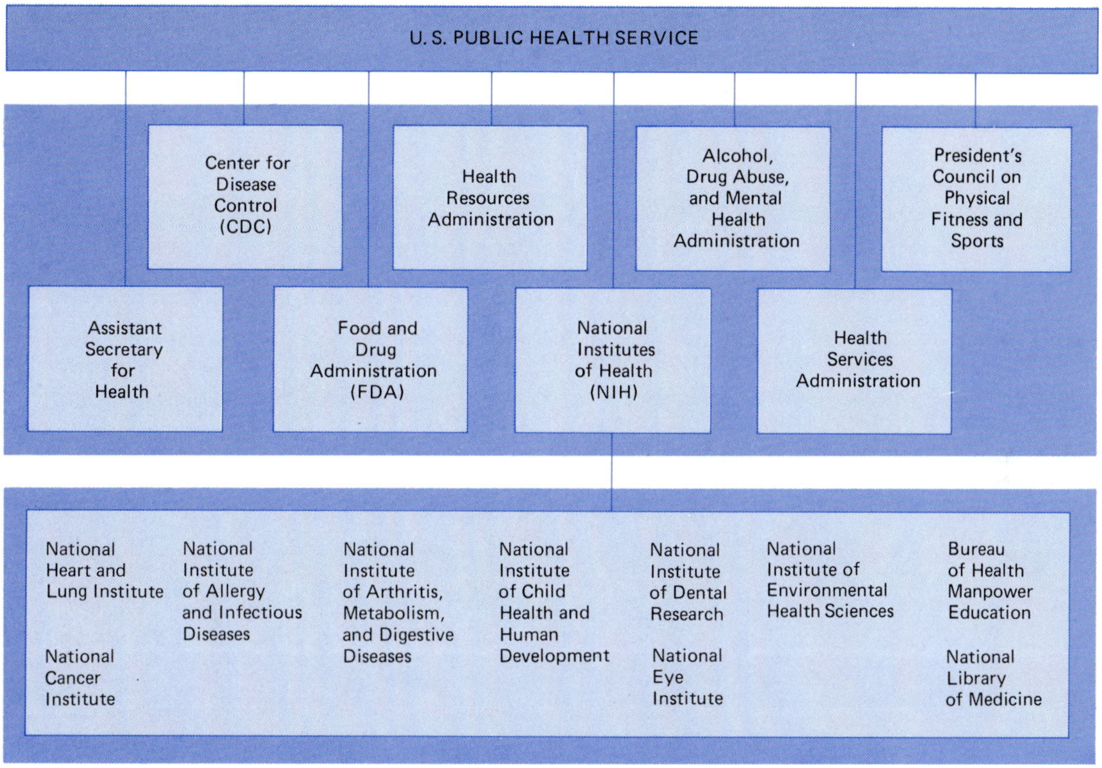

FIGURE 25.1 Divisions of the U.S. Public Health Service, under the Department of Health, Education, and Welfare.

cals, artificial organs, medical instruments, hospital equipment, and supplies are inevitably involved in research leading to medical progress, in testing products for safety and effectiveness, and in educating the public—though sometimes that education reflects as much self-interest as public interest.

Organized Medicine

The American Medical Association, the American Hospital Association (AHA), and hundreds of smaller professional medical organizations have two major interests: (1) to maintain and improve the status of their members, (2) to improve health care. Critics claim that some of these groups emphasize the first goal over the second and have failed to adequately censure those who fail to meet high standards of professionalism.

The Consumer

The person most affected by the health care system has until recently had little or no voice in its operations. Thanks to pressure from consumer advocates, consumers in the 1970s serve on boards of many health organizations including hospitals, have helped found and administer some health maintenance organizations (HMOs), are represented on health systems agencies (HSAs) and other local and regional planning groups, and sit on committees to evaluate medical services. They work

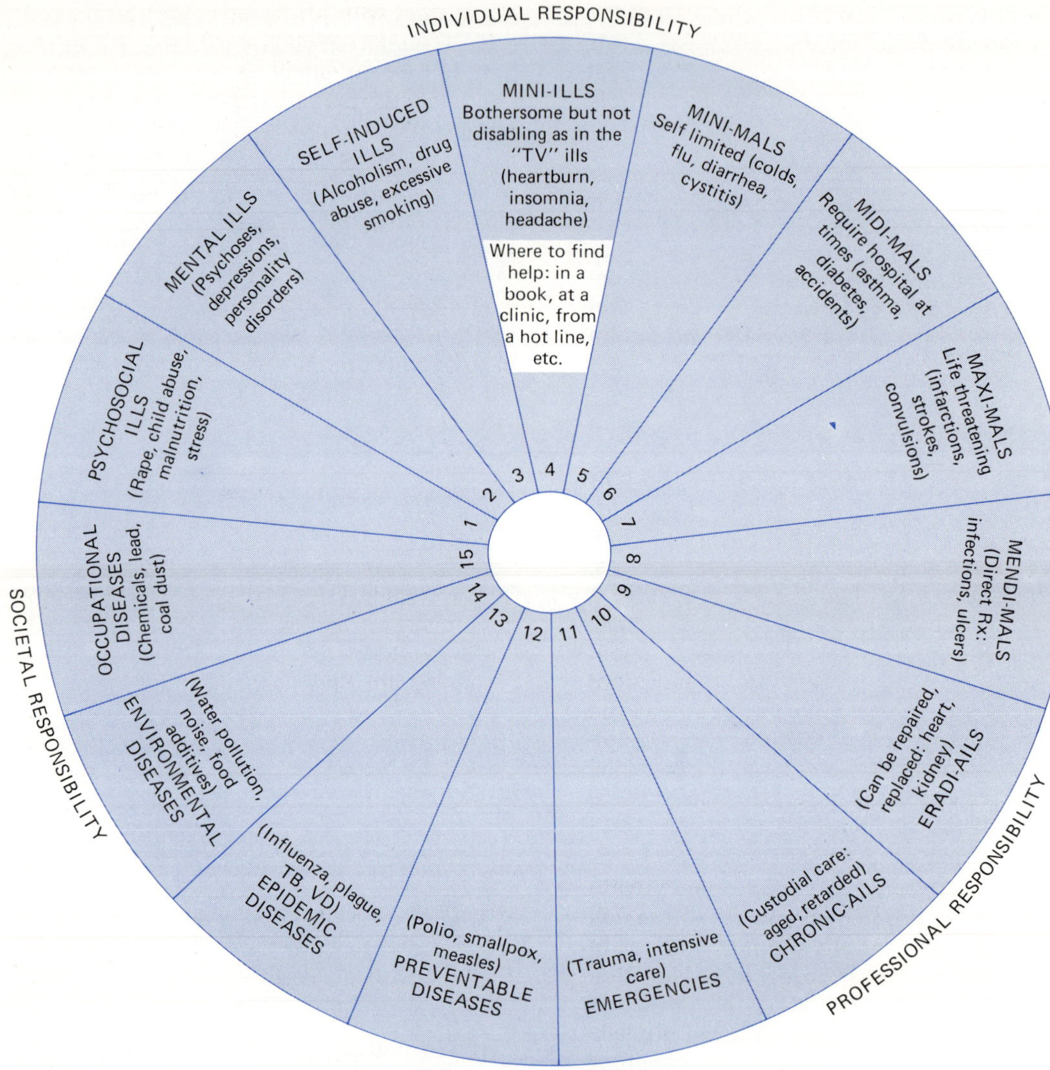

FIGURE 25.2 The wheel of health. Entering the health care system would be a great deal easier if the wheel of health, as suggested by Dr. Keith Sehnert, were adopted by local communities. Sehnert suggests that such an informational wheel, constantly updated with specific resources that can help with specific health problems (examples as shown), should be placed at conspicuous, convenient locations in every city, town, and village. Citizens would need only to spin the wheel to the area of immediate concern to learn where to turn for help. [*After Sehnert, p. 592.*]

in partnership with the other segments of the establishment to guard consumer interests and attempt to strike a balance of the best possible medical care at the lowest possible cost.

DELIVERY OF HEALTH CARE

Our pluralistic, many-faceted health care establishment has many separate, distinct, yet often overlapping, ways of delivering health care to the American patient.

The Private Practitioner

The American health care system is built on a foundation of physicians in business for themselves—some 200,000 private practitioners in solo practices, partnerships, groups, and corporations. Physicians working in a group practice share equipment, expenses, and staff, as well as office space, and benefit from joint consultation and lightened night and weekend workloads. Groups may be single-specialty (two internists or three pediatricians, for example) or multi-specialty practices offering patients complete medical care.

Some physicians have a team practice, efficiently organized to utilize allied health professionals: physicians' assistants (PAs), nurse-clinicians, or nurse-practitioners to handle health histories, physical examinations, well-patient care, and uncomplicated illnesses; and social workers or psychologists to give counseling. Auxiliary personnel allow the physician to give more time to patients who require it.

Health Maintenance Organizations

The health maintenance organization appeared in the 1970s with strong federal support as a new way of providing total health care, prevention included. An HMO has four elements: (1) an organized health care delivery system with physicians, supporting staff, and treatment facilities; (2) a membership that enrolls in advance for services; (3) a financial plan providing services on a prepaid basis; (4) a management branch. In a variation of the HMO, the individual practice association (IPA), patients see physicians in their offices rather than in a central facility. Major corporations are now experimenting with HMOs and IPAs as ways to deliver quality health care to employees at reduced cost. In 1977, the average monthly cost of belonging to such a group was lower in many areas than the cost of hospitalization insurance alone (Sullivan).

Federally Delivered Health Care

Millions of Americans receive health care directly from the government through the Public Health Service, Veterans' Administration, military hospitals and clinics, physicians under contract to the government, and the Indian Health Service. This last service, and thus the health of the population it serves, has been less than satisfactory, in part because of physicians' unwillingness to serve in isolated posts.

Hospital-Delivered Care

In 1976 there were 7156 hospitals with a total of more than 1.5 million beds registered with the American Hospital Association. Of these, 382 were federally owned and operated, 775 were investor-owned (by physicians or hospital chains), 2800 were nonprofit (voluntary) hospitals, and 1840 were run by state or local governments. These hospitals provide a broad spectrum of services, from emergency to surgery, to people at every income level. Increasingly, patients are treated on an outpatient basis when possible, rather than admitted to the hospital.

Selecting a hospital About 75 percent of all hospitals meet the minimal standards for ac-

Gilles Peress/Magnum

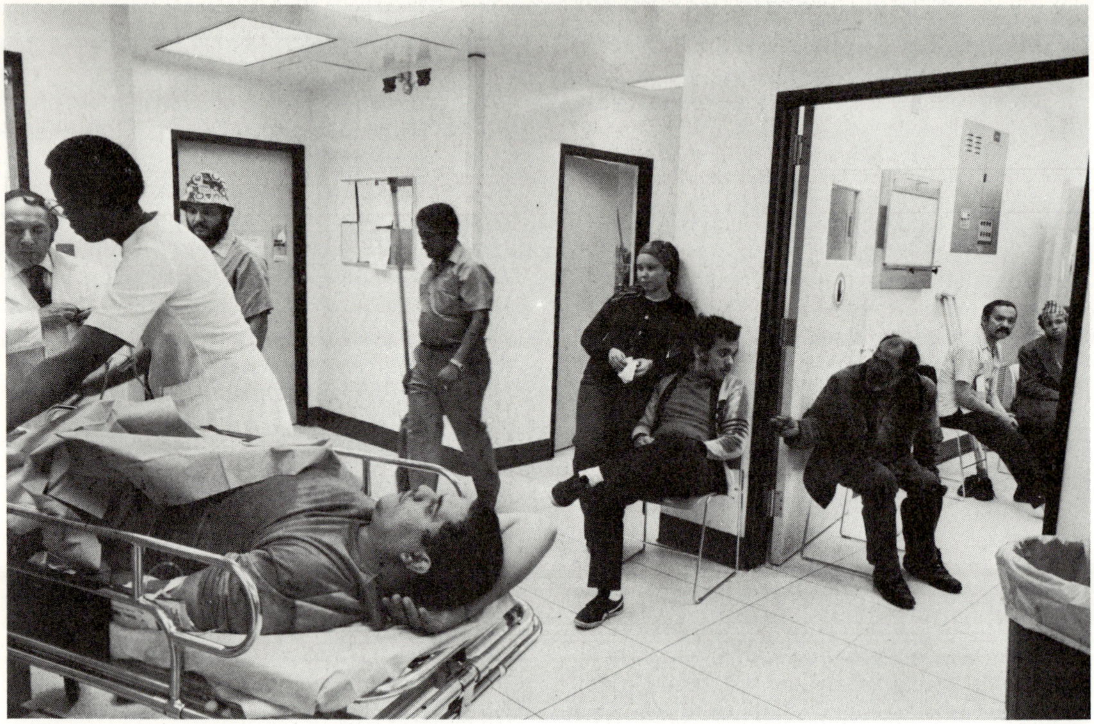

Hospitals provide a broad spectrum of services—from emergency to surgery—to people at every income level.

creditation by the Joint Commission on the Accreditation of Hospitals (JCAH), sponsored by the AMA, the AHA, and the American College of Surgeons. The facilities of many hospitals far exceed these standards. In selecting a hospital (when there is a choice), a patient should consider the following: (1) accreditation and general reputation, (2) special facilities for the medical problem being treated, (3) convenience of location, (4) whether or not one's own physician has practice privileges there.

Hospitals and patients A hospital can be a frightening place. Things go on that are unexplained, questions go unanswered, people in white (or blue or green) are everywhere, but the patient often feels alone. Activated health consumers, however, may fare better. They ask questions and expect answers: "Why must I take that sleeping pill?" "Do I *have* to be awakened every morning at 5:30?" And when they sense something is wrong, they say so. One woman who did not speak up nearly died when two nurses gave her insulin shots twice within 20 minutes.

In response to patient activation, many hospitals have appointed representatives who act as advocates for the patient in complaints about hospital staff, billing department, and so on. To further protect the patient, the American Hospital Association adopted "A Patient's Bill of Rights," which some hospitals have accepted as a guideline.

Free Clinics

The "free" in free clinics does not only mean

without cost. It means free from hassle, red tape, conventional value systems and labels, and from moralizing or talking down. The first free clinic opened its doors in Haight-Ashbury in 1967, when large numbers of young "street people" were cut off from or unable to afford the usual outlets for medical care. By 1977, there were more than 500 free clinics providing more than 3 million patient visits per year. Today, free clinic patient populations include not only the original street people and their children, but also unemployed workers and their families, minority group members, and middle-class individuals with VD or drug problems who are embarrassed to see their own family physicians.

Nursing and Convalescent Homes

We often think of nursing homes as warehouses for the elderly, but they provide care for those of any age unable to tend to themselves or recuperating from illness and in need of more skilled care than they can receive at home. Such facilities usually fall into two categories: facilities providing passive care for patients beyond medical help (such as those in a comatose state) and facilities providing active care for patients, often including the elderly with chronic diseases who can still benefit from treatment.

Other Dispensers of Health Care

Other facilities providing health care include medical centers and teaching hospitals, research centers, schools and colleges, industries. Care may also be delivered, particularly in rural areas or inner cities, by physicians' assistants (PAs), nurse-practitioners, nurse-midwives, emergency medical technicians (EMTs), and other trained medical personnel.

PAYING FOR HEALTH CARE

The $162 billion spent on health care in the United States in 1977, far more than the total defense budget, raises several questions: Who should pay for medical care? How? Can rapidly rising costs be stemmed and more and better care be provided at the same time?

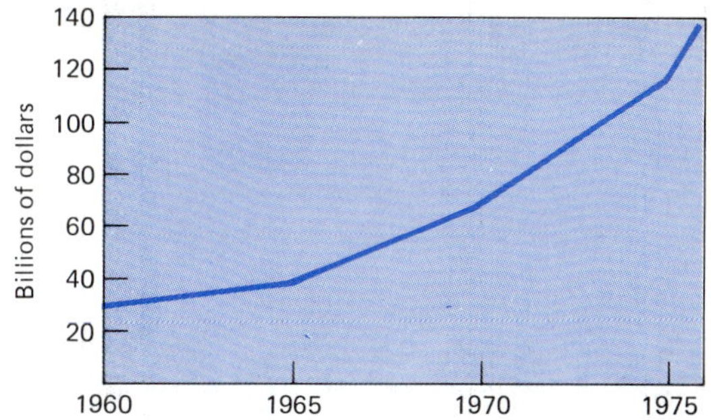

FIGURE 25.3 Cost of health care: combined public and private expenditures, rounded to nearest billion. In less than a generation, health care costs have nearly quintupled, totaling \$162.6 billion in 1977. Physician costs make up almost 20 percent of the total expenditure and hospital costs nearly 40 percent, making them the highest single category of health spending. [*U.S. Social Security Administration.*]

Rising Costs

In the 1970s, health care costs rose more rapidly than other costs (see Figure 25.3).

Reasons for higher costs Fingers have been pointed at many causes of the upward dance of health costs: inflation; higher salaries for low-paid hospital employees; poor management of some health facilities; enormous increases in malpractice insurance costs and in exhaustive testing that is part of "defensive medicine" to avoid lawsuits; building and staffing of new hospitals; and rapid technological advances in medicine often requiring costly apparatus, drugs, and equipment. Medicare and Medicaid have proved to be far more costly than originally envisioned by planners and legislators. Costs of all health insurance, federal and private, are boosted by

A Patient's Bill of Rights*

The American Hospital Association presents a Patient's Bill of Rights with the expectation that observance of these rights will contribute to more effective patient care and greater satisfaction for the patient, his physician, and the hospital organization. Further, the Association presents these rights in the expectation that they will be supported by the hospital on behalf of its patients, as an integral part of the healing process. It is recognized that a personal relationship between the physician and the patient is essential for the provision of proper medical care. The traditional physician-patient relationship takes on a new dimension when care is rendered within an organizational structure. Legal precedent has established that the institution itself also has a responsibility to the patient. It is in recognition of these factors that these rights are affirmed.

1 The patient has the right to considerate and respectful care.

2 The patient has the right to obtain from his physician complete current information concerning his diagnosis, treatment, and prognosis in terms the patient can be reasonably expected to understand. When it is not medically advisable to give such information to the patient, the information should be made available to an appropriate person in his behalf. He has the right to know by name, the physician responsible for coordinating his care.

3 The patient has the right to receive from his physician information necessary to give informed consent prior to the start of any procedure and/or treatment. Except in emergencies, such information for informed consent, should include but not necessarily be limited to the specific procedure and/or treatment, the medically significant risks involved, and the probable duration of incapacitation. Where medically significant alternatives for care or treatment exist, or when the patient requests information concerning medical alternatives, the patient has the right to such information. The patient also has the right to know the name of the person responsible for the procedures and/or treatment.

4 The patient has the right to refuse treatment to the extent permitted by law, and to be informed of the medical consequences of his action.

5 The patient has the right to every consideration of his privacy concerning his own medical care program. Case discussion, consultation, examination, and treatment are confidential and should be conducted discreetly. Those not directly involved in his care must have the permission of the patient to be present.

6 The patient has the right to expect that all communications and records pertaining to his care should be treated as confidential.

7 The patient has the right to expect that within its capacity a hospital must make reasonable response to the request of a patient for services. The hospital must provide evaluation, service, and/or referral as indicated by the urgency of the case. When medically permissible a patient may be transferred to another facility only after he has received complete information and explanation concerning the needs for and alternatives to such a transfer. The institution to which the patient is to be transferred must first have accepted the patient for transfer.

8 The patient has the right to obtain information as to any relationship of his hospital to other health care and educational institutions insofar as his care is concerned. The patient has the right to obtain information as to the existence of any professional relationships among individuals, by name, who are treating him.

9 The patient has the right to be advised if the hospital proposes to engage in or perform human experimentation affecting his care or treatment. The patient has the right to refuse to participate in such research projects.

10 The patient has the right to expect reasonable continuity of care. He has the right to know in advance

*Approved by the House of Delegates of the American Hospital Association, Feb. 6, 1973.

Source: Reprinted with the permission of the American Hospital Association.

what appointment times and physicians are available and where. The patient has the right to expect that the hospital will provide a mechanism whereby he is informed by his physician or a delegate of the physician of the patient's continuing health care requirements following discharge.

11 The patient has the right to examine and receive an explanation of his bill regardless of source of payment.

12 The patient has the right to know what hospital rules and regulations apply to his conduct as a patient.

No catalogue of rights can gurantee for the patient the kind of treatment he has a right to expect. A hospital has many functions to perform, including the prevention and treatment of disease, the education of both health professionals and patients, and the conduct of clinical research. All these activities must be conducted with an overriding concern for the patient, and, above all, the recognition of his dignity as a human being. Success in achieving this recognition assures success in the defense of the rights of the patient.

the minority of patients and physicians who abuse the programs.

Reducing health care costs Should costs continue their steep rise, it is estimated they will reach a staggering $1.6 trillion by 1994 (Ellwood). Some changes and suggested changes aimed at cutting these costs without cutting, and sometimes while improving, health services include:

HEALTH CONSUMER TIP

Evaluating a Nursing Home

- *Is this nursing home the right type of facility for the patient?* Does it offer skilled nursing care, rehabilitation, and a program of activities? Or simply custodial care? Is it acceptable to the patient's insurance provider? Are the hours flexible and the location convenient so that friends, relatives, and the patient's personal physician can visit easily? Is the home accredited by the JCAH?
- *Is the physical plant adequate?* Is the home well located in a pleasant area away from excessive noise without being totally isolated from the rest of the world? Does the building meet fire safety codes and have adequate fire exits? Are the rooms large and bright, with closets, drawers, a table, and comfortable chairs? Are there sufficient toilet facilities? Are there emergency call buttons at bedside, in bathrooms, and in other areas? Are public rooms attractive and well equipped? Are there opportunities for privacy for those who may desire it for sexual or other reasons? Are linens changed regularly?
- *How good is the nursing care?* Is the staff composed of a sufficient number of trained registered or licensed nurses? Do they appear to be experienced and capable, clean, courteous, contented, interested in patients, and informed about their conditions? Is there little staff turnover? Is there equipment and trained personnel to administer physical therapy?
- *Is the food service of high quality?* (Visit at mealtime.) Is the food appetizing, balanced, varied? (Taste it!) Is it prepared in a clean kitchen? Are portions adequate and neatly served? Are special diets carefully attended to?
- *What is the condition of the patients?* Do the patients appear happy, clean, and reasonably busy? Are there planned indoor and outdoor recreation activities, reading materials, games, crafts, television, excursions for those who are mobile? Are religious services available?

WHO'S WHO IN HEALTH CARE

The Health Care Team

- *Registered nurses (RNs)* Assist physicians in patient care and treatment in hospitals, clinics, doctors' offices; in industry, schools, and public health services; and as private-duty nurses. *Requirements:* A diploma from a hospital program, or an associate or baccalaureate degree in nursing plus passing a licensing examination.*†
- *Nurse-practitioners* Provide independent patient care in clinics, hospitals, doctors' offices, etc. *Requirements*: RN, baccalaureate, or master's plus specialty training, e.g., in pediatrics, midwifery.
- *Physicians' assistants* Work interdependently with doctors to provide patient care. *Requirements*: Usually two years of training in an approved program (one year for ex-medical corpsmen); certificate, or associate or baccalaureate degree. Previous health experience and/or college may be required. Certification by professional organization.
- *Licensed practical nurses (LPNs)* Provide skilled nursing care under physician or RN supervision as well as private-duty and baby nursing. *Requirements:* Passing an approved course and a licensing examination.
- *Nurses' aides, orderlies, attendants* Assist in patient care, e.g., feeding, bedmaking, transportation, etc. *Requirements*: Usually a high school diploma and on-the-job training.
- *Physiotherapists* Help rehabilitate those disabled by disease, injury, heredity. *Requirements*: Bachelors degree or certification plus licensing examination.†
- *Speech therapists* Rehabilitate people with speech defects. *Requirements*: A master's degree in many states; teacher's license in some states for work in schools.
- *Occupational therapists* Train or retrain the disabled for productivity. *Requirements*: Usually college training.†
- *Medical assistants* Assist with simple patient care and preparation in doctors' offices, keep records, deal with patients. *Requirements*: On-the-job training or a course at a junior college or vocational institute.
- *Medical record clerks or technicians* Process medical records in hospitals and other health care facilities. *Requirements*: A college or hospital program of 10 months to 2 years; accreditation certificate for supervisory positions.
- *Medical technologists or technicians* Work in labs, ORs, hospitals, etc., operating sophisticated machinery (x-ray, EEG, ECG, etc.). *Requirements*: Vary from on-the-job training to advanced college degrees depending upon complexity and level of responsibility.
- *Health administrators* Manage health facilities. *Requirements*: A two- or four-year college degree, master's, or Ph.D., depending upon the type of facility and level of responsibilty.

*Baccalaureate or advanced degree usually required for advancement.

†Advanced degrees usually necessary for administration, research, teaching.

- Increase outpatient procedures, including simple surgery performed in doctors' offices and same-day surgery in special surgical centers or hospital facilities, reducing the need for overnight stays
- Willingness of more insurance companies to pay for these less costly treatments under hospitalization policies
- Preadmission testing on an outpatient basis, instead of admitting a patient into the

hospital a day or two in advance of surgery for tests

- Increased home care, with visiting nurses and needed equipment and training to families supplied
- Self- or minimal-care units in hospitals for patients who are not seriously ill
- Reduction of duplication of equipment and services in local communities through crackdowns on hospital construction and expansion by the new health systems agencies (see page 567)
- Increased reliance on second opinions to reduce unnecessary surgery, tests, and treatment
- Careful audits of Medicare and Medicaid programs to cut the high cost of fraud and abuse
- Increased patient self-care and practice of preventive medicine, as described in this book

How Health Care Is Paid For Today

Americans pay the bill for health care in as many diverse ways as it is delivered. These are the common methods of payment.

Fee for service Most people pay their doctor a fee for each service the physician or an assistant performs.

Prepaid group Others pay nothing for individual visits. Their health care is paid for in advance through a prepaid group. An annual premium covers all medical needs, from camp physicals for the children to intensive care for coronary patients, from routine blood pressure checks to long-term use of a kidney dialysis machine. Every study of prepaid patients seems to show they have fewer sick days and spend less time in the hospital than fee-for-service patients. Premiums are often paid in full or in part by an employer, and physicians are paid by the group (usually an annual salary, but sometimes on the basis of workload carried).

Direct federal health care Uncle Sam pays the bills for such groups as the military, Indians, and veterans with service-incurred disabilities.

Private insurance Many persons who pay their physician for office visits carry health insurance for extraordinary expenses such as hospitalization (Blue Cross, for example) and in-hospital doctors' services and aftercare (Blue Shield). By 1980, it is anticipated that 9 out of 10 Americans will be carrying such private insurance coverage.

Government-sponsored health insurance Perhaps the most enduring programs of Lyndon B. Johnson's Great Society were Title XVIII and Title XIX, the 1965 amendments to the Social Security Act setting up Medicare and Medicaid. The former, price-tagged at $17.8 billion in 1976, was originally conceived as providing almost free hospital and other health care for those over 65. Rising costs have imposed a steadily rising "voluntary contribution" on the elderly. In 1978, for example, the patient was to pay $144 for the first 60 days of hospital care, $36 a day until day 90, and $72 a day after that.

Medicaid, designed to meet the health needs of families in a financial crunch, cost $15.3 billion in 1976, with costs shared by federal and state governments. Basically, the states must provide five services: outpatient and inpatient hospital care, diagnostic tests, physicians' services, and nursing home care. Optionally, they may also provide home health care, private-duty nursing, and dental and other services. In theory, Medicaid was to allow the indigent to go to the physician of their choice, and to receive care in the finest hospitals instead of county or municipal wards. Conditions and care have been greatly improved, but the dream exceeded the reality. Many private practitioners do not accept Medicaid patients because of slow pay, heavy paperwork, and shrinking fees. Fast-buck, fast-turnover Medicaid mills and overcrowded hospital emergency rooms and outpatient

HEALTH CONSUMER TIP

Selecting Health Insurance Coverage

Those in need of health insurance face a bewildering selection of policies and promises—what Herbert Denenberg calls a "uniform non-uniformity." Knowing what to look for will help:

Types of policies

- *Hospital, medical, and surgical* This basic health insurance policy covers hospital room and services, and doctors' and surgeons' fees while in the hospital (Blue Cross and Blue Shield coverage are an example). Some policies cover nearly all health costs, others only a small part of them. Payments are usually made in one of two ways: (1) on a flat-fee or indemnity basis, in which the insured gets a fixed sum for each day in the hospital and for each kind of illness, no matter what the actual cost is and even if costs rise; (2) on a service benefits basis (usually more costly), in which the insured gets a proportion (often 80 percent) of *all* the actual costs. If costs go up, so do benefits.
- *Major Medical* This is a backup type of policy for really serious illnesses, accidents, or miscellaneous expenses that might not be covered in a basic policy. There is usually a deductible, an amount that the insured must pay before payments begin, but the deductible is often covered by the basic policy. Payments are usually a percentage of total costs (often 75 to 85 percent), and there may be a maximum. Premiums are relatively low because chances are slight that a person will actually come down with a major illness.
- *Medicare supplements* Some persons take this insurance to cover costs that may not be covered by Medicare.

Important features to look for

- *Broad coverage* that includes illness *and* accident, diagnostic tests, drugs, out-of-hospital care, dental care, private-duty nurses, treatment for alcoholism and mental illness, payments for sterilization, abortions, family counseling, and preventive and maintenance care and evaluation, if possible.
- *Long-term coverage* that won't run out just when you need it most.
- *General coverage* that includes more than one or two catastrophic illnesses.
- *Pregnancy and childbirth coverage*, if you need it.
- *Full family protection*, including newborns at birth.
- *Adequate flat rates* if the policy is of the indemnity type so that payments will cover a major portion of costs.
- *Group coverage* which will usually offer broader protection at lower cost than individual policies (this may be available if you join a lodge or other organization).
- *A minimum number of conditions* such as waiting periods (during which new and/or preexisting illnesses are not covered)* and *few* exclusions.

Checking the insurance carrier Select an insurance company with a good reputation; check with friends, your physician, the state insurance department, and Best's Insurance which rates companies. A company that has a high loss ratio,† that is, pays a high percentage of premiums back to policyholders in payments, and has few complaints against it is a good one to consider.

*Waiting periods of from eight months to a year on maternity benefits are found in almost all policies.

†Fifty percent or higher is best.

clinics have, in many cases, become family physicians to the poor.

Workers' compensation When injured on the job, a worker is paid a weekly or lump-sum award covering both loss of wages and needed medical care, though often not rehabilitation. The cost of "workers' comp" insurance is borne by employers. Since the cost depends upon the firm's safety record, employers have a built-in incentive to improve working conditions.

Paying for Tomorrow's Health Care: The Options

Even with all these methods of funding, there are still millions of Americans who cannot afford adequate health care and yet do not fit under the Medicaid-Medicare umbrella. Judging from the number of bills introduced in Congress, everyone seems to have a solution, but no one knows how to shepherd conflicting power blocs into a workable compromise. Those in organized medicine have opposed plans that smack of national health insurance because they believe it will lead to a total takeover of medicine by the government, followed by an abrupt decline in quality of care. They warn that "free" medical care means higher taxes and predict an overload of the system, with the kind of short shrift in office visits and long waits for surgery that plague the British system of "socialized medicine." But some people believe that only National Health Insurance will ease the health care burden on individuals and bring modern medicine to all Americans.

Evaluating Suggested National Health Insurance Plans

Any national health insurance plan will involve trade-offs between cost and quality. Among questions to be explored before a decision is made are these:

- Who will be covered?
- What services should be covered?
- Should there be deductibles?
- Will people have to carry additional insurance to cover extras?
- Will there be waiting periods, time limits, or other limitations?
- Will catastrophic illnesses be covered? (Most see this as the area of greatest urgency.)
- Who will control quality of care?
- Will patients have "freedom of choice" of physician?
- How will physicians and other providers of care be reimbursed: through fee-for-service, an annual salary, or an annual "capitation" payment for each patient on their treatment list?
- How will the insurance be financed: by a payroll tax on employers, employees, or both; by a credit against income tax; from general tax revenues; or in some other way?
- Who will administer the program—private insurance carriers, specially created agencies, the states, or the federal government?
- How will abuses be prevented and efficient operations encouraged?
- Will private practice be stifled? Will health maintenance organizations be cultivated?
- Is a change in the style of delivery of health care inevitable, and, if so, will it be an improvement?

QUALITY OF HEALTH CARE

Many, if not most, Americans enjoy a higher standard of health than even a decade or two ago. Many once life-threatening diseases have virtually vanished. Treatment for several chronic diseases has improved. Sick days for employees (a useful yardstick of national health) have dropped. We have come a long way. But though we spend more money on health care than any nation on earth, we nevertheless do not rank number 1 in at least two important areas: infant mortality and life

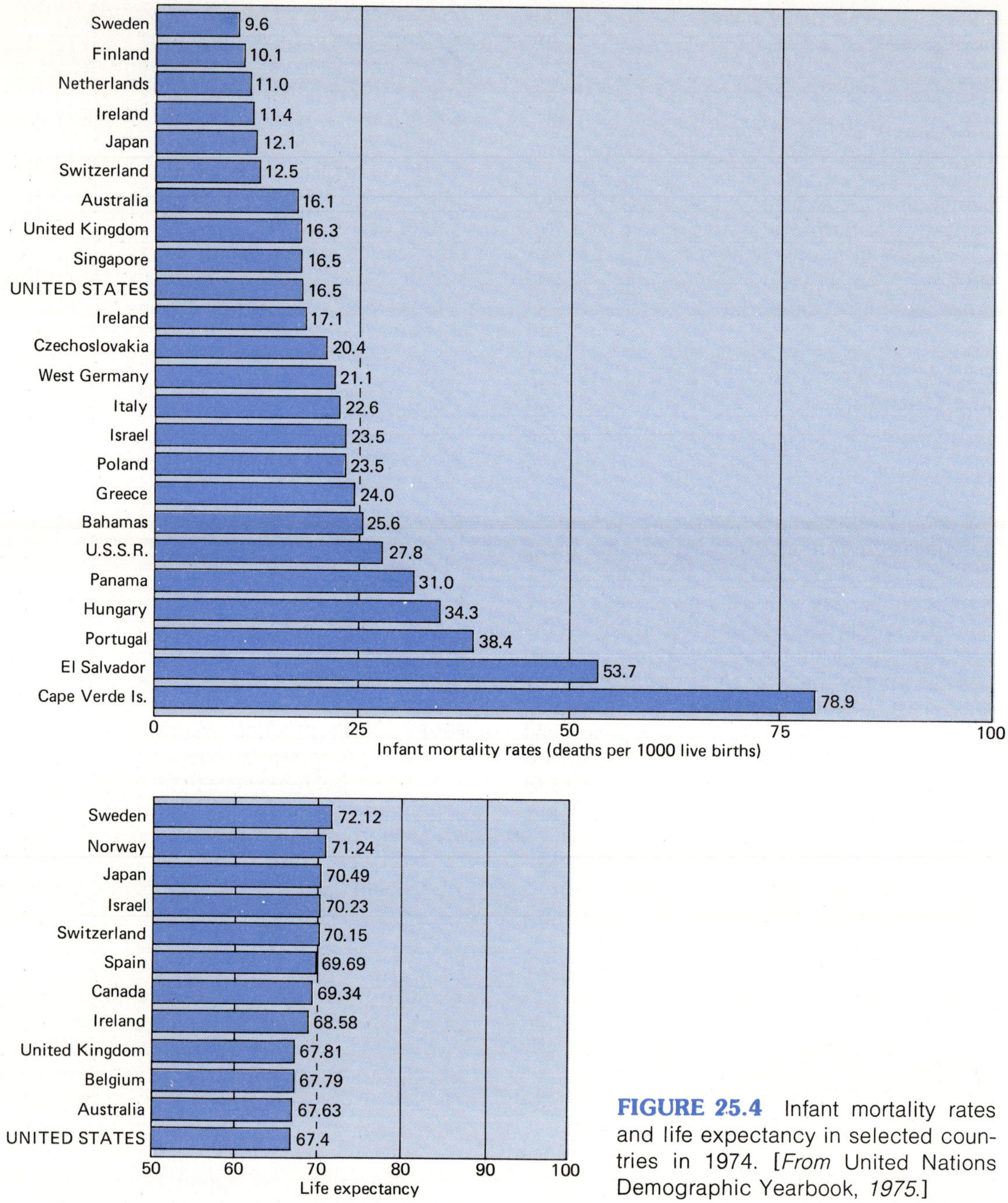

FIGURE 25.4 Infant mortality rates and life expectancy in selected countries in 1974. [*From* United Nations Demographic Yearbook, *1975.*]

expectancy (see Figure 25.4). People still fall ill and die of preventable diseases. Many people get no care at all.

Reasons for Less-than-Perfect Health Care

Among the reasons health care is not what it might be in this country are some we have already discussed: values and priorities, disorganized system, lack of coverage for some persons. But failure to transmit new medical advances to local physicians, use of outdated techniques, and lack of quality supervision and standards also contribute to the problem. Another major difficulty is the maldistribution of medical care: a glut of physicians in the prosperous suburbs, an undersupply in rural areas and inner cities.

Mechanisms for Improving Health Care

Hundreds of ways to improve health care services have been suggested, and some have been implemented. Proposals have included:

- Periodic relicensing examinations for all health professionals, such as those now imposed every six months on members of the American Academy of Family Physicians
- Required continuing education for physicians, now mandatory in Oregon
- Uniform licensing examinations for physicians throughout the United States
- Appointment of laypeople to sit on medical review boards
- Closer supervision of licensing of foreign medical doctors, some of whom are poorly trained
- Mandated service for medical school graduates in areas that are short of doctors
- Creation of incentives to attract physicians to such regions
- Increased support for and attention to preventive medicine

Already in action with the goal of improving health care and systematizing it are PSROs and HSAs. The PSRO (Professional Standards Review Organization), created by legislation in 1972, provides for a nationwide network of 203 generally physician-led organizations to set standards for and to monitor care paid for by Medicare or Medicaid. It is hoped that monitoring will extend to all patient care eventually. HSAs (health systems agencies), regional health planning units, with a minimum of 51 percent consumer representation on their boards, were created by Congress in 1975 to combat undisciplined health facility sprawl, in part through a tough administrative weapon known as the *certificate of need.* Before a health care facility can add a wing or purchase costly new equipment, it will have to convince its area HSA that an urgent need exists. Certificate-of-need laws may slow health care progress a bit, but they just might make it more affordable.

Malpractice and the Quality of Care

A carpenter topples off a roof at a construction site. He is rushed by ambulance to the nearest hospital, where a neurosurgeon treats him. Paralysis nevertheless sets in, and the patient is doomed to spend the rest of his life in a wheelchair. Five years later, a sympathetic jury decides that the surgeon is guilty of malpractice (literally, "bad" practice) and awards almost $1 million to the carpenter, at least 25 percent of which, and possibly more, goes to his attorney.

American doctors are being hit with some 20,000 such claims each year, with the number rising at about 10 percent annually. Patients, or their survivors, are suing physicians (anesthesiologists for administering overdoses, pediatricians for failure to recognize concussion, surgeons for slips of the scalpel), hospitals, and occasionally pharmacists or other health care workers. Multi-million-dollar awards have helped fuel the trend.

United Press International

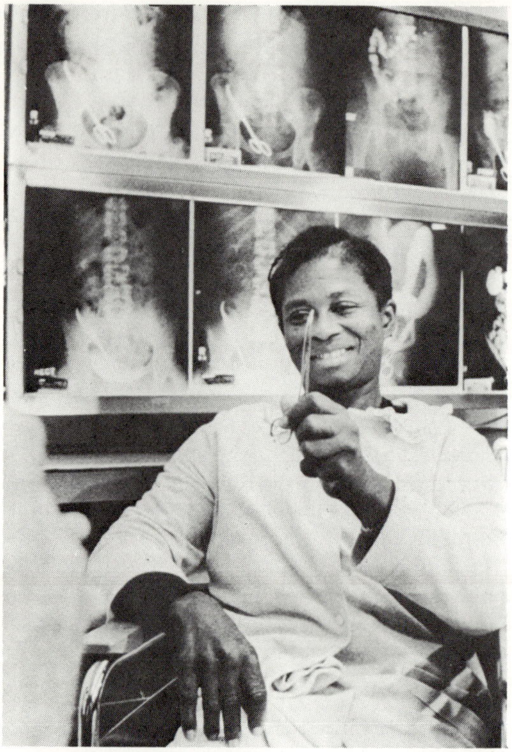

Elizabeth Collier displays a pair of forceps accidentally left in her stomach during an operation. Such incidents are among the many reasons for the surge of malpractice suits against American doctors.

Most malpractice suits, however, are settled out of court for relatively small cash sums (patients who file suits have only a 17 percent chance of collecting anything at all in malpractice cases) or lost at trial because the medical practitioner is judged not to be at fault or to have acted according to prevailing standards of care. The courts recognize that every "bad result" is not necessarily the result of physician error or ineptitude. Nevertheless, the surge of suits has led to massive increases in the malpractice insurance premiums doctors pay to protect themselves. In high-risk specialties like neurosurgery and orthopedic surgery, premiums have multiplied fivefold and more, jumping in high-occurrence states like California from $5000 to $25,000 a year and more. Much of the cost is passed on to the patients.

The malpractice crisis has affected quality of health care. In California, physicians went on strike against the high cost of insurance, refusing to provide any but emergency care. Many doctors are practicing defensive medicine: taking expensive series of x-rays after examining a minor accident patient "just in case," avoiding new or hazardous surgery or experimental drugs that might help otherwise hopeless patients, and performing simple office surgery in the hospital where costs are higher.

A few physicians have gone "bare"—practicing without insurance. Some have retired early, entered the military, or switched to less hazardous specialties (from anesthesiology to family practice, for example). Some have moved from high-risk states to those like Indiana, where legislation limits physician liability.

But the barrage of suits has had some positive effects, forcing medicine to put its house in order by disciplining negligent physicians and influencing individual practitioners to be more cautious.

Easing the Malpractice Crisis

Both patients and professionals suffer from the malpractice crisis, and scores of suggestions have been made to defuse it.

- *Patients should take greater responsibility.* An activated and informed patient makes a treatment error less likely. In a California case that resulted in a $4 million verdict, a young boy became a helpless paraplegic after a playground accident, when the diagnosis of head injury was missed in a busy hospital emergency room. He might still be in good health today if a parent or neighbor had recognized the easily spotted symptoms of concussion.

A 1977 California study of some 81,000 patients' hospital charts determined that 970 PCEs (potentially compensable events) had occurred, and that about 72 percent had taken place in operating rooms. The well-informed patient, who insists on a second opinion before surgery, who chooses only a highly recommended and respected surgeon, and who makes careful inquiries about the anesthesiologist and hospital, can reduce the risk. Similarly, the activated patient is more likely to avoid the 19 percent of PCEs caused by medications (see page 332).

- *Physicians should inform patients thoroughly.* Obtaining the patient's informed consent about benefits and risks of surgery, medications, and therapies, before surgery is performed, tests are made, or drugs given, is a vital part of the partnership between doctor and patient and insures both parties against bad results.
- *Arbitration should be instituted.* Either voluntary or compulsory, this process could eliminate the delays and costs of court proceedings. Malpractice arbitration panels exist in some states but have been declared unconstitutional in others because they "come between a citizen and his day in court." In arbitration, the patient and doctor each choose an attorney to represent them, and these two select a third arbitrator to avoid deadlocks. Some predict that a form of modified no-fault insurance will be developed, with doctors paying premiums and patients paying surcharges on their hospital bills. All injured patients would be compensated, but awards would tend to be smaller than some of the "jackpot" payments recently recorded.
- *Finally, the medical profession should do more to weed out "bad apples," the malpractitioners.* In 1974, in a Sacramento, California, courtroom, 84 witnesses paraded through 22 weeks of trial and exposed a series of horrors (an amputated leg, a broken back, repeated unnecessary surgeries) perpetrated by one physician. What most startled observers was that none of the physician's colleagues admitted so much as a suspicion of malpractice, and none had ever filed a complaint or inquiry.

Such revelations, as well as pressures from consumer groups and alarmed physicians themselves, along with concern over Medicaid and Medicare abuses, have led to a closer scrutiny of methods used to supervise and evaluate physicians. More physicians have begun to speak out against incompetent colleagues, or those disabled by drugs, alcohol, or mental illness, both in court and behind the closed doors of state medical boards responsible for disciplining doctors. A majority of states now have legislation enabling health officials to discipline and treat disabled physicians, and suspensions of incompetent practitioners have increased.

ETHICAL ISSUES IN HEALTH

The question of doctors cracking down on inept or exploitive colleagues is just one of many ethical issues in health. Medical ethics has been described as "the science of how medicine *ought* to be practiced." But exactly what "ought" to be has become rather difficult to decide. Should a single individual's life be lengthened by six months with a transplanted heart, or sustained by kidney dialysis, at a cost of tens of thousands of dollars—dollars that might be allocated to help hundreds of persons with lesser health problems instead? Should health resources focus on lowering the world rate of infant mortality and reducing the number of abortions, when half of those saved will later die of starvation and malnutrition anyway? Exploration of such questions is critical if individual and community decision making are to be soundly based. Some major issues are discussed below.

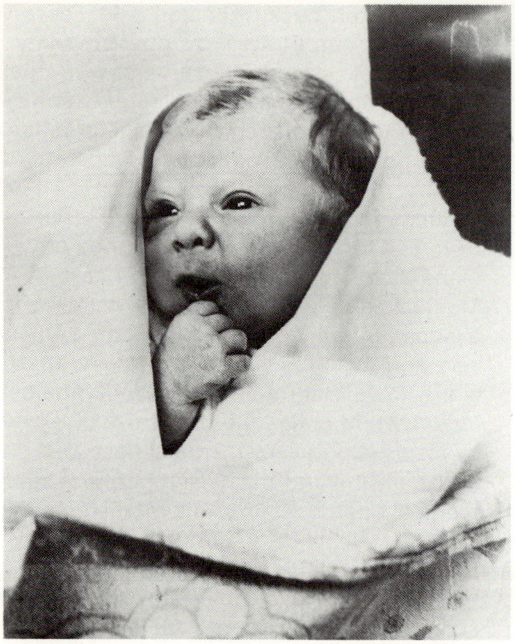

Louise Joy Brown. The successful birth of a "test-tube" baby offers hope to many women who cannot have children because of blocked fallopian tubes. But for some, it raises ethical issues.

Genetic Engineering

The words "genetic engineering" conjure up alarming images of the baby factories in Aldous Huxley's *Brave New World*. The scientist, however, sees another picture: a world without the tragedy of genetic diseases, where serious infectious illnesses are easily cured, where cancer is a disease of the past. Both visions probably exaggerate the possibilities of genetic engineering; even modest progress in these directions is a long way off.

However, some real work is already being done in controlling the genetic makeup of children through genetic counseling and testing of parents, testing of fetuses, and therapeutic abortion when the fetus has a fatal or disabling defect (see Chapter 23). Areas of research include the following.

Cloning This process involves the exact duplication of a living organism by transplanting the nucleus of a cell from that organism into a reproductive cell. It has been quite successful in reproducing carrots and works about 3 percent of the time in frogs. Because of the minute size of mammal eggs, however, mammal cloning has proved more difficult. Practical uses of cloning might some day include reproduction of especially fine beef and dairy cattle, the best-laying hens, and prize-winning racehorses. Claims of successful cloning of humans are unsubstantiated.

In vitro fertilization The creation of "test-tube babies" offers hope to women who cannot have babies because their fallopian tubes (where egg and sperm ordinarily meet) are blocked. In this type of fertilization, the egg is taken from the woman's ovary and placed in a test tube. Millions of her husband's sperm cells are added. If fertilization takes place, the rapidly developing cluster of cells is implanted in the woman's uterus. The first successful use of this procedure in humans resulted in the birth, in 1978, of a baby girl. The event raised hopes among infertile couples, but the technique is useful only when a woman's fallopian tubes are damaged or blocked. Success every time is not yet assured. In animal studies there is a high rate of deformity in such births.

Some believe the procedure is immoral, but many scientists believe that, if the process is perfected, not only can some childless couples be helped but eventually birth defects could be spotted at conception and eliminated. They believe that to bypass this path of study would be immoral. Indeed, they are pressing for more research funds.

Recombinant DNA Also called *gene splicing*, this is the actual manipulation of genetic makeup through the transfer of genes (the material of heredity) from one organism to another or the use of synthetic DNA to program the cells. Although recently scientists successfully transferred a gene controlling insulin production into a bacterium, much more must be done before such work yields practical dividends. Supporters envision tremendous benefits: the elimination of genetic disease, the development of plentiful supplies of insulin, antibiotics, human growth hormone (to prevent dwarfism), and a variety of other hormones and enzymes, and the creation of antibodies against serious infectious disease.

But much of this type of experimentation utilizes bacteria as hosts and viruses as the transmitting agents. Manipulating the genetic makeup of these microorganisms could unleash cancer-causing viruses or germs previously unknown, for which no human being or animal has any resistance. Opponents ask: Is progress worth the risk?

Strict guidelines for such research have been formulated to minimize the possible dangers of recombinant DNA research, but these guidelines do not extend to industrial and military research. Even if the research can be carried on safely, will researchers be able to cope with the ethical issues involved in manipulating the very foundations of life?

Use of Human Subjects in Scientific Research

The phrase "human guinea pig" has a harsh ring. Yet because of thousands of human subjects in scientific investigations, countless other human lives have been saved or improved over the years. Clinical trials on humans are not attempted until successful preliminary research has been carried out on animals or on human or animal tissue cells. But there is a catch: The fact that animal experiments were successful does not mean that human investigations will be, too. Thus, the human guinea pig always faces some potential danger.

Guidelines The first steps toward protecting human subjects were taken when international guidelines were set forth after the war crimes trials in Nuremburg, Germany, to prevent a repetition of the barbaric and senseless medical investigations by Nazi physicians during World War II.

But not until reports of questionable experiments in the early 1960s, including one in which two federally financed investigators injected live cancer cells into 250 uninformed patients, were enforceable guidelines drawn for researchers in the United States. Promulgated in 1971, these guidelines were refined and expanded, spurred on by the exposure in 1972 of the Tuskegee study. Begun in 1932 by the Public Health Service, this experiment allowed a group of 431 black men already infected with syphilis to live out their days without treatment so that the natural course of the disease could be observed.

Informed consent There is little controversy over whether a mature, competent adult can consent to participate in a medical investigation, if: (1) consent is given freely and without duress, (2) everything possible is done to protect the subject, (3) the risks and alternatives are fully and clearly explained, (4) the subject stands to benefit from the study.

Difficulties most frequently arise when the subjects are (1) *children,* (2) *mental patients,* (3) *the poor and uneducated,* and (4) *prisoners.* The latter may not feel free to refuse or may be anxious for benefits they believe may come from cooperating, such as money, better living conditions, earlier parole.

It has been suggested that all of us, young and old, rich and poor, have an obligation to contribute to the benefit of the human community, and that most Americans, by allowing research to be done primarily on the foreign poor, have evaded this responsibility. It has been suggested that we cannot "reap the benefits of research without accepting the risks of experimentation. The U.S. cannot simply impose these risks on people in other countries."

Fetal research The fetus certainly cannot give consent, and fetal research, partly be-

Questions to Consider in Discussing Human Experimentation

1 Does the experiment increase the person's anguish and suffering and deprive him or her of continued experience of life?
2 Does it brutalize the people who carry it out?
3 Does it increase the grief of those who care about the person?
4 Does it establish a pattern that will eventually harm all of society?

cause of its indirect link to abortion, has become a subject of controversy. In the past, nonviable (nonliving) fetuses, aborted either spontaneously or intentionally in order to save the mother's life, were used routinely for a wide variety of scientific projects including those that led to the discovery of the polio vaccine. But when the U.S. Supreme Court legalized nontherapeutic abortion, questions arose about the use of the aborted fetus for research. Federal guidelines were devised under which such research could continue. They included the need for the consent of the mother and, where appropriate, the father; strict protection of the fetus in its mother's uterus; and the use of alternatives to fetal research where practicable.

The Rights of Mental Patients

Does a parent have the right to commit a "troublesome" teenager to a mental institution? Do children have the right to commit aging parents who have become "difficult"? Should a person be committed for behaving in a way that is different, or annoying, or eccentric—though he or she may be no threat to self or others? Does a person who is diagnosed as mentally ill have the right to refuse treatment? Once committed to an institution, do such individuals have a right to treatment, or can they just be "warehoused" indefinitely?

These questions are complicated by the fact that mental illness is often characterized by the inability to make rational judgments or perceive reality. Thus, a patient often does not recognize the need for treatment and may have to be forced to accept it (as occurs in 1 out of 3 hospital admissions for mental disorders). In addition, the diagnosis of mental illness (discussed in Chapter 3) is not always clear-cut, and occasionally this results in the involuntary commitment of a well person.

Presently only a few states protect the rights of mental patients by insisting upon treatment for all those hospitalized and assuring the right of appeal against involuntary commitment and regular follow-up review of their legal and medical status.

Nonvoluntary Sterilization

"Lucy," said Dr. Benton, "when I deliver your baby, you should have your tubes tied."

"What does that mean?" asked Lucy. Her six grades in Belson County Elementary, still all black, had given her an even poorer education than the average white Tennesseean.

"You don't need no more chillen, Lucy. Tying your tubes will fix that." Dr. Benton's word was usually unquestioned, but this time Lucy knew something wasn't right.

"Lucy, you want me to deliver this baby, don't you? . . . Unless I let you use my office to get your Medicaid, you ain't gonna have no doctor. And unless you let me tie your tubes, I ain't gonna deliver your baby."

"But, Dr. Benton. . . ."

"Look, Lucy, if you don't agree, I'll get a court bond order and I'll see to it that your welfare is cut off."

To Become a Donor

Studies have shown that most Americans are willing to donate organs for use after death. But few make advance arrangements to do so, thus leaving the difficult decision up to next of kin. Since all 50 states have passed the Uniform Anatomical Gift Act that makes a donor card legally binding, all a potential donor now has to do is to fill out such a card and carry it at all times. In most states a card is routinely received with driver's license renewals. Cards can also be obtained from the National Kidney Foundation, 116 East 27th Street, New York, NY 10016. On the card, it is possible to specify a donation of a specific organ (kidneys, heart, eyes), of the complete body, or of "any needed parts."

Should those who are poor, illiterate, mentally retarded, or mentally ill be sterilized so that they will not be able to reproduce, for the benefit of society and "for their own benefit"? Can such persons really give informed consent to sterilization? What standards should be used in deciding who is competent to raise children and who is not? Should persons with serious hereditary disorders be sterilized?

These are serious questions raised by documented reports of incidents such as the one above, in which individuals have been coerced into sterilization procedures without wanting or fully understanding them. A decision handed down by a federal judge in 1974 declared that the Department of Health, Education, and Welfare does not have statutory power to sterilize mentally incompetent individuals or minors and ordered sterilization guidelines to be redrawn, to require that individuals be clearly informed before a sterilization decision is made and to ensure that federal benefits not be withheld if surgery is refused. The judge ordered, too, that guidelines indicate clearly who has the right to approve sterilization of a mentally incompetent person. Many state laws, however, do not protect against involuntary sterilization, and the procedure has many supporters.

Transplantation

The art of transplantation of organs and other human parts is still in its infancy, but it has raised many questions, among them: If we decide to save a single life, which one? Should the hard-to-get organs, when available, go to the young, the famous, the brilliant, the rich, the powerful? Should selection be on the basis of how valuable a person is to society, on how much the person can benefit, or simply through a random lottery?

Transplantation from the dead The sticky question that arises is when does death occur, a question which is not as easy to answer as it seems. When a British surgeon opened the abdomen of what he believed to be the corpse of a 64-year-old man in order to remove a kidney for transplantation, the victim, whose brain had been injured beyond repair, coughed and twitched his feet. The surgeon closed the incision, and the "corpse" lived another 15 hours (see Chapter 13).

Physicians must walk a tightrope. If they remove the organ before the patient is legally dead, they commit a crime and possibly an unethical act. If they wait too long, the organ they need to save another life may "die," too.

Transplantation from live donors Is it right to ask one person to surrender a part of himself for another—an eye or kidney, for example? According to the courts, an adult with normal mental capacity may volunteer to donate such a part, and many do. But children, the mentally retarded, or otherwise incompetent adults cannot have such a decision made for them.

HEROES AND QUACKS

When William Withering began prescribing digitalis, a derivative of the foxglove plant, to heart patients in Birmingham, England, in 1775, he was labeled a quack. So was a Chicago doctor some 200 years later when he claimed a new cure for diabetes. When Ignaz Semmelweis declared in 1848 that physicians should wash their hands between an autopsy and a baby delivery, colleagues considered him a wild-eyed madman, and he was driven from his post at a Vienna hospital. Daniel David Palmer, too, was considered a fanatic when in 1895 he came up with *the* single answer for all illnesses: spinal manipulation.

Withering and Semmelweis went on to become medical heroes, with their discoveries among medicine's most important. The other two ended up in jail—the Chicago physician because the diabetes "cure" he promoted could be deadly, and Palmer, the creator of chiropractic, for practicing medicine without a license.

The differences between quack treatments and monumental new discoveries are not always immediately clear. Sometimes a truly well-intentioned physician, or even an entire medical community, can use a treatment that later proves as dangerous as a quack's. X-rays, for example, were used very freely until it was discovered that heavy use could cause cancer. Because medicine is such an inexact science, there is probably no way that such things can be entirely prevented. But exploitation by charlatans *can* be avoided.

Recognizing the Quack

How can you tell the difference between a responsible physician or therapist and a quack? The American Medical Association suggests several common characteristics in those engaged in deceiving and defrauding the public:

1 Quacks often use special "secret" formulas or machines they claim can cure disease.
2 They may promise or imply quick or easy cures or talk about "pepping up" your health.
3 They advertise, using "case histories" and testimonials from "patients."
4 They refuse to accept tried and proved methods of medical research and evidence. While inviting "medical investigation" and recognition, they avoid testing or stop short of providing the data needed for scientific evaluation.
5 They claim physicians are persecuting them or fear competition.
6 They claim their methods of treatment are superior to surgery, x-rays, or accepted drugs.

Of course, not every physician who takes a viewpoint different from the establishment or who tries something new is a quack. As you have seen throughout this book, there are many unknowns and uncertainties in medicine, and honest scientists may disagree. One physician may prescribe vitamin C for colds, another may scoff. But when a physician, or especially a nonphysician, exhibits many of the signs in the list above, there is cause for alarm. Suggestions for expensive shots, drugs, or courses of treatments should ring the alarm even louder.

Why People Turn to Quacks

Medicine does not have all the answers. But when the body is painfully crippled by arthritis or a child is doomed to die of cancer, it is difficult to accept that nothing can be done. Somewhere, somehow, "there must be someone. . . ."

And so, the desperate turn to charlatans. William Nolen, author and surgeon, suggests in his book *Healing* that people also turn to quacks because they may offer more comfort and compassion than busy physicians. And finally, people turn to quacks because they have heard, or believe they have seen with their own eyes, that they *do* help.

Quack Cures: Are They for Real?

A California physician hooked up nearly every patient who entered his office to a complex metal box that he called an "electric diagnostic machine." In almost every case, the lights and gauges "diagnosed" some dread disease—which, fortunately, the doctor could "cure." He administered "Koch" shots, supposed to contain a drug called Glyoxylide 12X, but later analyzed as distilled water. It was not until a patient came in who really had a serious illness—cancer—and the "treatment" did not work, that the physician was exposed and prosecuted.

Thus, one way for a quack to effect a cure is to diagnose a nonexistent disease. However, most apparent cures achieved by quacks deal with real illnesses. And often, in a sense, the cure too is real. The patient does get well, for reasons like these:

1 About 70 percent of human ailments are self-limiting; they cure themselves after a period of time. It is easy for the quack to appear to have cured them.

2 Many illnesses (ulcers, for example), are related to tension and anxiety. Reduction of tension often relieves symptoms. The relaxation can come through a therapist, an understanding physician, changes in the environment, and sometimes through a quack whose powers of suggestions are strong enough to help a "believer."

3 Similar to the functional illnesses are the hysterical ones: a woman is unable to walk after being trapped in a fire; a man, fearful of losing his job, suddenly finds the vision in his right eye is gone; a student, pushed into a premed career and petrified over having to take the MCATs (Medical College Aptitude Tests), suddenly finds he cannot lift his right arm. A large proportion of cures achieved by faith healers, using a combination of suggestion and hypnosis, may fall into this category.

4 In almost all chronic diseases, there are rare instances of remission and regression in which the patient inexplicably becomes well. In cancer, spontaneous regression has been estimated to occur anywhere from 1 in 10,000 to 1 in 100,000 cases. A faith healer who sees tens of thousands of people a year may very well be able to claim a few cases of cured cancer or other chronic illnesses.

Why Are Quacks So Dangerous?

If the quack is not administering a dangerous drug or using hazardous equipment (some do), then the major risk to the patient is the substitution of hocus-pocus for science. Most people turn away from legitimate medical care, their only real hope when they turn to quackery.

Often the temporary success of quack treatment leads to disaster. A quack's treatment relieves a woman's headaches for several months, just long enough to allow the tumor growing in her brain to spread to inoperable proportions. Or it relieves an arthritic's pain, while his disease, untreated, continues to worsen, and he becomes permanently crippled.

The other major danger of quack treatment is damage to the pocketbook. Quacks almost invariably charge large fees because they know that desperate people will pay any price.

Beauty Quackery

Appearance is so intimately linked to one's feelings about oneself that the pursuit of beauty is equated with the pursuit of happiness in many minds. People seeking beauty, like those seeking cure of disease, are often willing to go anywhere for help, even to practitioners with dubious credentials. The list of beauty frauds is long and includes diet mills (see page 124), some beauty spas that promise more than they can deliver, "inches-

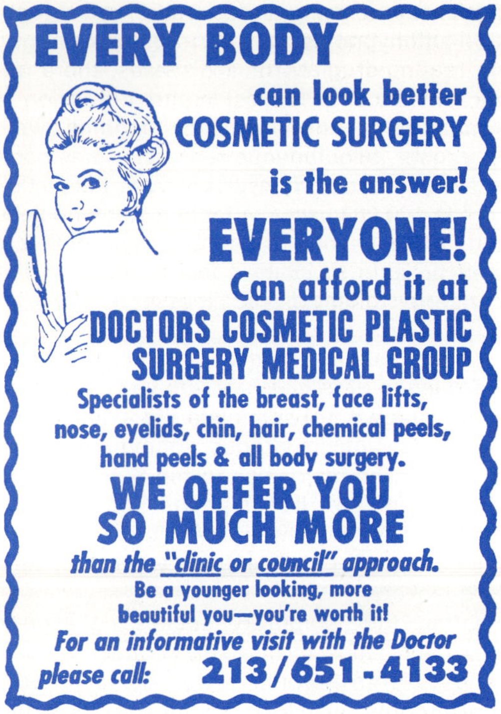
EVERY BODY
can look better
COSMETIC SURGERY
is the answer!
EVERYONE!
Can afford it at
DOCTORS COSMETIC PLASTIC
SURGERY MEDICAL GROUP
Specialists of the breast, face lifts,
nose, eyelids, chin, hair, chemical peels,
hand peels & all body surgery.
WE OFFER YOU
SO MUCH MORE
than the "clinic or council" approach.
Be a younger looking, more
beautiful you—you're worth it!
For an informative visit with the Doctor
please call: 213/651-4133

A major area of quackery and abuse is cosmetic surgery.

off'' devices, breast developers, and assorted cosmetics of doubtful value and not inconsiderable cost. A major area of abuse is cosmetic surgery.

Women anxious to increase breast size have been frequent victims. A recent example is that of women who traveled to Mexico for silicone injections (the material is also used in waxes, car polishes, and synthetic rubber) that promised them fuller breasts. These injections, banned in the United States in 1971 after several deaths, cases of blindness, and breast losses, are estimated to cause tragic results in 70 to 100 percent of women receiving them. Many women are at first pleased with their new shapes, but eventually silicone rot sets in. Once begun, it is difficult to halt without removal of the breast.

Safe breast enlargement is, however, possible with the use of silicone implants, sealed plastic bags of semisolid silicone gel implanted over chest muscles behind the natural breast tissue. The silicone never comes in direct contact with breast tissue. Many reputable surgeons will not attempt this increasingly popular augmentation mammoplasty on women who believe that larger breasts will save a shaky marriage or bring instant popularity. Breast augmentation is most effective for women who suffer from *micromastia* (*micro* = small + *mastia* = breast), or a lack of breast development, or for those with breasts of different sizes. Breast reduction surgery for women with inordinately large and heavy breasts can help the patient both psychologically and physically; heavy breasts are more than an embarrassment, as their weight can be painful and disfiguring.

To be certain that one does not fall victim to an unscrupulous or unqualified cosmetic surgeon, a person interested in such a procedure can contact the American Board of Plastic Surgery or the family physician for the name of a plastic surgeon skilled in the subspecialty of cosmetic surgery. Some types of plastic surgery (removal of moles or scar tissue, or dermabrasion for acne, for example) may also be handled by dermatologists. (For factors to consider in making a decision to undergo cosmetic surgery, see page 296.)

Unconventional Care

Most people at one time or another are faced with the question of whether or not to seek unorthodox forms of health care. In order to make an intelligent decision, they need to know something about such approaches.

Acupuncture Since far back into antiquity, the Chinese have used needles placed into carefully mapped points in the human body to treat disease. After President Nixon's first trip to China in 1972, acupuncture centers sprang up like bean sprouts all over the United States, promising, or at least implying, that acupuncture could cure almost anything from psoriasis to nerve deafness. Inevitably, some centers were staffed by unqualified personnel. Many charged large fees and encouraged repeated visits. Some patients endorsed them enthusiastically, but complaints of fraud and failure were filed by others, and several centers were closed or brought under state supervision, with physicians required to supervise the staff.

Is acupuncture, as some physicians termed it, "mere quackupuncture," or does it have some medical value? Apparently, the needle-twirling therapy does, indeed, relieve or reduce pain in some cases, and it can be used as an anesthetic in surgery, again in some patients and some procedures. There is some indication that acupuncture may be of value in treating drug abuse, depression, and obesity, but the case is far from proved. Reports that it can cure nerve deafness or multiple sclerosis have been explored but, so far, appear to be totally without foundation.

The mechanism by which acupuncture works is not understood. Some suggest it is merely hypnosis. But recent NIH studies point to a physiological mechanism, possibly involving the autonomic nervous system or direct stimulation of the brain. From present knowledge, it is likely that acupuncture may one day have a legitimate place in American

From present knowledge, it is likely that acupuncture may one day have a legitimate place in American health care, but it is equally clear that it is no panacea.

Charles Gatewood

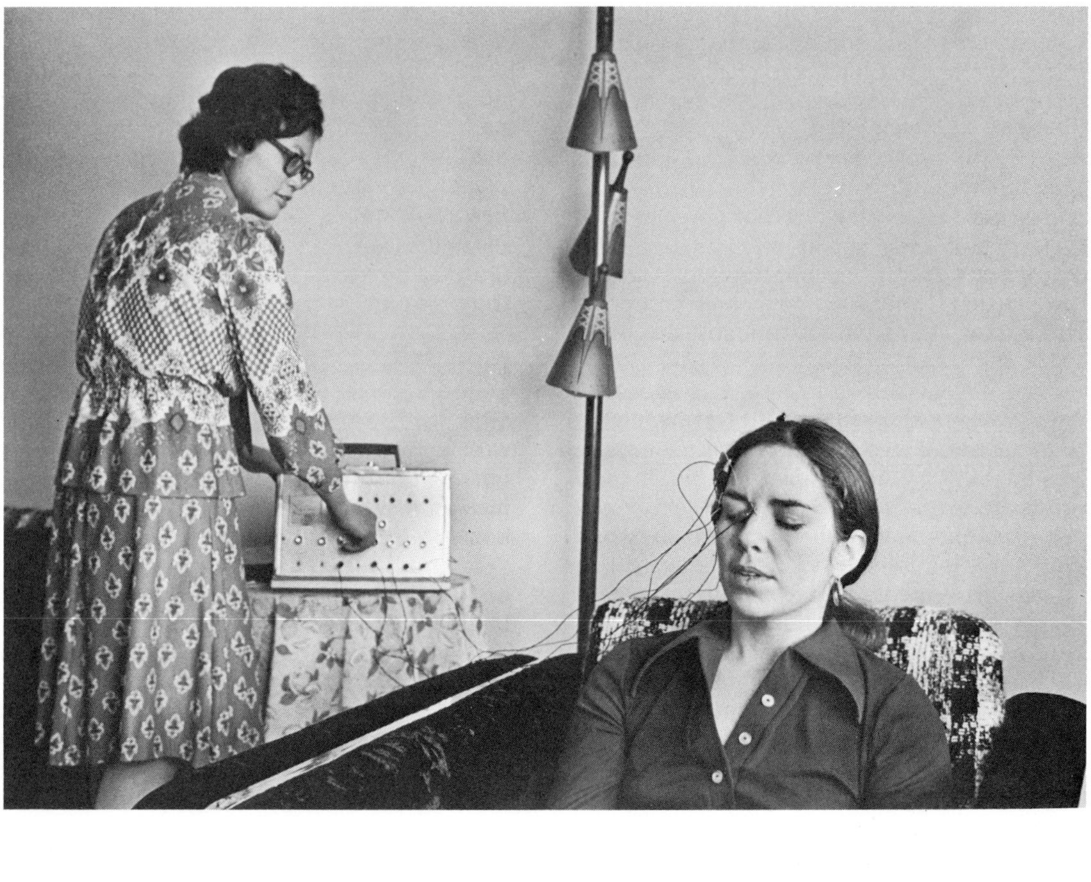

health care, but equally clear is that it is no panacea.

Hypnosis A useful tool in the hands of qualified medical personnel, hypnosis is, however, no miracle cure. Although most children are easily hypnotized, only about 1 in 4 adults is. Administered by a well-trained therapist (physician, psychologist, dentist) hypnosis may help a reasonably well-adjusted patient who understands its limitations. Hypnosis has successfully relieved pain, helped women go through childbirth without drugs, alleviated some nervous skin conditions, and reinforced the resolve of those anxious to give up smoking, drugs, and overeating. When poorly controlled, however, hypnosis can be dangerous.

Chiropractic Just before the turn of this century, a grocer-fishmonger in Iowa, Daniel David Palmer, who dabbled in such things as healing through personal magnetism (a crude form of hypnosis) theorized that all disease stems from dislocated spinal bones and can be cured by realignment of the spine. Today, the more than 20,000 chiropractors in active practice in the United States are divided into two chief groups: the "straights," who still believe that only spinal manipulation and massage should be used to treat disease and the "mixers," who also advocate the use of water, heat, light, and diet therapy.

The direction of the International Chiropractic Association is toward respectability. Once trained in months or not at all, chiropractors today study at four-year institutions that meet accrediting standards for federal funds. Pressure from vocal supporters (many of them appreciative patients, some in public office) has led to licensing programs in all 50 states, to payments toward chiropractic care by many insurance companies, by Medicare, and, in most states, by Medicaid and workmen's compensation. On paper, at least, the major chiropractic organizations now concede that there can be causes of disease other than dislocation (subluxation) of vertebrae.

Whether or not these changes will end the controversy that has been tied to chiropractic in the past, only time will tell. Extensive debates revolving around horror stories, as well as testimonials to chiropractic effectiveness, continue. Of course, neither viewpoint represents scientific evidence. Presently, there is no documented evidence either to support or to disprove the chiropractic hypothesis. Federally financed studies are under way to try to determine finally whether or not there is any scientific basis for the theory.

Meanwhile, the organized medical community continues to take a negative position on the subject, though some individual physicians refer an occasional patient to a chiropractor. A survey of 827 physicians found that some 53 percent of them believed that chiropractic had occasional value to patients. An additional 19 percent cited the placebo effect as valuable.

Millions of Americans seek the assistance of a chiropractor every year. Those who do should bear in mind: (1) the chiropractor is not a medical doctor, has no medical training, and cannot serve as a family physician or diagnose illness. (2) Frequent x-rays, customary with some chiropractors, can be hazardous. (3) Manipulation of the spine cannot cure disease, though it may relieve some skeletal problems. (4) Any persistent symptoms should be checked by a physician.

Faith healing The physician was gentle and compassionate as he examined the unhappy young woman. He listened to her pour out her tale of pain and woe. Quietly he reassured her, made a few positive suggestions about how she might handle her problems. The doctor was only doing what physicians sometimes refer to as "laying on hands." But the patient left feeling much better; the headache she had had for a week was gone.

Faith healing is not solely the province of the flamboyant tent preacher. Because of the power of mind over body, many pains and ills seem to melt away with not much more than the power of charismatic suggestion. But there are many things that cannot be cured by faith alone.[1] Faith could not cure the little boy with kidney disease who died when his life-saving medication was replaced with acupuncture, or the 11-year-old diabetic whose parents threw away his insulin, believing prayer and anointing would heal him, or the little girl who succumbed to diphtheria after her parents refused to allow vaccination and treatment.

Some faith healers are sincere in their efforts to help others; some are sincerely trying to get rich quick. Either type can do great harm if substituted for proper medical care.

Homeopathy Homeopathy (*homeo* = same + *pathy* = disease) is a form of medicine practiced exclusively by a handful of physicians and combined with traditional medicine by some 5000 others. It is based on the concept that "like cures like." Thus, a medication that can cause symptoms in a healthy person can cure the same symptoms in a sick person. Homeopaths believe that "disease is primarily a disturbance in the vital force, or guiding energy which governs and regulates all of the organs. . . ." Treatment, often stressing diet, is aimed at stimulating this vital force to heal itself.

Naturopathy Naturopathic medicine is the prevention and treatment of disease by such "natural" methods as corrective nutrition, body mechanics (manipulations, exercise, prosthetics), physiotherapy (ultrasound, light, water, heat, electricity), and remedial psychology. Its practitioners (an estimated 5000 in the United States, with the number apparently decreasing) are only rarely physicians. Although licensed to practice in a limited way in several states, none but the few who are physicians have hospital privileges.

[1]Some religious persons do believe that, when all else fails, faith may cure.

LOOKING BACK

REVIEWING CONCEPTS IN CHAPTER 25

- In effect, each nation chooses the level of health care it is willing to pay for. Health must compete with other necessities (education, housing, the courts), as well as luxuries (cosmetics, pet foods, color telephones), for financial resources.
- The health care system in the United States was not carefully preplanned and structured; it just grew as needs were defined. Government (federal, state, local), private enterprise, nonprofit voluntary agencies, and a professional medical community all play major roles in this sprawling establishment.
- The consumer has only recently become a factor in health care but can effectively work in partnership with the other sectors to improve it.
- Health care delivery is as loosely structured as the medical establishment. Care may be delivered by private physicians (practicing solo, with partners, or in groups), by physician-extenders (physicians' assistants, nurse-practitioners), by prepaid health maintenance organizations, by the federal government, in hospital outpatient facilities, in free clinics, in nursing and convalescent homes, at school health services, etc.
- Hospitals have changed greatly in recent years, and now deliver more outpatient

and other services than ever before. Patients are demanding consumer rights in hospitals.

- Many ways have been proposed to halt the rise of health care costs, but they keep going up. Medical payment methods include: fee-for-service by the patient or insurance company, prepayment, government funding, workmen's compensation.
- Many national health insurance plans have been proposed, but none has won universal approval.
- The quality of health care is not directly related to the amount of money spent on it. Many factors contribute to inadequate health care, and the many suggestions for improving it include continuing education for professionals, better review of care, promotion of self-care, patient education, and more attention to prevention.
- Malpractice suits against health professionals and hospitals have affected both the quality (possibly improving it) of care and its cost (raising it). The crisis might be eased by patients assuming more responsibility for their own care, by physicians better informing patients of risks, by better weeding out of "bad apples" by physicians themselves, and through some form of arbitration being substituted for adversary proceedings in court.
- Many ethical issues confront both the medical community and the individual today. They include the pros and cons of genetic engineering; the propriety of research on humans (especially those unable to give informed consent); the rights of mental patients; nonvoluntary sterilization of the poor, the retarded, or the incompetent; the timing of organ transplantation from live or deceased donors.
- Quackery preys on the desperate. There are useful guidelines for recognizing the quack.

26

CAN WE SURVIVE? THE ENVIRONMENTAL CHALLENGE

WHAT'S AHEAD IN CHAPTER 26 Why is it possible that health activation and better medical care may not be enough to keep the human race flourishing? How has human tampering with the ecological balance, in the form of progress, had an impact on health? How safe can we make the environment? What difficulties stand in the way of improving environmental safety? In what two basic ways can an individual consumer participate? How do the decisions we make every day affect the environment?

The rise of health activation in this country can go a long way toward improving levels of health and increasing potential lifespans via the many routes discussed in this book: changes in lifestyle (with respect to eating, exercise, smoking, drinking, other drug use), more and better medical care, and greater patient participation in preventing, detecting, and treating disease. But these measures may not be enough.

In 1974, a list of endangered species was published in the *New York Times*. It included the white-fronted wallaby, the straight-horned markhor, and the helmeted honey-eater, as well as the more familiar American alligator, the green turtle, and the chimpanzee. Of the more than 700 species listed, one—*Homo sapiens*, the human animal—was conspicuously missing, but many authorities agree that humans, too, face the threat of extinction. Even those, like microbiologist René Dubos, who believe that humans are capable of adaptation to any conditions, fear that the quality of life is threatened.

The menace to human existence at the root of this concern is "progress"—progress that has led to a disturbance of the ecological balance of the earth and contamination of our environment. Factory smokestacks, the burning of wastes by municipalities, and the burning of leaves by homeowners pollute the air. So do emissions of automobiles, trucks, buses, cigars, cigarettes, and pipes. Industrial and human wastes, oil spills, and agricultural pesticides foul our water. Colorings, thickenings, fresheners, and flavorings adulterate foodstuffs. Empty bottles, cans, and plastic containers add to solid waste disposal problems. Innumerable substances befoul our working places: asbestos fibers, vinyl chloride, chemicals, coal dust, and so on (see Chapter 7). Even modern medical treatment (use of radiation and antibiotics, for example) can upset ecological balance and add hazards to the environment.

In addition, nearly everything an individual in an industrialized society does—flushing a toilet, spraying deodorant, driving a car, walking a dog, smoking a cigarette, discarding food wrap, doing laundry, flicking a light switch—has impact on the environment. Without careful planning, good controls, cooperation of groups and individuals, business and industry, farmers and lawmakers, the impact will be all bad, and the end result will be, or rather, will continue to be, a serious menace to human health and the quality of life.

As pollution depletes breathable air, drinkable water, edible fish, and living space,

Homo sapiens—endangered species?

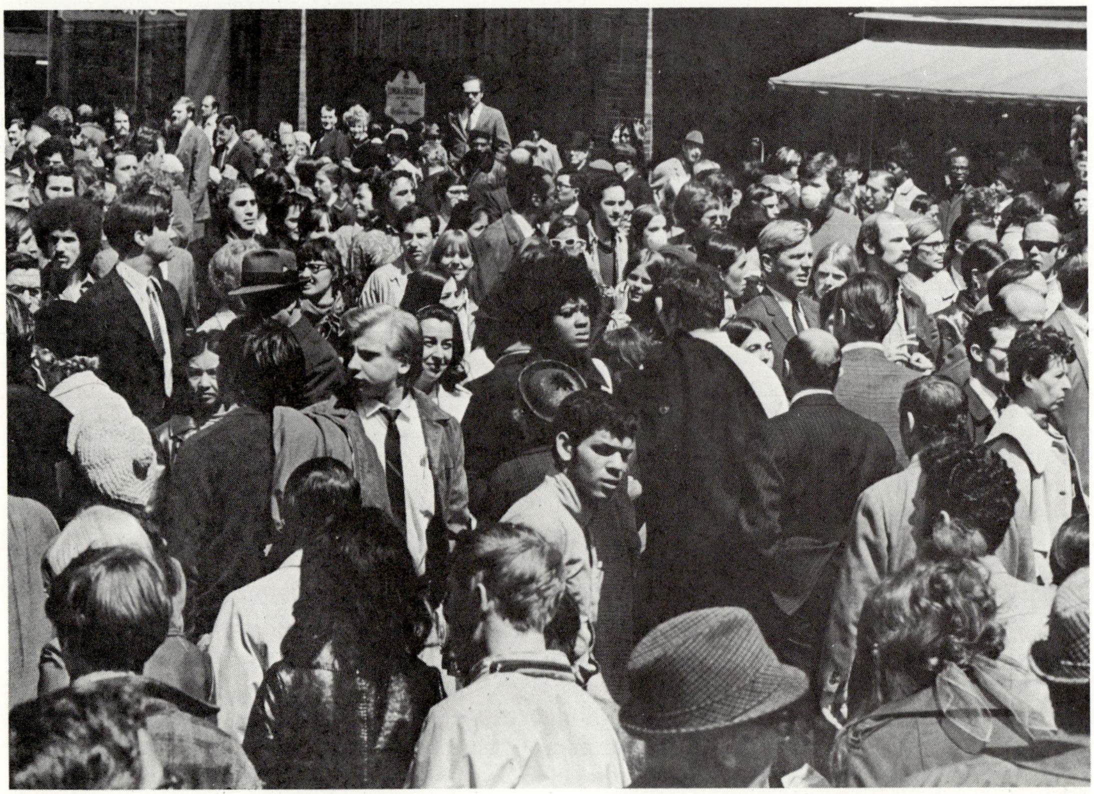

Fujihira/Monkmeyer

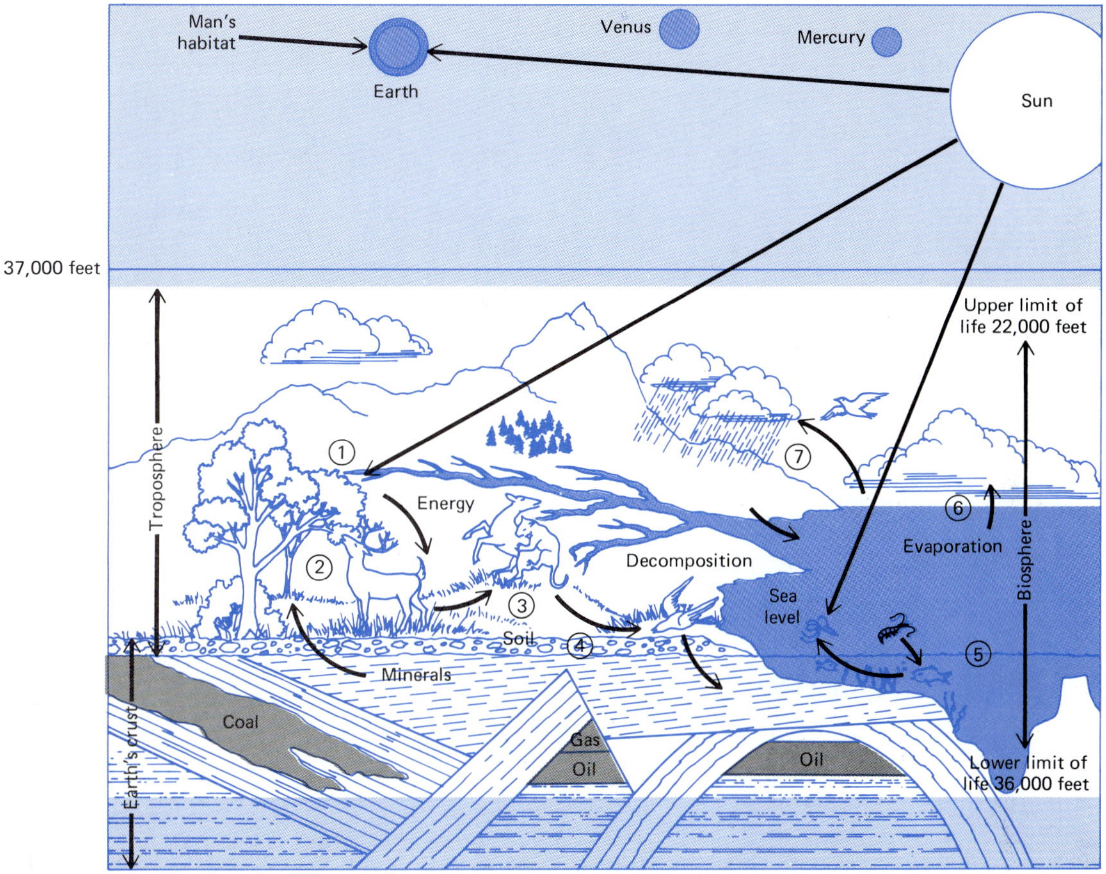

FIGURE 26.1 The interrelatedness of life on earth. *Energy cycle:* (1) plants bind solar energy into food; (2) herbivores eat plants sustained by soil nutrients; (3) carnivores feed on herbivores; and (4) carnivores are ultimately eaten by scavengers, the end result being decomposition and the return of nutrients to the soil. *Water cycle:* (5) bodies of water evaporate; (6) water returns to soil and ultimately to waterways via rains and snows.

This ingenious blueprint of our earth in its natural state provided for a prudent balance between consumption and disposal involving all living and nonliving things, as can be seen above. Then, millennia ago, a creature that lived not simply by instinct but by creative thought and crude logic, a creature able to utilize the interrelationships of living things to its own ends and needs, came along. The delicate balance of the ecosystem was upset. The creature guilty of perpetrating this ecocatastrophe was, of course, *Homo sapiens*. And the disaster that at first seemed to threaten only "nature" soon became recognized as a threat to its authors as well. [*Schematic drawing by Engle, p. 33.*]

TABLE 26.1 Humans threaten the environment

	SOURCES OF DANGER	POLLUTANTS PRODUCED	EFFECTS ON LIFE AND HEALTH
	AIR		
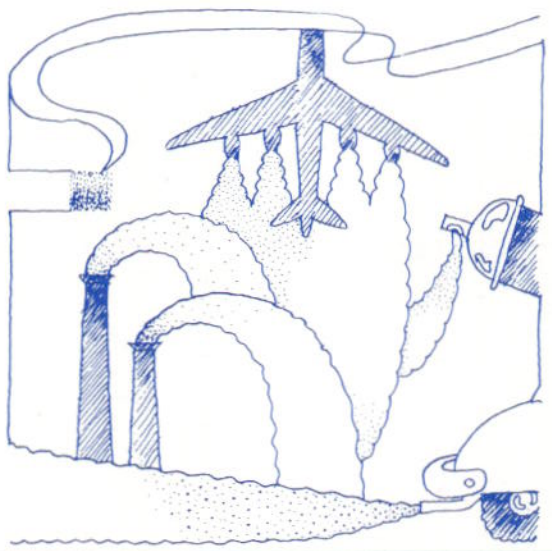	Automobile and other vehicle exhausts	Lead, unburned hydrocarbons, CO, nitrogen oxides	Lung disorders Increased heart disease
	Jet efflux	Kerosene, unburned fuel, soot	Neurological damage
	Steam boilers, diesels	Gaseous and particulate matter	Cancers
	Industrial plants, power plants	Chemicals, heat	Genetic damage
	Nuclear weapons, tests, accidents	Radiation, fire, fallout	Danger to fetus
	X-ray, other electronic gear	Radiation	Skin cancers and disorders
	Aerosol sprays	Fluorocarbons	Climate changes (from heat pollution and damage to ozone)
	Cigarettes, cigars, pipes	Tars, nicotine, CO, etc.	
	Pesticide sprays	Toxic residues	
	WATER		
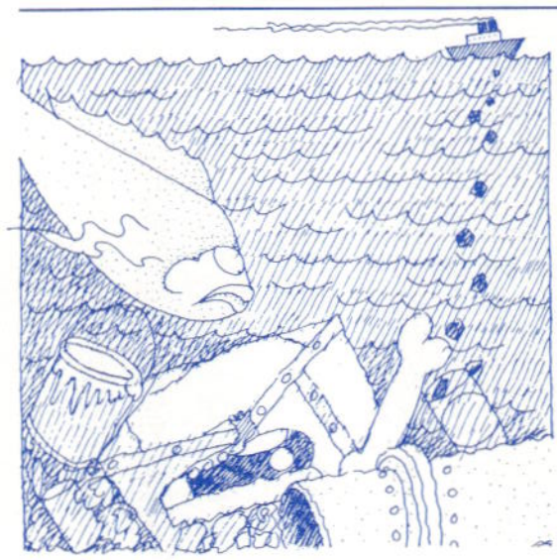	Nuclear plant wastes dumped	Heat, radioactivity	Great reduction in available food supply from oceans, rivers, etc.
	Industrial wastes dumped	Chemicals, heat, toxic metals	
	Treated and untreated sewage dumped	Germs, algae, oxygen reduction	
	Refinery and chemical plant wastes	Heat, liquid refuse, chemicals	Toxic chemicals in drinking water that might cause illness
	Fertilizers, pesticides	Chemicals seep into waters	
	Ships accidentally losing cargo	Oil spills, other refuse	
	Mineral exploration	Upset to ocean floor life	Toxic chemicals in fish, likewise
	Accumulation of refuse	Blockage of sunlight	
	Corroded pipes	Lead, other elements	Restriction of waterways for recreation
	LAND		
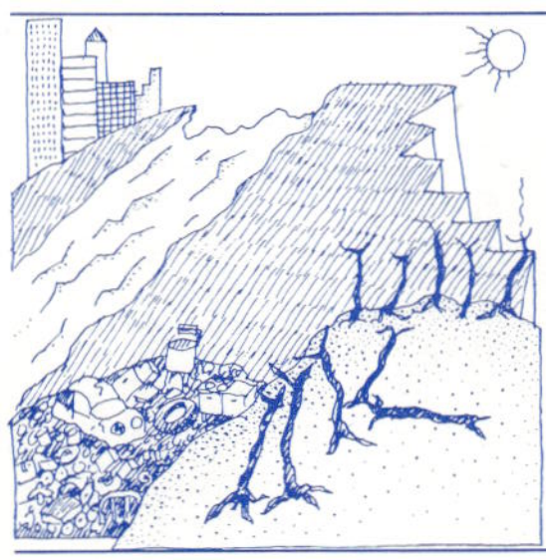	Coal stripping, quarrying	Contributions of various sorts to the breakdown of ecological balances and natural life cycles and food chains	Eventual shortage of needed natural resources
	Dumping of nonbiodegradable garbage		
	Destruction of timberland		
	Flood control, swamp drainage		
	Pesticides		Damage to crops
	Construction of cities, towns	Ugliness	Less esthetic atmosphere to live in

	Sources	Hazards	Possible effects
	NOISE		
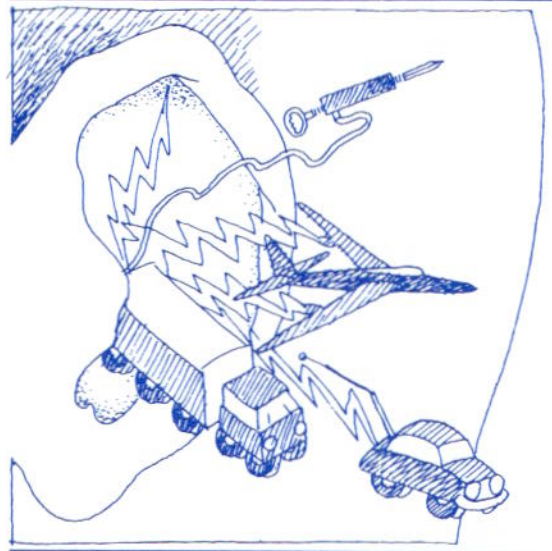	Jet airplanes Automobiles, trucks, other traffic Mechanical appliances Industrial noise Rock music CB radios	Continuous sound at 90 decibels or more Intermittent sound at 120 decibels Continuous din at lower decibels	Hearing disorders Frazzled nerves Poorer performance Poorer learning Headache Irritability
	WORKING PLACES*		
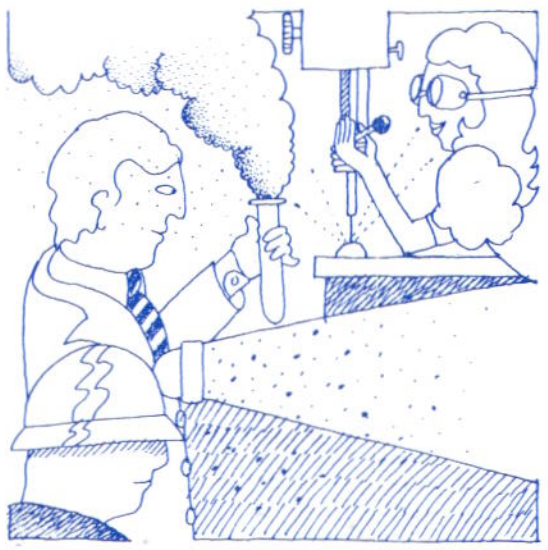	X-ray facilities Nuclear power plants Industrial plants Medical facilities Scientific laboratories Mines Farms	Radiation Chemicals, gases Coal dusts, etc.	Genetic, fetal damage Radiation sickness Cancers Neurological disorders Sterility Wide range of illnesses Lung disorders
	FOOD		
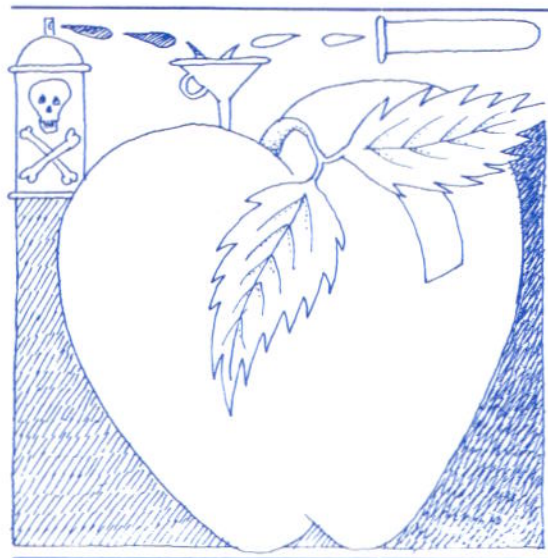	Pesticide, herbicide use Industrial wastes in water Chemical food additives Poor food storage, preparation Lead paints or other accidental toxic elements	Contamination of foodstuffs Contamination of fish, seafood Toxic chemicals in food Toxic organisms in food	Immediate illness Possible long-term damage such as cancer Slow poisoning Food poisoning

*See also Table 7.1.

Pollution: Nothing New

Pollution is the result of modern technology, right? Not entirely. In about 535 A.D., Aetios wrote: "Irritations of the eyes, which are caused by smoke, over-heating, dust, or similar injury, are easy to heal; the patient being advised first of all to avoid the irritating causes. . . ." And about 700 years later, when the population of England began to swell, a royal commission found "the air . . . infested and corrupted" in industrial areas. In 1307, pollution controls and penalties were enacted. The excessive population growth was cut back by famines and the Black Death in the fourteenth century, and air pollution was not considered a serious hazard again until the mid-seventeenth century.

world population continues to multiply dramatically. We are haunted by predictions of early nineteenth-century economist Thomas Malthus that unchecked population will increase faster than the necessities of subsistence with a resultant "war of extermination, sickly seasons, epidemics, pestilence and plague. . . . Should success still be incomplete: gigantic inevitable famine." This is the kind of leveling-out process that nature arranges when overpopulation of a particular species threatens the smooth operation of

Population Pollution

There have been many dire warnings about the population explosion, suggesting that if it is not dealt with reasonably, it will truly explode: explode in suffering, explode in violence, explode in humanity.*

But just what is a "reasonable"—and also effective—way of dealing with the population problem? The concept that birth control could be spread around the globe merely by distributing condoms or Pills has proven a failure. It did not take into account reasons for the high birth rate in underdeveloped nations that go beyond lack of birth control know-how: poverty and ill health. When parents know that they will have to produce about seven live offspring in order to assure two sons who will survive to care for them in their old age, limiting births is not appealing. It can only make sense to parents who can be relatively certain that all children born will reach maturity in good health.

India's new incentive program, in effect, combines pressures for sterilization (permanent birth control) with financial benefits or other "payoffs" that may help to raise living standards: a clean new house in the suburbs in return for a vasectomy, a better job or education for one's children in return for permanent birth control. The program, aimed at families with two or more children, has been criticized as being overly coercive. But the Indian government, after 20 years of being unable to stop the baby boom, obviously considers the situation critical.

The effects of the population explosion on health are most clearly seen in world food supplies, for such supplies do not increase as rapidly as population. But hunger and starvation are not the only results of overpopulation. It contributes, too, to overcrowded cities where physical and mental illness breed, to abuse and misuse of available land, to strains on health, education, and other resources, and in general, to a decline in the quality of life.

*Most recent census reports indicate a slowing of the population spiral.

United Nations/ILO

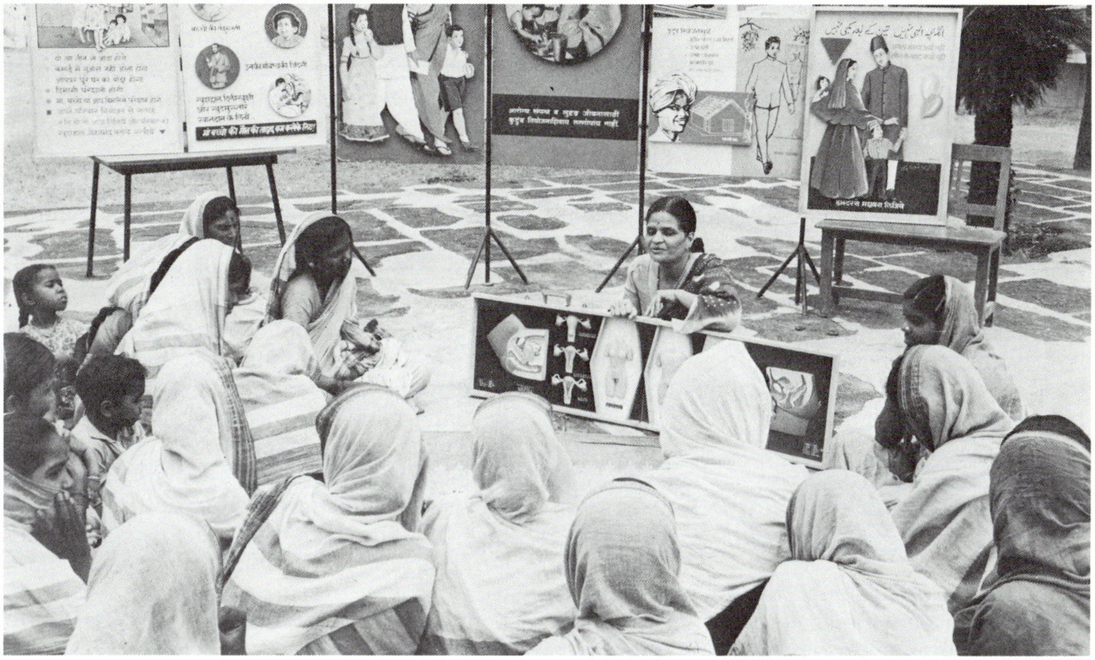

United Nations/ILO

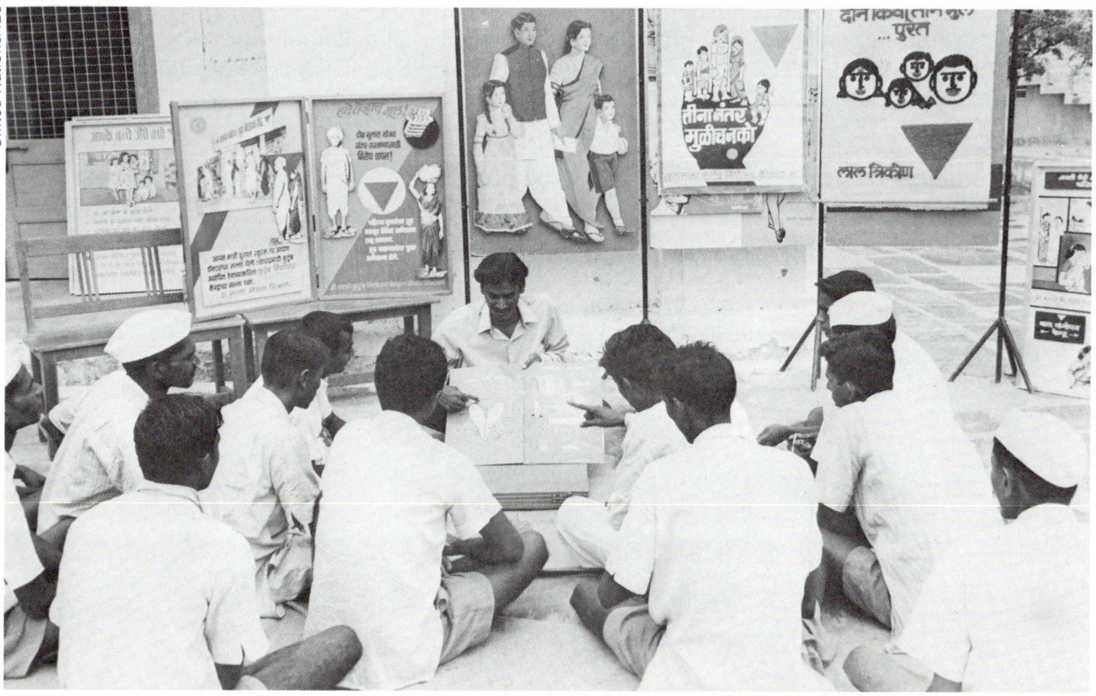

the ecosystem. One question remains unanswered: Can human beings, with all their ingenuity, beat the system?

Certainly society has been successful in other massive drives to improve health—vaccination programs, public sewer systems, water purification, and milk pasteurization among them. The challenge today is to continue to do so when many of the steps that must be taken to protect human health from environmental hazards will impinge not only on the economic system by raising production costs, but on our pleasures, our comforts, and even on things we have come to think of as necessities.

PERSPECTIVES ON ENVIRONMENTAL ISSUES

In the fairy tale, Sleeping Beauty's father tries to make his daughter safe from the witch's curse by putting a torch to every spinning wheel in his kingdom. He sets the Industrial Revolution back considerably, but still Beauty manages to find the only one left, pricks her finger, and begins a 100-year nap.

Today our chances of making our environment *totally* safe are about as good as the king's chances. Life without risk is impossible. In dealing with environmental questions, our goal is not total elimination of hazard, but reduction to the lowest level possible at which we can still enjoy the benefits of progress. This requires constantly and judiciously weighing risks against benefits and the application of personal and community values to decision making.

But are the benefits worth the cost? The costs may be economic (loss of jobs, increases in costs of goods) or social (reduced travel or entertainment), or may be in terms of personal convenience (fewer convenience products, fewer energy-consuming appliances and tools, returnable bottles) or comfort (keeping temperatures lower in winter, higher in summer). When do we reach a point where the costs are no longer worth the benefits? Delaware Governor Pierre S. du Pont has explained it this way:

> . . . There's no question that you reach a point of very small return for a very large investment. In other words, it may be reasonable to get the first

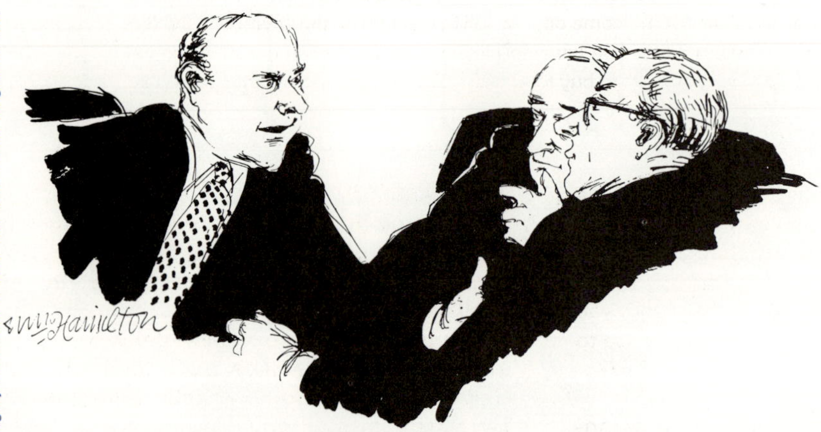

"I mean, you can have the cleanest air in the world but if you can't manufacture anything what the hell good is it?"

Opinions on the Environment

Man's health is intimately linked to his environment. Long-term, low-level exposures to many chemical, biological and physical environmental agents are known to adversely affect man's health. (David P. Rall, Director, National Institute of Environmental Health Sciences, p. 1061)

I'm beginning to wonder if so many things are harmful why we don't all stay in bed. But then we'd all get bed sores. (A cynical consumer in Brozan, p. 29)

Look at the values which galvanize energies and allocate resources in the business system: pursuit of money, enrichment of self, exploitation of man—and of nature—to generate still more money. Is it surprising that a system seeking to turn everything into gold ends up turning everything into garbage? (Editors of *Ramparts,* p. ix)

Control of the environment . . . is a very important but sensitive area because you begin to have to choose very often . . . what's most important—work, the economy, health. And if you want to start trading them off, you get into a very inappropriate discussion. Health outcomes, if you want to measure health status, depend upon being productively employed, being able to eat, having adequate shelter. No culture is pure. We have to have some form of compromise with our environment in order to work. The compromise doesn't have to be excessive but how to grasp that is an important public policy issue. (Theodore Cooper, former Assistant Secretary of Health)

The economic impact [of pollution controls] . . . will drastically change the competitive posture of many of the major basic industries. . . . It would be difficult to find a more effective method for bringing econom c growth to a halt. (Presidents of major corporations, in G. Smith, p. 1)

Top executives should be required to live within 200 yards of their plant gates and the water used in their homes should be piped in from downstream of plants that dump wastes in rivers. (Zamecnik, p. 28)

Everybody's for a clean environment, clean rivers, and clean air. And I'm for that. Strongly. . . . But when you walk over to that switch and your light doesn't come on, and when you turn on the thermostat and the heat doesn't come up . . . then is it important that we have absolutely pure water and pure air, when we don't have any jobs for our people . . . no money to buy food with? (South Carolina Governor James B. Edwards, p. 5)

> 95 percent of the pollutants out [in cleaning up a manufacturing plant's discharge], but the cost of getting that last 5 percent may be three times as much as the cost of getting the first 95 percent out. And I think when you get to that point, you have to stop and ask whether it makes sense to go further. (p. 5)

Finally, the long-term effects of environmental protection plans, as well as other projects that affect the environment, must be considered. Careful planning, thorough research, and the avoidance of hasty action are needed to keep us from jumping from the frying pan of one hazard into the fire of another. For example, when manganese was suggested as a cheap fuel additive and antiknock agent to replace toxic lead and cut down black carbon particle emission, a University of California researcher quickly pointed out that manganese could create "invisible pollution" leading eventually to "symptoms of nerve impairment similar to Parkinson's Disease" (Hughes).

It is important to keep in mind that progress is not *all* bad. In spite of the many perils of the machine age, humans who live in it are healthier and live longer on the average than any earlier people. And fear that progress will have negative effects is not new. Around the turn of the century, a congressional hearing was held on legislation to require a bathtub in every house. The perfume industry testified against it, declaring it would be put out of business. Change does upset the order of things. But when it is well planned, the disorder is temporary and, in fact, may benefit even those most worried about being injured.

THE INDIVIDUAL AND THE ENVIRONMENT

The battle against environmental problems is one in which the little guy or gal may feel powerless. So much seems to rest in the hands of government, industry, big business. In fact, however, as with other health-related issues, everyone can play an important role in improving the environment and thus prevent the health hazards resulting from its abuse.

True, isolated effort is often wasted. When China was faced with an epidemic of debilitating shistosomiasis, millions of people reportedly turned out to clean up rivers and ponds, ridding them of the small snails that harbor the disease-causing organisms. If just one family had made the effort, the epidemic certainly would not been have stemmed. However, one family's example might have given others the idea.

A massive effort by Americans to clean up the environment has yet to be made. Many do not perceive a threat. ("The problems are exaggerated.") Some would like to see changes made, but not at the expense of their own comfort, convenience, or effort. Still others are willing to give up certain conveniences but are unwilling to take any active steps themselves. ("*They* should stop manufacturing dangerous products.")

But many Americans are beginning to recognize that they can make a difference. ("If I stop buying dangerous products, maybe *they* will stop making them!") And indeed, they have been successful. When consumers began looking for substitutes for aerosol deodorants, many manufacturers began producing and promoting nonaerosols.

Environmental Decision Making

Probably the vast majority of Americans rarely think about environmental issues one way or another. Still they make scores of decisions daily that directly or indirectly affect the environment.

Power use The production of power to run our electrically oriented lives, whether by burning oil, gas, or coal or by nuclear energy, adds to environmental hazards and to the depletion of resources. Each unnecessary flick of a light switch adds to the problems of pollution. So does washing a half-load of dishes, drying "just a few little things" in the dryer, setting the heat at 72°F in winter and air conditioning at 70°F in the summer, leaving a TV set running when no one is watching, or using power equipment when hand tools will do the job.

Transportation use Slide into the car to get to the pizzeria a mile from campus, drive alone to the football game 10 miles away or downtown to shop? Or hike to the pizza shop, car-pool to the stadium, take the bus downtown? Those who opt for walking or bicycling get the added benefit of physical exercise, but everyone benefits from cleaner air every time a car key goes into a pocket or purse rather than into an ignition lock.

Waste disposal In Egypt, there are entire villages made up of refuse pickers: families that pay for the privilege of carting away the

United Press International

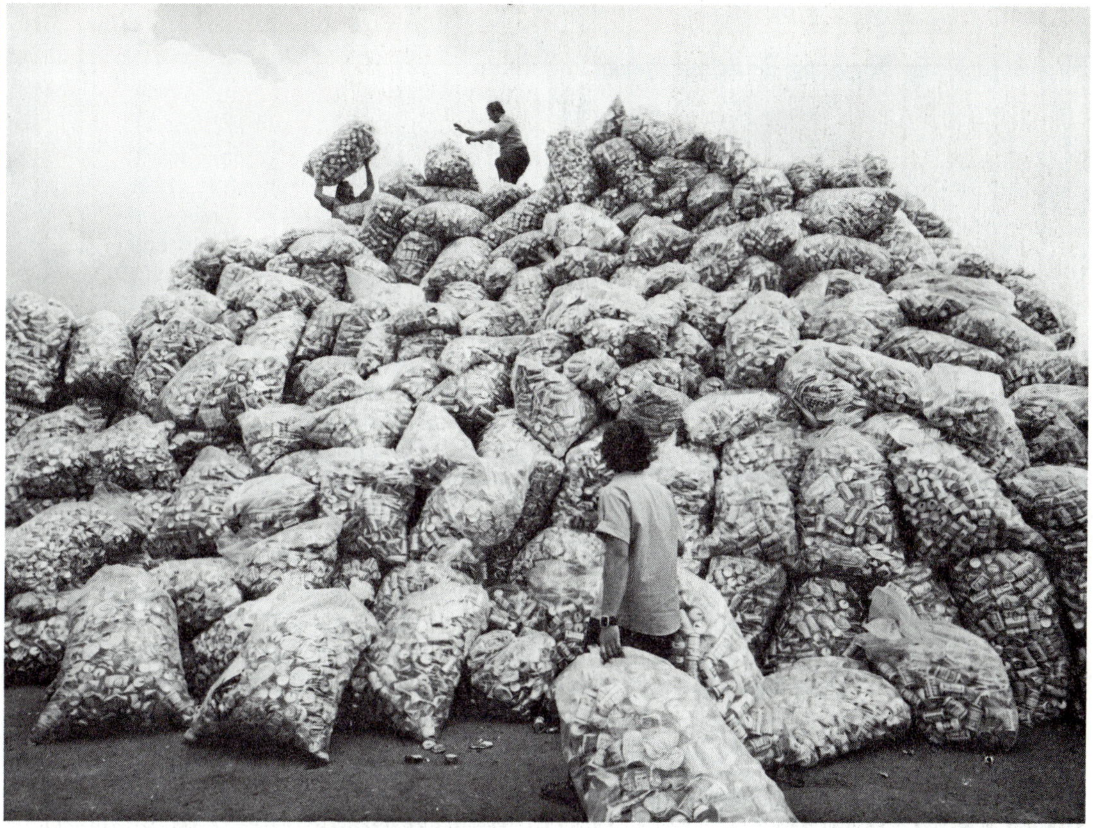

Decisions we make as individuals can help cut down the waste of resources.

garbage of city dwellers and earn their pittah bread by sorting out the recyclable glass, plastics, and metals dumped therein. Our more affluent society has not yet come to that, but some commercial firms and communities have done it profitably on a larger scale, and decisions we make as individuals can help cut down the waste of resources.

Among them: should we buy soda pop in aluminum cans and throwaway bottles or in refillables? If throwaways, should we save them for recycling? Should we rely on paper cups, plates, and napkins that devour precious trees, nonbiodegradable plastic disposables, or on china and linens that must be washed and in the process consume water and power and spew detergent residues? Paper towels or sponge to mop up spills? Bulk cheese or individually wrapped slices?

Clean air Pipes, cigars, and cigarettes are undoubtedly the chief culprits in indoor air pollution (see Chapter 17). Smokers' antipollution alternatives include quitting, cutting down, or only smoking outdoors. Nonsmokers must decide how much unpopularity they can take if they answer unexpectedly, "Yes, I *do* mind if you smoke!" and whether or not to ban smoking in rooms or homes, as so many have already successfully done. Other clean

HEALTH CONSUMER TIPS

Reducing Noise Pollution

Consumers concerned about the hazards of noise can reduce noise pollution in many ways. They can look for and purchase products with reduced noise levels: major and minor household appliances, lawn mowers, and power tools. They can replace metal trash cans with plastic, use carpeting instead of hard-surfaced flooring, install sound-absorbing surfaces such as cork and fabric in rooms that tend to be noisy. Dogs can be trained not to bark indiscriminately. Humans can learn to avoid shouting, to put things down gently rather than dropping them, to close doors instead of slamming them, to play radios, TV sets, and stereo systems at moderate levels. Earplugs or muffs can protect hearing when noisy machinery is operating.

Dishwashers, clothes washers, and other appliances can be run when family members are out or in another part of the house. It is also useful to install appliances with sound-absorbing cushioning, to keep them in good repair (they will be quieter), to be sure bolts and screws are always tightly fastened. Finally, concerned consumers can join in community efforts to reduce noise pollution.

air questions include: "Should I use aerosol cans, or alternatives?" Should I burn leaves and trash, or bag them, or use them to enrich the environment by recycling them in a compost heap?"

Resource conservation As the number of people moving into the industrial age spirals upward, so does use of natural resources. And, for many of these resources, "use" means "use up." Oil and other mineral deposits took billions of years to develop naturally. Little more than 200 years of industrial revolution has brought us to the point of worrying about their depletion. Timber resources, too, are being used more rapidly than we can replenish them. And though we see "water, water everywhere," supplies that are safe to drink are dwindling.

So we are presented with decisions: Should we switch to showers instead of baths? (Run a test and you find that short showers use less water than baths.) Do we ignore dripping faucets and long-running toilets? Should we let the water gush relentlessly while brushing our teeth or washing the dishes? Should we go to the bother of stacking and tying newspapers for recycling? Should we save the blank sides of scrap paper for reuse in rough drafts? Should we make an effort to buy books, cards, and napkins made from recycled paper?

LOOKING BACK

REVIEWING CONCEPTS IN CHAPTER 26

- An increase in health activation and better health care may not be enough to keep the human race flourishing.
- Many authorities believe that the species *homo sapiens* may be marked for extinction because of careless treatment of the environment. Others believe that human life will survive, but that its quality will be diminished.
- Tampering with the earth's ecological balance in the name of progress has been both harmful (polluting the air with chemicals and toxic gases, contaminating water, etc.) and beneficial (controlling disease-causing microorganisms, increasing agricultural productivity, etc.). Nearly every human act has some impact on the environment.
- It is impossible to make our environment totally safe. But we can use technology, know-how, and common sense to decrease risks and increase benefits.
- Two major barriers stand in the way of efforts toward improving environmental safety: economics and public apathy.
- Individuals can play a role in environmental control in two ways: (1) by trying to influence government and industry through voting and purchasing power, and (2) by making decisions in their daily lives that will reduce harm to the environment without wholly eliminating creature comforts.
- Decision making on environmental issues is complicated by the fact that even steps aimed at improving the environment can have a negative impact.

IN CONCLUSION

You have finished this book and, presumably, the course in health as well. We hope that you have come away with a lot more than facts and figures. We hope that you understand yourself, and what keeps you "alive and well," better. We are sure you understand now why we quoted Nobel prizewinner Alexis Carrel at the beginning of the book:

> Every man is a fluid that becomes a solid . . . a history in the making, a personality that is being created. And our progress or our disintegration depends on physical, chemical, and physiological factors, on viruses, and bacteria, on psychological influences and, finally, *on our own will.*

APPENDIX

HEALTH TABLES

Personal medical history

Name ______________________ Date of birth ______________________

Address ______________________ Telephone ______________

In case of emergency notify ______________________

Address ______________________ Telephone ______________

Physician ______________________ Address ______________________

Dentist ______________________ Address ______________________

Therapist ______________________ Address ______________________

Other treating health professionals ______________________

____

Place of work or school ______________________

Insurance coverage ______________________

Blood type ______________________ Rh factor: ______________________

Chronic illnesses: Diabetes __________ Asthma __________ Bronchitis __________

Epilepsy __________ TB __________ Heart disease __________

Other __________ __________ __________

Medications taken regularly ______________________ Dose ______________

______________ Dose __________ ______________ Dose __________

Allergies: Drug (penicillin, aspirin, etc.) ______________________

____

Food ______________________

Other ______________________

Eyeglass prescription ______________________

Physical examinations*

	DATE	RESULTS	DATE	RESULTS	DATE	RESULTS
Height						
Weight						
Blood pressure						
Pulse						
Temperature						
Vital lung capacity						
Exercise recovery index						
Eyes						
Hearing						
Other ____________						
____________						
Breasts (females)						
Testes (males)						
Hematocrit						
Cholesterol						
Sugar, blood						
Wassermann/VDRL						
Gonorrhea						
Pap smear (females)						
Other lab work						
Sugar, urine						
ECGs						
X-rays						
Dental:						
Teeth						
Gums						

*Complete with the help of a physician or other health professional.

Immunization history*

	DATE	DATE	DATE	DATE	DATE	DATE
ACTIVE IMMUNIZATIONS						
Whooping cough (pertussis)†						
Tetanus toxoid†						
Diphtheria toxoid†						
Poliomyelitis (specify type)						
Influenza						
Measles						
Smallpox						
Tuberculosis (Bcg)						
PASSIVE IMMUNIZATIONS						
Tetanus antitoxin‡						
Diphtheria antitoxin‡						

*Insert date of latest immunizations; add immunizations or boosters as received. See page 191 for recommended schedule.
†Generally given in combined dose as DPT.
‡These immunizations, which are prepared with horse serum, are given following exposure to the diseases and should not be confused with toxoids given routinely.

Illness history

DATE	COMPLAINT	DOCTOR	DIAGNOSIS	TREATMENT

Common home remedies

REMEDY	RECOMMENDED FOR	HOW-TO-DO-IT
Cold applications	Reducing local circulation	
Dry	Controlling bleeding under the skin in bruises and sprains and minor cuts*	Use an ice bag, several ice cubes in a plastic bag, or a solidly frozen juice or vegetable package; place over injury.
Cold soak (wet)	Ankle, feet, hand, and wrist injuries*	Place a tray or two of ice cubes in a basin (a styrofoam bucket or cooler is best); add cold water; immerse the injured part; repeat as needed.
Cold compresses	Reducing swellings or bruises*	Dip a soft cloth in a basin of ice cubes and cold water; wring and place over affected site; rechill when cold dissipates.
Ice, orally	Cut lips, inner cheeks, etc.*	Suck on a frozen juice cube, a popsicle, or an ice cube.
Constricting band	Poisonous insect or snake bites	Use rag, tie, sash, etc. and tie between wound and heart, 2 to 4 inches from wound. Do not tie too tightly. If pulse cannot be felt below band, loosen slightly.
Cooling baths	Reducing fever* (see also Sponge bath)	Place the patient in a tub of tepid water; after a few minutes, lower water temperature gradually by adding ice cubes (stop immediately if shivering begins). Cool showers may also be useful.
Gargle	Post-nasal drip, sore throat	Dissolve 1 teaspoon salt in 8 ounces hot water (not so hot it burns) and gargle for 5 minutes; repeat as needed or every 2 hours.
Heat applications	Increasing blood flow, dilating blood vessels, improving drainage	
Dry heat	Superficial muscle pain, tension, and bruises and sprains after the first 24 hours	Use heating pad directly over affected area.
Hot soaks (wet)	Relaxing muscles, easing pain, reducing tension, treating bruises and sprains after the first 24 hours*	Wet towel thoroughly in warm water; wring and place over affected site; cover the towel completely with two pieces of plastic bag; place a heating pad over the plastic at medium setting (be certain that it is not touching the wet towel); keep on for 1 hour, twice daily. (A plug-in radio nearby will crackle a warning static if the pad is getting wet.)
Warm soaks	Scratchy eyes, discharging eyes*	Use a cloth dipped in *warm* (not hot) water (test on inner forearm); apply to eye for 5 to 10 minutes every 3 hours.

*Your health care professional may recommend these remedies for other ailments as well.

REMEDY	RECOMMENDED FOR	HOW-TO-DO-IT
Hot and cold compresses, alternating	Sinusitis	Apply a hot soak to forehead and/or cheeks until heat dissipates (about 30 seconds); then apply cold compress until cold dissipates; continue alternating heat and cold for 10 minutes; 4 times daily.
Inhalation	Croup, cough, respiratory distress*	Use a standard humidifier or vaporizer or a steaming kettle; prepare a tent by draping a sheet over an open umbrella and a chair back; place the humidifier on the chair; the patient should spend 40 minutes 3 or 4 times daily under the tent and if possible sleep under it. (Be careful to avoid burns.)
	Emergency treatment of croup*	Turn the cold water faucet of the shower on full blast and let the room fill with humidity; stay with the child in the humid room until croupiness is relieved.
Meat tenderizer	Insect stings	Wash site with warm water and soap; sprinkle meat tenderizer on wet handkerchief or 4 × 4 gauze pad; apply to sting.
Sitz bath	Hemorrhoids, genital area cysts, other rectal pain, vaginal pain*	Sit in enough hot water (hotter than usual bath) to cover affected areas for 20 to 30 minutes 3 or 4 times a day or as directed by physician. A folded towel under each buttock may make the patient more comfortable.
Special drink (GI drink)†	Fluid replacement in diarrhea, vomiting, heat exhaustion, etc., of respiratory illness*	Combine 1 quart boiled water, 1 level teaspoon salt, 1 heaping teaspoon baking soda, and 4 rounded teaspoons sugar. Stir until clear. Add 1 package sugarless Kool-Aid or similar flavoring product. Store in refrigerator. Make fresh daily.
Sponge bath	Fever (when it is difficult to move the patient to bathtub)*	Place a plastic sheet under the patient and apply cold towels (soaked in 2 quarts water, 1 pint rubbing alcohol, and 1 quart ice cubes) to the naked body; avoid making the patient shiver.
Baking soda and ammonia	Relief of itching*	Make a paste of ½ cup baking soda with enough household ammonia to make a paste; apply to itching skin.

*Your health care professional may recommend these remedies for other ailments as well.
†From *Patient Care*, Apr. 15, 1974.

BIBLIOGRAPHY

Abelson, H., and R. B. Atkinson: *Public Experience with Psychoactive Substances*, Response Analysis Corp., Princeton, N.J., August 1975.

———, H. R. Cohen, and D. Schrager: *Marihuana: A Signal of Misunderstanding*, National Commission on Marihuana and Drug Abuse, Washington, D.C., Appendix to vol. II, 1972.

——— et al.: *Drug Use in America: Problem in Perspective*, National Commission on Marihuana and Drug Abuse, Washington, D.C., Appendix to vol. I, 1973.

Ackerman, Nathan: In N. Lobsenz, "Living Together," *Redbook*, June 1974, p. 87.

Adams, Junius: *Drink to Your Health*, Harper's Magazine Press, Harper & Row, New York, 1976.

Alberra, Robert: In "Sure I've Got Responsibilities—But One of Them Is *Me*," *Medical Economics*, Mar. 8, 1976, p. 96.

Allergy Foundation of America (*a*): *Allergic Diseases*, E-27410.

——— (*b*): *Allergy in Children*, C-47410.

American Academy of Periodontology: *Effective Hygiene.*

American Cancer Society (*a*): *The Dangers of Smoking, the Benefits of Quitting*, 1972.

——— (*b*): *Cancer Facts*, 1978.

American Dental Association (*a*): *They're Your Teeth . . . You Can Keep Them*, 1971.

——— (*b*): *Your Child's Teeth*, 1973.

——— (*c*): "Can Americans Get the Dental Care They Need?" *New York Times*, Oct. 5, 1975, (advertising supplement).

——— (*d*): Personal interview, June 1, 1978.

American Health Foundation: *It's Possible to Quit Smoking.*

American Heart Association (*a*): *Coronary Risk Handbook*, 1973.

———(*b*): *Heart Facts,* 1976.

American Medical Association (*a*): "Zen Macrobiotic Diets." Council on Foods and Nutrition, *Journal of the American Medical Association.* vol. 218, no. 3, Oct. 8, 1971, p. 397.

——— (*b*): "A Critique of Low-Carbohydrate Ketogenic Weight Reduction Regimens: A Review of Dr. Atkins' Diet Revolution," *Journal of the American Medical Association*, vol. 224, no. 10, June 4, 1973, pp. 1415–1419.

American Optometric Association: *Contact Lenses: White Paper*, January 1972, revised March 1974.

Ames, B. N., H. O. Kammen, and E. Yamasaki: "Hair Dyes Are Mutagenic: Identification of a Variety of Mutagenic Ingredients," *Proceedings of National Academy of Science*, vol. 72, no. 6, June 1975, pp. 2423–2427.

Anderson, Dave: "Danny Thompson," *New York Times*, June 13, 1976, p. V, 5.

Anderson, O. W., with J. J. Feldman: *Family Medical Costs and Voluntary Health Insurance: A Nationwide Survey*, McGraw-Hill, Blakiston Division, New York, 1956.

Andry, R. G.: *Parental and Maternal Roles and Delinquincy in Deprivation and Maternal Care: A Reassessment of Its Effects*, World Health Organization, Geneva, 1962.

Apgar, Virginia, and Joan Beck: *Is My Baby Alright?* Trident Press, New York, 1973.

Ardell, Don B.: *High Level Wellness: An Alternative to Doctors, Drugs, and Disease*, Rodale, Emmaus, Pa., 1977.

Arntzen, F. I.: "Some Psychological Aspects of Nictotinism," *American Journal of Psychology*, vol. 61, 1948, p. 425.

Aronow, W. S.: "Effect of Passive Smoking on the Cardiovascular and Respiratory Systems," Presented at Third World Conference on Smoking and Health, New York, June 3, 1975.

——— and J. Cassidy: "Effect of Smoking Marijuana and of a High-Nicotine Cigarette on Angina Pectoris," *Clinical Pharmacology and Therapeutics*, vol. 17, no. 5, May 1975, pp. 549–554.

Ash, P.: "The Reliability of Psychiatric Diagnosis," *Journal of Abnormal Psychology,* vol. 44, 1949, pp. 272–276.

Ashley, Richard: *Heroin, the Myths and Facts*, St. Martins, New York, 1972.

Auerbach, O., et. al.: "Relation of Smoking to Age and Emphysema," *New England Journal of Medicine*, vol. 286, Apr. 20, 1972, pp. 853–857.

Bach, George R., and Peter Wyden: *The Intimate Enemy*, William Morrow, New York, 1970.

Baker, Susan P.: "Injury Control," in P. Sartwell (ed.), *Preventive Medicine and Public Health*, Appleton-Century-Crofts, New York, 1972.

Baltes, Paul B.: "You're Never Too Old to Learn," *Story Ideas from Penn State*, September 1976.

Barber, Bernard: *Drugs and Society*, Russel Sage Foundation, New York, 1967.

Bardwick, Judith M.: *Psychology of Women*, Harper & Row, New York, 1971.

Basowitz, H., et al.: *Anxiety and Stress*, McGraw-Hill, New York, 1955.

Bates, Richard (*a*): "The Case for Conventional Sexual Morality," *Medical Economics*, June 10, 1968, p. 152.

——— (*b*): "Thumbs Down on the Methadone Thing," *Medical Economics*, June 7, 1971, p. 139–151.

Baudrey, Francis, and Alfred Weiner: "A Woman's Choice: Pregnancy or Abortion," *Mademoiselle*, April 1974, p. 34.

Bauman, Richard: "Why I Don't Wear Seat Belts," *Highway Patrolman*, October 1973, p. 16.

Beach, F. A., and L. Jordan: "Sexual Exhaustion and Recovery in the Male Rat," *Quarterly Journal of Experimental Psychology*, vol. 8, 1956, pp. 121–133.

Belloc, Nedra: "Relationship of Health Practices and Mortality," *Preventive Medicine*, vol. 2, 1973, pp. 67–81.

———and Lester Breslow: "Relationship of Physical Health Status and Health Practices," *Preventive Medicine*, vol. 3, 1972, pp. 409–421.

Belsky, Marvin S., and Leonard Gross: *How to Choose and Use Your Doctor*, Arbor House, New York, 1975.

Benendo, Franciszek: In "Of Coitus and Babies' Sex," *Medical World News*, vol. 12, no. 30. Aug. 13, 1971, p. 50H.

Benenson, Abram S.: *Control of Communicable Diseases in Man*, 11th ed., American Public Health Association, New York, 1970.

Benet, Sula: *How to Live to Be 100: The Life-style of the People of the Caucasus*, Dial, New York, 1976.

Benjamin, H.: "Tranvestism and Transexualism in the Male and Female," *Journal of Sex Research*, vol. 3, 1967, pp. 107–127.

Benson, Herbert: *Relaxation Response*, Morrow, New York, 1975.

Benson, Leonard: *Fatherhood, a Sociological Perspective*, Random House, New York, 1968.

Berendes, Heinz, Chief of Contraceptive Evaluation Branch: National Institute of Child Health and Human Development, personal interview, July 1974.

Bernstein, Gerald S.: "Conventional Methods of Contraception: Condom, Diaphragm, and Vaginal Foam," *Clinical Obstetrics and Gynecology*, vol. 17, no. 1, March 1974, pp. 21–33.

Besharov, Douglas: In "U. S. Finds Epidemic Child Abuse Rate," *New York Times*, Nov. 30, 1975, p. 44.

Bieber, Irving: In "The Issue is Subtle, the Debate Still On," *New York Times,* Dec. 23, 1973, IV, 5:1.

——— et al.: *Homosexuality: A Psychoanalytic Study of Male Homosexuals*, Basic Books, New York, 1962.

Bieber, Toby: in "Is Homosexuality Pathologic or a Normal Variant of Sexuality?" *Medical Aspects of Human Sexuality*, December 1973, p. 18.

Bieri, John G., Chief of Section on Nutritional Biochemistry: National Institute on Arthritis, Metabolic and Digestive Disorders, personal interview, July 1974.

Blackman, Ann: "Why They're Living Together on Campus," *Rockland Journal-News*, New York, (AP), May 6, 1974, p. 11A.

Blaine, Graham B. (*a*): "Why Intelligent Young People Take Drugs," lecture delivered at Annual Meeting of Iowa Medical Society, 1968 (reprinted by the New York State Narcotics Addiction Control Commission).

——— (*b*): In "Teenage Sex: Letting the Pendulum Swing," *Time*, Aug. 21, 1972, p. 38.

——— and Charles C. McArthur: *Emotional Problems of Students*, Appleton-Century-Crofts, New York, 1971.

Blanton, Smiley: *Love or Perish*, Simon & Schuster, New York, 1965.

Blinn, Johna: "Our Top Food Watcher Likes Simple Meals," *Rockland Journal-News*, New York, (Gannett), Sept. 11, 1974, p. 3C.

Block, Bartley C.: *Man, Microbes, and Matter*, McGraw-Hill, New York, 1975.

Block, Marvin A.: *Alcoholism, Its Facets and Phases*, John Day, New York, 1962.

Bloomquist, Edward R.: *Marijuana, The Second Trip*, Glencoe, Beverly Hills, Calif., 1971.

Blount, J.: CDC, personal interview, September 1978.

Blum, Richard H., and Associates: *Society and Drugs, Drugs I*, Jossey-Bass, San Francisco, 1970.

Blum, Sam: "Marijuana Clouds the Generation Gap," *New York Times Magazine*, Aug. 23, 1970, p. 28.

Bogen, Emil: In Haven Emerson (ed.), *Alcohol and Man,* Macmillan, 1932, pp. 126–152.

Bonadonna, G., E. Brusamolino, and P. Valagussa: "Combination Chemotherapy as an Adjuvant Treatment in Operable Breast Cancer," *New England Journal of Medicine*, vol. 294, no. 8, Feb. 19, 1976, pp. 405–410.

Bond, Julian: Letter, Southern Poverty Law Center, 1974.

Bonica, John J., Director: University of Washington Pain Clinic, personal interview, July 1974.

Borowitz, Eugene B.: *Choosing a Sex Ethic: A Jewish Inquiry*, Schocken, New York, 1969.

Bowen, William: "The Search for a Caries Vaccine," presented to Federal Focus on Health, Washington, D.C., July 11, 1974.

Branson, Roy: "Challenging Kübler-Ross," *Pediatric News*, October 1975, pp. 30–31.

Braun, P., and E. Druckman: "Vinyl Chloride: Can the Worker Be Protected?" *New England Journal of Medicine*, vol. 294, no. 12, Mar. 19, 1976, p. 653.

Brecher, Edward, and Editors of Consumer Reports: *Licit and Illicit Drugs*, Consumer Reports, Little Brown, Boston, 1972.

Breslow, Lester: In D. Ardell.

Briggs, George: In "High Price of Sugar May Lead Consumers to Better Nutrition," *UC Clip Sheet*, Dec. 17, 1974.

Briody, Bernard A.: *Microbiology and Infectious-Disease*, McGraw-Hill, New York, 1974.

Brody, Jane (*a*): "How a Mother Affects Her Unborn Baby," *Woman's Day*, July 1970, p. 12.

——— (*b*): "Chiropractic Long Ignored as 'Unscientific,' Now Is Increasingly Scrutinized by Health Specialists," *New York Times*, Oct. 1, 1975, p. 25:1.

——— (*c*): "Incompetent Surgery Is Found Not Isolated," *New York Times*, Jan. 27, 1976, p. 1.

——— (*d*): "Cancer Project Shows Home Care for Dying Child Helps Families," *New York Times*, Apr. 7, 1977, p. 20:3.

Brown, Bertram S.: In G. Luce (*a*).

Brown, D. G.: "Transvestism and Sex Role Inversion" in A. Ellis and A. Arbanel (eds.), *Encyclopedia of Sexual Behavior*, Hawthorn, New York, 1973, pp. 1012–1022.

Brown, Howard: Response to "Paul Jay Fink on Homosexuality," *Hospital Physician*, December 1974, p. 32.

Brown, J. W., et al.: "Turning Off: Cessation of Marijuana Use After College," *Social Problems*, vol. 21, no. 4, 1974, pp. 527–538.

Brozan, Nadine: "Aerosol Can Controversy: Effects Are Filtering Down to the Beauty Salon," *New York Times*, May 12, 1976, p. 29:1.

Buck, Pearl S.: Forward to *The Terrible Choice: The Abortion Dilemma*, an interpretive analysis of the International Conference on Abortion, Bantam, New York, 1968.

Buonocore, Michael G.: "Adhesives in the Prevention of Caries," *Journal of the American Dental Association*, Special Issue, vol. 87, October 1973, pp. 1000–1005.

Burgess, Ann, and Lynda Lytle Holstrom: *Victims of Crisis*, R. J. Brady, Bowee, Md., 1974.

Burgess, Ernest W., and Leonard Cottrell: *Predicting Success or Failure in Marriage*, Prentice-Hall, Englewood Cliffs, N. J., 1939.

Burkitt, Denis Parsons: "Fibre: Depleted Carbohydrates and Disease," *Community Health* (Bristol, England), vol. 6, no. 4, January–February 1975, pp. 190–194.

Burnet, Sir Frank MacFarlane (*a*): In *Harvard Medical Area Newsletter and Focus*, vol. 2, no. 10, Nov. 20, 1975, p. 1.

———(*b*) In Immunological Parallel Seen in Cancer and Rheumatoid Disease," *Medical Tribune*, Jan. 7, 1976, p. 9.

Burton, Benjamin T.: *Human Nutrition*, 3d ed., McGraw-Hill (Heinz), New York, 1976.

Busse, Ewald W., and Eric Pfeiffer (eds.): *Behavior and Adaptation in Late Life*, Little Brown,Boston, 1969.

Butler, N. R.: "A National Long-term Study of Perinatal Hazards," presented at Sixth World Congress of Gynecology and Obstetrics, New York, Apr. 12–18, 1970.

———, H. Goldstein, and E. M. Ross: Cigarette Smoking in Pregnancy: Its Influence on Birth Weight and Perinatal Mortality," *British Medical Journal*, vol. 2, Apr. 15, 1972, pp. 127–130.

Butler, Robert N.: *Why Survive? Being Old in America*, Harper & Row, New York, 1975.

Cairns, John: "The Cancer Problem," *Scientific American*, November 1975, pp. 64–78.

Calderone, Mary (*a*): In R. Collins, "College Sex Is a Cop Out," unpublished, pp. 3, 4.

——— (*b*): In N. Brozan, "For Decades a Voice of Reason on Sex," *New York Times*, June 28, 1974, p. 39.

Calloway, Nathaniel O.: In "Nutrition's Importance May Hit Peak in Perinatal Period," *Pediatric News*, May 1974, p. 22.

Campbell, Angus, Philip E. Converse, and Willard L. Rodgers: *The Quality of American Life*, Russel Sage Foundation, New York, 1976

Cancer Care, Inc., and the National Cancer Foundation, Inc. (*a*): "The Impact, Costs, and Consequences of Catastrophic Illness on Patients and Families," in *Annual Report*, 1972–1973.

——— and ——— (*b*): "Sharing Care During Crisis at Home," in *Annual Report*, 1972–1973.

Carlos, James P., and Herschel S. Horowitz: National Caries Program, National Institute of Dental Research, personal interview, July, 1974.

Carnegie Commission on Higher Education: *New Students and New Places: Policies for the Future Development of American Higher Education*, McGraw-Hill, New York, 1971.

Carpenter, Philip L.: *Microbiology*, W. B. Saunders, McGraw-Hill, New York, 1963.

Castelli, W. P., et al.: "HDL cholesterol and Other Lipids in Coronary Heart Disease: The Cooperative Lipoprotein Phenotyping Study," *Circulation*, vol. 55, no. 5, May 1977, pp. 767–772.

Cates, W., Jr., and R. W. Rochat: "Illegal Abortions in the United States 1972–74," *Family Planning Perspectives*, vol. 8, no. 2, March–April 1976, pp. 86–92.

Central Conference of American Rabbis: In Guttmacher, p. 127.

Chafetz, Morris (*a*): "Problems of Reaching Youth," presented at the session on Alcohol and the Adolescent, at the 44th Annual American School Health Association, San Francisco, Jan. 13, 1972.

——— (*b*): Statement before Subcommittee on Special Studies of House Committee on Government Operations, July 10, 1972.

Chapple, P. A. L.: "Cannabis: A Toxic and Dangerous Substance: A Study of Eighty Takers," *British Journal of Addiction*, August 1966, p. 271.

Charren, Peggy, and Evelyn Sarson: In testimony before U.S. Senate Select Committee on Nutrition and Human Needs, March 1973.

Cheek, F. E., et al.: "Four Patterns of Campus Marijuana Use: Part I, Drug Use," *International Journal of the Addictions*, vol. 8, 1973, pp. 13–31.

Chein, Isador: In Oliver Gillie, p. 76.

Chickering, Arthur W.: *Education and Identity*, Jossey-Bass, San Francisco, 1971.

Christiensen, Harold T.: In Vance Packard.

Claridge, Gordon: *Drugs and Human Behavior*, Praeger, New York, 1970.

Clarke, Kenneth S. (*a*): *Drug Testing in Sports—An Editorial*, unpublished.

——— (*b*): Personal communications, 1974–1977.

Clatworthy, Nancy Moore: "Living Together," in N. G. Malbin (ed.), *Old Family/New Family*, Van Nostrand, New York, 1975.

Cohen, Aharon: In Jean Mayer (e), p. 166.

Cohen, Allan Y.: *Alternatives to Drug Abuse: Steps Toward Prevention*, National Institute on Drug Abuse, publ. no. 14, 1973.

Cohen, Benjamin E.: In "Vitamin A May Enhance Immune Responses," *Medical World News*, Dec. 14, 1973, p. 21.

Coleman, James: *Psychology and Effective Behavior*, Scott Foresman, Chicago, 1969.

Comfort, Alex (*a*): *A Good Age*, Crown, New York, 1976.

——— (*b*): Personal interview, October 1977.

Constantine, Larry, and Joan Constantine: *Group Marriage*, Macmillan, New York, 1973.

Consumer Product Safety Commission: Annual Report, Fiscal Year 1976.

Consumers Reports (*a*): *The Medicine Show*, Pantheon, New York, 1974.

——— (*b*): "Too Much Sugar?," March 1978, p. 136.

Consumer's Guide to Dentistry, Connecticut Citizen Action Group in Concert with Connecticut State Dental Association, 1974

Cook, Joan: "Child Abusers Seek Help," *New York Times*, Oct. 27, 1974, p. 84:4.

Cooper, David: *The Death of the Family*, Pantheon, New York, 1971.

Cooper, Kenneth H.: *The New Aerobics*, M. Evans, Philadelphia, 1970.

Cooper, M. H., and A. J. Culyer (eds.): *Health Economics*, Penguin, Harmondsworth, Middlesex, England, 1973.

Cooper, Theodore: Personal interview, October 1978.

Coopersmith, Stanley: *Antecedents of Self-Esteem*, W. H. Freeman, San Francisco, 1967.

Corfman, Philip: "The Medical Effects of Vasectomy and Contraceptive Device Development," Center for Population Research Science Writers' Seminar, Bethesda, Md., Sept. 18, 1973.

Crile, George, Jr.: "Kicking the Fee-for-Service Habit," *Hospital Physician*, October 1975, p. 34.

Croce, Philip: "Bargaining: A System of Marital Counseling for the Family Practitioner," *Journal of the Maine Medical Association*, vol. 64, October 1973, pp. 224–225.

Cumming, Elaine: "Further Thoughts on the Theory of Disengagement," *International Social Science Journal*, vol. 15, 1963, pp. 377–393.

Curley, Suzanne: "Dining with 5 Nutritionists—Separate Checks, Please!" *Parade*, Oct. 7, 1973, p. 26.

Curtin, Sharon: "Grandparents," *New York Times Magazine*, Dec. 2, 1973, p. 12.

Dalton, Katherina (*a*): *The Premenstrual Syndrome*, Charles C Thomas, Springfield, Ill., 1964.

——— (*b*): "Menstruation and Examinations," *Lancet*, vol. 2, 1968, p. 164.

Dement, William C.: *Some Must Watch, While Some Must Sleep*, W. F. Freeman, San Francisco, 1972.

Dempsey, David: "Noise," *New York Times Magazine*, Nov. 23, 1975, p. 31.

Denenberg, Herbert S. (*a*): *A Shopper's Guide to Health Insurance*, Pennsylvania Insurance Department, Harrisburg, Pa., 1973.

——— (*b*): *A Shopper's Guide to Surgery*, Pennsylvania Insurance Department, Harrisburg, Pa.

Despert, J. Louise: *Children of Divorce*, Doubleday, Garden City, N.Y., 1962.

Dickason, Elizabeth J., and Martha Olsen Schult: *Maternal and Infant Care*, McGraw-Hill, Blakiston Division, New York, 1975.

Diehl, Harold: *Tobacco and Your Health*, McGraw-Hill, New York, 1969.

Dilley, James W.: "Smoking on Campus," *Journal of the American College Health Association*, vol. 19, no. 4, April 1971, pp. 230–234.

Divoky, Diane (ed.): *How Old Will You Be in 1984?* Avon Books, New York, 1969.

Dobson, Rodney H.: "Seat Belt Users: An Analysis of Who They Are and Why," presented at the midyear meeting of the Society of Automotive Engineers, Detroit, May 18–22, 1970.

Doutt, Richard L., Professor Emeritus, UCLA: Personal interview, October 1978.

Downey, Gregg W.: "Crip Lib: The Disabled Fight for Their Own Cause," *Modern Health Care*, February 1975, p. 21.

Dretchen, Kenneth: "Over-the-Counter Medicine and You," Georgetown University, interview notes, May 1975.

Driver, Caroline: "What a Dying Man Taught Doctors About Caring," *Medical Economics*, Jan. 22, 1973, p. 81.

Drug Enforcement Administration of U.S. Department of Justice and National Institute on Drug Abuse of U.S. Department of Health, Education, and Welfare: Unpublished data from Project DAWN V (drug abuse warning network), May 1976–April 1977.

Drug Topics: "Drug Store Sales in 1977," June 20, 1978, p. 36.

Drugs of Abuse: Drug Enforcement Administration, U. S. Department of Justice, JUS-437.

Duberman, Lucile: *Marriage and Its Alternatives*, Praeger, New York, 1974.

Dubos, René Jules: *Man Adapting*, Yale, New Haven, Conn., 1965.

DuPont, Robert L. (*a*): *Drug Abuse Prevention Report*, vol. 1, no. 5, 1974.

——— (*b*): In *Marijuana and Health: In Perspective*, National Institute of Drug Abuse, 1975.

DuPont, Pierre S.: In I. S. Carey, "The States and the Environment," *Context*, no. 2, 1977, p. 5.

Duvall, Evelyn Ruth Millis: *Faith in Families*, Rand McNally, New York, 1970.

Dyer, Robert: in R. Jones, "Comment," *New Scientist*, vol. 68, Dec. 11, 1975, p. 618.

Edelman, Gerald: In Edson, p. 11.

Edelson, Ed: "The Dark Side of Wonder Drugs," *Family Health*, October 1974, p. 22.

Editors of *Ramparts*: *Eco-Catastrophe*, Harper & Row, New York, 1970.

Edson, Lee: "A Secret Weapon," *New York Times Magazine*, Feb. 17, 1974, p. 10.

Edwards, James B.: In I. S. Carey, "The States and the Environment," *Context*, no. 2, 1977, p. 5.

Eiger, M. S., and S. W. Olds: *The Complete Book of Breast Feeding*, Bantam, New York, 1973.

Eisenberg, Arlene, and Howard Eisenberg: "Asleep at the Wheel," *Family Safety*, Fall 1973, p. 4.

——— and ———: "The Heart Fitness Test that Could Save Your Life," *Parade*, May 12, 1974, p. 4.

——— and ———: "Acupuncture Probe: What Works, What Doesn't," *Parade*, Oct. 20, 1974, p. 22.

——— and ———: "All about Pacemakers," *Parade*, Sept. 28, 1975, p. 18.

——— and ———: "Around the World in a Wheelchair," *Parade*, Aug. 29, 1976, p. 10.

Eisenberg, Howard: "Challenging Fee for Service: The Free-Clinic Movement," *Medical Economics*, Oct. 9, 1972, p. 24.

Elisa, Louis A.: In U. S. DHEW (*g*).

Ellis, Albert: *The Search for Sexual Enjoyment*, McFadden-Bartell, New York, 1966.

Ellwood, Paul M.: "$1.6 Trillion a Year for Health Care?" *Medical Economics*, June 12, 1978, p. 17.

Elson, Lawrence M.: *It's Your Body*, Mc-Graw Hill, New York, 1975.

Engle, Robin: Schematic drawing, *New York Times*, Apr. 20, 1970, p. 33.

Epstein, Franklin H., M.D.: "No, It's Our Duty to

Keep Patients Alive," *Medical Economics*, Apr. 2, 1973, p. 97.

Epstein, Joseph: In Enid Nemy, "For the Divorced Man, Too, It's a Wrenching Experience," *New York Times*, Aug. 12, 1974, p. 29.

Erikson, Erik Bomburger (*a*): *Young Man Luther, A Study in Psychoanalysis and History*, Norton, New York, 1958.

——— (*b*): *Identity, Youth and Crisis*, Norton, New York, 1968.

Faigel, Harris: "Rehabilitation and the Self-destructive Adolescent," presented before the Ambulatory Pediatric Association, Washington, D.C., Apr. 29, 1974.

Farnsworth, Dana L. (*a*): "The Drug Problem Among Young People," *Oklahoma State Medical Association Journal*, September 1968, p. 461.

——— (*b*): "Drugs—Do They Produce Open or Closed Minds?" *Medical Insight*, vol. 2, July 1970, pp. 33–44, August 1970, pp. 22–31, reprinted in *Resource Book for Drug Abuse Information*, National Clearing House for Drug Abuse Information, Rockville, Md., pp. 3–8.

——— (*c*): "Young Adult: An Overview," *American Journal of Psychiatry*, vol. 131.8, August 1974, pp. 845–851.

——— (*d*): "Adverse Drug Reaction in the United States," *Medical Tribune*, Feb. 26, 1975, p. 5.

Farquhar, J. W., et al.: "Community Education for Cardiovascular Health," *Lancet*, vol. I (8023), June 4, 1977, pp. 1192–1195.

Federal Register: "Protection of Human Subjects," Aug. 8, 1975, pp. 33526–33552.

Feldman, David M.: *Marital Relations, Birth Control, and Abortion in Jewish Law*, Schocken Books, New York, 1975.

Ferguson, Alexander C.: "Report on Depressed Cellular Immunity and Malnutrition," presented to the Canadian Pediatric Society, St. John's, Newfoundland, September 1974.

Fink, Paul Jay: "Paul J. Fink on Homosexuality," *Hospital Physician*, December 1974, p. 22.

Fisher, Seymour: *The Female Orgasm: Psychology, Physiology, Fantasy*, Basic Books, New York, 1973.

Flamant, R., et al.: "Differences in Sex Ratio According to Cancer Site and Possible Relationship with Use of Tobacco and Alcohol; Review of 65,000 Cases," *Journal of the National Cancer Institute*, vol. 32, 1964, pp. 1309–1316.

Fleischer, Nathan: Personal interview, 1958.

Fletcher, C. M., and D. Horn: "Smoking and Health," *Who* (World Health Organization) *Chronicle*, vol. 24, no. 8, Aug. 19, 1970, pp. 345–370.

Ford, C. S., and F. A. Beach: *Patterns of Sexual Behavior*, Harper & Row, New York, 1951.

Fort, Joel: *The Pleasure Seekers*, Bobbs-Merrill, Indianapolis, 1969.

Fraiberg, Selma: *Every Child's Birthright: In Defense of Mothering*, Basic Books, New York, 1977.

Frazier, Claude A.: *Coping with Food Allergy*, Quandrangle, New York Times Book Co., New York, 1975.

Frederick, Calvin J. (*a*): "The School Guidance Counselor as a Preventive Agent to Self-destructive Behavior," *Journal of Personnnel and Guidance*, New York State Branch APGA, vol. 5, no. 1, June 1970, pp. 1–10.

——— (*b*): "The Present Suicide Taboo in the U.S." *Mental Hygiene*, vol. 55, no. 2, April 1971, pp. 178–183.

——— (*c*): Assistant Chief, Center for Suicide Prevention, NIMH, Personal interview, July 1974.

——— and Louise Lague: "Dealing with the Crisis of Suicide," Public Affairs Pamphlet No. 406A, Public Affairs Committee, New York, 1972

Fredericks, Carlton, and Herman Goodman: *Low Blood Sugar and You*, Grosset and Dunlap, New York, 1969.

Freedman, Mervin B.: *The College Experience*, Jossey-Bass, San Francisco, 1967.

French, Ruth M.: *The Dynamics of Health Care*, McGraw-Hill, New York, 1974.

Freud, Sigmund: "Three Essays on the Theory of Sexuality," in *The Standard Edition of the Complete Psychological Works of Sigmund Freud*, Macmillan, New York, 1953.

Freund, Paul A. (ed.): *Experimentation with Human Subjects*, George Braziller, New York, 1970.

Friedan, Betty: "New Marriages Make Their Own Rules," *McCall's*, May 1973, p. 67.

Friedman, A., and S. Frazier with Dodi Schultz: *The Headache Book*, Dodd, Mead, New York, 1973.

Friedman, M., and R. Rosenman: *Type A Behavior and Your Heart*, Knopf, New York, 1974.

Fromm, Erich: *The Art of Loving*, Harper & Row, New York, 1956.

Fuchs, Lawrence H.: *Family Matters*, Random House, New York, 1972.

Fuchs, Victor: "The Jungle or the Zoo: What Price Health?" *Medical Economics*, Apr. 28, 1975, p. 160, condensed from *Who Shall Live? Health Economics and Social Choice*, Basic Books, New York, 1974.

Gadpaille, Warren (*a*): "Could that Youngster Become a Homosexual?" *Medical Economics*, Nov. 24, 1969, p. 250.

——— (*b*): In Lucy Freeman (ed.), *The Cycles of Sex*, Scribner's, New York, 1975.

Galanter et al.: "Marijuana and Social Behavior—A Controlled Study," *Archives of General Psychology*, vol. 30, April 1974, pp. 518–521.

Gallagher, Tom: "Can Death Ever Be Merciful? Yes," *Good Housekeeping*, June 1972, p. 90.

Garner, Craig: "All They Need Is a Chance," *Context*, no. 1, 1978, p. 15.

Geacintov, Martha: "Abortion Was Not Their Answer," *Rockland Journal-News*, New York, Oct. 4, 1974, p. 7A.

Gebhard, P. H., et al.: *Sex Offenders*, Harper, New York, 1965.

Geis, Gilbert: *Not the Law's Business? An Examination of Homosexuality, Abortion, Prostitution, Narcotics, and Gambling in the U.S.*, National Institute of Mental Health, Center for Studies of Crime and Delinquency, Washington, D. C., 1972.

Gelatt, H. B., B. Varenhorst, and R. Carey: *Deciding: A Leader's Guide,* Palo Alto, Calif.

Gerich, J. E.: "Plasma Glucagon and Analine Responses to Acute Insulin Deficiency in Man," *Journal of Clinical Endocrinology and Metabolism*, vol. 40, no. 3, March 1975, pp. 526–529.

Gillie, Oliver: "Drug Addiction—Facts and Folklore," *Science Journal*, vol. 5A, no. 6, December 1969, pp. 75–80.

Glaser, Barney, and Anselm Strauss: "Dying in Hospitals," in Anselm Strauss (ed.), p. 119.

Glasser, William: *Reality Therapy, A New Approach to Psychiatry*, Harper & Row, New York, 1965.

Globetti, G.: "Social Adjustment of High School Students and Problem Drinking," *Journal of Alcohol Education*, vol. 13, no. 2, Fall 1967, pp. 21–29.

Goldman, Rachel: In "The Hazards of Hashish," *Interface*, February–March 1976, p. 2.

Goldman, Ralph: *Principles of Medical Science*, McGraw-Hill, Blakiston Division, New York, 1973.

Goldstein, Bernard: *Human Sexuality*, McGraw-Hill, New York, 1976.

Goode, Erich: *The Marijuana Smokers*, Basic Books, New York, 1970.

Goodwin, Frederick: Alcohol, Drug Abuse, and Mental Health Administration, personal communication, Oct. 11, 1978.

Goro, Herb: *The Block*, Vintage Books, New York, 1970.

Gould Medical Dictionary, 3d ed. (A. Osol, ed.), McGraw-Hill, Blakiston Division, New York, 1972.

Gould, Robert: "A Psychiatrist Answers Teen Questions About Homosexuality," *Seventeen*, vol. 36, September 1977, p. 152.

Gould, Roger: "Adult Life Stages: Growth Toward Self-Tolerance," *Psychology Today*, February 1975, p. 74–78.

Green, Leslie: "Why I Miss Being Married," *Woman's Day*, November 1974, pp. 51.

Grossman, Herbert J.: *Manual on Terminology and Classification in Mental Retardation*, Special Publication no. 2, American Association on Mental Deficiency, Washington, D.C., 1973 rev., p. 18.

Guerin, Gilbert R.: "Early Classroom Un-Conditioning: A Rehearsal for Non-Drug Behavior," in M. Nellis (ed.), *Resource Book for Drug Abuse Education* (excerpted from a talk, "Life Without Drugs," given at the San Francisco Conference of Drug Abuse Project, 1968), National Clearing House for Drug Abuse Information, Rockville, Md., 1972, p. 80.

Guilford, Joan S.: "Prediction of Accidents in a Standardized Home Environment," *Journal of Applied Psychology*, vol. 57, no. 3, June 1973, pp. 306–313.

Guttmacher, Alan, with Winfield Best and Frederick S. Jaffe: *Birth Control and Love*, Macmillan, New York, 1969.

Hackett, Thomas P. (*a*): "How to Help the Dying Patient," *Medical Economics*, June 27, 1966, p. 148.

——— (*b*): "Grief—Good or Bad? Here's What to Watch For," *Medical Economics*, Nov. 26, 1973, p. 93.

——— (*c*): "Let's Remember that Dying Is a Family Event," *Medical Economics*, Feb. 21, 1977, p. 131.

——— (*d*): Personal interview, 1976.

Halberstam, Michael: *The Pills in Your Life*, Grosset & Dunlap, New York, 1972.

Halpern, Milton, and Y. M. Rho: "Deaths from Narcotism in NYC," *New York State Journal of Medicine*, Sept. 15, 1966, pp. 2402–2403.

Hammond, E. C. (*a*): "Smoking in Relation to Mortality and Morbidity," *Journal of the National Cancer Institute*, vol. 32, no. 5, May 1964, pp. 1161–1187.

——— (*b*): "Life Expectancy of American Men in Relation to Their Smoking Habits," presented at World Conference on Smoking and Health, New York City, Sept. 11–13, 1967.

——— and D. Horn: "Smoking and Death Rates," *Journal of The American Medical Association*, vol. 155, August 1954, pp. 1316–1328, and vol. 166, March 1958, pp. 1159–1294.

——— et al.: "Effects of Cigarette Smoking on Dogs," *Archives of Environmental Health*, December 1970, p. 752.

Harper, Robert, and Walter R. Stokes: *45 Levels to Sexual Understanding and Enjoyment*, Prentice-Hall, Englewood Cliffs, N.J., 1971.

Harris Survey (*a*): "Public Attitudes Toward Drinking and Alcohol Abuse," survey prepared for the National Institute on Alcohol Abuse and Alcoholism, New York, 1972–1974.

——— (*b*): "Public Attitudes Toward Legalization and Decriminalization of Marijuana," New York, 1977.

Harris, Thomas A.: *I'm Okay, You're Okay*, Harper & Row, New York, 1967.

Hartmann, Ernest: *The Functions of Sleep*, Yale, New Haven, Conn., 1973.

Hatterer, Lawrence J.: "What Makes a Homosexual?" *McCall's*, July 1971, p. 32.

Heath, Douglas H.: *Growing Up in College*, Jossey-Bass, San Francisco, 1968.

Hechtman, Lilly: In "Hyperactive Children Are Found to 'Catch Up as They Grow Up,'" *Pediatric News*, February 1967, p. 67.

Henderson, John: *Emergency Medical Guide*, 3d ed., McGraw-Hill, New York, 1973.

Henrie, W. J. Bryan, Personal communications, 1968, 1969.

Henry, Jules: "How One's Family and Peers Serve the Development of Identity," presented to the U.S. DHEW Conference on Identity in a Troubled World, June 20–21, 1968.

Hetherington, E. Mavis (*a*): "Effects of Paternal Absence on Sex-typed Behavior in Negro and White Preadolescent Males," *Journal of Personality and Social Psychology*, vol. 4, no. 1, 1966, pp. 87–91.

——— (*b*): "Effects of Father Absence on Personality Development in Adolescent Daughters," *Developmental Psychology*, vol. 7, no. 3, 1972, pp. 313–326.

HIS (Health Interview Survey): "Current Estimates from the HIS, U.S., 1974," *Vital and Health Statistics*, ser. 10, no. 100, U.S. DHEW publ. no. (HRA) 76-1527.

Hochman, J. S., and N. Q. Brill: "Chronic Marihuana Use and Psycho-Social Adaptation," *American Journal of Psychiatry*, vol. 130, February 1973, pp. 132–140.

Hoffman, La Roche, with David A. Hamburg, consultant: "This Question of Coping" in *Medical Tribune*, "Introduction," Jan. 2, 1974, pp. 13–20; "Competent Coping," Feb. 13, 1974, pp. 13–20; "The Development of Coping Behavior," Feb. 27, 1974, pp. 13–20; "Anxiety and Coping Behavior," Mar. 13, 1974, pp. 13–20; "Coping with Cancer," Apr. 10, 1974, pp. 15–26.

Hollister, Leo E.: "Psychopharmacology for Older Patients," presented to the press at Concepts of Health Care for the Aging, Washington, D.C., sponsored by the Veteran's Administration, Mar. 24, 1976.

Horn, Daniel: "Current Needs of Dealing with Cigarette Smoking," presented to the Commission on Smoking Policy of the American Cancer Society, Los Angeles, Mar. 22, 1977.

Horowitz, Herschel S. (*a*): "A Review of Systemic and Topical Fluorides for the Prevention of Dental Caries," *Community Dentistry and Oral Epidemiology*, vol. 1, 1973, pp. 104–114.

——— (*b*): "Fluoride: Research on Clinical and Public Health Applications," *Journal of the*

American Dental Association, Special Issue, vol. 87, October 1973, pp. 1013–1018.

Horvath, Peter N.: "What You Should Know About Hair Transplants," Georgetown University, Washington, D.C., interview notes, July 1973.

Hovel, Cleo: In Charren and Sarson.

Hubbard, Ellen: "How We Solve Breast Feeding Problems," *RN*, vol. 33, no. 3, March 1970, p. 46.

Hughes, Langston: *The Panther and the Lash*, Knopf, New York, 1974.

Hunt, Morton: *Sexual Behavior in the 1970s*, Playboy Press, New York, 1974.

Huyck, Margaret Hellie: *Growing Older*, Prentice-Hall, Englewood Cliffs, N.J., 1974.

Ingelfinger, F. J.: "Cancer! Alarm! Cancer!" *New England Journal of Medicine*, vol. 293, no. 23, Dec. 18, 1975, pp. 1319–1320.

Ishmael, William K., and Howard B. Shorbe: *Care of the Back*, Lippincott, Philadelphia, 1969.

Jaffe, Jerome H.: In Martha Lear, p. 19.

Jaffin, Alvin R.: In Martha Lear, p. 91.

Jain, A. K. (*a*): "Safety and Effectiveness of Intrauterine Devices," *Contraception*, vol. 11, 1975, p. 243.

——— (*b*): "Mortality Risk Associated with Use of Oral Contraceptives," *Studies in Family Planning*, vol. 8, no. 3, March 1977, pp. 50–55.

Janus, Samuel S.: In "Not a Laughing Matter," *New York Times*, May 28, 1974, p. 41:7.

Jarvik, Lissy F.: "Thoughts on the Psychobiology of Aging," *American Psychology*, vol. 30, no. 5, May 1975, pp. 576–585.

Jarvik, Murray: In Martha Lear, p. 19.

Jessor, R., and S. L. Jessor: "Problem Drinking in Youth: Personality, Social and Behavioral Antecedents and Correlates," Publication no. 144, Institute of Behavioral Science, University of Colorado, Boulder, 1973.

Joffe, J.: *Prenatal Determinants of Behavior*, Pergamon Press, New York, 1969.

Johnson, Ralph E.: in "Total Body Radiation Produces Remissions in Chronic Leukemia," *Medical Tribune*, July 16, 1975, p. 19.

Johnson, Sharon: in "In California, Teenagers Get Counseling First, Married Later," *New York Times*, Aug. 6, 1975, p. 21:1.

Jones, Ben Morgan, and O. A. Parsons: "Alcohol and Consciousness; Getting High, Coming Down," *Psychology Today*, vol. 8, January 1975, pp. 53–58.

Jones, Kenneth L., et al.: "Outcome in Offspring of Chronic Alcoholic Women," *Lancet*, June 1, 1974, pp. 1076–1078.

Jones, Reese: "Marijuana Induced High: Influence of Expectation and Setting and Previous Drug Experience," *Pharmacological Reviews*, vol. 23, December 1971, pp. 359–369.

Journal of Pediatrics: "On the Pediatric Approach to Geriatrics," vol. 63, no. 1, October 1963, pp. 685–688.

Kaiser-Permanente: The Walnut Creek Contraceptive Drug Study, Center for Population Research, DHEW, 1975.

Kales, Anthony: In Maggie Scarf.

Kallman, F. J.: "Comparative Twin Studies of the Genetic Aspects of Male Homosexuality," *Journal of Nervous and Mental Diseases*, vol. 115, 1952, pp. 286–294.

Kameny, Franklin: "Gay Liberation and Psychiatry," *Psychiatric Opinion*, February 1971, pp. 18–27.

Kaminester, Lewis H.: "When Friends or Patients Ask About . . . Acne," *Journal of the American Medical Association*, vol. 239, no. 20, May 19, 1978, pp. 2171–2172.

Kandel, D., and R. Faust: "Sequence and Stages in Patterns of Adolescent Drug Use Patterns," *Journal of Counseling Psychology*, vol. 21, no. 5, 1974, pp. 440–445.

Kanin, E. J.: "Sex Agression by College Men," *Medical Aspects of Human Sexuality*, vol. 4, no. 9, 1970, pp. 25–40.

——— and D. H. Howard: "Postmarital Consequences of Premarital Sex Adjustments," *American Sociological Review*, vol. 23, 1958, pp. 556–562.

Kantner, John F., and Marvin Zelnik (*a*): "Sexuality, Contraception, and Pregnancy Among Young Unwed Females in the United States," in C. F. Westoff and R. Parke, Jr. (eds.), *Demographic and Social Aspects of Population Growth*, vol. I of Commission Research Reports, Washington, D. C., 1972.

——— and ——— (*b*): "Contraception and Pregnancy: Experiences of Young Unmarried Women in the United States," *Family Planning Perspectives*, vol. 5, 1973, p. 21.

——— and ——— (*c*): "Sexual and Contraceptive Experience in Young Unmarried Women in the United States," *Family Planning Perspectives*, vol. 9, no. 2, March/April 1977, p. 55.

Kaplan, Norman M.: "Gross Obesity: New Therapies for an Old Problem," *Hospital Physician*, November 1974, pp. 64–71.

Kaplan, John: *Marijuana—The New Prohibition*, World, Cleveland, 1970.

Karel, Irving: School of Dental and Oral Surgery, Columbia Univerisity, personal interview, 1976.

Karp, L. E., et al.: "Prenatal Diagnosis of Genetic Diseases," *University of Washington Medicine*, vol. 1, no. 1, Spring 1974, pp. 5–13.

Kasindorf, Jeanie: "The Pill that Produces Unwanted Babies," *McCall's,* August 1973, p. 33.

Kelly, George A.: *The Catholic Marriage Manual*, New York Archdiocese, 1958.

Kelly, Orville E.: In J. Brody, "A Cancer Patient Has Social Woes," *New York Times*, March 31, 1976, p. 9:1.

Kenrick, Margaret M.: "Short Cuts to Exercise," Georgetown University, Washington, D.C., interview notes, July 1973.

———, F. M. Ball, and J. J. Canary: "Exercise, Weight Reduction and Obesity," *Archives of Physical Medicine and Rehabilitation*, vol. 53, 1972, p. 323.

Kilbourne, E. D., and W. G. Smillie (eds.): *Human Ecology and Public Health*, Macmillan, New York, 1969.

Kinsey, A. C., et al. (*a*): *Sexual Behavior in the Human Male*, Saunders, Philadelphia, 1948.

———, et al. (*b*): *Sexual Behavior in the Human Female*, Saunders, Philadelphia, 1953.

Kirk, Cameron: *Ohhh! My Back*, The Economics Press, Fairfield, N.J., 1960.

Kissin, Benjamin J.: In "Alcoholism: Is It a Treatable Disease?" *Modern Medicine*, Oct. 1, 1973, p. 33.

Klaw, Spencer: *The Great American Medicine Show*, Viking, New York, 1975.

Klein, David: "Some Social Characteristics of Accident Victims: Why Some Risk Takers Get Killed and Others Never Get Injured," *Traffic Safety*, April 1974, p. 8.

Klein, Edmund: Roswell Park Memorial Comprehensive Cancer Center, personal interview, October 1978

Klemesrud, Judy: "The Bisexuals," *New York*, Apr. 1, 1974, p. 37.

Kline, Nathan: *From Sad to Glad: Kline on Depression*, Putnam, New York, 1975.

Klopf, George C.: "Does Boredom Cause Accidents?" *National Safety News*, February 1973, pp. 61–62.

Kolansky, Harold, and William T. Moore: "Marijuana, Can it Hurt You?" *Journal of the American Medical Association,* vol. 232, no. 9, June 2, 1975, p. 923.

Kolodney, Robert C., et al: Depression of Plasma Testosterone Levels After Chronic Intensive Marihuana Use, *New England Journal of Medicine*, vol. 290, Apr. 18, 1974, pp. 872–874.

Konopka, Gisela: Personal interview, 1972.

Kraus, Hans: *The Cause, Prevention, and Treatment of Backache*, Pocket Books, New York, 1972.

Kremer, Malvina: "Identity Formation in Male and Female Adolescent Homosexuals," in *Science and Psychoanalysis,* vol. XV, Jules H. Masserman (ed.), *Dynamics of Deviant Sexuality*, Grune and Stratton, New York, 1969, p. 51.

Kübler-Ross, Elizabeth (*a*): *On Death and Dying*, Macmillan, New York, 1970.

——— (*b*): "Quizzing the Expert, Kübler-Ross on Coping with a Job You Dread," *Hospital Physician*, April 1973, pp. 30–39.

——— (*c*): In J. Lavin, "There Is Life After Death," *Fate*, February 1977, pp. 67–70.

Kupfer, Carl: In "All About Your Eyes and How to Save Them," *U.S. News and World Report*, June 11, 1973, p. 66.

Kupperman, Herbert S.: "Treating Menopausal Women and Climacteric Men," *Medical World News*, June 28, 1974, p. 42.

LaBarre, Harriet: *Beauty You can Buy,* Holt, Rhinehart, and Winston, New York, 1970.

Lader, Lawrence: *Fool Proof Birth Control: Male and Female Sterilization*, Beacon Press, Boston, 1972.

Lake, Alice: "The Right to Say No," *Seventeen*, June 1974, p. 110.

Lally, James J.: *The Modern Home Guide to Signs and Symptoms of Human Illness*, Parker, West Nyack, N.Y., 1970.

Landis, Judson T., and Mary G. Landis: *Building a*

Successful Marriage, Prentice-Hall, Englewood Cliffs, N.J., 1973.

Lang, Theo: *The Difference Between a Man and a Woman*, John Day, New York, 1971.

Larson, L. A.: *International Guide to Fitness and Health*, Crown, New York, 1973.

Lasagna, Louis: "Dr. Lasagna Writes on Colds and Antibiotics," *Medical Tribune*, Nov. 19, 1975; Responses Feb. 4, 1976 and Jan. 28, 1976.

Lauer, B., E. tenBroek, and M. Grossman: "Battered Child Syndrome: A Review of 130 Patients with Controls," *Pediatrics*, vol. 54, July 1974, pp. 67–70.

Laufer, Rob: "Handicapped Amendment Praised," *Rockland Journal-News*, New York, Nov. 26, 1974, p. 1B.

Lavin, John H., and Linda C. Bucek: "What Makes Americans So Operation Happy?" *Medical Economics*, Jan. 8, 1973, p. 67–75.

Lazlo, Maurice H.: In "Health Sciences," U. of Health Sciences, Chicago Medical School, Spring 1978, p. 4.

Lear, Martha Weinman: "All the Warnings Gone Up in Smoke," *New York Times Magazine*, Mar. 10, 1974, p. 18.

Leboyer, Frederick: *Birth Without Violence*, Knopf, New York, 1975.

Leech, Peter: In Gregg Downey.

Leeson, Lewis J.: "Generic Drugs Labeled 'Caution'?" *New York Times*, June 5, 1977, p. N.J.28.

LeFevre, Perry: In "What Are the Psychological Effects of Premarital Intercourse?" *Medical Aspects of Human Sexuality*, April 1968, pp. 22–27.

Lehmann, Phyllis: "Occupational Cancer," *Job Safety and Health*, vol. 3, no. 7, July 1975, pp. 5–13.

Lemon, Henry M.: "Estriol Prevention of Mammary Carcinoma Induced by 7,12-dimethylbenzanthracena and procarbazine," *CA Research*, vol. 35, no. 5, May 1975, pp. 1341–1353.

Lenoski, Edward: "Physical Child Abuse and the Abusing Parent," paper delivered to 101st annual meeting of the Public Health Association, San Francisco, Nov. 5, 1973.

LeShan, Eda J.: *The Wonderful Crisis of Middle Age*, David McKay, New York, 1973.

Leuchtenberger, C., R. Leuchtenberger, and A. Schneider: "Effects of Marihuana and Tobacco Smoke on Human Lung Physiology," *Nature*, vol. 241, Jan. 12, 1973, pp. 137–139.

Levine, M. S., and E. P. Radford: "Fire Victims Medical Outcomes and Demographic Characteristics," *American Journal of Public Health*, November 1977, p. 1077.

Levy, Hilton B., et al.: "Report on Study of Interferon Inducers in Primates," presented at First International Congress of the International Association of Microbiological Societies, Tokyo, Sept. 1–7, 1974.

Levy, Norman J.: "The Use of Drugs by Teenagers for Sanctuary and Illusion," *American Journal of Psychoanalysis*, vol. 28, no. 1, 1968, pp. 48–58.

Lieberman, James E., and Ellen Peck: *Sex and Birth Control: A Guide For the Young*, Crowell, New York, 1973.

Lief, Harold: In "Yesterday's Perversion—Tomorrow's Variation," *Ob. Gyn. News*, vol. 9, no. 10, May 15, 1974, p. 3.

Lipscomb, David M.: *Noise: The Unwanted Sounds*, Nelson-Hall, Chicago, 1974.

Lobsenz, Norman: "Sex and the Senior Citizen," *New York Times Magazine*, Jan. 20, 1974, p. 8.

Logan, Josh: Personal communication, October 1978.

"Logical Lines to Acne Control," *Patient Care*, Apr. 15, 1975, p. 108.

Long, Esmond R.: *A History of Pathology*, Dover, New York, 1965.

Louria, Donald B.: *Overcoming Drugs*, McGraw-Hill, New York, 1971.

Low: See Recovery, Inc.

Lowenthal, Marjorie F., and David Chiraboga: "Transition to the Empty Nest: Crisis, Challenge, or Relief?" *Archives of General Psychiatry*, vol. 26, January 1972, pp. 8–14.

Luce, Gay Gaer (*a*): *Biological Rhythms in Psychiatry and Medicine*, U.S. DHEW, PHS publ. no. 2088, 1970.

——— (*b*): *Current Research on Sleep and Dreams*, U.S. DHEW, HSM-73-9153, 1973.

Luy, Mary Lynn M.: "The Roughage Rage: Would More Fiber in the Diet Improve Health?" *Modern Medicine*, Apr. 1, 1976, pp. 76–80.

McBride, Angela Barron: *Growth and Development of Mothers*, Harper & Row, New York, 1973.

McCary, James Leslie: *Human Sexuality*, Van Nostrand Reinhold, New York, 1973.

McCormack, William M.: "Sexually Transmissible Conditions Other Than Gonorrhea and Syphilis," *Practice of Medicine*, vol. 3, ch. 20, 1974.

McCormick, Richard A. (*a*): "To Save or Let Die, the Dilemma of Modern Medicine," *Journal of the American Medical Association*, vol. 229, no. 2, July 8, 1974, pp. 172–176.

——— (*b*): In *Federal Register*.

MacFarland, J. W., and J. A. Clausen: "The Effect of Childhood Influences Upon Intelligence, Personality, and Mental Health," prepared by H. Yahraes, Mental Health Program Reports, no. 3, Public Health Service, January 1969.

McGinnis, Tom: *Your First Year of Marriage*, Doubleday, Garden City, N.Y., 1967.

McIntire, Roger: "Licensing Proposal for Parenthood," *Science News*, vol. 103, May 12, 1973, p. 305.

McTaggart, Aubrey C.: *The Health Care Dilemma*, Holbrook, Boston, 1971.

Madison, Peter: *Personality Development in College*, Addison-Wesley, Reading, Mass., 1969.

Mainardi, Pat: "The Politics of Housework," in Robin Morgan (ed.), *Sisterhood is Powerful*, Vintage, New York, 1970, pp. 447–454.

Malfetti, James L.: "Attitudes and Safety in Recreation," *Public Health Reports*, vol. 78, no. 6, June 1973, pp. 477–484.

Mann, William A.: "Difficulties in Changing Human Behavior," *National Safety Congress Transactions*, vol. 2, 1968.

Manual for Law Enforcement Officers, Smith, Kline, and French, Philadelphia, revised 1968.

Markovitz, Andrew S.: "How to Gain Weight," *Mechanics Illustrated*, November 1973, p. 86.

Marmor, Judd: In "Is Homosexuality Pathologic or a Normal Variant of Sexuality?" *Medical Aspects of Human Sexuality*, December 1973, pp. 10, 15.

Maslow, Abraham: *Toward a Psychology of Being*, Van Nostrand, New York, 1962.

Masters, William H., and Virginia E. Johnson (*a*): *Human Sexual Response*, Little Brown, Boston, 1966.

——— and ——— (*b*): *Human Sexual Inadequacy*, Little, Brown, Boston, 1970.

——— and ——— (*c*) (in association with Robert Levin): *The Pleasure Bond*, Little, Brown, Boston, 1970.

Mastroianni, Luigi, Jr.: "Rhythm: Systematized Chance-Taking," *Family Planning Perspectives*, vol. 6, no. 4, Fall 1974, pp. 209–212.

Mau, G., and P. Netter (*a*): "Die Auswir Kungen des vaterlichen zigaretten-Komsum auf die perinatale sterblichkeit und die Missbildungshaufigkeit," *Dtch. Med. Wachenschr*, vol. 99, May 24, 1974, pp. 1113–1118.

——— and ——— (*b*): "Kaffee-Und Alkohol Konsum—Risik of ackturen in der Schwangerschaft?" *Geburtschilfe Frauenheilkd*, vol. 34, no. 12, December 1974 (English abstract), pp. 1018–1022.

Mayer, Jean (*a*): *Overweight: Causes, Cost and Control*, Prentice-Hall, Englewood Cliffs, N.J., 1968.

——— (*b*): *Human Nutrition*, Charles C Thomas, Springfield, Ill., 1972.

——— (*c*): In "Diet Is Stressed as Longevity Aid," *New York Times*, June 19, 1974, p. 9:1.

——— (*d*): *A Diet for Living*, McKay, New York, 1975.

Mead, Beverly T. (*a*): In "What Are the Psychological Effects of Premarital Intercourse?" *Medical Aspects of Human Sexuality*, April 1968, pp. 22–27.

——— (*b*): "Reactive Depression in Young Adults," in A. J. Enelow (ed.), *Depression in Medical Practice*, Merck, Sharp & Dohme, West Point, Pa., 1970.

Medea, Andrea, and Kathleen Thompson: *Against Rape*, Farrar, Strauss, and Giroux, New York, 1974.

Medical Tribune: "In Suffering, Terminal Patients: 77 Percent of U.S. Family Physicians Would Consider Passive Euthanasia," May 26, 1976, p. 1.

Medical World News (*a*): "Sex Counseling and the Primary Physician," Mar. 2, 1973, p. 35.

——— (*b*): "Treating Menopausal Women—and Climacteric Men," June 28, 1974, p. 32.

——— (*c*): "Dealing with Food Poisoning," Aug. 25, 1975, p. 74.

Mendelson, J. H., and N. K. Mello: "The Significance of Alcohol-Induced Hypertriglyceridemia in Patients with Type IV Hyperlipoproteinemia," *Annals of Internal Medicine*, vol. 80, February 1974, pp. 270–271.

Menning, Barbara Eck: *Infertility, A Guide for the Childless Couple*, Prentice-Hall, Englewood Cliffs, N.J., 1977.

Menninger, Karl (*a*), with Martin Mayman and Paul Pruyser: *The Vital Balance, The Life Process in Mental Health and Illness*, Viking, New York, 1963.

——— (*b*): *Whatever Became of Sin?* Hawthorn, New York, 1973.

——— (*c*): "Sheer Verbal Mickey Mouse," *International Journal of Psychiatry*, vol. 7, no. 6, 1969, p. 415.

Merigan, Thomas C., S. E. Reed, T. S. Hall, et al.: "Inhibition of Respiratory Virus Infection by Locally Applied Interferon," *Lancet*, vol. 1, Mar. 17, 1973, pp. 563–567.

Merritt, Allen T.: Perinatologist, personal interview, July 1974

Messolonghites, Louisa (ed.): *Alternative Pursuits for America's 3rd Century, A Resource Book on Alternatives*, National Institute on Drug Abuse, 1974.

Meyer, Jon K.: In response to "Paul Jay Fink on Homosexuality," *Hospital Physician*, December 1974, p. 37.

Milt, Harry: *Basic Handbook in Mental Illness*, Scribners, New York, 1974.

Mirkin, G.: "Carbohydrate Loading: A Dangerous Practice," *Journal of the American Medical Association*, vol. 223, 1973, pp. 1511–1512.

Mishell, Daniel R., Jr.: "Assessing the Intrauterine Device," *Family Planning Perspectives*, vol. 7, no. 3, May–June 1975, p. 103.

Monahan, Thomas P.: "Does Age at Marriage Matter in Divorce?" *Social Forces*, vol. 32, October 1953, p. 81.

Money, John: In "Categorizes Homosexuality as Intractable," *Pediatric News*, September 1974, p. 24.

Montagu, Ashley (*a*): *Sex, Man and Society*, Putnam, New York, 1969.

——— (*b*): *Touching, The Human Significance of the Skin*, Columbia University, New York, 1971.

Morbidity and Mortality Weekly Report (MMWR) (*a*): vol. 26, no. 27, July 8, 1977.

——— (*b*): vol. 27, no. 21, May 26, 1978.

——— (*c*): vol. 27, no. 16, Apr. 21, 1978.

Morris, Terry: "Can Death Ever Be Merciful? No." *Good Housekeeping*, June 1972, p. 91.

Moss, Bertram B. (*a*): "Facts and Fiction About Caring for the Aged," *Resident and Staff Physicians*, October 1971, p. 41.

——— (*b*): "Normal Aging," *Chicago Medical School Quarterly*, vol. 32, nos. 1–4, 1973, pp. 90–93.

——— (*c*): "Your Patients' Care," *Nursing Homes*, November 1970, p. 33.

Mowrer, O. Hobart: *The Crisis in Psychiatry and Religion*, Van Nostrand, Princeton, N.J., 1961.

National Clearing House for Smoking and Health: "Smoker's Self-testing Kit," U.S. Public Health Service, U. S. DHEW 73-8716, 1973.

National Conference of Catholic Bishops and U.S. Catholic Conference: *In Response to Supreme Court Decision on Abortion*, U. S. Catholic conference, 1973.

National Council on Alcoholism: "What Are the Signs of Alcoholism?" New York, March 1973.

National Council of Churches: In Guttmacher.

Nation's Business: "Strong Protest Against Early Retirement," July 1976, pp. 14–15.

Nelkin, Dorothy: *Methadone Maintenance: A Technological Fix*, Braziller, New York, 1973.

Nelson, Ralph A.: "What Should Athletes Eat? Unmixing Folly and Facts," *Physician and Sports Medicine*, September 1975, pp. 67–72.

Neu, Carlos, and Alberto Dimascio: "Variations in the Menstrual Cycle," *Medical Aspects of Human Sexuality*, February 1974, p. 164.

Neufeld, Elizabeth: National Institute of Arthritis, Metabolism, and Digestive Diseases, personal interview, July 1974.

New York State Department of Motor Vehicles: *Pilot Study of Driver Attitude Toward Seat Belts*.

New York Times: "Rare and Endangered Wildlife," Nov. 2, 1974, p. 29.

Newsweek: "Is It Time for a Change in Our Laws?" Sept. 7, 1970, p. 20.

Nicoli, Armand, M.: "A New Dimension of the Youth Culture," *American Journal of Psychiatry*, vol. 131, no. 4, April 1974, pp. 396–401.

Nolen, William A.: *Healing: A Doctor in Search of a Miracle*, Random House, New York, 1974.

Nutrition in Japan 1960, Ministry of Health and Welfare, Tokyo, November 1960.

Ochsner, Alton: *Smoking: Your Choice Between Life and Death*, Simon & Schuster, New York, 1970.

O'Connor, Timothy: National Cancer Institute, personal interview, July 1974.

O'Donnell, T. J.: "To Live—To Die," *Journal of the American Medical Association*, vol. 228, Apr. 22, 1974, p. 501.

Ossofsky, Jack: Statement of the National Council of the Aging to Subcommittee on Equal Opportunity, Committee on Education and Labor, U.S. House of Representatives, Sept. 14, 1976.

Ostfeld, Adrian M., and Don C. Gibson (eds.): *Epidemiology of Aging*, U.S. DHEW publ. no. (NIH) 75-711, 1972.

Packard, Vance: *The Sexual Wilderness*, McKay, New York, 1968.

Paffenbarger, Ralph S., Jr., et al.: "Work Energy Levels, Personal Characteristics, and Fatal Heart Attack: A Birth Cohort Effect," *American Journal of Epidemiology*, vol. 105, no. 3, March 1977, pp. 200–213.

Patient Care (*a*): "The Mechanics of Blood Pressure," Nov. 15, 1973, p. 45.

——— (*b*): "Why COPD Patient Gets in Trouble," Feb. 15, 1974, p. 119.

——— (*c*): "Summer Syndrome: Help for Your Sunburn Prone Patients," July 1, 1974, p. 56–69.

——— (*d*): "Basic Life-Support Techniques for Witnessed Cardiac Arrest," Dec. 1, 1974, p. 67.

Payne, Howard J.: In "Jejunoileal Bypass for Gross Obesity: Yes or No?" *Medical World News*, Apr. 19, 1974, p. 62.

Peck, Ellen: "Obituary Motherhood," *New York Times*, May 13, 1972, p. 31:1.

Pedersen, Frank A., and Kenneth S. Robson: "Father Participation in Infancy," *American Journal of Orthopsychiatry*, vol. 39, no. 3, April 1969, pp. 466–472.

——— et al. "Father Absence in Infancy," prepared for presentation at the 1973 meeting of the Society for Research in Child Development, Philadelphia, Mar. 29–Apr. 1, 1973.

Pediatric News: "Return to Breast Feeding Said to Halt 30 Year Trend," February 1976, p. 26.

Perper, Joshua, pathologist: Personal interview, October 1978.

Perrine, M. W., et al.: "Alcohol and Highway Safety: Behavior and Medical Aspects," *National Highway Traffic Safety Administration Technical Report*, DOT HS-800-599, 1971.

Perry, William: Harvard Bureau of Study Counseling, Cambridge, Mass., personal interview, 1975.

Petite, Michael T.: Georgetown University, Washington, D.C., personal interview, January 1974.

Planned Parenthood: *Abortion: A Woman's Guide*, Pocket Books, New York, 1975.

Pogrebin, Letty Cottin: In "Would You Have Another Abortion?" *Rockland Journal-News*, New York, Sept. 17, 1974, p. 6A.

Popenoe, Paul: "The New Morality is Bunk," *McCall's*, December 1971, p. 118b.

Pops, Martin A., and Arthur D. Schwabe: In "Mystery Starvation Malady," U.C. Clip Sheet, Apr. 26, 1977.

Population and the American Future, report of the Commission on Population Growth and the American Future, Washington, D.C., 1972.

Powelson, Harvey: "U.C. Psychiatrist Sees Some Lasting Harm in Using Pot," *U.C. Clip Sheet*, May 12, 1970.

Prehn, R. T.: "Do Tumors Grow Because of the Immune Response of the Host?" *Transplant Review*, vol. 28, pp. 34–42, 1976.

Protection of Human Subjects, Federal Register, no. 33526-52, Aug. 8, 1975.

Proxmire, William: *You Can Do It!* Simon & Schuster, New York, 1973.

Public Law 91-513, Ninety-first Congress, H.R. 18583, Oct. 27, 1970.

"The Pursuit of High," *Medical Economics*, Special Issue, Apr. 20, 1970.

Rabbinical Alliance of America: In Guttmacher.

Rabbinical Assembly of America: In Guttmacher.

Rada, Richard: "Alcoholism and Forcible Rape," *American Journal of Psychiatry*, vol. 132, no. 4, April 1975, pp. 444–446.

Rall, David P.: In U.S. Senate Appropriation Hearings, part 4, 1975.

Raper, Nancy R., and Mary M. Hill: "Vegetarian Diets," *Nutrition Program News*, U.S. Department of Agriculture, July–August 1973, reprinted in Nutrition Reviews Supplement, July 1974, pp. 29–33.

Rawls, John: *A Theory of Justice*, Harvard University (Belknap Press), Cambridge, Mass., 1971.

RDA (Recommended Dietary Allowances): National Academy of Sciences, Food and Nutrition Board, Washington, D.C., 1974.

Read, Merrill S.: *Malnutrition and Learning*, U.S. DHEW, no. 724-798/59, 1973; adapted from *American Education*, vol. 5, no. 10, December 1969, pp. 11–14.

Recovery, Inc.: What It Is and How It Developed, Recovery, Inc., Chicago, 1973.

Reiss, Ira L.: *Premarital Sexual Standards in America*, Free Press, New York, 1960.

Rensberger, Boyce: "Abuse of Prescription Drugs: A Hidden, but Serious Problem," *New York Times*, Apr. 19, 1978, p. A12:3.

Rifkind, Basil M.: National Heart and Lung Institute, personal interview, July 1974.

Roberts, Guy: *Personal Growth and Adjustment*, Holbrook, Boston, 1968.

Roelfs, Pamela J.: "Teaching and Counseling Older Students," *ETS Findings*, vol. 2, no. 1, 1975.

Roesler, Thomas, and Robert W. Deisher: "Youthful Male Homosexuality," *Journal of the American Medical Association*, vol. 219, no. 8, Feb. 21, 1972, pp. 1018–1023.

Roper Organization: "Survey of the Attitudes of Women on Marriage, Divorce, the Family, and America's Changing Sexual Morality," for Virginia Slims (Philip Morris), Washington, D.C., 1974.

Rosebury, Theodor: *Microbes and Morals*, Viking, New York, 1971.

Rosenhan, D. L.: "On Being Sane In Insane Places," *Science*, vol. 179, Jan. 19, 1973, pp. 250–258.

Rosenthal, Mitchell S., and Ira Mothner: *Drugs, Parents and Children—The Three Way Connection*, Houghton Mifflin, Boston, 1972.

Ross, Walter Sanford: "Peggy Was Dying," *Ladies Home Journal*, July 1965, p. 50.

Rostand, Jean: In *The First Days of Human Life*, Canadian Catholic Conference, Ottawa, Canada, 1971.

Rothman, K., and A. Keller: "The Effect of Joint Exposure to Alcohol and Tobacco on Risk of Cancer of the Mouth and Pharynx," *Journal of Chronic Diseases*, vol. 25, 1972, pp. 711–716.

Royal College of General Practitioners, Oral Contraceptives and Health, An Interim Report, Pitman Medical, London, 1974.

Rubin, I.: "The New Kinsey Report," *Sexology*, February 1966, pp. 443–446.

Ruebsaat, Helmut J., and Raymond Hull: *The Male Climacteric*, Hawthorn, New York, 1975.

Rundles, R. Wayne: *Cancer 78*, Duke University Comprehensive Cancer Center, April 1978.

Rush, Benjamin: *An Inquiry into the Effects of Ardent Spirits Upon the Human Mind and Body*, 8th ed., Merriam, Brookfield, 1814.

Ryan, Kenneth J., and Don C. Gibson (eds.): *Menopause and Aging*, U.S. DHEW, NIH 73-319, 1973.

Sackett, Walter W., Jr.: "I've Let Hundreds of Patients Die, Shouldn't You?" *Medical Economics*, Apr. 2, 1973, p. 93.

Saghir, Marcel T., and Eli Robins: *Male and Female Homosexuality*, Williams & Wilkins, Baltimore, 1973.

St. John, Adela Rogers: In "Beauty Can Be a Terrible Problem for Women," *Rockland Journal-News* (United Features), New York, Dec. 17, 1973, p. 12A.

Santulli, Thomas V., et al.: "Acute Necrotizing Enterocolitis in Infancy, A Review of 64 Cases," *Pediatrics*, vol. 55, no. 3, March 1975, pp. 376–387.

Sarrel, Philip, and Lorna Sarrel (*a*): "Health and Sex," *Glamour*, December 1971, p. 181.

——— and ——— (*b*): "Health and Sex," *Glamour*, June 1972.

Scanzoni, Letha, and John Scanzoni: *Men, Women, and Change, A Sociology of Marriage and the Family*, McGraw-Hill, New York, 1976.

Scarf, Maggie: "Oh, for a Decent Night's Sleep!" *New York Times Magazine*, Oct. 21, 1973, p. 36.

Schacter, Stanley: In Neil Solomon, pp. 67ff.

Scherp, Henry W.: "Dental Caries: Prospects for Prevention," *Science*, vol. 173, September 1971, pp. 1199–1205.

Schmeck, Harold M.: "Panel Cites Doubt On Cold Remedies," *New York Times*, Feb. 15, 1976, p. 18:1

Schmidt, Alexander: *FDA report to the White House Focus on Health,* July 10, 1974.

Schneiderman, M.: Paper presented at American Cancer Society seminar for science writers, St. Petersburg, Fla., Mar. 28, 1976.

Searcy, Laurel: "Nursing Care of the Laryngectomy Patient, *RN*, October 1972, p. 35.

Sehnert, Keith W.: "The Wheel of Health," *Delaware Medical Journal,* October 1975, p. 592.

——— and Howard Eisenberg: *How to Be Your Own Doctor—Sometimes*, Grosset and Dunlap, New York, 1975.

Selikoff, Irving J.: *Testimony Before Senate Commerce Subcommittee on the Environment*, Aug. 20, 1975.

Selye, Hans (*a*): *The Stress of Life*, McGraw-Hill, New York, 1956.

——— (*b*): *Stress Without Distress*, Lippincott, Philadelphia, 1974.

Senate Select Committee on Nutrition and Human Needs: *Dietary Goals for the United States*, 1978.

Settel, Edward M.: "Use of Female Hormones Topically to Treat Baldness in Men," presented to American Academy of Family Physicians, Chicago, September 1975.

Sex Information and Education Council (SEICUS): *Sexuality and Man*, Scribner's, New York, 1970.

Shalita, Alan R.: "Acne Vulgaris: Not Curable, But Treatable," *Modern Medicine*, Aug. 1, 1975, pp. 66–76.

Shapiro, Eli: "Destructive Cultism," *American Family Physician*, vol. 15, no. 2, February 1977, pp. 80–83.

Sheridan, Edward J.: "When Your Child Needs You Most," Georgetown University, Washington, D.C., interview notes, March 1974.

Shimkin, Michael B.: *Science and Cancer*, U.S. DHEW, NCI no. 1162, 1969.

Shope, D. F., and C. B. Broderick: "Level of Sexual Experience and Predicted Adjustment in Marriage," *Journal of Marriage and the Family*, vol. 29, no. 3, August 1967, pp. 424–427.

Shulman, Alix Kates: "Up from Under," August-September 1970, p. 32.

Simmons, H. E., and P. D. Stolley: "This Is Medical Progress?" *Journal of the American Medical Association*, March 4, 1974, pp. 1023–1028.

Smith, Gene: "Chemical Paper and Metal Industry Say Economy Will Be Hurt by Cost of Achieving Zero Pollution," *New York Times*, Dec. 8, 1975, p. 1.

Smith, Ralph Lee: *At Your Own Risk: The Case Against Chiropractic*, Pocket Books, New York, 1969.

Smitson, Walter S.: "The Meaning of Emotional Maturity," *Mental Hygiene,* vol. 58, Winter 1974, pp. 9–11.

Snyder, John A.: "The Use of Gatekeepers in Crisis Management," *Bulletin of Suicidology*, NIMH no. 8, Fall 1971, pp. 39–44.

Socarides, Charles W. (*a*): "Homosexuality and Medicine," *Journal of the American Medical Association*, vol. 212, no. 7, May 18, 1970, pp. 1199–1202.

——— (*b*): "Homosexuality—Basic Concepts and Psychodynamics," *International Journal of Psychiatry*, vol. 10, no. 1, 1972, pp. 118–125.

——— (*c*): "Homosexuality," in Silvano Arieti (ed.), *American Handbook of Psychiatry*, Basic Books, New York, 1974.

——— et al.: "Homosexuality in the Male: A Report of a Psychiatric Study Group," *International Journal of Psychiatry*, vol. 11, no. 4, 1973, pp. 460–479.

Solomon, Neil, with Sally Sheppard: *The Truth About Weight Control*, Stein & Day, New York, 1971.

Somers, Anne R. (ed.): *Promoting Health: Consumer Education and National Policy*, Aspen, Germantown, Md., 1976.

Sorensen, Robert C.: *Adolescent Sexuality in Contemporary America*, World, New York, 1973.

Spitzer, Robert L. (*a*): In "The Issue Is Subtle, the Debate Still On," *New York Times*, Dec. 23, 1973, p. IV, 5:1.

——— (*b*): Personal interview, September 1978.

Stent, G. S.: "The Multiplication of Bacterial Viruses," *Scientific American*, vol. 188, no. 5, May 1953, pp. 36–39.

Stokes, Bruce: "Birth Control: More People Are Turning to Sterilization," *New York Times*, May 22, 1977, p. IV, 7:4.

Stonecypher, D. D., Jr.: *Getting Older and Staying Younger*, Norton, New York, 1974.

Strauss, Anselm L.: *Chronic Illness and the Quality of Life*, Mosby, St. Louis, 1975.

Streshinsky, Shirley: "Beyond Love: The Special Rewards of Marriage," *Redbook*, May 1974, p. 169.

Strickland, Stephen P.: *U.S. Health Care, What's*

Wrong and What's Right, Universe Books, New York, 1972.

Stuelke, Richard: Duke University Fat Clinic, Durham, N.C., personal interview, January 1974.

Stunkard, Albert J. (*a*): "The Obese," in J. Mayer (ed.), *U.S. Nutrition Policy for the Seventies*, Freeman, San Francisco, 1973, pp. 29–36.

——— (*b*): In "At the AMA Scientific Sessions: A New Approach to Dieting," *Medical World News*, June 14, 1974, p. 22.

Styron, William: In Martha Lear.

Sullivan, Ronald: In "Health Maintenance Groups Take Growing Role as Resistance Eases," *New York Times*, May 21, 1978, p. 1.

Suomi, John D.: "Prevention and Control of Periodontal Disease," *Journal of the American Dental Association,* vol. 83, no. 6, December 1971, pp. 1271–1287.

Szasz, Thomas S.: *The Manufacture of Madness*, Harper & Row, New York, 1970.

Tashkin, Donald: "Marijuana May Prove More Harmful than Tobacco," *U.C. Clip Sheet*, July 11, 1978.

Thomas, Caroline Bedell, et al.: "What Becomes of Medical Students: The Dark Side," *Johns Hopkins Medical Journal*, vol. 138, no. 5, May 1976, pp. 185–195.

Thomas, John L. (*a*): "Romance and Reality," Georgetown University, Washington, D.C., interview notes, September 1973.

——— (*b*): "How to Do Nothing Better," Georgetown University, Washington, D.C., interview notes, March 1974.

——— (*c*): "Marital Failure and Duration," *Social Order*, vol. 3, 1953, pp. 211–229.

——— (*d*): In "What Are the Psychological Effects of Premarital Intercourse?" *Medical Aspects of Human Sexuality*, April 1968, pp. 22–27.

Thomas, Piri: "Problems of Identity in Adolescence for Selected Classes of Youth: Low-Income, Negro, Indian, Puerto Rican, Mexican-American," paper presented at Conference on Iden tity in a Troubled World, Washington, D.C., June 20–21, 1968.

Tietze, Christopher (*a*): "The Effect of Legalization of Abortion on Population Growth and Public Health," *Family Planning Perspectives*, vol. 7, no. 3, May–June 1975, pp. 123–127.

——— (*b*): "New Estimates of Mortality Associated with Fertility Control," *Family Planning Perspectives*, vol. 9, no. 2, March–April 1977, pp. 74–76.

Tiger, Lionel: "Male Dominance? Yes, Alas. A Sexist Plot? No." *New York Times Magazine*, Oct. 25, 1970, p. 134.

Tjossem, T.: National Institute of Child Health and Human Development, personal interview, July 1974.

Tobin, Charles E.: *Basic Human Anatomy*, McGraw-Hill, New York, 1972.

——— and Ng.: "Visual Principles of Elementary Human Anatomy," F. A. Davis, 1965.

Toffler, Alvin: *Future Shock*, Random House, New York, 1970.

Torrance, E. Paul: *Constructive Behavior: Stress, Personality, and Mental Health*, Wadsworth, Belmont, Calif., 1965.

Torrey, E. Fuller: *The Death of Psychiatry*, Chilton, Radnor, Pa., 1974.

Trout, Marda Z.: "Problems of Alcoholic Children," *Washington Post*, July 15, 1973, p. A22.

Underwood, K: "The Church, the University, and Social Policy," Danforth Study of Campus Ministries, 1968, quoted in Chickering, pp. 130–132.

United Nations Demographic Yearbook, New York, 1975.

U.S. Consumer Product Safety Commission: *Annual Report*, fiscal year 1976, Washington, D.C., Government Printing Office, October 1976.

U.S. Department of Agriculture: *Keeping Food Safe to Eat*, Home and Garden Bulletin no. 162, 1971.

U.S. Department of Commerce: *Statistical Abstracts*, Bureau of the Census, 1978.

U.S. Department of Health, Education and Welfare (DHEW) (*a*): *Smoking and Health*, a report of the Advisory Committee to the Surgeon General of the Public Health Service, Jan. 11, 1964.

——— (*b*): "Cellular Aspects of Immune Response," a report by the Anatomical Sciences Training Committee of the National Institute of General Medical Sciences, NIH, 1967.

——— (*c*): *The Health Consequences of Smoking*, PHS 1696, 1967.

——— (*d*): *Tracking Diseases from Nature to Man*, PHS 1675, March 1968.

——— (*e*): *Better Care for Mental Patients*, PHS 1896, February 1969.

——— (*f*): *The Mental Health of Urban America*, PHS 1906, April 1969.

——— (*g*): *Identity in a Troubled World*, 469-1970, a summary of the Conference on Identity, Washington, D.C., June 20–21, 1968.

——— (*h*): *Oral Disease: Target for the 70s*, NIDR, December 1970.

——— (*i*): *Research Explores Dental Decay*, PHS 1483, 1970.

——— (*j*): *Research Explores Pyorrhea and Other Gum Diseases: Periodontal Disease*, PHS 1482, 1970.

——— (*k*): *The Health Consequences of Smoking*, a report to the Surgeon General, HSM 71-7513, 1971.

——— (*l*): *Current Concepts in Amphetamine Abuse*, HSM 72-9085, 1972.

——— (*m*): *Mental Retardation: Its Biological Factors*, NIH 72-155, 1972.

——— (*n*): *Task Force on Homosexuality*, final report and background papers, 1972.

——— (*o*): *Hearing Loss—Hope Through Research*, NIH 73-157, 1973.

——— (*p*): *How Children Grow—Clinical Research Advances in Human Growth and Development*, NIH 73-166, 1973.

——— (*q*): *Immunology Research: An Introduction*, NIH 73-529, 1973.

——— (*r*): *Learning About Depressive Illnesses*, HSM 73-9134, 1973.

——— (*s*): *Mental Retardation: The First Decade*, a report to the National Advisory Child Health and Development Council, NICHHD, Mar. 23, 1973.

——— (*t*): *Diagnosis and Treatment of Adverse Reactions to Sedative Hypnotics*, ADM 4-24, 1974.

——— (*u*): *If You Must Smoke*, CDC 74-8706, 1974.

——— (*v*): *The Health Consequences of Smoking*, 1974.

——— (*w*): *Infectious Disease Research: Venereal Disease*, NIH 74-532, 1974.

——— (*x*): *Marihuana and Health*, third annual report to the United States Congress, 1973, ADM 74-50, 1974.

——— (*y*): *National Caries Program*, status report, 1972, NIH 74-394, 1974.

——— (*z*): *A National View of Mental Health*, NIH 74-661, 1974.

——— (*aa*): *What Are the Facts About Genetic Disease?* NIH 74-370, 1974.

——— (*bb*): *Alcohol and Health*, second special report to the U.S. Congress, June 19, 1974, ADM 75-212, 1975.

——— (*cc*): *Marijuana and Health*, fourth annual report to the U.S. Congress, ADM 75-181, 1975.

——— (*dd*): *Report on Adult Use of Tobacco in the U.S.*, 1975.

——— (*ee*): *Alcohol and Health*, first special report to the U.S. Congress, ADM 76-359, 1976 (reprinted).

——— (*ff*): *Marijuana and Health*, fifth annual report to the U.S. Congress, 1975, ADM 76-314, 1976.

——— (*gg*): *Health United States, 1976–1977*, HRA 77-1232, 1977.

——— (*hh*): *Your Eye Care*, Consumer Information Series No. 4, NEI, prepublication.

U.S. News and World Report: "Rise of the Singles," Oct. 7, 1974, p. 54.

The Use of Chemicals in Food Production, Processing, Storage, and Distribution, National Academy of Sciences, Washington, D.C., 1973.

Vaillant, George: "The Normal Boy in Later Life: How Adaptation Fosters Growth," *Harvard Magazine*, November-December 1977, p. 46.

Verrett, Jacqueline, and Jean Carper: *Eating May Be Hazardous to Your Health*, Simon & Schuster, New York, 1974.

Vessey, M., et al.: "A Long Term Follow-up Study of Women Using Different Methods of Contraception—an Interim Report," *Journal of Biosocial Science*, vol. 8, 1976, p. 373.

Vidal, Gore: "Drugs: Case for Legalizing Marihuana," *New York Times*, Sept. 26, 1970, p. 29:1.

Vincent, Clark E.: *Sexual and Marital Health*, McGraw-Hill, New York, 1973.

Voth, Harold M.: In "Is Homosexuality Pathologic or a Normal Variant of Sexuality?" *Medical Aspects of Human Sexuality*, December 1973, p. 16.

Vreeland, R., and C. Bidwell: "Organizational Effects on Student Attitudes: A Study of the Harvard Houses," *Sociology of Education*, vol. 38, no. 3, 1965, pp. 233–250.

Wain, Harry: *A History of Preventive Medicine*, Charles C Thomas, Springfield, Ill., 1970.

Wallace, Daniel J.: "The Biology of Aging: 1976, An Overview," *Journal of the American Geriatric Society*, vol. 25, no. 3, March 1977, pp. 104–111.

Waller, J. A.: "Factors Associated with Alcohol and Responsibility for Fatal Highway Crashes," *Quarterly Journal of Studies on Alcohol*, vol. 33, 1972, pp. 160–170.

Watson, James D.: In "Biologist Assays Cancer Research," *New York Times*, May 6, 1975, p. 10:1.

Wechsler, H., and M. McFadden: "Sex Differences in Adolescent Alcohol and Drug Use: A Disappearing Phenomenon," *Journal of Studies on Alcohol*, vol. 37, no. 9, September 1976, pp. 291–130.

Weil, A. T., N. E. Zinberg, and J. Nelson: "Clinical and Psychological Effects of Marijuana in Man," *Science*, Dec. 13, 1968, pp. 1234–1242.

Weinberg, Martin S., and Colin J. Williams: *Male Homosexuals, Their Problems and Adaptations*, Oxford, New York, 1974.

Weinstock, E., et al.: "Legal Abortions in the United States Since the 1973 Supreme Court Decision," *Family Planning Perspectives*, vol. 7, no. 1, January–February 1975, pp. 23–31.

———: "Abortion Needs and Services in the United States, 1974–75," *Family Planning Perspectives*, vol. 8, no. 2, March–April 1976, pp. 58–69.

Weiss, N. S., D. R. Szekely, and D. F. Austin: "Increasing Evidence of Endometrial Cancer in the U.S.," *New England Journal of Medicine*, vol 294, no. 23, June 3, 1976, pp. 1259–1262.

Wesley, John: *Primitive Remedies*, Woodbridge Press, Beverly Hills, Calif., 1973.

Westoff, Charles F., and Elise F. Jones: "Contraception and Sterilization in the United States, 1965–1975," *Family Planning Perspective*, vol. 9, no. 4, July–August 1977, pp. 153–157.

——— and Ronald R. Rindfuss: "Sex Preselection in the US: Some Implications," *Science*, vol. 184, May 10, 1974, pp. 633–636.

Whelan, Elizabeth M., and Fredrick J. Stare: *Panic in the Pantry*, Atheneum, New York, 1975.

White, R. W.: *The Enterprise of Living: Growth and Organization in Personality*, Holt, Rhinehart, & Winston, New York, 1972.

Whitehurst, Robert: "The Double Standard and Male Dominance in Non-marital Living Arrangements: A Preliminary Statement," presented at meetings of the American Orthopsychiatric Association, New York, 1969.

Wicker, Tom: "Another Report on Pot," *New York Times*, Feb. 9, 1971, p. 39:1.

Wilner, D. M., R. P. Walkley, and L. S. Goerke: *Introduction to Public Health*, Macmillan, New York, 1973.

Winkelman, E. I., et al.: In "Jejunoileal Bypass Surgery for Gross Obesity: Yes or No?" *Medical World News*, Apr. 19, 1974, p. 62.

Wittman, Karl S.: *Basic Sciences for Health Careers*, McGraw-Hill, Gregg Division, New York, 1976.

Wohl, Michael Gerson: In Robert Goodhart and Maurice E. Shils (eds.), *Modern Nutrition in Health and Disease*, Lea and Febiger, Philadelphia, 1973.

Woodward, Kenneth, and Betty Woodward: "Why Young People Are Turning Away from Casual Sex," *McCall's*, April 1974, p. 83.

World Health Organization (WHO): *The Etiology and Prevention of Dental Caries*, WHO Technical Report Series No. 494, Geneva, 1972.

Wotman, Stephen: School of Dental and Oral Surgery, Columbia University, New York, personal interview, 1977.

Wright, Jim: "The Sweet Taste of Excess: Is Sugar America's New Energy Within?" *New Times*, Apr. 15, 1977, p. 28.

Wright, William F.: National Institute of Dental Research, personal interview, July 1974.

Wurmser, Leon: "Drug Abuse: Nemesis of Psychiatry," *American Scholar*, vol. 41, no. 3, Summer 1972, pp. 393–407.

Wyden, Peter, and Barbara Wyden: *Growing Up Straight*, Stein and Day, New York, 1968.

Wynder, Ernest: In Martha Lear.

Yankelovich, Daniel: *The New Morality: A Profile of American Youth in the 70s*, McGraw-Hill, New York, 1974.

Yarrow, Leon J.: "Enrichment and Deprivation: Towards a Conceptual and Empirical Differentiation of the Early Environment," in *Determinants of Behavioral Development*, Academic Press, New York and London, 1972.

Yevtushenko, Yevgeny: *Selected Poems*, Penguin, Baltimore, 1964.

Yolles, Stanley: In "Pop Drugs: The High As a Way of Life," *Time*, Sept. 26, 1969, p. 69.

Yudkin, John: *Sweet and Dangerous: The New Facts about the Sugar You Eat as a Cause of Heart Disease, Diabetes, and Other Killers*, Wyden, New York, 1972.

Zamecnik, John P.: Letter to the Editor, *New York Times*, Dec. 6, 1975, p. 28:6.

Zohman, Lenore R.: *Beyond Diet . . . Exercise Your Way to Fitness and Heart Health*, Mazola Public Service, CPC International, Englewood Cliffs, N.J., 1974.

Zuidema, George: "Study of Surgical Services in the U.S. and the Outlook for American Surgery," *Annals of Surgery*, vol. 182, no. 4, October 1975, pp. 531–537.

Zuti, William Z., and Lawrence A. Golding: "Weight Reduction Regimens Found Enhanced by Exercise," *Medical Tribune*, Apr. 3, 1974, p. 23.

ACKNOWLEDGMENTS

Chapter 1

Table 1.1 From "Relationship of Health Practices and Mortality," by N. B. Belloc, PREVENTIVE MEDICINE, vol. 2, 1973, pp. 67–81. Reprinted with permission of Preventive Medicine.

Health Hazard Appraisal Adapted from HOW TO BE YOUR OWN DOCTOR—SOMETIMES, by Keith W. Sehnert, M.D., with Howard Eisenberg. Copyright © 1975 by Keith W. Sehnert, M.D., and Howard Eisenberg. Used by permission of Grosset & Dunlap, Inc.

Chapter 2

Quotation from PERSONALITY DEVELOPMENT IN COLLEGE, by Peter Madison Reprinted with permission of Peter Madison.

Excerpt from poem "Zima Junction," by Yevgeny Yevtushenko Reprinted with permission of Penguin Books Ltd. from Yevtushenko: SELECTED POEMS, translated by Robin Milner-Gulland and Peter Levi, S.J. (Penguin Modern European Poets, 1963), pp. 24–25. Copyright © 1962 by Robin Milner-Gulland and Peter Levi.

Chapter 3

Table 3.1 Adapted from THE VITAL BALANCE, by Karl Menninger, M.D., with Martin Mayman and Paul Pruyser, pp. 153ff. Copyright © 1963 by Karl Menninger, M.D. Used by permission of The Viking Press.

Chapter 4

Quotation, Health Consumer Tip (questioning the physician), and Figure 4.1 From HOW TO BE YOUR OWN DOCTOR—SOMETIMES, by Keith W. Sehnert, M.D., with Howard Eisenberg. Copyright © 1975 by Keith W. Sehnert, M.D., and Howard Eisenberg. Used by permission of Grosset & Dunlap, Inc.

Figures 4.6, 4.8, and 4.10 Adapted from EXERCISE YOUR WAY TO FITNESS AND HEART HEALTH, by Lenore Zohman, M.D. Copyright ©

CPC International, Englewood Cliffs, N.J. Single copies available gratis from Mazola Exercise Book, Box 307, Dept. ZD, Coventry, Conn. 06238.

Chapter 5

Tables 5.4 and 5.5 From material in A DIET FOR LIVING, by Jean Mayer, pp. 260ff. and pp. 265ff. Copyright © 1975 by Jean Mayer. Used by permission of the David McKay Company, Inc. And from material in HUMAN NUTRITION, by Benjamin Burton, pp. 127ff. Copyright © 1976 by the H. J. Heinz Company. Used with permission of McGraw-Hill Book Company.

Table 5.7 Reprinted from HUMAN NUTRITION, by Benjamin Burton, p. 245. Copyright © 1976 by the H. J. Heinz Company. Used with permission of McGraw-Hill Book Company.

Table 5.9 Reprinted from FAMILY CIRCLE MAGAZINE, 1971, copyright © 1971, The Family Circle, Inc. All Rights Reserved.

Chapter 6

Figure 6.3 (periodontal disease) Adapted from THEY'RE YOUR TEETH . . . YOU CAN KEEP THEM, American Dental Association, 1971. Used with permission.

Figures 6.4 and 6.5 Adapted from EFFECTIVE ORAL HYGIENE, American Academy of Periodontology. Used with permission.

Figure 6.9 Redrawn from IT'S YOUR BODY, by Lawrence M. Elson, p. 367. Copyright © 1976 by McGraw-Hill, Inc. Used with permission of McGraw-Hill Book Company.

Figure 6.10 Redrawn from BACKACHE, STRESS AND TENSION, by Hans Kraus. Copyright © 1965 by Simon & Schuster, Inc. Used by permission of Simon & Schuster, a Division of Gulf & Western Corporation.

Figure 6.11 Redrawn from OHHH! MY BACK, by Cameron Kirk. Used with permission of The Economics Press, Inc.

Chapter 7

Figure 7.2 Used with permission from the WORLD HEALTH ORGANIZATION, 1967 data.

Chapter 8

Figure 8.1 From "The Multiplication of Bacterial Viruses," by Gunther S. Stent, in SCIENTIFIC AMERICAN, May 1953. Copyright © 1953 by Scientific American, Inc. All Rights Reserved.

Figure 8.2 From MAN, MICROBES, AND MATTER, by Bartley C. Block. Copyright © 1975 by McGraw-Hill, Inc. Used with permission of McGraw-Hill Book Company.

Figure 8.4 From HUMAN ECOLOGY AND PUBLIC HEALTH, p. 14, by Edwin D. Kilbourne and Wilson G. Smillie. Copyright © 1969 by Macmillan Publishing Co., Inc. Used with permission of Macmillan Publishing Co., Inc.

Opinions on antibiotic use From MEDICAL TRIBUNE, November 1975.

Chapter 9

Figures 9.2 and 9.7 Adapted from BLAKISTON'S GOULD MEDICAL DICTIONARY. Copyright © 1972 by McGraw-Hill, Inc. Used with permission of McGraw-Hill Book Company.

Figure 9.4 Redrawn from IT'S YOUR BODY, by Lawrence M. Elson, p. 367. Copyright © 1976 by McGraw-Hill, Inc. Used with permission of McGraw-Hill Book Company. And from drawing in NEWSWEEK by Roy Doty. Used with permission of Roy Doty, Newsweek.

Chapter 10

Table 10.1 From CORONARY RISK HANDBOOK, copyright © 1976. Used with permission of the American Heart Association.

Figure 10.4 From PATIENT CARE (R), Nov. 15, 1973. Copyright © 1973, 1974, Patient Care Publications, Inc., Darien, Conn. All Rights Reserved.

Figure 10.5 From HEART FACTS, copyright © 1976. Used with permission of the American Heart Association.

Figure 10.7 From METROPOLITAN LIFE information piece. Used with permission, courtesy of Metropolitan Life Insurance Company.

Figure 10.8 From PATIENT CARE (R), Dec. 1, 1974. Copyright © 1973, 1974, Patient Care Publications, Inc., Darien, Conn. All Rights Reserved.

Figures 10.9 and 10.10 From "The Cancer Problem," by John Cairns, SCIENTIFIC AMERICAN, vol. 233, no. 5, pp. 68–69 and 78. Copyrights © 1975 by Scientific American, Inc. All Rights Reserved.

Table 10.2 From CANCER FACTS AND FIGURES, 1978. Reprinted by permission of the American Cancer Society.

Quote from Orville E. Kelly From THE NEW YORK TIMES, Mar. 31, 1976. Copyright © 1976 by The New York Times Company. Reprinted by permission.

Chapter 11

Figure 11.2 Redrawn with permission from the May 1978 issue of GOOD HOUSEKEEPING MAGAZINE. Copyright © 1978 by the Hearst Corporation.

Figures 11.5 and 11.6 Adapted from THE LIFELINE publication. Copyright © 1977 International Group Plans, Inc. Used by courtesy of International Group Plans, Inc., Sylvia Laurenti.

Chapter 12

Table 12.1 From THE IMPACT, COSTS AND CONSEQUENCES OF CATASTROPHIC ILLNESS ON PATIENTS AND FAMILIES: A Report of a Social Research Study of Selected Families Stricken by Advanced Cancer. Copyright © 1973 by the National Cancer Foundation, Inc., and Cancer Care, Inc. SHARING CARE DURING CRISIS AT HOME: Annual Report of Cancer Care, Inc., and the National Cancer Foundation, Inc., 1972–73.

Chapter 13

Figure 13.1 Reprinted with permission of CONCERN FOR DYING, 250 West 57th Street, New York, N.Y., 10019.

Excerpt by Jane Brody From THE NEW YORK TIMES, Apr. 7, 1977. Copyright © 1977 by The New York Times Company. Reprinted by permission.

Chapter 15

Lyrics from "Mother's Little Helper," by Mick Jagger and Keith Richard Copyright © 1966 ABKO Music, Inc. All Rights Reserved. International copyright secured. Reprinted by permission.

Poem by Nancy Ernst Reprinted from HOW OLD WILL YOU BE IN 1984? edited by Diane Divoky. Copyright © 1969 by Avon Books. Reprinted with permission of Avon Books, New York.

Chapter 16

Signs of Alcoholism Adapted in part from THE MODERN APPROACH TO ALCOHOLISM, 1972, Good Reading Communications, Inc. Prepared in cooperation with the Labor Management Staff of the National Council on Alcoholism. Used with permission of Employee Communications Div., National Research Bureau, Burlington, Iowa.

Table 16.2 From ALCOHOL AND HEALTH, 1974, DHEW. Reprinted with permission of R. Flamant from JOURNAL OF THE NATIONAL CANCER INSTITUTE, vol. 32, 1964, pp. 1309–1316.

Table 16.3 From ALCOHOL AND HEALTH, 1974, DHEW. Reprinted with permission of K. Rothman and A. Keller from JOURNAL OF CHRONIC DISEASES, vol. 25, 1972, pp. 711–716, Pergamon Press, Ltd.

Chapter 17

Table 17.1 From JOURNAL OF THE AMERICAN COLLEGE HEALTH ASSOCIATION, vol. 19, no. 4, April 1971. Used with permission from the Journal of the American College Health Association.

Table 17.3 Adapted from O. Auerbach et al., "Relationship of Smoking to Age and Emphysema," NEW ENGLAND JOURNAL OF MEDICINE, vol. 286, Apr. 20, 1977, pp. 853–857. Reprinted by permission from the New England Journal of Medicine.

Figure 17.1 From "The Cancer Problem," by John Cairns, SCIENTIFIC AMERICAN, vol. 233, no. 5, November 1975, p. 72. Copyright © 1975 by Scientific American, Inc. All Rights Reserved.

Figure 17.3 From PATIENT CARE (R) magazine. Copyright © 1974, Patient Care Publications, Inc., Darien, Conn. All Rights Reserved.

It's Possible to Quit Smoking Adapted from AMERICAN HEALTH FOUNDATION literature. Reprinted by permission of the American Health Foundation.

Chapter 18

Poem "Motto" by Langston Hughes From THE PANTHER AND THE LASH: POEMS OF OUR TIMES. Copyright 1951 by Langston Hughes. Reprinted by permission of Alfred A. Knopf, Inc.

Chapter 19

Figure 19.1 Modified from VISUAL PRINCIPLES OF ELEMENTARY HUMAN ANATOMY, by Tobin and Ng. Copyright © 1965 by F. A. Davis Co.

Figure 19.4 Adapted from BLAKISTON'S GOULD MEDICAL DICTIONARY. Copyright © 1972 by McGraw-Hill, Inc. Used with permission of McGraw-Hill Book Company.

Figure 19.6 Redrawn from HUMAN SEXUALITY, by B. Goldstein. Copyright © 1976 by McGraw-Hill, Inc. Used with permission of McGraw-Hill Book Company.

Figure 19.7 Redrawn from IT'S YOUR BODY by Lawrence M. Elson. Copyright © 1976 by McGraw-Hill, Inc. Used with permission of McGraw-Hill Book Company.

Chapter 20

Table 20.1 From ADOLESCENT SEXUALITY IN CONTEMPORARY AMERICA, by Robert C. Sorensen. Copyright © 1972 by Robert C. Sorensen. Reprinted by permission of Harry N. Abrams, Inc.

Figure 20.1 From SEXUAL BEHAVIOR IN THE HUMAN MALE, by Alfred C. Kinsey et al., pp. 638–643, W. B. Saunders, 1948. Used by permission of The Institute for Sex Research.

Chapter 21

Figure 21.1a–d From BUILDING A SUCCESSFUL MARRIAGE, 7th ed., by Judson T. Landis and Mary G. Landis. Adapted by permission of Prentice-Hall, Inc., Englewood Cliffs, N.J.

Figure 21.1e From PREDICTING SUCCESS OR FAILURE IN MARRIAGE, by Ernest W. Burgess and Leonard Cottrell. Reprinted with permission of Leonard S. Cottrell, Jr.

Marriage Agreement Used by permission of Alix Kates Shulman. Copyright © 1970, 1971 by Alix Shulman.

Quotation from Philip and Lorna Sarrel Reprinted with permission of Dr. Philip M. Sarrel.

Chapter 22

Figure 22.5 Used with permission of the ASSOCIATION FOR VOLUNTARY STERILIZATION, Inc.

Chapter 23

Opinions on motherhood Excerpted from "Obituary Motherhood," by Ellen Peck, THE NEW YORK TIMES, May 13, 1972. Copyright © 1972 by The New York Times Company. Reprinted by permission.

Figure 23.7 From UNIVERSITY OF WASHINGTON MEDICINE, vol. 1, no. 1, Spring 1974. Used by permission of the University of Washington Medicine.

Table 23.5 From MANUAL ON TERMINOLOGY AND CLASSIFICATION IN MENTAL RETARDATION, 1973 revision. Reprinted with permission from the American Association on Mental Deficiency and the author, Herbert J. Grossman.

Chapter 24

Excerpt by D. D. Stonecypher, Jr., M.D. From GETTING OLDER AND STAYING YOUNGER, copyright © 1974 by David Stonecypher. Reprinted with permission of W. W. Norton & Company, Inc.

Chapter 25

The Wheel of Health By Keith W. Sehnert, in DELAWARE MEDICAL JOURNAL, October 1975. Modified from Rushmer: DESIGN AND ANALYSIS OF PRIMARY CARE ADVANCES IN PRIMARY CARE, 1974. Reprinted with permission of Keith W. Sehnert, INTERSTUDY (Vice President and Director, Health Promotion Group).

Chapter 26

Quotation from John P. Zamecnik Letter to the editor, THE NEW YORK TIMES, Dec. 6, 1975. Copyright © 1975 by The New York Times Company. Reprinted by permission.

INDEX

INDEX

HOW TO USE THIS INDEX

This index-glossary is designed for quick and easy pinpointing of information in *Alive and Well.* Particularly important terms are defined right in the index. Entries referring to material found in tables and figures are labeled in *italic t.* and *f.,* respectively: 12*t.,* 103*f.* When material is found both in the text and in the table or figure, it is referenced in parenthesis: 12*(t.)* 103 *(f.).* Material found only in a footnote is labeled *n.:* 436*n.* Photos that do not appear on the same page as text material and are particularly instructive are referenced with an *i.* for "illustration." Health care professionals not entered separately are listed under the "Who's Who in Health Care" sidebar listings. There are similar special listings under the headings: "Health Consumer Tips," "Self-Care," "When to Seek Help," "Where to Find Help," and "Opinions."

*Some entries found in text of figures rather than sidebars.